PUBLIC HEALTH POLICY AND ADMINISTRATION

PUBLIC HEALTH POLICY AND ADMINISTRATION

DR. S.L. GOEL
Professor of Public Administration (Retd.)
DCS, Panjab University, Chandigarh
Emeritus Fellow, University Grants Commission
Director, State Bank of India (Local Board), Chandigarh
Director, National Horticulture Board, Ministry of Horticulture,
Government of India, New Delhi
Formerly Member UGC, Member Distance Education Council
and Member All India Board of Management, AICTE

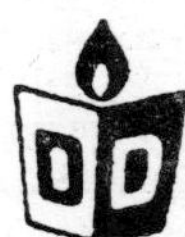

DEEP & DEEP PUBLICATIONS PVT. LTD.
F-159, Rajouri Garden, New Delhi-110027

PUBLIC HEALTH POLICY AND ADMINISTRATION

ISBN 81-7629-595-7

Typeset by ASHISH TECHNOGRAPHICS,
3190, Mohindra Park, Shakur Basti, Delhi-110034.

Printed in India at ELEGANT PRINTERS,
A-38/2, Maya Puri, Phase-I, New Delhi-110064.

Published by DEEP & DEEP PUBLICATIONS PVT. LTD.,
F-159, Rajouri Garden, New Delhi-110027.
Phones: 25435369, 25440916
E-mail: ddpbooks@yahoo.co.in • deep98@del3.vsnl.net.in
Showroom:
2/13, Ansari Road, Daryaganj, New Delhi-110002 • Telefax: 23245122

Contents

Preface vii

PART I

ECOLOGY, PRINCIPLES AND MODERN TRENDS

1. Social Development, Social Services and Health Care 5
2. Nature and Scope of Public Health Administration 17
3. Challenges of Health and Hospital Administration in New Millennium 47
4. Administration of Environmental Health Programmes 91

PART II

POPULATION POLICY, CONTROL AND HEALTH DEVELOPMENT

5. Administration of Family Planning Programme 121
6. Reproductive and Child Health Programme 155
7. Information, Education and Communication 187

PART III

POLICY-MAKING AND PLANNING

8. Policy-Making for Health Administration 211
9. Planning for Health Care Administration 223
10. Planning Nursing Education and Administration 241

PART IV

ORGANISATIONAL FRAMEWORK FOR IMPLEMENTATION OF HEALTH POLICY

11. Administration of Primary Health Care 285

12. Health Care Administration at the Union Level: Organisation and Working of Ministry of Health and Family Welfare 319

13. Health Care Administration at the State Level 343

14. District Health Care Administration 363

15. Block Level Health Care Administration: Community Health Centres 397

16. Organisation and Working of Primary Health Centres 419

17. International Health Care Administration: Role of the World Health Organisation (WHO) 441

PART V

INNOVATION IN HEALTH AND HOSPITAL SERVICES

18. Administration of Hospital Services 469

19. Health Education and Health Development 511

20. Modernising Health and Hospital Administration 539

Appendices:
I. National Health Policy 560
II. Draft Health Policy 576
III. National Population Policy: 2000 581
IV. Health Resources Indicators 597
V. National Health Policy, 2002 608

Bibliography 638

Index 645

Preface

Promotion of health is basic to national progress. Nothing could be of greater significance than the health of the people in terms of resources for socio-economic development. In spite of this realisation, the people living in the developing world and especially 80 per cent of them who live in rural areas have little or no access to modern medicine and health care. Inevitably this results in morbidity and high rate of mortality from preventable diseases. This state of hopelessness and frustration among the people is not because of the lack of professional knowledge or competence but due to poor administration of health services. Administration can provide the means whereby, the most effective use can be made of the knowledge and skills of the personnel responsible for the health care delivery system. The benefits of modern science and technology can reach the people only if such services are properly planned and effectively implemented.

The design of an administrative system is a basic aid to the achievement of its primary objectives; if the design is unsound, the achievement of objectives is likely to fall short of expectations. This requires the capabilities to design and manage the health care administration. To quote from a recently published book, "in the field of health we rarely have consciously trained executives . . . We have expected a vast army of professional care-givers to fill individual human needs, mainly on a *laissez-faire* basis, mostly without planning, without coordination, without sufficient concern for those who either do not look for care, cannot afford it or cannot get to it".

The development of health and medical services has been promoted greatly by advances which have been made in professional skills and technical proficiencies, but it seems apparent that the parallel advance has not been made in the art and science of public health administration.

The education and training of personnel responsible for the delivery of health care, in the art and science of Health Care Administration is of great significance as most of them devote 20 per cent to 80 per cent of their time in various aspects of health care Administration. Besides, a large number of health personnel have the primary responsibility of administering a health complex whether administering the health services from the state headquarters or administering a district health centre complex or a primary health centre complex. Many of the intermediary functionaries of health care are responsible for supervision, coordination and control of health care. The key health administrators are exclusively responsible for policy-making, planning and designing administrative structures to provide the best health care to all.

In the rural area, services are provided through a network of integrated health and family welfare delivery system. As on 31st March 2001 an extensive network of 3,043 Community Health Centres, 22,842 Primary Health Centres and 1,37,311 sub-centres had been set-up to provide primary health care at the grass-root level. One sub-centre manned by one female and a male multi-purpose worker covers a population of 5,000 in plane areas and 3,000 in hilly, tribal and backward/difficult terrain areas. One Primary Health Centre covers a population of 30,000 in the plane areas and 20,000 in tribal and difficult terrain areas. One Community Health Centre covers 80,000 to 1,20,000 population. It has 30 indoor beds, well-equipped laboratory and X-ray facility.

At present all those functionaries have been discharging these administrative responsibilities without proper education or training in administration with special reference to health care administration, obviously resulting in poor health care delivery systems. Dr. H. Mahler, former Director-General of WHO, rightly remarked at the Post-graduate Institute of Medical Education and Research, Chandigarh: "It is a pity that a country like India with its rich intellectual background has still to grapple with basic health problems even 30 years after independence." This holds true of most of the countries in the developing world. Unless the training of the health and medical professionals includes a study of the principles, practice and philosophy of public health administration, they are ill-prepared for the jobs for which they are appointed.

The question arises as to how we can develop the administrative skill and capability along with professional competence among the personnel responsible for health care administration? This can be made possible by two methods. The first is to incorporate the teaching and research of health care administration in the syllabus of under-graduate and post-graduate medical education. The second method is to impart training to the personnel already engaged in health care administration, especially the arranging of executive development programmes. A few steps have been taken in this direction, such as the setting up of the National Institute of Health and Family Welfare for the training of personnel in health and family welfare administration; starting of MS in Hospital Administration, starting of diploma course in Health and Hospital Administration; arranging seminars on various aspects of Health Administration, etc.

The success of these methods depends upon the availability of well prepared literature in health care administration based on the researches and case studies. The literature in this form is non-existent. Most of the available literature relating to the health care administration has tended to be historical or broadly descriptive. In a publication from Pittsburgh University it has been remarked that "In health administration, there are few theoreticians, few training centres, few books, and an almost absolute dearth of strict scientific investigations."

Whatever scanty literature is available on Health Care Administration is in the context of the developed world and hence totally unsuited to the different political, social, economic and cultural milieu in the developing world. Conventional health practices designed on the basis of Western models have proved inappropriate and beyond the capacity of the developing world.

Why has Health Care Administration literature not been developed for such a long time? A contributory factor in this regard has been the dichotomy between Public Health and Medical Care specialists and social scientists. Both worked in their narrow grooves without benefiting each other. Fortunately, in recent years this dichotomy has been disappearing progressively. Even in the WHO there has been a growing consciousness that the social scientists have an increasing role to play in regard to the formulation of curative, preventive, promotive and rehabilitative health policies and programmes along with the medical scientists to solve the complex health care problems of a rapidly increasing population. A healthy trend is emerging wherein some health administrators are feeling interested in learning the social sciences relevant and useful to the understanding of their field. Some of the social scientists are feeling motivated to analyse the whole process of health care administration to help these experts in finding solutions to various problems outside their domain. Encouraged by such trends, the author has written earlier three books on Health Care Administration and four Volumes on Hospital Administration and Family Planning Administration and Beyond.

The present book "Public Health Policy and Administration" divided into 20 chapters deals with the nature, scope, role of health care administration and its relationship with socio-economic development. It analyses the challenges of health and hospital care administration in the context of the developing countries with special reference to South-East Asia. The problem of population explosion has been engaging the attention of policy-makers, planners and administrators since the last five decades without much success. The population policy and the family planning programmes have been examined to bring about the changes in the programmes to make its success time bound. A careful study of quantitative elements indicate that they interact continuously, while quantitative performance is necessary on the basis of effective performance, it is in itself of little value unless a high qualitative standard is achieved. When the quantitative shortcomings are glaring, it is easy to isolate them and pick them out. But often they elude an objective assessment. The author has, however, made an enquiry into the quality and adequacy of arrangements made for motivating the family planning programmes as a way of life.

It also analyses the process of policy-making and planning for health care administration. It discusses the role of different agencies and stages in the formulation of health policy and plan. It has been rightly said that among the elements relating to the development of administration, policy-making and planning are the most important and yet the least developed. The formulation of realistic and scientific health policy and plans based upon our realistic assessment and understanding of our health needs and problems will go a long way towards the best utilisation of our resources. Besides, the issues and problems connected with the education and administration of nursing services have been dealt with.

It further analyses the organisational and administrative aspects of health care administration. It examines the role of UN System—WHO, UNICEF, etc. "The International Cooperation which is implicit in the very concept of WHO is the alchemy which has translated the goodwill and good sense of nations into actions directed to making this world a healthier and more decent place for all mankind." The issues and problems concerned with multi-lateral technical assistance provided through these agencies has been examined quantitatively and qualitatively to assess their impact on the health status of the people inhabiting this world. After this, the role of health administration at the Federal/Union level has been assessed in order to improve its administrative set-up to subserve the needs of the society. The real authority to deal with health care is vested in regional/State governments. It needs innovative measures to improve the functioning of health departments at the State level. The most serious problem is of adequate coverage of health services in the fields for which we have introduced the machinery of PHCs, Subsidiary Health Centres, Sub-centres and Community Health Workers' Scheme. The success of this structural pyramid depends upon the efficiency of PHCs which has been analysed in depth. In this book, the newly introduced Community Health Workers' Schemes has also been examined in light of the International Conference on Primary Health Care, Alma-Ata, USSR (6-12 September 1978) prevalent in different parts of the world and how this experience can be useful to India.

Besides, the descriptions, statements, arguments and analyses have been reinforced with the help of well-prepared Charts, Tables for the easy comprehension of the subject.

The impetus and encouragements to write this book came from the study of WHO and UNICEF literature connected with Health Care Administration and especially the articles and addresses of Dr. Mahler, former Director-General of WHO. Besides, the literature on health care administration from the Ministry of Health and Family Welfare, Government of India, State Departments of Health, autonomous organisations, and institutes have been quite useful in providing the basic facts and information. In addition to this, teaching and guiding research in health care administration involving post-graduate and doctoral students of the university for over three decades, teaching senior health and medical personnel enrolled for the Diploma in Health and Hospital Administration jointly run by the University and the PGI, Chandigarh; teaching the students of M.Sc. and B.Sc., Nursing in the PGI for many years has enabled me to gauge deeply the subtle intricacies of health care administration. Finally, a lot of empirical data based on field research through survey methods has been collected to support and reinforce the arguments. The method of case study was used to examine the impact of the variety of factors operating within a unit as an integrated whole in many chapters of this book. The author's participation in many training courses, especially the Training Course in NIHFW on "Fourth Country Course on Health Planning" has been quite useful as these provided the opportunity to discuss during the training period the different aspects of health care administration with the senior health experts staying in the hostel. This apart, the personal discussions with the health policy-makers, planners and administrators at all levels, general administrators interested in health care administration, legislators, members of panchayats and municipal committees and ordinary citizens as beneficiaries of health care delivery system, have helped in the examination of the various issues connected with Health Care Administration.

It is hoped that this book "Public Health Policy and Administration" would make a modest contribution to the knowledge and existing literature on this expanding field. Besides, this would help the academicians, national health officials, public health administrators, medical research workers and the policy-makers and planners in the proper understanding of health care delivery system. I will consider my labour well rewarded if the findings of the study are translated to provide decent health care to the millions of people living in rural areas, urban slums and tribal areas. Comments and suggestions from the readers would always be welcome.

Chandigarh S.L. GOEL

PART I

ECOLOGY, PRINCIPLES AND MODERN TRENDS

CHAPTER I

SOCIAL DEVELOPMENT, SOCIAL SERVICES AND HEALTH CARE

> Economic growth without specifically attuned to human needs, is not worth very much. Once more you hear every where people speaking about nuclear energy, oil energy, solar energy, wind energy and everybody seems to be overlooking the fact that without human energy, there would be no kind of progress either socially or economically.
>
> —Dr. H. Mahler
> Former Director General,
> World Health Organisation

Social Development, Social Services and Health Care

GOALS AND ASPECTS OF DEVELOPMENT AND THEIR INTER-RELATIONSHIP

Meaning and Goals of Development (See Chart 1.1)

The word 'development' is so often used in our daily life that we hardly care to think of its real meaning. The meaning of the term 'develop' is to unfold itself or to grow into a fuller or mature condition, and 'ment' stands for instrument of action, an act or process. So, in simple words, development is to discover or unfold any hidden field. Development can be defined as a process of directed change towards some objectives which are accepted as desirable goals. Development implies progressive improvements in the living conditions and quality of life enjoyed by society and shared by its members. It is a continuing process that takes place in all societies.

As stated in Dag Hammarskjold Report, entitled What Now, the goal of development is to ensure:

> "Development of every man and woman . . . and not just the growth of things, which are merely means 'for' development geared to the satisfaction of needs beginning with the basic needs of the poor . . . 'and for' development to ensure the humanisation of man by the satisfaction of his needs for expression, creativity, conviviality, and for deciding his own destiny."

Development is a process of growth in the direction of modernity, especially towards nation-building and socio-economic progress. It has been stressed that "development is the rational process of organising and

CHART 1.1

Administrative Law
Administrative Procedures
Administrative Culture
Administrative System
Administrative Philosophy
Cultural System
Political System
Administrative System
Social System
Technical
Natural
Resources
Capital
Human
Socio-economic Development
Structural
Population Situation
Growth Rate
Communi-cation
Trade
Process of Development
Urbanisa-tion
Industriali-sation
Education
Health
Standard of Living
Social Services
Housing

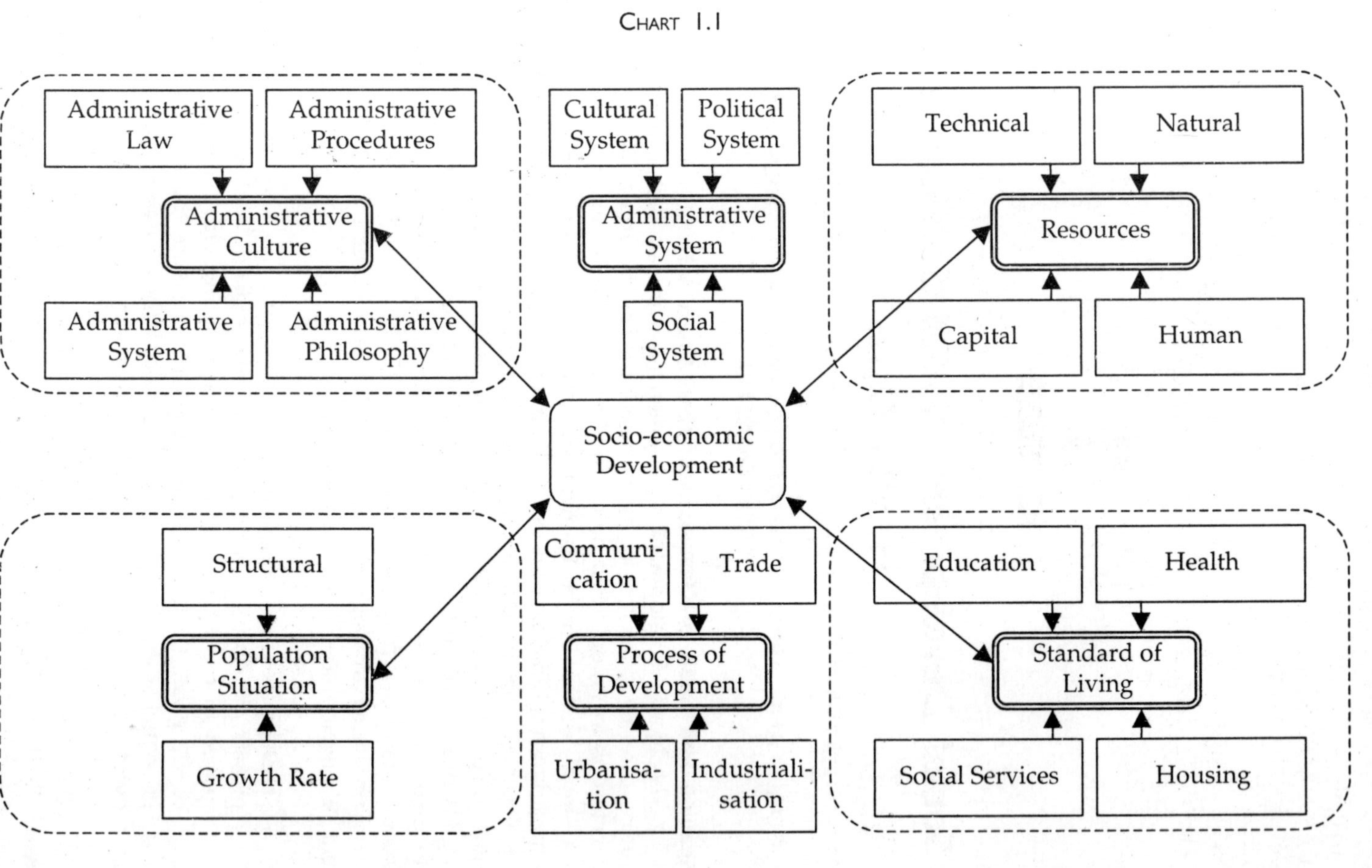

carrying out prudently conceived and staffed programmes or projects as one would organize and carry out military or engineering operations." Development has been defined in the same report, what now published by the Dag Hammarskjold Foundation, Uppasala, Sweden. It states,

> "Development is a whole; it is an integral, value loaded, cultural process; it encompasses the natural environment, social relations, education, production, consumption and well-being . . . Development is endogenous; it brings from the heart of each society, which relies first on its own strength and resources and defines in sovereignty the vision of its future, cooperating with societies sharing its problems and aspirations."[1]

We must be clear that the development is indeed a dynamic concept. Development implies growth plus social change. Nevertheless, development has often been conceived of primarily in economic terms, since sustained economic changes are necessary for the achievement of many social goals. This is not wholly correct. According to Dr. Candua, former Director-General of the WHO:

> "Amongst the objectives of the development are health and productivity. They are reciprocal and complementary. Without health, productivity can hardly flourish. On the other hand, productivity may increase means and opportunities for better health."[2]

Only a man who is healthy, enjoys working and is rewarded by a high degree of productivity.

Health Care Administration as a Component of Socio-Economic Development

In this work, we shall deal with one of the social services, i.e., health services. The health component and other components of the socio-economic system necessarily interact. Health not only affects the remainder of the socio-economic complex, but is also affected by it, sometimes favourably, sometimes unfavourably. K.S. Dodzie, United Nations Director-General for Development and International Economic Cooperation in his article, "The UN Answers the Challenge" in *World Health* (November, 1979) has rightly said: "The promotion and protection of the health of the people is essential to sustained economic and social development and contributes to a better quality of life and to world peace." The major areas in which health affects socio-economic development include problems arising out of the rate of population growth, rapid industrialisation and urbanisation, mental stress and social instability, environmental pollution and the growing disparity of living standards within and among nations. It needs to be reiterated here that social development not only continuously interacts with economic development but that the various aspects of social development keep on interacting with one another. 'A sound mind in a sound body' is an old proverb. Thus, changes in one sector of social activity produce changes in the other. We must see that these chain reactions are conducive to the attainment of overall objective of social development. Myrdal has summed up the position very succinctly as:

> "Standards of both health and education depend, in turn, on the whole social milieu, especially the prevailing attitudes and institutions."

In an overall and integrated concept of social and economic development of a country health cannot be considered exclusively as an end in itself. One must take into account also its role as one of the social sectors in overall development and try to establish measurable relationships between health and the macroscopic variables, such as consumption, productivity and labour on which it depends or with which it is involved most directly. In other words, it is necessary to determine the investment in health required for development or the rate of development. The benefits acquiring from health programmes are less difficult to measure. It is rarely, if ever, possible to identify all the consequences of a health programme especially the long-term consequences. A health care is primarily a social service. Health programmes are mostly established because they contribute to the satisfaction of primary human needs, irrespective of economic considerations except in so far as they can be afforded and constitute an asset for the future. For this and other reasons the cost and other data required to evaluate the contribution made by health programmes to development are rarely completely available, even when it would be feasible to obtain them.

To plan for health, that is, to meet the basic needs of the community and, at the same time, to satisfy the requirements of the overall pace for development is a complex process. It will be possible to achieve it fully when the economic benefits obtained with a specific health measure can be expressed in quantitative terms and when it is possible to measure precisely the degree of benefit to health from activities which are carried on outside this direct operational sphere. While health planners have always assumed that there is a good correlation between health and socio-economic development, doubts have been expressed by the general planners regarding such a correlation. Research is still in its infancy in this area. H. Leibenstein has rightly said that data on general relationship indicated that health and education were the most evident among the large 'residual' of factors that proved statistically more important than the usual economic indicators in explaining economic development.[3] Prof. D. Banerji stresses the role of health as a contributor to economic growth and the need to integrate health activities into general economic activities so that the former don't interfere with the latter or *vice-versa*. Dr. E.J. Thierry in his article, "Laying the Foundations", succinctly remarked that:

> "Health is man's most precious possession; it influences all his activities; it shapes the destinies of people. Without it, there can be no solid foundation for man's happiness. Nevertheless, all too often, social planners, forget this simple truth and leave health out of account. Integration of health schemes in overall development plans are of paramount importance."[4]

The tasks assigned to health economists in cooperation with planners include the development of instruments for measuring social phenomenon; the identification of the fields of health where the maximum results can be obtained with the available resources and provision of and in improving the management of health services (e.g., in hospital establishment).[5]

Though progress has been made in the analysis and estimation of costs and benefits in public programmes, but cost-benefit analysis in public health area has lagged behind.

The economics of health is a newer term than medical economics: it encompasses the medical care industry, extends into such fields as the analysis of the economic costs of diseases and the benefits of control programmes, return from investment in education and training, etc. Many have tried to evaluate man or, in other words, to put a price upon his economic worth. One of the earliest attempts was that of Sir William Petty (1623-87) who originated many ideas later used by the political economists. Adam Smith used in his *Wealth of Nations* and other works; Dublin Lotka and Spiegelman have attempted to translate the figures of life expectancy into terms of financial values to the community. It was observed that the period of infancy and early childhood represent a drain upon family and community resources. This investment made towards a productive age is therefore a loss to the community, not only in the investment made but also of future earnings of the individual. But, loss due to sickness, on the other hand, is limited to the duration of illness when the individual remains unproductive or under-productive from ill-health. Let us now mention the possible direct and positive effects of health on socio-economic development.

1. Many uninhabitable areas can be made fit for settlement and thus it can help in the exploitation of idle resources of that area, e.g., in Haryana, an area of Pehowa Block was made fit through the Malaria Eradication Programme. The area was infested with malarial parasites and was unfit for human settlement. Various studies have indicated the useful

consequences of disease eradication programmes on agricultural development and ultimately economic growth.
2. It can help in the lowering of absenteeism rate resulting from poor health caused by diseases. Here, we must be cautious about its limitations in the developing countries where there is widespread unemployment or underemployment and where a sick person is readily replaceable without affecting the socio-economic conditions in these countries.[6]
3. Good health can promote good labour morale and productivity, i.e., a healthy worker can work full-time and has a greater productivity potential. According to Benjamin, in these countries "where health conditions are worst that relatively simple and low-cost health programmes can produce dramatic lessening of the ability and disability of the labaour force.[7]
4. Good health affects intelligence, improper nutrition and lack of mother-care can cause mental retardation and other mental problems. A study carried out by Correa and Cummins in "Contribution of Nutrition to Economic Growth covering 18 Countries for the period 1950-62", reveals that in 9 countries of Latin America, there was an increase in the national product, whereas the contribution was zero in the economically developed countries. The poorer the country, the greater the role of improved nutrition in its development.[8]
5. Good health is a basic right and produces civic consciousness. We should not look at health only as a means of economic development. What is more important is to view economic growth as contributing to the betterment of the health of people, as it must be recognized that health is a basic human right. Thanis Kraivixien, the Prime Minister of Thailand, rightly said in his inaugural address to the 30th WHO Regional Committee for South-East Asia, held at Bankok, Thailand (2-8 August, 1977).
   "A society should consider that a high quality of life, and I dare say happiness of the people, which can only be obtained through a sufficient level of health, is not only a basic prerequisite to development but should be the basic objective of any development effort."[9]
6. Better health is generally associated with better capability and leadership. In a study by ILO on qualitative difference in the labour force, health was found to be the factor mostly clearly related to difference in economic growth.[10] According to Myrdal: "The required personal qualities are certainly multiple and probably have a synergistic action. However, there can be no doubt that health plays an essential part."[11]
7. Better health induces positive attitudes conducive to economic

growth and modernisation. The individuals become better citizens as they hope for future betterment and work hard to make the future more pleasant and enjoyable. Improved health may induce in the people to increase productivity and motivation to reduce family size. The people with good health are generally enthusiastic and try to achieve higher and higher goals in life.

Let us now review some studies which have analysed the loss resulting from poor health or diseases. Sinton (1936)[12] made an assessment of the financial loss due to malaria to the individual and the family alone at not less than Rs. 11,000 lakhs annually. In this conservative estimate of the annual financial loss to the country due to malaria, Sinton arrived at the figures of Rs. 1,000 crores. He stated:

> "It constitutes one of the most important causes of economic misfortune engendering poverty, diminishing the quantity and quality of food supply, lowering the physical and intellectual standards of the nation and hampering increased prosperity and economic progress in every way."[13]

Tuberculosis is a widespread and contagious disease. A study was carried out by Dr. A.S. Sen and Dr. R.N. Basu, Consultant and Senior Research Officer, Planning Commission, Government of India, to measure the cost of tuberculosis in India.[14] They found that the total losses from mortality, morbidity and the direct cost[15] of the disease amounted to Rs. 420.4 crores, Rs. 288.58 crores and Rs. 29.68 crores respectively. The production loss due to mortality and morbidity from tuberculosis has been very large. As compared to these losses, the amount of direct expenditure which is being incurred on the control programme is very small. The annual direct cost for a population of about six million works out at Rs. 0.49 per person per annum. Hence, the eradication of tuberculosis is not only a social welfare activity but an ultimate economic gain.

Because of this inter-relationship, economic development cannot be isolated from the social context. Health programmes cannot be related unilaterally to either the economic or the social spheres, as they influence both and are influenced by both. Thus, there is a need to promote, encourage and support research on the standardisation of nomenclature, systems of health statistics, indices of health and socio-economic development, evaluation methods, and health economics theory and practice. The World Health Assembly Technical Discussion on the contribution of Health Programmes to socio-economic development (1972) arrived at the following general agreement:[16]

"It was recognised as a basic principle that health programmes are

> rarely ever justified solely on economic grounds, but rather as the means of maintaining and improving health, which is perhaps the most important single factor in improving the quality of human life. It was accepted without question that health is an objective in its own right and represents one of the most important manifestations of social progress.

Thus, there is a clear indication of the needs for knitting together social and economic components of development plans to attain intended objectives of development among the people within a time schedule and a resource schedule.

All the countries of Asia, Africa and Latin America should apply development planning to accelerate socio-economic development guided by social justice. Development planning relates to a "teleologically-determined manipulation of policy measures and instruments devised so as to stimulate the authors of the socio-economic scene to act in the way most conducive to the achievement of the national socio-economic development objectives and goals.[17] T.T. Thahane defines it as

> "a process of organizing national economic and social effort for the promotion or achievement of clearly defined national development goals."[18]

The process of Development Planning can help us to get the benefits of modernization which depends upon

> "the Systematic, sustained and purposeful application of human energies to the rational control of man's physical and social environment for various human purposes."[19]

The people inhabiting the developing world expect their governments to pull them out of the morass of distressing under development. This would be possible only provided the efforts of the Governments are comprehensive, selective, coordinated and sustained. Besides, timely action, backed by a strong will and determination at all decision-making and operational levels, can change the complexion of our socio-economic scene.

Notes and References

1. Milton J. Esman, "The Politics of Development Administration", in Montgomery and Stiffin, (eds.); *Approaches to Department Politics, Administration and Change,* (New York, McGraw Hill, 1965), p. 9.
2. Message from Dr. M.G. Candua, Director General of the WHO in the *World Health,* March 1969, p. 5.
3. H. Leibenstin, "Population" Theories, Non-traditional Inputs and Interpretation of Economic History in P. Deprez (eds.) *Population and Economic Proceedings* of Section

V of the Fourth Congress of the Economic History Association Winnipg, University of Manitoba, 1968.

4. Dr. F.J. Theirry, "Laying the Foundation" in *World Health,* March 1969, p. 13.
5. Banerji, D.C. (1967), "Health Economics in Developing Countries", *Indian Medical Journal,* Ass. 49, 471-72.
6. WHO, *Public Health Papers,* No. 64, p. 20.
7. B. Benjamin, "Social and Economic Factors Affecting Mortality" in *Confluence: Surveys of Research in the Social Services,* Vol. V, (Hague, Mauton 49, p. 47).
8. H. Corea and G. Communis, Contribution of Nutrition to Economic Growth, *American Journal,* Clin-Nutr, 23, 560-63, in PHP, 49, p. 47.
9. WHO, SEARO:SEA/RC. 30/p. 64.
10. Galenson and G. Pyatt, "The Quality of Labour and Economic Development in Certain Countries", Geneva, ILO, 1964.
11. G. Myrdal, Asian Drama—An Inquiry into the Poverty of Nation, New York, Pantheon, 1968.
12. M. Periman, "On Health, Population Change, and Economic Development", in M. Perlman and Other (eds.), *Spatial, Regional and Population Economics,* Essays in Honour of Edgar, M. Hoover (New York and Breach, 1972), pp. 293-310.
13. J.A. Sinton, "What Malaria Costs in India Nationally, Socially and Economically — condensed and reprinted in *Health Bulletin* in 1958, No. 26, Government of India Press, 125.
14. A.S. Sen and B.N. Basu, Economics of Health—The Cost of Tuberculosis, Planning Commission, Government of India, Health Division, 1968, No. 26, Government of India Press, p. 125.
15. Direct Cost means expenditure on hospitals, clinics, durgs, research, training, BCG vaccination, etc.
16. WHO: World Health Assembly, 1972, A/25, Technical Discussion 66, p. 6.
17. UN: Proceedings of the Inter-regional Seminar on Organization and Administration of Development Planning Agencies, Vol. I, p. 113 (Sales No. E-74, II.H.2).
18. T.T. Thahane, "Planning for Development in John Barratt and others, (eds.), Accelerated Development in Southern Africa, London, Macmillan, 1974, p. 451.
19. Quoted in Marrico, B. Jansen, ed., Changing Japanese Attitude Towards Modernization, Princeton, 1965, pp. 23-24.

CHAPTER 2

NATURE AND SCOPE OF PUBLIC HEALTH ADMINISTRATION

> Health is a positive state of well-being in which harmonious development of mental and physical capacities of the individuals lead to the enjoyment of a rich and full life. It implies adjustment of the individual to his total environment—physical and social.
>
> —First Five Year Plan,
> Planning Commission,
> GOI, New Delhi

Nature and Scope of Public Health Administration

SIGNIFICANCE OF HEALTH

Good health is a prerequisite to human productivity and the "development" process. It is essential to economic and technological development. A healthy community is the infrastructure upon which to build an economically viable society. The progress of society greatly depends on the quality of its people. Unhealthy people can hardly be expected to make any valid contribution towards development programmes. Health is man's greatest possession, for it lays a solid foundation for his happiness. Charaka, the renowned Ayurvedic physicians is known to have said: "Health was vital for ethical, artistic, material and spiritual development of man."

Buddha has said that of all the gains, the gains of health are the highest and the best. Health is not only basic to leading a happily life for an individual but it is also necessary for all productive activities in the society. Who would deny that a soldier who is not keeping good health cannot be expected to defend the frontiers of his country even when he is provided with the latest sophisticated weapons? Similarly, who would deny that an unhealthy farmer with the best possible technological know-how would not succeed in producing the best that can be expected of him? Obviously what is true to an unhealthy soldier or an unhealthy farmer is also true of other categories of workers. Thus, no industry can expect the optimum output if it does not employ healthy workers or does not make and provide adequate facilities for proper maintenance of their health. Undoubtedly, professional efficiency, good health and productivity are inter-related. Yet, health cannot be bestowed upon people if they themselves do not make any effort to maintain a proper balance between their external and internal environments.

Whatever one may say, a disease-stricken society can hardly hope to extricate itself from the clutches of poverty and ignorance that keep it backward and underdeveloped in many areas of life. A nation can become truly healthy only when it succeeds in overcoming all these deficiencies stemming from cultural, social, economic and other causes. A nation that is ill-fed can hardly afford to exhibit efficiency in any field. In fact, an epidemic or endemic disease in any part of the world can pose a potential danger to all mankind and even a challenge to modern science. The Planning Commission has stressed the vital importance of public health in the enrichment of community life. It has been stated:

> "Health is fundamental to the national progress in any sphere. In terms of resources for economic development, nothing can be considered of higher importance than the health of the people which is a measure of their energy and capacity as well as of the potential man-hours for productive work in relation to the total number of persons maintained by the nation. For the efficiency of industry and of agriculture, the health of the worker is an essential consideration."

In his address to 3lst Session of WHO Regional Committee for South-East Asia held at Ulan Botor, Mongolia (22-28 Aug., 1978), Dr. Nyam-Osor, Minister of Public Health, Mongolia read a passage from a poem by Dashdorjiin Natragdorj, which glorifies "Health." It is being reproduced below.[1]

> "Happiness, happiness, happiness
> It may be of different origin on this earth
> But the happiness of being healthy
> Is the real happiness."

Thus, there can be no two opinions that health is basic to national progress and in terms of resources for economic development nothing could be of greater significance than the health of the people. To quote Herophilas, C., 300 B.C.

> "When health is absent
> Wisdom cannot reveal itself
> Art cannot manifest
> Strength cannot fight,
> Wealth becomes useless
> And Intelligence cannot be applied."

As such, good health must be a primary objective of national development programmes. It is a precursor to improving the quality of life for a major portion of mankind.

MEANING OF HEALTH

Health is viewed differently by different people all over the world. The World Health Organisation defined health as "a state of complete physical; mental, social and spiritual well-being and not merely an absence of disease or infirmity."

Thus, good health is a synthesis of physical, mental and social well-being. As stated in the First Five Year Plan,

> "Health is a positive state of well-being in which harmonious development of mental and physical capacities of the individuals lead to the enjoyment of a rich and full life . . . It implies adjustment of the individuals to his total environment—physical and social.[2]

Some people even define it as a condition under which an individual is able to mobilise all his resources intellectual—emotional and physical—for optimum living. Thus health is not static; on the contrary, it fluctuates on a scale which ranges between optimum health as defined by WHO to complete lack of health.

Dr. E. Berthet, Secretary-General of the International Union for Health Education, Paris, defines health as follows:

> "We no longer ought to define health only in terms of sickness, but rather in relation to the harmonious development of every individual's personality. After all, it represents a balanced measure of a person's total potential—whether biological, psychological and social; and to the nation of individual health we should add the concepts of family and community health."[3]

S.C. Seal, in his presidential address, defined health as:

> "flexible state of body and mind which may be described in terms of a range within which a person may sway from the condition wherein he is at the peak of enjoyment of physical, mental and emotional experiences, having regard to environment, age, sex and other biological characteristics due to the operation of internal or external stimuli and can regain that position without outside aid.[4]

"Health" has found an important place in the constitutions of all states and the UN agencies. Of the 30 Articles of the Universal Declaration of Human Rights, Art. 25 is particularly concerned with the right to health. Everyone has the right to a standard of living adequate for the health and well-being of himself and of his family, including food, clothing, housing and medical care and necessary services and the right to security in the event of unemployment, sickness, disability; widowhood, old age or other lack of the livelihood, in circumstances beyond his control. Motherhood and childhood are entitled to special care and assistance. All children whether born in or out of wedlock shall enjoy the same social protection.

The preamble to the WHO Constitution also states that the enjoyment of the highest attainable standard of health is a fundamental right of every human being and that governments are responsible for the health of their people and can fulfil that responsibility by taking appropriate health and social welfare measures.

FACTORS INFLUENCING HEALTH

A variety of factors influence human development both favourably and unfavourably. Some of these factors are: environmental/natural or man-made; physical, chemical, biological and social; economic, cultural factors: education, genetic factors; prenatal health development factors and nutritional factors. Thus, the promotion of health cannot be achieved by measures that derive from any single health discipline, nor can health measures be considered independently of the broader educational, social, economic and administrative factors that are crucial to human development. Obviously, the relationship between socio-economic development and progress of health is of extreme importance. In fact, every aspect of economy has a health component which has an important bearing on the overall socio-economic development. Thus, as stated in a WHO paper on public health: "The health component and other components of the total system necessarily interact. Health not only affects the remainder of the socio-economic complex but is also affected by it, sometimes unfavourably."[5]

Because of this intimate relationship, it has been mentioned in the First Five-Year Plan, "If this subject is regarded in the proper light as one which is concerned with everything affecting the health of the community, it must be admitted to be the biggest and the most important problem of India.[6]

Socio-economic development consists of various components related to the productive shares of activities. Health programmes cannot be related unilaterally to either the economic or the social spheres as they influence both and are influenced by both.

There, obviously, is a need for a unified, integrated approach to public health, i.e., to combine services for nutrition improvement, communicable disease-control, better maternal and child-health and family-welfare. Thus, conventional linear planning and the execution of separate programmes cannot meet the needs of human development. As stated by T. Adeoye Lambo in his article, 'Total Health' in *World Health*,

"It is now apparent that a more balanced consideration of the biological, social and cultural aspects of health is needed. Life is a process and not a substance—a living system based upon the primacy of continuity and inter-relatedness throughout the universe . . . If man and his family are to remain in empathy with the emerging necessities in the developing milieu, an adequate design of inter-disciplinary tools will have to be made to assist in this task of providing a total health package."[7]

In general, the factors influencing health could be classified into three broad categories: hereditary, environmental and personal. Similarly, the various conditions which play a vital role in determining one's health status can be put under three major areas, viz., mental health, spiritual health and physical health.

PRINCIPLES FOR HEALTH CARE ADMINISTRATORS

The Health Care administrators need to be aware of certain basic principles for the formulation of health policies. Some of the principles are stated below:

(a) Health opportunities need not be related to the purchasing power of the people.
(b) While planning Public Health Programmes for the benefit of the whole community, care should be taken to see that medical facilities are accessible to the poor people inhabiting the rural areas, urban slums and tribal areas.
(c) Investment on preventive as well as curative health programmes and activities should be considered as beneficial. However, the priority may be given to the preventive health care as we know that prevention is better than cure.
(d) Doctors should be trained to act as social physicians as well to promote healthy and happier life.
(e) Health should not be considered in isolation from other socio-economic factors.
(f) Health consciousness should be fostered through health education and by providing opportunities for the participation of the individuals in the health programme.
(g) Sound Health Administrative structures may be designed for the implementation of the health policy.
(h) All the systems of medicine must be encouraged to provide decent health to the people in a coordinated fashion.
(i) Utilize community resources and encourage local participation to promote self-help programmes at the village level.
(j) Ensure basic health services available, accessible and acceptable to the people.

MEANING OF HEALTH ADMINISTRATION

We have already defined the term 'Health'. Let us define the term 'Administration'. Administration is at the centre of all human affairs. Its principal aspects are formulation of policy and its implementation for the attainment in an optimum manner of stated ends in the 'shape of services or products. Administration is an activity which demands correct analysis and accurate orientation. According to Simon, "In its broadest sense, administration can be defined as the activities of groups cooperating to accomplish common goals."[8] In the words of Marx:

> "Administration is determined action taken in the pursuit of a conscious purpose . . . It is the systematic ordering of affairs and the calculated use of resources aimed at making those things happen which one wants to happen—and forestalling everything to the contrary."[9]

In simple words, administration may be defined as the management of affairs with the use of well thoughtout principles and practices and rationalized techniques to achieve certain objectives. Pfiffner and Presthus define administration as "the organization and direction of human and material resources to achieve desired ends."[10]

Administration consists of a structure or an organization of various institutions essential for its functioning; the processes, procedures and interaction of various constituents; and the techniques and skills of human relation. It is the management of human affairs concerned with the needs of carrying out specific objectives. Administration is involved in all fields of human endeavour where there is a planned effort. It is a force which lays down the objectives which an organization and its management are to strive for and the broad policies under which to operate. Administration provides the means whereby the most effective use can be made of the knowledge and skills of those giving the service. It is a way of conceptual thinking for attaining pre-determined goals through group efforts.

Now let us define the term 'Health Administration'. It is a branch of Public Administration which deals with matters relating to the promotion of health, preventive services, medical care, rehabilitation, the delivery of health services, the development of health manpower and the medical education and training. The purpose of Public Health Administration is to provide total health services to the people with economy and efficiency. Health Administration must use the knowledge of health economics to achieve economy. Three French teachers of Health Economics (Professor P. Bonamour, F. Guyot and D. Jolly) defined Health Economics as:

"that branch of knowledge which seeks to optimize medical action, that is, to study ways of spreading the available resources so as to ensure the best possible state of health for the population, within the limited means."[11]

Efficiency in health administration can be achieved through proper policy formulation and its implementation. Health administration is the force which can help the health system in the formulation of sound health policy and its implementation. One of the best definitions of Health Administration is given by C.E.A. Winslow who defined it as: "The science and art of preventing diseases; prolonging life, promoting health efficiency through organized community effort for the sanitation of the environment, the control of communicable diseases, the education of the individual in personal hygiene, the organization of medical and nursing services for the early diagnosis and preventive treatment of disease, the development of social machinery to ensure to every citizen a standard of living adequate for the maintenance of health, so organizing these benefits as to enable every citizen to realize his birth right of health and longevity."[12] Thus, Public Health Administration is the application of administrative processes and methods which are used in carrying out the objectives of health in an organized community. The term community refers to the entire population of functionally defined geographic area that has developed common interests, activities and inter-relations.

According to Beaton:

"Public Health is the planning, carrying out and evaluation of health measures and systems services that both maintain and improve the health of a population group and prevent and control diseases within that population group.[13]

There has been an increase in the variety, number and complexity of functions that have to be performed by the health administration, because of scientific and technological advancement. The health administration has not been modernised correspondingly to make use of the new technology. A serious imbalance exists between aspirations and performances. There is a widespread belief prevalent among the experts in the field of Health Administration that there is an urgent need for better management of health services if higher standards of health and health care are to be achieved.

The following are typical of the symptoms that demonstrate the need for better management:

(a) Overlapping, conflicting and competing organisations within the health 'system.' Where the system is composed of translated parts, it is not possible to manage a coherent health programme because no administrative structure can execute it.

(b) Widely scattered funding mechanism with little control over costs. Many health services have little idea of the true cost of some of their facilities or services.

(c) Decisions on the mixture of facilities and services without reference to population needs and with no information about those who do not use the services. Medical management thus tends to be based on currently met demand, not a need.[14]

Good management provides the surplus investment which nourish the processes of industrialization and modernization of society. Good administration furnishes the infrastructure of services which secure the order, stability and security which are the prerequisites of economic and social development. Carefully recruited and periodically trained or re-trained personnel are needed for both spheres of operation.

We would, therefore, like to conclude with Charles Beard, who wrote at the end of his long career:

> "There is no subject more important than this subject of Public Administration. The future of civilised government, and even, I think of civilisation itself, rests upon our ability to develop a science, philosophy and practice of administration competent to discharge the public functions of a civilized society.[15]

There is no doubt that medicine has accumulated a long list of triumphs as regards the care containment, or amelioration of established somatic diseases: Yet, it knows almost nothing of social aspects of disease and its treatment. In the past not much attention has been paid by the medical and other scientists to such causes of social disease as parental inadequacy, overcrowding, poverty, malnutrition, inadequate occupational and educational opportunities, the non-therapeutic uses of leisures, the misuse of mass media or the suppression of underprivileged section of the community. Medicine today with all its success or failures and the kind of demand it faces, is increasingly becoming a part of longer societal concern. The health administrators have to become aware of the fact that the obligatory relationship of social, mental and somatic disease requires looking afresh, at medicine's expanding role. They have to think in terms of planning and execution of comprehensive medical care programmes, including preservation of health and prevention as well as cure of disease. Already, continuity of home care has become a new slogan in the medical circle, particularly in the developing countries. While all these aims appear laudable, they are rarely achieved except for the 'cure of disease part.' Obviously, as the successes of medical science pile up, the sub-division of medical labour increases with its attendant technical incompetence, discontinuity of care and high cost. These considerations coupled with the present defensive isolation of the medical world in the bastion of acute curative, specialized and technical medicine, the hospitals prevent the giving of comprehensive care and the development of the true 'health centre' as a focal point for community health care. All this must be studied as the most crucial area of health administration.

In the developing countries in particular, the emphasis has changed from the physical environment to preventive medicine. A great deal of attention is now being paid to man's relationship with his total complex social environment. The occurrence and spread of disease is being looked at in relation to numerous interacting factors in man's physical, biological, socio-economic and cultural environment. Thus, the discipline of health administration is faced with many new challenges and nothing much can be achieved by it without looking at health problems from a holistic point of view.

One of the basic principles of public health administration relevant both to developed and developing countries should be that scarce sources, including that of medical manpower, should not be utilized only for the purpose of creating high power clinical establishments to treat rare diseases rather than using them for the successful functioning of public health services to combat common health problems, particularly of vulnerable groups, like, pregnant women, lactating mothers and young children. Similarly, medical education can be reoriented and medical services reorganised with; the involvement and cooperation of political and social scientists.

OBJECTIVES OF PUBLIC HEALTH ADMINISTRATION

There are numerous objectives of public health administration. The following deserve special attention:

(a) Increasing the average length of human life.
(b) Decreasing the mortality rate, particularly infant mortality rate and maternal mortality rate due to those diseases which can be easily prevented or remedied.
(c) Decreasing the morbidity rate.
(d) Increasing the physical, mental and social well-being of the individual.
(e) Increasing the pace of adjustment, of individual to his environment.
(f) Providing total health care to enrich quality of life.

The important activities in the domain of Health which need the attention of health administration has been well-enshrined in the 'Charter of Health' adopted by the Regional Committee for South-East Asia. The objectives of the Charter include:

(a) The provision of primary health care services to the rural population and under-served groups in urban areas, aiming at full coverage.
(b) The development of health manpower which will maintain its sensitivity and relevance to the health service delivery system.
(c) The provision of safe water to rural and urban communities and improvement of the facilities for waste-water disposal and basic sanitation.
(d) The reduction of mortality and morbidity among infants, children and mothers; and the regulation of fertility so as to achieve a balance between population growth and economic development.
(e) The implementation of effective measures for the surveillance, prevention and control of the major communicable diseases, with prevention and control of malaria being given the highest priority and due importance being given to an integrated multi-immunization programme.
(f) The promotion and formulation of national and regional food and nutrition policies and the development of common programmes jointly with the other economic and social sectors concerned.

The Health Charter should serve as a spring board to renewed activities, for the health and happiness of humanity.[15a] It is beautifully expressed in the Vedic benediction:

May all humanity be happy
May all be without disease
May all witness auspicious sights
May none have to undergo suffering

In practice, it is difficult to achieve the ideals of public health as mentioned in the Constitution of World Health Organisation. Even the most advanced countries have not been able to meet this ideal. So, the Health administrators in the developing countries must focus their attention on achieving a level of health which they can afford. They must proceed gradually in the pursuit of this idea. "Health Administration, whether in developed or developing countries, are faced with a number of managerial problems ranging from the provision of the most basic health and sanitary measures to the best use of finite resources in elaborate medical care system. All countries, however, have one basic problem in common—how can one best improve the health status of the population? This problem has become more pressing owing to changes in the needs and expectations of communities to developments in health and other technologies, and to the urgent need to link health improvement with socio-economic development."[16]

The purpose of public health administration is to enrich the quality of life 'leading to ethical, artistic, material and spiritual development of man'.

If the ideal of health administration is to provide better medical care to the people then we shall have to see that in a given situation we make the best possible use of our resources in terms of personnel and finance to achieve optimum results. For instance, in a developing country like India, the health administrator should normally be concerned with the following:

(a) that the patients are treated as close to their homes as possible in the smallest, cheapest and simply equipped unit such as a sub-centre which is capable of looking after them adequately;
(b) that the medical services should be organised and administered in such a way that the quality of medical care improves gradually;
(c) that medical care services should be organised from the bottom-up and not from the top-down.
(d) that the services planned should meet the needs of the people;
(e) that all members of the health and medical personnel function as a well-knit team; and
(f) that new categories of health personnel such as multi-purpose health workers and community health workers should be given suitable training to provide simple medical care and preventive services to large sections of the community.

In the case of virtual epidemic of behavioural disorders, modern health care must place a new emphasis on solving the human side of medicine. As stated by Maureen A. Backy, "The crucial link between the person providing health care and the persons receiving it, is often very weak indeed. Modern medicine tends to emphasize technical solution and to overlook the value of close personal contact and relationship."[17]

NATURE

Health administration is becoming complex day-by-day. Man is acquiring undreamt of powers, for scientific progress makes him everyday more capable of shaping the world and his destiny. He has the potentiality to bring about socio-economic revolution for the harmonious and healthy development of the people. The world has the resources and know-how to achieve a significant improvement in health care. But improved health will not percolate to the majority of the people as a natural consequence of economic growth. It requires an efficient administrative and managerial system to translate the benefits of science and technology of the people. Unfortunately, developing countries have failed to produce the expected system. The weakness, ineptitude and general inefficiency of their governmental systems are massive obstacles not only in their development but even in their survival.[18] These deficiencies prevent the vast flood of money, talent and material from achieving their objective. It is accepted that inability to manage efficiently or utilise effectively the available and potential resources is the common ill of all the less-developed countries. It follows that successful development demands a sound programme for managerial improvement.[19] Thus, the administrative inadequacies in a national government have a retarding influence on socio-economic development. Charles F. Nicklas, Public Administration Advisor to the Philippines Government, remarked:

> "The success of management improvement efforts and indeed the quality of public administration depends to a very great and undeniable extent upon the concepts, philosophies, interests and characteristics of key officials at the top echelons of the government hierarchy. Without the proper attitude and impetus at these levels, the cause of improved management and operation in government faced constant frustration. . . . It is, therefore, essential in the interest of progress that the individuals be endowed with the desire to see that the public service is administered in the most efficient, effective and economic manner possible and possess the knowledge and breadth of understanding necessary to fulfil that desire."[20]

Public health administration is an area of activity which calls for specialized knowledge and techniques which can help the people to achieve the health care. Until and unless, we understand all the implications of such an administration, we may not be able to reap the potential benefits of health organisations. This is a definite art which can be learnt and practiced to produce pre-designed output. Health administration is an art as it can help to direct and guide the efforts of those involved in such an enterprise towards some specific ends or objectives efficiently. There is a great need to make this art perfect and professional. A professionally efficient and competent administration is able to serve the people better. Besides, the health personnel must be dedicated to their profession.

Dr. H. Mahler is very critical about the inability of health workers in contemporary society to influence those social and environmental factors which truly determine public health. He states:

> "There persist widespread negative attitudes among health professionals towards the health care of the poorest strata in the rural and urban populations in the developing countries. Most of these attitudes imply—with a repetitiveness of an old gramophone

record caught in a narrow, arrogant, condescending and indifferent groove—that these poor people are too apathetic, too superstitious, too illiterate to benefit from the health care potentially available to them . . . Health professionals and those who train them should be much more radical in accepting a social responsibility for the health needs of the people in these poor rural and urban communities so that they can act as agents for change.[21]

Thus, we can say that there is a need to train health administrators and workers in the new art of Public Health Administration so that they can take the benefits of the modern science to the common man and maintain the spirit of Geneva Declaration."[22]

"Now being admitted to the profession of Medicine, I solemnly pledge to concentrate my life to the service of humanity. I will give respect and gratitude to my deserving teacher. I will practice medicine with conscience and dignity. The health and life of my patients will be my first consideration. I will hold in confidence all that my patriot confides in me. I will maintain the honour and noble traditions of the medical profession. My colleagues will be my brothers. I will not permit considerations of race, religion, nationality, party politics or social standing to intervene between my duty and my patient. I will maintain the utmost respect of human life. Even under threat I will not use my knowledge contrary to the laws of humanity. These promises I make freely and upon my honour."

The same feeling has been expressed in the Tokyo Declaration. To quote the preamble to the Declaration of Tokyo:

"It is the privilege of the medical doctor to practice medicine in the service of humanity, to preserve and restore bodily and mental health without distinction as to persons, to comfort and to ease the sufferings of his or her patients."[23]

Prof. J.S. Neki has rightly said in this connection that "to help, to heal, to reconstruct, to comfort—and all along the line to act with compassion—all these bear testimony to the moral consciousness of the doctor. Whatever the new strains imposed upon medical ethics, this structure will survive and continue to guide doctors in their professional conduct . . . Legal and judicial obligations they have, of necessity, to fulfil. But these are not genuine ethics. Genuine ethics has to be ingrained into character and does not have to depend upon external controls."[24]

Now the question arises whether public health administration is a science or not. It is definitely not a science like the physical sciences as it cannot claim certainty. It is a science similar to other Social Sciences like Economics, Sociology, etc. We are applying scientific methods in health administration for careful planning, analysis and the design of the procedures. We can make the instruments of Health Care Administration more perfect through careful practice and research and thus reach definite universal principles. We should be clear here that the universal principles in human organisations would differ to a great extent depending upon the ecological differences prevalent in different areas. We can say that scientific societies, and the exchange of knowledge and hypotheses by natural scientists have advanced the exactness of knowledge in the domain of natural science, so we may expect administrative societies, and the exchanges among administrators to advance the exactness of knowledge in the domain of administration."

Thus, public health administration is both a science and an art. In order to advance the cause of this budding discipline for the present and the future academic scholars and practitioners, we may concentrate on its principles, philosophy and practice. The developing world is faced with the problems of limited resources, infinite needs and competing demands in the domain of health. In order to provide the health services (preventive, promotive, curative and rehabilitative) to the total population—sick and the healthy, the developing world would have to provide an effective system of health administration. If these components are combined fruitfully, it is sure that the health administration can deliver the desired goods and services to its constituents.

SCOPE OF HEALTH CARE ADMINISTRATION (Chart 2.1)

In order to translate the aims and objectives of the public health organisations, the scope of health administration is expanding. Besides curative, preventive, promotive aspects, Health Administration studies social medicine which is concerned with the study of man as a total individual for the understanding of health and disease. The British Medical Association considers this concept from the angle:

> "That the health of the people depends primarily upon the social and environmental conditions under which they live and work, upon security against fear and want, upon nutritional standards, upon educational facilities and upon the facilities for exercise and leisure."

Social medicine includes social anatomy, social psychology, social pathology and social therapy.

There is also a new term, i.e. Medical Geography-linking medicine with geography. Medical Geography views disease as maladjustment to the environment to which numerous factors contribute; disease, therefore, becomes an anthropological phenomenon with geographical distribution.

TABLE 2.1

Development of Medical Science up to the year 2000

	Empirical Health Era *1950*	*Basic Science Era* *1900*	*Clinical Science Era* *1950*	*Public Health Science Era* *1975*	*Political Health Science Era* *2000*
Purpose and Philosophy	Symptom-centred	Bacteria or Disease-centred	Patient-centred	Community centred	People-centred
	Empirical diagnosis and treatment of symptoms	Diagnosis and treatment of disease	Diagnosis and treatment of the individual	Diagnosis and treatment of community	Diagnosis and treatment of total body politic
Education	Lectures Authoritarian instruction	Laboratory instruction	Clinical instruction besides teaching	Clinical public health instruction. Community side teaching	Social experience learning.Social and economic under-standing. Manager-ial acumen. Politi-cal psychology and process. Country health programme
Research	Hisotrical	Basic Laboratory Development of new tools	Clinical Development of clinical techniques	Community Develop-ment of the community Measurement and criteria Planning techniques	Social and economic indices for health development. Subjective indices for quality of life. Intersectoral activity process. Network process
Behavioural Unknown	Unknown	Not needed	Ancillary Social Sciences an adjunct to medicine speciality group necessary	Integrated Social Sciences. Sophisticated skills co-equal with public health science. Inter-disciplinary team	Inter-related Social, health, economic and political sciences. Inter-sectoral team

Source: WHO: *World Health*, July 1979, p. 14 (from the articles by W.L. Barton).

CHART 2.1

Scope of Health
Preventive
Curative
Promotive
Rehabilitative
Primary Care
Secondary Care
Tertiary Care
Immunization
Yogic Exercise
Mental Health
Social Medicine
Balanced Diet
Environmental Sanitation
Personal Hygiene
Social and Psychological
Vocational
Medical
Interated Research
Social Medicine
Health Care
Population Control
Health Economics
Health and Medical Education
Sex Education
Nutrition

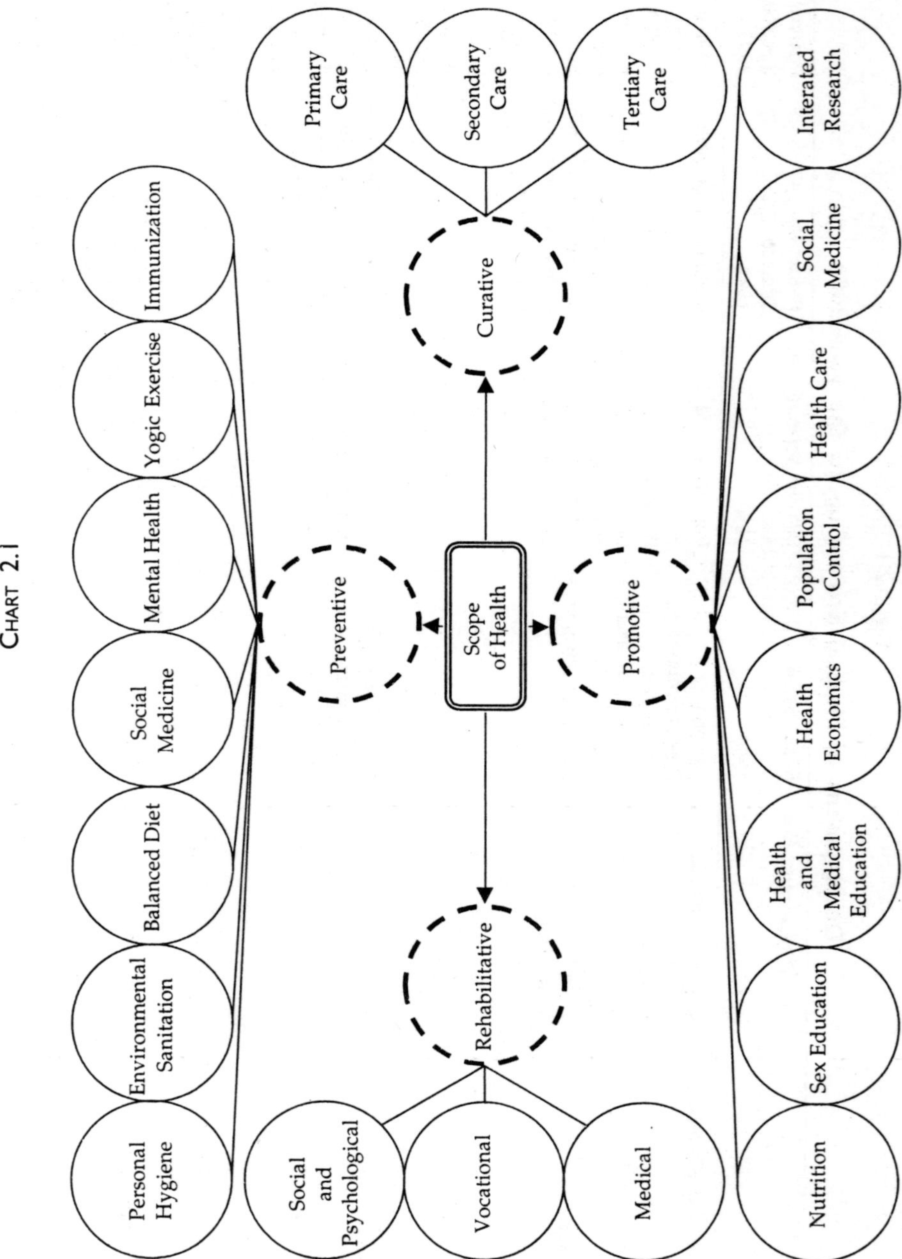

CHART 2.2

Promotion of the Concept of Total Health

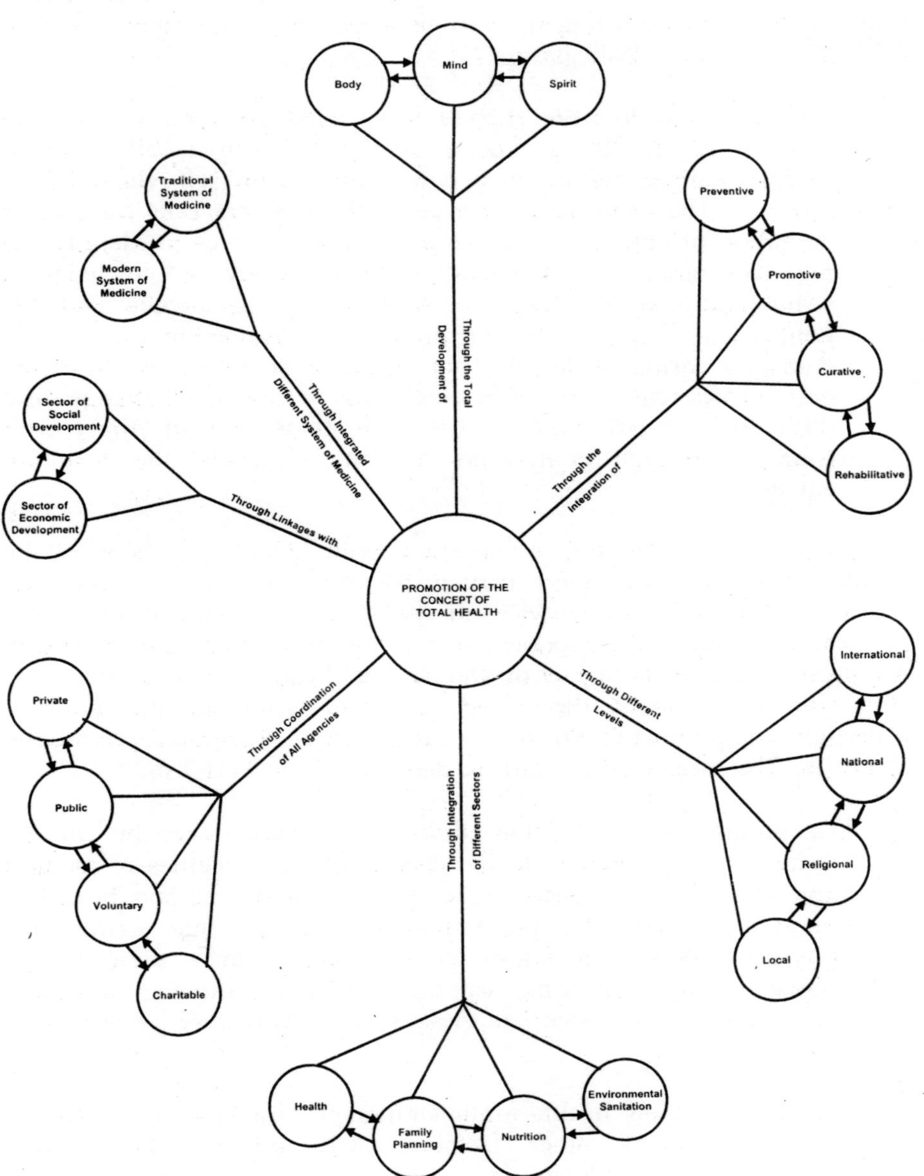

Thus, to understand the implications of health, it is necessary to have knowledge of the ecology of man: Such understanding would throw a flood of light on problems of diagnosis and treatment.

We can see the expanding and diversified field of medical science from the Table 2.1 depicting the various stages of the development from 1850-2000. To quote, W.L. Barton:

> "If this era is to have success there must be a move from the concept of health as being the total responsibility of a professionalized service to a new emphasis on self-reliant health care . . . The engineering science of the new era calls for a clear definition of objective, purpose and function, so as to identify the required competence, distinctive skills and body of knowledge in terms that can be clearly understood by the people and the politicians, as well as by the professional leadership involved. It demands daring leadership, not afraid to step forward from the basic professions from which they came, to face the challenges and difficulties of education in the new fields and to direct with courage, through competence in public health, the team of equals:"[25]

Health administration is concerned with 'what' and 'how' of the health. 'What' is the subject matter, covering preventive, promotive, curative and rehabilitative services. It also covers professional training of the health and medical personnel and the role of the International Health Administration and its impact on the national health administration. It is very difficult to classify the subject matter of health administration in watertight compartments. We have to focus on an integrated philosophy of health. The term medical care is defined by the WHO as:

> "a programme of services that should make available to the individual, and thereby to the community, all facilities of medical and allied sciences necessary to promote and maintain health of mind and body. This programme should take into account the physical, social and family environment, with a view to the prevention of disease, the restoration of health and the alleviation of disability. The extent of these services will vary according to local conditions."[26]

We have to view health administration from a broader viewpoint. It encompasses many other factors which influence health care administration. The broadening scope of health care administration can be seen from the chart given on previous page.

The various activities which can come under each sub-head can be seen from this chart entitled "Promotion of the concept of total health."(See Chart 2.2)

As regards 'how', it is the technique of management, i.e. the principles of management which can make the health administration successful and fruitful.

These principles have been classified by different management experts into a number of functions. Clough[27] gives only two—making decisions and providing leadership. R.C. Davis[28] gives three—planning, organising and controlling. Newman, Summer and Warrens[29] list four—organising, planning, leading and controlling. Terry[30] notes planning, organising, actuating and controlling.

Koontz and O'Donell[31] list five functions: planning, organising, staff, direction and control. Hicks[32] covers six functions: creating, planning, organising, motivating, communicating and controlling. Dale[33] goes one step further, i.e. seven functions—planning, organizing, staffing, direction, control, innovation and representation.

Many experts on Administrative Management feel that management is a basic operative force in all complex, purposive organisations. It is the function of executive leadership anywhere. It means that management skills are transferable. But there are writers who argue that there are fundamental differences between managing one organisation and the other. Earnest Dale; for instance, says that the universality of management principles is contradicted by observed examples of the difficulties faced by managers who work in widely different types of organisation from the one in which they were successful. As such, we should be careful in applying the general principles of management to health organisations within the peculiar environment surrounding them.

We must understand the difference between administration and management, though, we have used the term interchangeably. Orday Tead has made a distinction between these two terms in the following words: "Administration is the process and agency which is responsible for the determination of the aims for which an organisation and its management are to strive, which establishes the broad policies under which they are to operate, and which gives general oversight to the continuing effectiveness of the total operation in reaching the objectives sought." And he goes on to say that "management is the process and agency which directs and guides the operations of an organisation in the realising of established aims.[34]

To quote Mcfarland: "In government agencies administration is preferred over managements, although in recent years the term management has become widely used in government agencies. Another possible distinction refers to the levels of organisation. In business, the term administration refers to the activities of the higher levels in the managerial ranks. Still another distinction related to organizational level is that administration refers to the determination of major aims and policies, while management to the carrying out of the operations designed to accomplish the aims and effectuate the policies. Here, again, the distinction is not only widely followed but it exists."[35]

Peter F. Drucker has rightly observed: "Our society has become, within an incredibly short fifty years, a society of institutions. It has become a pluralist society in which every major social task has been entrusted to large organizations from producing economic goods and services to health care, from social security and welfare to education, from the search for new knowledge to the protection of the natural environments."

Now let us discuss some of the definitions of management which can be understood and applied by Health Administrators and managers.

"Management may be defined as the art of securing maximum results with a minimum of effort so as to secure maximum prosperity and happiness for both employer and employee and give the public the best possible service."[36]

Peter F. Drucker has rightly pointed out that, "Management is the crucial factor in economic and social development. It was obvious that the economists' traditional view of development as function of savings and capital investment do not produce management and economic development. On the contrary, management produces—economic and social development, and with it savings and capital investment. It becomes apparent that the developing countries are not underdeveloped, they are under managed."[37]

Massive says that, "Management is defined as the process by which a cooperative group directs action towards common goals."[38]

Terry has rightly said that, "management is a distinct process consisting of planning, organising, actuating, and controlling, performed to determine and accomplish the objectives by the use of people and resources."[39]

According to A. Dasgupta, "Management is the creation and control of technological and human environment of an organisation in which human skill and capacities of individuals and groups find full scope for their effective use in order to accomplish the objectives for which an enterprise has been set-up. It is involved in the relationship of the individual, group, the organisation and the environment."[40]

To Stanely Vance, "Management is simply the process of decision-making and control over the action of human beings for the express purpose of attaining predetermined goals."[41]

According to Lundy, "Management is principally the task of planning, coordinating, motivating and controlling the efforts of others towards a specific objective."[42]

The health sector has wide and varied relationships with other sectors of the social system. Individual and community health depend on a multiplicity of factors, such as nutrition and other basic biological requirements, personal and psychological security, culturally supported behavioural patterns, legislation, education, opportunity for participation of the community in planning and implementation, protection against exposure to pathogens, and accessibility of treatment 'to reduce the impact of disease. Indeed, it is hard to think of a community activity that has no relationship to health.' This view makes health the result of occurrences in many sectors of the social system; it implies that what occurs in those sectors may support, negate or offset the preventive and therapeutic interventions of the health sector. These considerations have enlarged the objectives of health administration from the mere provisions of health services to the improvement of community health by all available means.

The health administration studies all aspects for the delivery of health care services. In this context health administration studies the role of public, private, and voluntary efforts in meeting health challenges. Health administration also studies the structure and functioning of international health administration, government administration at all levels, private administration and voluntary administration which help the people in improving their health status. A recent development in health administration has been the encouragement to the traditional medical systems to help the needy people. According to Dr. P.N.V. Kurup, Adviser to the Government of India for indigenous system of medicine,

> "In our anxiety to make an effective comprehensive health service available as soon as possible to the maximum number of people the available material, financial and manpower resources that are rooted in traditional medical practices should not be overlooked. Against this background the traditional systems of medicine can play a vital role as an additional or alternative approach in a country's Health Delivery Programme."[43]

China has used this system with definite results. Thus, health administration studies the role of all the systems of medicine which help in the improvement of the health status of the people.

However, in order to make a really good contribution it has to adopt a multi-disciplinary approach. In the West, the health administrators are increasingly relying on the application of behavioural administrative sciences—anthropology, sociology, social psychology and public administration—in the identification and solution of administrative problems in the area of health. Thus, this needs to be achieved with a much greater pace in a developing country like India. It cannot be delayed in view of the kind of problems we face today. In the present context, the health administrator has to acquire a broad outlook and a strong will and determination to grapple with the existing mind-boggling health problems.

RESEARCH AND MONITORING IN HEALTH ADMINISTRATION

There is a need for conducting systematic research on many aspects of health care administration. By using operational research methods and techniques one can assess the extent to which scientific knowledge is utilized for bringing, about improvement in the health level of the bulk of the people at the lowest cost. Research in health administration is concerned with administrative, economic and organisational aspects of the delivery of health and medical services. Success of health care administration depends not only on research investigations in the medical field but also on the researches in other allied fields and particularly on the application of the procedures and practices as evolved in these fields. It may be stressed that operational research has special relevance to health administration in India because of inadequacy of organising health services as well as of several shortcomings of policy-making. However, nothing much can be achieved without providing the necessary training to personnel engaged in public health programmes and activities. The Central and the state ministries of health and family welfare have to play a special role in this regard. There is a definite need for studying the patterns of utilization of health services both in the rural and urban areas. By identifying factors affecting delivery of health care services, they can possibly plan to overcome them. The Union Government has already done a good job in this direction by instituting an Institute of Family and Health Welfare Administration which is actively engaged in various types of researches relating to health and hospital administration. Some universities are also teaching an independent paper on health administration. It would be suggested that the universities must be encouraged to take up research projects in health and hospital administration as the dichotomy between the social scientists and medical personnel is fast fading.

MONITORING AND SURVIELLANCE IN HEALTH ADMINISTRATION

Unplanned development in the area of health has led to many unforeseen problems, which are directly or indirectly related to certain deficiencies in the planning processes. Thus, there is a great need to develop specific guidelines for monitoring the public health programmes and activities so as to yield maximum benefits to the largest number of people. The governments both at the Centre and the state levels need to be made aware of malfunctioning of health organisations in time so that remedial measures could be adopted in all communities where a central organisation exists, there are some devices to keep Government informed about the health of the people they govern. There is a need to examine these devices so that these could be further modified to yield the desired results. By applying modified devices one could provide a sensitive indication of trends in health and development to the health planners for taking appropriate decisions regarding adoption of remedial measures.

Health surveillance is the comparison and interpretation of data generated through monitoring or from any other sources to determine the impact of health measures on the health status of populations:

> "Surveillance means the epidemiological study of a disease as a dynamic process involving the ecology of the infectious agent, the host, the reservoirs, the vectors, and the environment as well as the complex mechanisms concerned in the spread of infection and the extent to which the spread occurs."[44]

INDICATORS MEASURING IMPACT OF HEALTH CARE ADMINISTRATION

Health is generally referred to as a measurable quantity, but the concept is elusive and words cannot define it with precision. A WHO study indicated that among the problems of measurement of levels of living, that of the measurement of health levels occupies a central position. Health, a very broad concept, lend itself poorly to objective measurement; direct measurement of healthy status is often impossible and, in practice, indicators concern states that deviate from health but can be measured—indicators of the health status of individuals or groups; indicators of environmental conditions that may have an effect on health status; and the indicators of the activities of health services.[45] The distinction between 'health' and 'sickness' is not always well-defined. Most people would agree that it is desirable to prevent illness and premature death. However the prevalent indices are:

Crude Death Rate

All over the world death rates have been coming down and the average age at death has been moving up. It has come down from 25.1 in 1951 to 12.5 in 1981, 9.8 in 1991 and 8.4 in 2001.

Infant Mortality Rate

It means the number of infants who die under one year of age out of every 1,000 who are born alive. It has been going down. It has come down from 146 in 1951 to 110 in 1981, 80 in 1991 and 66 in 2001.

Incidence and Prevalence of Disease

In most countries of the world a system operates that enables both the local and the central health administration to know fairly and quickly about variations in the occurrence of the notifiable infectious diseases and about the outbreak of epidemics. The system has come in for heavy criticism because reporting is often patchy, incomplete and unreliable. But with all these limitations these statistics, looked at over the years do provide an enormously useful record of the long-term gradual decline of many infectious diseases as well as of sudden epidemics, their rise and fall, and their passage from one community to another or from one country to another.

Admission Rate of Patients to the Hospitals in the Area

Hospitalization statistics are essential for administering a hospital service and for planning and evaluating the services. They cannot provide a full and undistorted picture of the health or ill-health, of the population served. However, with experience health statisticians and health administrators learn to interpret the statistics and can often determine what is going on in the community.

Surveys and Special Enquiries

Such health surveys or morbidity surveys can be of various kinds. They may involve medical examinations or special disease finding (surveys) tests or they may be performed through household visits and enquiries. National sickness surveys have been carried out in many countries including Canada, Denmark, Japan, India, UK, USA, for the past 20 years. However, although continuous health surveys have great value within a country, something less elaborate is needed for comparing levels of health in different places and for recognizing important changes over the course of time. It would be good if we could devise a simple but general health index that would summarise the state of health of a population in one single figure that would be easy to monitor and interpret—something like the GNP in the economic field. But so far this has not been possible as health is not a readily quantifiable entity or attribute.

Proportional Mortality Ratio

It is defined as the number of deaths at the ages of 50 and over as the percentage of total deaths. If all persons survive up to 50 years of age, then the index would be 100, if no one reaches this age, the index would be zero.

Expectation of Life

The expectation of life at birth is generally considered to be the single indicator of the health status of a population.[46] Life expectancy has increased from 37.2 in 1951 to 63.8 in 2001, a spectacular achievement.

Limitations of Health Administration

Health is concerned with qualitative improvement and it is not subject to exact measurement. Any health organisation can be successful if the following facts, peculiar to health management, are taken into consideration:[47]

(a) The nature of the object being managed;

(b) Public attitudes to that object;
(c) The difficulty of placing a value on 'health';
(d) The multiplicity of aims and objectives and of the criteria applied to them;
(e) The long interval between decision and outcome and the associated uncertainty surrounding decision-making; .
(f) Orientation to 'service' rather than 'production';
(g) The involvement of several professions in the management process;
(h) Political intervention;
(i) The scope for public involvement; and
(j) The need to coordinate many different agencies, official, private and voluntary.

All these factors must be taken into consideration while administering the health development. Health administrators should be sensitive to all these limitations and plan and administer health services most conducive to the satisfaction of the population. It is really difficult to have a single model to solve the health problems in a country or area. A single model has not been devised for the solution of health problems. However, we can design any workable model suitable to a given area.

The ideal index which combines the effect of a number of components measured independently, is yet to be developed, although it can be stated that such an index should satisfy the following requirements:[48]

(a) Availability

It should be possible to obtain the data required without special and complex investigations.

(b) Completeness of Coverage

The index should be derived from data covering the population of an entire country or that part of it to which the index is supposed to refer.

(c) Quality

The national data should not vary with time and place in such a way as to have any substantial effect on the index.

(d) Universality

The index should, as far as possible, be the expression of a group of factors that determine and affect the level of health.

(e) Calculation

The index should be calculated in as simple a manner as possible and the calculation should not be costly in terms of the resources required.

(f) Acceptance

The index should be widely accepted and used and no doubts should exist in respect of the methods employed for developing the index or for interpreting it.

(g) Specificity

The index should reflect changes only in those phenomena of which it is the expression.

(h) Reproductibility

When the index is used by different specialists under different conditions at different times the results should be identical.

(i) Sensitivity

The index should be sensitive to changes in the phenomena concerned. Allowance should be made for the effect of inflation of the index.

(j) Validity

The index should be a true expression of the factors of which it is supposed to be a measure. Some form of independent external evidence of this should be provided.

Moreover, health cannot be measured in isolation. It is a part of much broader spectrum of inter-related and inter-dependent conditions, and no picture of health status can be complete without also taking account of the socio-economic and environmental circumstances—income, education, housing, environment, clothing, food, climate, pollution and still other facts that influence levels of health and disease at least as much as the activities of the health services themselves.

Notes and References

1. WHO, SEARO, S.E.A./RC/31/p. 59.
2. Government of India, First Five Year Plan, p. 488.
3. WHO, *World Health*, May 1979, p. 23.
4. Seal S.C. (1963), Presidential Address, Seth Science Congress, Delhi.
5. WHO, *Public Health Papers*, 1-10, 49; 1973, p. 9.
6. Government of India, First Five Year Plan, p. 511.
7. WHO, *World Health*, December 1975, p. 3.
8. Simon H., *et al.*, Public Administration, p. 3.
9. Marx (ed.), Elements of Public Administration, p. 3.
10. Pfiffner and Presthus, Public Administration, New York, p. 3.
11. WHO, *World Health*, May 1979, p. 14.
12. Hanlon, J.J. (1964), Principles of Public Health Administration, C.V. Mosby.
13. Beaton, G.H. (1974), *Canad J. Public Health*, 65, 463.
14. WHO, *Public Health Papers*, 55, Geneva, 1974, p. 8.
15. Dimock and Dimock, Public Administration, p. 2.

15a. Gunaratne, Therat V., Challenges and Responses: Health in South-East Asia Region, Tata McGraw-Hill, New Delhi, 1977, pp. 44-46.
16. WHO, Technical Report Series (596), "Application of System Analysis to Health Management, Geneva", 1996, pp. 5-6.
17. WHO, *World Health*, December 1975, p. 6.
18. David Brown, S., "Improving the Administrative Capability of the Aid Receiving Countries," *Public Administration Review*, June 1964, p. 64.
19. Iboko, J.I., "Developing the Administration in a Developing Country", *International Review of Administrative Science*, Vol. XXXVIII, No. 2, 1972, p. 293.
20. Charles, Nicklas, F., In the book Approaches to Development: Policies, Administration and Change, Edited by Montgomery and Siffin, New York, 1966, p. 188.
21. Text of Address by Dr. H. Mahler, Director General, WHO to Thirtieth Session of WHO. Regional Committee for South-East Asia, 2-8 August, 1977, Bangkok, Thailand, published in South-East Asia, Region Office; Final Report and Minutes of the Meeting of the Thirtieth Session, New Delhi, September 1977, pp. 69-70.
22. Geneva Declaration.
23. "I Swear by Apollo" by Christians Viedma, *World Health*, the magazine of the WHO, July 1979, p. 28.
24. Medical Ethics: "A viewpoint from the developing world", by J.S. Neki, *World Health*, July 1979.
25. "Alma-Ata: Signpost to a new health era", by W.L. Barton, *World Health*, July 1979, p. 14.
26. WHO, *Technical Report Series*, No. 176.
27. Clough, Donald J., Concepts in Management Science, Prentice-Hall, Englewood Cliffs, N.J., 1963, p. 2.
28. Davis, Ralph C., Industrial Organisation and Management, Harper, New York, 1956, p. 54.
29. Newman, Summer and Warren, The Process of Management, Prentice-Hall, Englewood Cliffs, N.J., 1967, p. 10.
30. Terry, George R., Principles of Management (Homewood, Illinois, Irwin, 1965), p. 52.
31. Koontz and O'Donnell, Management—A Book of Readings, McGraw-Hill Book Co., London, 1968, p. 1.
32. Hicks, Herbert G., The Management of Organisations, McGraw-Hill, New York, 1967, p. 156.
33. Dale, Earnest, Management Theory and Practice, McGraw-Hill, New York, 1967, pp. 5-7.
34. Orday Tead, The Art of Administration, McGraw-Hill Book Company, Inc., New York, 1951, p. 101.
35. Dalton, Mcfarland, E., Management: Principles and Practice, IVth ed., 1970, p. 7.
36. John Mee, F., Management Thought in a Dynamic Economy, New York, 1963.
37. Peter, Drucker, F., *op. cit.*, pp. 13-14.
38. Joseph Massie, Essentials of Management, New Delhi, 1973.
39. George, Terry, R., Principles of Management, Homewood, Illinois 6, 1968, p. 4.
40. Dasgupta, A., Indian Business Management, Delhi, 1969, p. 60.
41. Stanely Vance, Industrial Administration, New York, 1959.
42. James, Lundy, L., Effective Industrial Management, New Delhi, 1968, p. 1 (Ed).
43. WHO, *World Health*, Nov. 1977, p. 15.
44. WHO, *WHO Chronicle*, 20, 315 (1966).
45. WHO, *Technical Report Series*, No. 137.
46. WHO, *World Health*, Nov., 1974.
47. WHO, *Public Health Papers*, Geneva, 1974, p. 17.
48. WHO, *Technical Report Series*, 472, p. 20.

CHAPTER 3

CHALLENGES OF HEALTH AND HOSPITAL ADMINISTRATION IN NEW MILLENNIUM

> A growing awareness has emerged of the need for a more efficient administration, management and delivery of health care delivery services in new millennium which will have to be more adopted to local conditions. The challenges are almost daunting and yet we cannot afford to fail. We must succeed.
>
> —*WHO*

Challenges of Health and Hospital Administration in New Millennium

PART I

HEALTH ADMINISTRATION

CHALLENGES OF PUBLIC HEALTH CARE IN NEW MILLENNIUM

Current problems faced by the health care services include: (Ninth Five Year Plan)

1. Persistent gaps in manpower and infrastructure especially at the primary health care level.
2. Sub-optimal functioning of the infrastructure; poor referral services.
3. Plethora of hospitals not having appropriate manpower, diagnostic and therapeutic services and drugs, in Government, voluntary and private sector.
4. Massive inter-state/inter-district differences in performance as assessed by health and demographic indices; availability and utilisation of services are poorest in the most needy states/ districts.
5. Sub-optimal inter-sectoral coordination.
6. Increasing dual disease burden of communicable and non-communicable diseases because of ongoing demographic, lifestyle and environmental transitions.
7. Technological advances which widen the spectrum of possible interventions.
8. Increasing awareness and expectations of the population regarding health care services.

9. Escalating costs of health care, ever widening gaps between what is possible and what the individual or the country can afford.

CHALLENGES OF HEALTH CARE ADMINISTRATION

We have examined the present health situation in the developing countries which is quite discouraging though hope-inspiring. There is a great potential in the developing countries to solve all the present and emerging health problems. This needs resolute determination to solve health problems based on proper planning. Health services have become more complex as the result of technological, social and economic advances. In order to reap the benefits of modernisation, a recent UN report has indicated that in both developed and developing countries, "a growing awareness has emerged for the need of a more efficient administration, management and delivery of health care services, which will have to be more adapted to local conditions."[1]

We shall discuss the challenges of health administration which need the attention of policy-makers, planners and health administrators, to provide adequate and effective health care to all at the earliest. This calls for strengthening the administration and management of the national health services.

> "Effective administration and management call for more intensive preparation and training of senior medical and non-medical administrative personnel, whose functions must be considered in the wider context of the national public administration and not just in the mere limited sphere of public health administration. The major share of national budgets in the future will most certainly go to the departments that develop and use the best systems of planning, performance and programmes—accountability."[2]

Let us now review some of the inadequacies of health administration which need immediate attention to provide decent health care to all.

The health care administration has been functioning with the following shortcomings:

(a) The inability of the health care system to make available the services required to meet the demands of those most in need, who are usually too poor or too geographically or socially remote to benefit from such facilities.
(b) Wide differences in resources distribution and service and a multiplicity of institutions which are unrelated and not functioning as a system.
(c) The placing of emphasis on medical rather than overall health

care. The curative aspect of care has been stressed with insufficient priority to promotive, preventive and rehabilitative care. This has resulted in a fragmentation of the care provided to the individual.

(d) Training of health personnel directed primarily towards medical and institutional care, and largely irrelevant to the tasks and functions required outside institutional settings.

(e) The education and training of health professionals in such a manner as to accentuate the social distance between health professionals and the population, resulting in an inability on the part of the providers of health services to identify with the consumers.

(f) A lack of recognition as well as a rejection of useful, traditional healing practices.

(g) An inadequate assessment of other community resources, imposing unnecessary limitations on the scope of action of health services and often preventing them from approaching major community needs in an effective manner.

(h) The people have rarely been given the opportunity to play an active role in deciding the types of activities they want and have not participated in the actual services they receive. Community interest and resources have too often been inadequately expressed and activated because there has been a failure to recognise that people will be most interested in and responsive to activities related to their own priority concerns.

We have discussed in detail some of these problems in the various chapters that would follow. We shall concentrate here only on some of the challenges of health care administration.

Lack of Coordination and Linkages

Coordination means bringing about consistent and harmonious action of persons and programmes with each other towards a common goal. The coordination is lacking in the field of health care administration resulting in poor delivery of health services. Professor Mofide (Iran) has rightly indicated the prevailing atmosphere when he states: "In the majority of countries with some or all of these problems (environmental) pollution, uncontrolled population growth; nutritional deficiencies; the high risk of disease; shortages and mal-distribution of trained staff; and insufficient financial, material and physical resources, there exists also a fragmentation of responsibilities for the delivery of health care, with overlapping, conflicting, and competing organisations within the health system and widely scattered funding mechanisms with little control over costs. Health services authorities give only token recognition to those segments of the services that are not under their direct executive or financial control, and often plan only for that part of the national budget that is said to be their responsibility. The state of affairs is unjustified and harmful."[3]

Resources for the health care delivery are limited in the developing world. An effective health approach and strategy requires the coordinated efforts of sectors and agencies that can contribute directly or indirectly to the promotion of health care. Such coordinated efforts would promote health services that will be more efficiently and effective from both the standpoint of the providers and that of the beneficiaries. The need of coordination is so great that according to Findlay, "It expresses the principles of organization in toto; nothing less."[4]

The first essential requisite to achieve coordination is to develop meaningful linkages with sectors of social and economic development which can influence the promotion of health care, e.g., agriculture, public works, housing, communication, education, etc.

The second step is to pool the efforts of all health agencies at all levels in a system to achieve maximum output—public and private; national and international; curative and promotive; peripheral, intermediate and central; western medicine and traditional medicine. This would avoid the dangers of dysfunctional attitudes.

Third, there is the need of welding different aspects of health services into a total health package, e.g., integration of maternal and child care, family planning, prevention of communicable diseases, health education, environmental sanitation.

Coordination and linkages on a systematic, rather than on *ad hoc* basis will definitely reduce costly duplications of effort and lead to increased health coverage of the needy population and neglected area, while making the optimum use of the resources. Most of the countries in their reply to the WHO admitted that the lack of coordination in health care delivery system is a serious challenge. To quote WHO:

> "The consensus of opinion is that the most important managerial problems are foreseen in the continued reduction of the imbalance of the system and the lack of integration in the distribution of care with the existence of parallel systems with different objectives. Fragmentation and division of responsibility between the different levels of care have led to a lack of effective communication between the health and social welfare agencies. . . . As there are several agencies providing medical care there is over-lapping and duplication of activities . . . The major managerial problems . . . is to recognise the various components of this system in a way that reflects complementarity, eliminates duplication, and minimizes waste of resources."[5]

This problem becomes more acute in a federal country like India where health is a State subject. It becomes important to coordinate the health programmes at the national level. The dilution of health standards in one State may affect adversely the whole country. There is a need, therefore, to give more powers to the central authority by making health a concurrent subject. One of the health experts went on to say: "The present health situation in developing countries, especially India, is in a chaotic condition as no scientific and realistic attempt is visible to coordinate the available inputs to produce maximum output. We can locate a large area without any health care facilities while in some areas, every third shop or house is providing medical care."[6]

How can we achieve effective coordination? According to Dr. White, its achievement may require:

> "The most delicate insights, the most mature wisdom, and perception of a truely artistic quality."[7]

It has to be achieved through formal as well as informal methods.

The effective co-ordination and linkages would automatically result from effective planning, policy-making, manpower planning.[8] After planning and policy-making, the effective instrument to achieve coordination is to design a sound organisation. Dr. White says:

> "An organisation characterised by clear lines of authority, adequate powers, well-understood allocation of functions, absence of overlapping and duplication of effort and proper delegation of work in itself reduce the necessities of coordination"[9]

Besides, if the organisational boundaries are properly demarcated, there would be little scope of confusion and misunderstanding and coordination would naturally flow from this inherent structure.

The coordination among different agencies, however, can be obtained through mutual consultation or information. This mutual consultation should be encouraged through setting up of inter-departmental agency/committees for joint planning, joint decision-making and joint action in areas concerning more than one agency. While achieving coordination, we may keep the cost factor in mind. Such inter or intra-agencies can serve a useful purpose when the members come duly prepared with a sense of urgency and commitment. According to Key, "a session of an inter-departmental committee tends to be a place where departmental representatives come well prepared to defend their positions and leave more convinced than before of the correctness of their attitudes."[10]

We are to take care that the benefits achieved through coordination should surpass the expenditure incurred to obtain coordination.

Besides formal methods, we should adopt informal methods which are as effective as the formal ones, e.g., the Central Council of Health and the Central Council of Family Welfare (India) uses the informal method to achieve coordination among the different States and between the Union Government and the State Governments. It is the most powerful cement in the whole executive structure.[11]

We must encourage such informal methods at all levels of Government.

We must try to achieve coordination to obtain coherency in all the agencies dealing directly or indirectly with health care, all the systems of medicines, all the persons responsible for health care team work and at all the levels through well designed formal and informal organisation with minimum costs to fulfil the goal—the betterment of the health of mankind irrespective of the status and location and to obtain optimum benefit from available and potential resources.

Lack of Equity of Distribution and Adequacy of Coverage in Relationship to Need

According to David Morley:

> "Three quarters of our population are rural, yet three quarters of our medical resources are spent in the towns where three quarters of our doctors live. Three quarters of the people die from diseases which could be prevented at low cost and yet three quarters of medical budgets are spent on curative services."

The large population of the people living in rural areas are not being provided even rudimentary health care in this age of modern medicine. The benefits of modern medicine are available only to the chosen few living in metropolitan cities, e.g., 10-20 per cent of the people are consuming 80 per cent of the resources invested in health care in India. What has happened during the last three decades is not in tune with the spirits of the Constitution of India. The Government must serve the millions of people who suffer from chronic poverty, ignorance, disease and inequality of opportunity. The Government must fulfil the aspirations of the people enshrined in the Constitution. Austin summed up the Constitution of India in the following words:

> "The Indian Constitution is first and foremost a social document. The majority of its provisions are either directly aimed at furthering the goals of the social revolution or attempt to foster this revolution by establishing the conditions necessary for its achievement. Yet despite the permeation of the entire constitution by the aim of national renaissance the core of commitment to the social revolution lies in Parts III and IV, in the Fundamental Rights and in the Directive Principles of State Policy. They are the conscience of the Constitution."[12]

Have we lived up to the expectations and aspirations of the people? The answer is plain and simple: certainly not. What can we do in future? We can devise technology and organisation objectives and structure that would benefit the largest number of the people and if possible to the last person as desired by Mahatma Gandhi. What is required is change of ideology, philosophy and priorities in favour of the poor people, i.e., any device to improve health care should ensure improvement in the health status of the whole population. This may be possible if our planning in future takes care of the following:

(a) We should attend to the needs of the largest groups rather than meet the demands of a particular group or section of society. We can ascertain the need of the target groups through epidemiological studies.
(b) We may provide that health care to the people through the technology that may reach all. We may not invest in highly sophisticated technology only to be used by the few. The dilemma can be best described as an attempt to ride two horses galloping in different directions. On the one hand is maintenance of the high standard of medical excellence taught in the West. The other is the problem of providing health care for the millions of poor who cannot possibly provide an economic support base for our Western-styled health systems. There is no particular merit in promoting the highest level of medical services when the direct result is medical care costed beyond the reach of four-fifths of the population.[13]

The Government of India is presently thinking of reviving short-term LSMF (Licentiate of the State Medical Faculty) to provide health care to the rural population in 580,000 villages. *The Tribune* Editorial has rightly mentioned:

"The Medical Council of India's opposition to the short-term medical course and the dubbing of Licentiate Doctors as half baked seems strange in view of the fact that in three decades we have failed to remove dichotomy of 85 per cent of the health resources being utilised for the benefit of less than 15 per cent of the country's population. On the contrary, the revival of the licentiate cadre may lessen the burden of the MBBS doctors, especially, general practitioners."[14]

Thus, we must train more and more health personnel of lower categories who can serve the people at large and restrict the few specialities only for referral services.

The United Nations in its 1974 Report on the world social situation reported that:

"Despite the generally greater availability of resources, most governments are faced with difficult choices, because of the recognised need to provide the best possible personnel health care to the rapidly growing population, on the one hand, and because of limitation created by the increase in costs, on the other. Even the most affluent countries have started encountering growing financial difficulties in responding to the health demands of their people. Governments are now paying closer attention to the amount they spend on health services and the value they get in return. They are considering new financing arrangements in the health care field with the objective of reducing the rate of cost escalation and enabling health authorities to achieve flexibility in determining priorities and in pursuing the most efficient and effective approaches to health care."[15]

Kenneth Hill is surprised to notice the opposition of the health experts in the use of Auxiliaries. He says, 'Although the use of intermediary personnel is on the increase, resistance to their recognition continues and this is often even stronger in developing countries than it is elsewhere. It is hard to understand the rationale of such opposition. It is true that there is a remote danger of people with less advanced training developing inflated ideas of their own capabilities, but such people can only be relatively few and they will be found at the fringe."

All this would be possible if the principles of socialism are put into practice. This would encourage political, economic and social democracy. Nehru, in his presidential address at the Lucknow session of AICC in April 1936, expressed his deep faith in the success of socialism. "I am convinced", he said, "the only key to the solution of world's problems and that of India's problems lies in socialism and when I use this word, I do so, not in vague humanitarian way but in the scientific-economic sense. Socialism, however, is something more than an economic doctrine, it is a philosophy of life . . . I see no way of ending poverty, the vast unemployment, the degradation and subjection of Indian people except through socialism."

If socialism is established in the real sense in the developing world, the entrenched disparities would go away benefiting the poor. This would automatically solve the problems in the field of health care administration as well.

Poor Financial Allocation to the Health Care Delivery and Improper Utilisation of Existing Resources

The developing countries give low priority in the allocation of resources to the health care of their people. We can see from the table given earlier that the expenditure has been very low. The health expenditure to the total expenditure has been very low in South-East Asian countries, i.e., 1.6 per cent in Indonesia, 2.1 per cent in India, 3.8 per cent in Bangladesh. Mongolia has been spending 10 per cent for the health care of its people. There is a need to raise the health allocations to improve the quality of life. Dr. White has rightly said that, "Nothing can be done without the expenditure of money . . . Available financial resources set a maximum limit on administrative activity as a whole and on each of its separate parts."[16]

A sound state of finance is of paramount importance to the political heath of a nation. . . . The soundness of public finance depends both upon the right policy and good organisation, but a great deal upon the latter.[17] The scarcity of resources affect all aspects of the health delivery system. There is a need to step up the health allocations to the minimum of 10 per cent of the total budget.

Secondly, there is maldistribution of health resources. Most of the health budgets (about 80 per cent) are being spent only on a few people (20 per cent). This deprives the people living in rural areas and urban slums. A WHO study group on the Financing of Health Services which met in Geneva from 21 to 25 November 1977, mentioned the following characteristics which reflect the situation in the developing countries.[18]

(a) Disproportionate concentration of expenditure on health services in urban areas compared with expenditure in rural areas.
(b) Heavy concentration of expenditure on secondary and tertiary care services compared with expenditure on primary care services.
(c) Heavy concentration of expenditure on curative services compared with expenditure on preventive services.

We can correct this imbalance through the innovative health policies developed in tune with the needs of the country rather than based on any foreign model.[19]

The third serious problem in this area is of inefficient use of expenditure and non-utilisation of actual and potential resources judiciously and properly. In the developing countries, huge resources are being wasted because of the selection of inappropriate technology,[20] inefficient management,[21] and unsatisfactory control mechanism.

> "It is necessary that public revenue should be raised is an equitable manner and spent economically so that the tax-payers may get full value for his money."[22]

The objects of financial control are to ensure—(i) that no wastage of resources occurs; (ii) that public money is not misused; and (iii) that intended results are obtained with the money spent. We can exploit the potential resources through careful planning and management. The traditional system of medicine can be of immense value to provide health care at a very low cost provided this is properly tapped by the designers of health services. It was reported in a recent UN Survey (1976) that, these adverse trends are despite the higher percentage of government expenditure being devoted to health, compared with 1960s and the fact that ratio of population to the number of beds and of medical personnel have moved favourably. Essentially, the continuance of poor health standards is indicative of a less-than-optimal use of resources available. Some aspects of this are the emphasis on curative, as opposed to preventive techniques embodied in the existing hospital systems, the inadequate development of indigenous medicine systems on which there is a continued reliance and the limited coverage of available medical facilities particularly in rural areas.[23]

In a paper presented by M. Siegel, Assistant Director-General, Department of Administration and Finance, WHO, Geneva, to the Advisory Group on Nursing Administration (16 December 1957) rightly remarked:

> "If the resources for health work, in trained persons and in finances, were unlimited, the need for constant attention to these factors would not be so great. But the limitation in the number of trained personnel and the lack of adequate financial resources are major obstacles to greatly improved health in the world today. We must, therefore, husband our resources carefully to accomplish as much as possible with what we have available."

The fourth serious challenge in this field is the rising cost of health services beyond the reach of most of the people inhabiting the developing societies. It is very difficult to afford the costly urban-based hospitals using highly sophisticated technology. A huge amount is being spent on costly buildings and equipment which the developing countries cannot afford. The only services which can meet the health needs of the people are low-cost services which should be efficient and effective. This is possible if we use methods and equipment appropriate to the socio-economic environment existing in a country, e.g., the people can contribute voluntary labour to maintain health services. This would reduce the cost. We must take decisions and think of alternative solutions to provide health care to the people as financing and decision-making are complementary functions. The health administrator should encourage the low-cost service programmes beneficial to the larger section of the community.

The fifth problem in this connection is the lack of coordination among different agencies financing health care services. This may result in wasteful duplication of efforts. Besides, many health services may not get the desired financial allocation because of this wastage. The situation can be improved through proper among such agencies.

Lack of Adequate Information Required for Health Planning, Implementation and Evaluation

Information is the life-blood of an organisation. According to R.R. Duersch, "it is a system which provides management with the information it requires to monitor progress, measure performance, detect trends, evaluate alternatives, make decisions and to take corrective action."[24]

There is no centralised department in the health organisations to collect, analyse, interpret, store and retrieve information. Confusion between 'Statistical data' and 'information' still prevails, with the result that many statistical services fail to provide public health administrators with the information they need for sound decision-making, planning and evaluation. In most of the health organisations, the data collected from the fields is either not of the required type or is not presented in a form or in time to be really useful to health administrators. Beside, the data is collected without a clear understanding about the use that such information will have. The routine collection of data which is neither reliable nor timely serves no purpose. These defects can be weeded out if we can design a scientific Health Information System or Management Information System (MIS). MIS is an analytical tool which facilitates more informal and better decision to be made and it helps to identify problem areas and to take timely remedial measures. It is in no case a substitute for management decisions but it is management's most important tool for decision-making. As Morton puts it:

> "Good management information system is no cure for bad management. Bad information always leads to bad management, but good information does not in itself ensure good management. Information is only a tool of management. The ability to put information to work is what determines a successful manager."[25]

Four basic processes involved in an information system are the collection of data, storing of data, processing of data and transmission of information. The term data is used to denote the input into the information system while information is the output. MIS should be designed to ensure smooth and proper flow of information into the desired channels. The information must be made available to the management at the required time and in right quantity and quality. It is also to be borne in mind that supplying unnecessary or unwanted information is also a sign of inefficiency of the system. To quote a UNICEF Report:

> "Information Services should be recast according to the priorities of the health system and should be aimed strictly at problem solving."[26]

Lack of Organisation Concept in Planning and Developing the System

The absence of a clear national health policy in most of the countries has created an environment in which fragmented health services have sprung up haphazardly. There is a need of a balanced health policy. Besides, the health planning though picking up, has yet to be adopted in the right earnest. The planning of health services and their expansion requires special skills and knowledge which must be cultivated among the personnel responsible for planning. Proper identification of the health needs and priorities of the general population is essential for the development of a comprehensive national health plan.[27]

Lack of a Sound Health Manpower Policy[28]

A sound health manpower policy is the main requirement for the development of any functionally effective health care system. Most of the countries in the developing world have never formulated or implemented such a policy.

> "The most crucial factor for the improvement of the World Health situation . . . is undoubtedly the development of health manpower that is properly attuned to the health problems of the people and suitably trained to respond to health programme and service need."[29]

We must find the method to achieve greater productivity, efficiency and cost-effectiveness in health manpower utilisation. No society, especially the developing, can long justify investing years of education and training in individuals who later on perform rudimentary duties that could be achieved satisfactorily by people trained in half that time. The critical decisions in health manpower planning concern the kinds of personnel required, the type and adequacy of education and training and financial resources necessary to produce them, their relationship to each other in the health team, and where and how they would practise.

Lack of Community Participation and Involvement

Merle Fainsod remarks: "The most favourable setting for progress in development administration exists where a politically influential and dynamic modernizing elite strongly desires development and can successfully project this attitude into both the bureaucracy and the population at large."[30]

Many well-intentioned and technically sound programmes aimed at solving health problems have been frustrated by a lack of popular acceptance and community participation. "It has been observed that such programmes are either not actively associated or passively ignored because they do not 'belong' to the population they are designed to help;

they are rather seen by the population as imposed external programmes that belong to the government and consequently deserve and require little, if any, of the population's attention, action, or other response."[31] We must be clear that health cannot be imposed; it can only be acquired. This requires participation based on enlightenment of the beneficiaries.[32]

Dr.. Madiou Toure, Director, Hygiene and Health Protection, Ministry of Public Health, Republic of Senegal, in his article, "The Health Revolution", in *World Health* (November, 1979) has rightly said: "The medicine of tomorrow will be shaped by the people for the people, because the people themselves will determine their own condition, their own destiny."

Lack of Administrative Capability and Competence

Administrative capability is *sine qua non* for the success of any programme. It is a major and crucial factor in the success or failure of development programmes. It is the scarcest of all resources in the developing world. The general administrator is fit only for the maintenance of law and order and he is not suitably equipped to deal with the problems of development and welfare economics.

According to K.N. Rao: "Unlike advanced countries there is no pool of experienced and well informed leaders of thought available as potential leaders for ministerial positions which greatly handicaps their assuming policy-making and decision-making responsibilities in the Government. This results in over-dependence on the Secretaries who are non-technical general administrators."[33]

The technical experts must be given training in public health administration to make them competent in the art of health planning and administration.

Highly Centralized: Need of Decentralization

The national health system, within whose structure the services required to deliver care to the urban, sub-urban and rural family nucleus must be organized, is a mechanism of such administrative complexity that it cannot possibly be run on a centralized basis. Hence, the need to decentralize the administrative process. This decentralization should include the extensive delegation of functions from the higher to the intermediate and local echelons, so as to produce effective decentralization in staff management, budgetary control, application of laws and regulations and if possible, financing as well. A consequence of this will be the need to provide administrative facilities at the regional level. An important factor supplementing the mechanisms of decentralization should be the participation of the community and of health professionals in the administration of the regional and local services.

In most countries there is a marked trend in the opposite direction, i.e., towards centralization of authority, and it is not always easy to convince the powers that be of the need to decentralize the health services. There are nevertheless many reasons that justify decentralization. One that has already been mentioned is the extent of the facilities needed to provide comprehensive preventive, curative and rehabilitative services to the whole population of a country. This requires a large multi-disciplinary staff which must deliver an enormous variety of services involving different technologies to a population composed of millions of individuals of widely differing cultural levels and with different health needs. The administrative machinery required to operate this gigantic service is so complex that its management cannot be centralized—furthermore, if planning and evaluation of these services is to be conducted locally, it is essential that the implementation of the health activities also be directed at the local level, with the effective participation of the suppliers and consumers of health services.

MEETING THE CHALLENGES

On the basis of our discussion and analysis the following suggestions are given in brief to revitalise the health care delivery system, to meet the challenges and fulfil the basic health needs of the people:

(i) Need of will and determination on the part of the political elite, to accept innovative measures to meet the population's health needs and priorities.
(ii) Identification and implementation of a clear and comprehensible National Health Policy.
(iii) Need of decentralised planning involving the participation of the target communities.
(iv) Mobilisation of existing and untapped resources—community, government (local and national), bilateral, multilateral and non-governmental to provide adequate health care for all.
(v) Establishment of appropriate administrative structures with necessary competence and capability and devolution of authority and responsibility for the implementation and development of the programme in a team spirit and a well-designed information system to help in planning, implementation and evaluation.
(vi) Manpower development for national health needs.
(vii) Strengthening existing rural establishment and graded extension of national administrative structures to provide adequate and accessible referral, supervisory, logistical and other supporting services to ensure the judicious use of health services.
(viii) More allocation of financial resources based on the principles of equitable distribution and maximum utility.

(ix) Encouraging integration and coordination.
(x) Reorientation of Medical Education to suit the needs of the community.
(xi) Designing health technology to suit the environment and making the best use of existing technology of traditional system of medicine.
(xii) Improving research and development capacity to solve health problems.
(xiii) Devising measures to promote the use of simple, standardised equipment and drugs, placing reliance on available local resources whenever possible to foster self-reliance.
(xiv) The preventive health measures are crucial for sustained improvement and must be intensified to attain:
  (a) Total coverage of the entire urban and rural population in the country with assured potable drinking water supply and sewerage;
  (b) The disposal of urban wastes should also be given a high priority to ensure clean environment;
  (c) For improving the environmental sanitation and hygiene, high priority must be given to town and country planning, provision of better working and living conditions, removal of congestion through the increased tempo of housing construction, slum clearance and prevention of water and air pollution;
  (d) The nutritional status of the population must be raised and total prevention of food adulteration and drugs control should be achieved through rigorous controls; and
  (e) Health education should be an integral part of all health programmes.

SUGGESTIONS GIVEN BY NINTH FIVE YEAR PLAN

(a) Creation of a functional, reliable health management information system and training and deployment of health manpower with requisite professional competence.
(b) Multi-professional education to promote team work.
(c) Skill upgradation of all categories of health personnel, as a part of structured continuing education.
(d) Improving operational efficiency through health services research.
(e) Increasing awareness of the community through health education.
(f) Increasing accountability and responsiveness to health needs of the people by increasing utilisation of the Panchayati Raj institutions in local planning and monitoring.

(g) Making use of available local and community resources so that operational efficiency and quality of services improve and the services are made more responsive to user's needs.

Approach During the Ninth Five Year Plan

The approach during the Ninth Plan will be:

(i) An absolute and total commitment to improve access to, and enhance the quality of primary health care in urban and rural areas by providing an optimally functioning primary health care system as a part of the Basic Minimum Services;

(ii) To improve the efficiency of existing health care infrastructure at primary, secondary and tertiary care settings through appropriate institutional strengthening, improvement of referral linkages and operationalisation of Health Management Information System (HMIS);

(iii) To promote the development of human resources for health, adequate in quantity and appropriate in quality so that access to essential health care services is available to all so that there is improvement in the health status of community, periodically organise programmes for continuing education in health sciences, update knowledge and upgrade skills of all workers and promote cohesive team work;

(iv) To improve the effectiveness of existing programmes for control of communicable diseases to achieve horizontal integration of ongoing vertical programmes at the district and below district level; to strengthen the disease surveillance with the focus on rapid recognition, reporting and response at district level; to promote production and distribution of appropriate vaccines of assured quality at affordable cost; to improve water quality and environmental sanitation; to improve hospital infection control and waste management;

(v) To develop and implement integrated non-communicable disease prevention and control programme within the existing health care infrastructure;

(vi) To undertake screening for common nutritional deficiencies especially in vulnerable groups and initiate appropriate remedial measures; to evolve and effectively implement programmes for improving nutritional status, including micronutrient status of the population;

(vii) To strengthen programmes for prevention, detection and management of health consequences of the continuing deterioration of the ecosystems; to improve linkage between data from ongoing environmental monitoring and that on health status of the population residing in the area including health in impact assessment as a part of environmental impact assessment in developmental projects;

(viii) To improve the safety of the work environment and worker's health in organised and unorganised industrial and agricultural sectors especially among vulnerable groups of the population;

(ix) To develop capabilities at all levels for emergency and disaster prevention and management; to implement appropriate management systems for emergency, disaster, accident and trauma care at all levels of health care;

(x) To ensure effective implementation of the provisions for food and drug safety; strengthen the food and drug administration both at the Centre and in the States;

(xi) To increase the involvement of ISM&H practitioners in meeting the health care needs of the population;

(xii) To enhance research capability with a view to strengthening basic, clinical and health systems research aimed at improving the quality and outreach of services at various levels of health care;

(xiii) To increase the involvement of voluntary, private organisations and self-help groups in the provision of health care and ensure inter-sectoral coordination in implementation of health programmes and health-related activities; and

(xiv) To unable the Panchayati Raj Institutions (PRIs) in planning and monitoring of health programmes at the local level so that there is greater responsiveness to health needs of the people and greater accountability; to promote inter-sctoral coordination and utilise local and community resources for health care.

It is hoped that the implementation of these suggestions would ensure wider and more evenly distributed health care based on social justice, greater involvement and satisfaction of the beneficiaries and more efficient and more economical health services.

PART II

HOSPITAL ADMINISTRATION

Hospital infrastructure has grown in both size and complexity as well as hospitals have grown both in size and direction, making its management a challenging task. With the coming in of poly clinics and big hospitals in private sector, the problems of hospitals administration have compounded. What are the problems that are likely to be encountered by hospitals in new millennium? What can be done to make them serve the cause of health of the community? How can we translate the definition of health given by WHO to make the lives of people healthier. Let us discuss some of the potential problems and their solution that the hospitals are likely to face in the new millennium. We may keep the following words in mind. We cannot continue doing what we have always done. Tomorrow cannot be just more of yesterday. We need flexibility and pragmatism as much as innovation. But the stress must invariably be on action.

In *World Health,* in an article, "Globalization and Public Health, a new challenge for WHO", (51st year No. 2, March-April, 1998), it was emphasized that it is important to note, however, that the implications of globalization for public health are not all negative. The diffusion of modern technologies and ideas between countries present promising opportunities for improving global health in the future. Recent advances in telecommunications technology, can be exploited for health purposes, which include: telemedicine, interactive health networks, disease surveillance systems, communication links between health workers, human resources development and continuing education, and distance learning.

In summary, a strong case can be made that the globalization of public health represents an important trend for the 21st century. Although some transnational health problems have historical precedents, many new issues are emerging which are unique to our time. The 1997 Kyoto conference on climate change under-scored the fragility of the world's ecosystem, and showed how interdependent the health of all of humanity has become. Shared global problems transcending state borders call into question conventional paradigms which divide countries into North and South, or developed and developing. Let us discuss important problems and their solutions.

I. COMPLEXITY OF HOSPITALS CREATED BY EVER INCREASING SOPHISTICATED DIAGNOSTIC TOOLS RESULTING INTO HIGH COSTS BEYOND BUDGETARY ALLOCATION: NEED OF ANALYSIS AND PLANNING

The developments in science and technology has resulted into the designing of complex medical equipments which can help medical experts in easy and accurate diagnosis and treatment. The development is so fast that old instruments become outdated after 3-4 years. All these equipments cost heavily and are mostly beyond the reach of many hospitals. Even if some hospitals acquire them, they have to cut on essential items, thus badly affecting the efficiency of hospital services. It is a paradox as to how to get the best of medical equipments as well as remain within financial constraints. This is a dilemma for many planners of the hospital. Based upon personnel observation, discussion and study, we suggest here some points to come over this serious problem.

(a) Need of Defining the Objective of the Hospitals

First of all, it is necessary to define the objective of the hospital, i.e. what level of health care is to be provided and to meet that care, what instrumentation and medical equipments are required? Upon the answers to this question would depend the purchase and use of equipment. What happens in practice, equipment available is not used, equipment needed is not available. It needs a thorough analysis before equipping the hospital with any new equipment.

(b) Need of Ensuring the Technical Manpower to Handle Costly Equipments

In most of the Government hospitals, equipments are lying idle and becoming junk because of not appointing the required technical personnel to handle the instrument. Even if the personnel are available, these become outdated and thus need be trained to make use of the latest knowledge.

(c) Need of Maintaining the Output to Ensure Benefits

Most of the equipment in Government hospitals either remain non-functional or work at lowest output resulting into highest per unit cost. It is done intentionally so that the patients may be referred to private laboratories to oblige/earn commissions. The technician's salary should be dependent and made conditional to the minimum output. His responsibility should be fixed and he should be held personally responsible for all the lapses. It may be mentioned here that he must be associated with the purchase of the machinery. He should be given necessary authority. Equipment should be used at least in two shifts and even private patients may be encouraged to use the services at some premium.

(d) Essential Use of these Equipments should be Encouraged but not a Routine Affair

It has been seen that it has become a fad with most of the specialists to prescribe unnecessary tests using complex instruments to make their false reputation and prestige resulting into wastage of resources both of the hospitals and the patients. It is suggested that doctors should prescribe only essential tests and move from simple to complex and not jump to complex examination. Doctors should be encouraged to develop more and more of their clinical sense.

Besides, costly equipment either not used or mostly remain non-functional causing losses worth crores of rupees. Let us illustrate with some examples reported by Poonam Bath in *The Tribune,* dated July 13, 2000. She stated that Machines worth lakhs of rupees are not being put to any use in the Department of Physiotherapy, PGI. While, some of them are out of order, a few other which are brand new, are yet to be used.

The department, which has been recently shifted to the new OPD block, has a daily OPD attendance of 100-150 patients. It offers patients at least five different forms of the therapy. This includes electro therapy, exercise therapy, heat therapy, hydro therapy and manual therapy. But the non-functionning machines are causing problems not only for the patients but for the doctors as well, who are forced to recommend an alternate therapy in the absence of the required therapy.

Sources reveal that a bio-tech machine worth Rs. 25 lakhs was purchased by the institute in 1997. But till today it is lying locked up in the department. Even a short wave diathermy machine, which is used for heat therapy, is out of order most of the time. Similarly, another machine for heat therapy, which is an essential equipment used to reduce the muscle spasm and various kinds of body pains, is not being put to its optimum use as half of its screen is damaged. One of the regular patients, who comes here for exercises, said earlier this machine was being used to give heat treatment to facilitate exercises, but this is not being used now.

(e) Private Laboratories may be Identified and Contracts Entered to Facilitate Cheap and Efficient Services

Even if the hospitals are overloaded or cannot provide the services, they may enter into contract with private laboratories to provide cheap and efficient services.

(f) Indigenous Equipment of Quality Need be Preferred

It has become a fashion to use imported equipments resulting into loss of foreign exchange and unemployment. Our equipment manufacturers can supply quality equipment provided corrupt practices are strictly dealt with and transparency in purchases is ensured.

2. DECLINING PROFESSIONAL ETHICS AMONG SPECIALISTS AND OTHER HOSPITAL STAFF—NEED OF DEVELOPING ETHICAL STANDARDS

The tendency to make money is on the increase in the profession. Medical professionals attend on priority the wealthy and influential people who can compensate them directly or indirectly while neglecting the common man. This tendency is on the increase and can become a big problem in new millennium.

Bertram M. Gross, an eminent Professor of Urban Affairs, Hunter College, City University of New York, has remarked: "One of the most important characteristic of a genuine profession—in addition to a recognized body of knowledge or skill and some organized provision for training, recruitment or certification—is a code of ethics. Professional codes of ethics, recognize the special power that may be exercised by someone with expert skill and knowledge. They are designed to protect clients against the abuse of such power by the professional—whether he be a doctor who penetrates bodily secrets of clients or a lawyer who learns the details of their private affairs."[34]

Large scale bureaucratic management, particularly when equipped with the most refined calculational techniques, can develop—to use Erich Fromm's words—a spirit "inhospitable to life, joy, independence, love, compassion, meaningful human relations, real intimacy and sharing between people." If the public administrators, managers and political leaders in developing countries cannot develop non-bureaucratic methods and institutions, "the result will be increasing loneliness, boredom, aggressiveness, competition, consumption—from cars to sex, liquor and drugs—and cruelty as the result of a lack of compassion."[35]

We can thus say that there is a need to develop both human and modern technology to improve efficiency. We must, however, give priority to human development.

As stated in a UN Report: "There are two aspects to development —technical and human. Organizations had usually been more sensitive to possibilities offered to them by the achievements of modern technology than to the refinements of human behaviour as revealed by the sciences of Sociology and Psychology. On the other hand, lessons drawn from experience showed that technical innovations derived from the engineering sciences encountered considerable resistance unless supported by corresponding changes in human attitudes and behaviour. In an era of rapid change, the improvement of management in its human aspect had become a critical issue. It was important to make full use of the findings of social sciences which endeavoured to be instrumental in giving guidance in behaviour of individuals and groups in varying circumstances. Organizations should, therefore, be conceived as complex, socio-technical systems whose management required both technical skills and insight into the motives of human behaviour."[36]

It is widely agreed that manipulation and lack of integrity produce strong negative side-effects and reduce organizational effectiveness. With this important value commitment the organization may shift their styles and climate from one of direction, control and surveillance to one of providing help, support and instruction. Mutuality and collaboration between the leaders and the led, self-control and mutual support are essential for creating an organic organization. Let the newcomers strive to set-up organized society with social democracy and high human values settings up ideal societal or public management institutions and if such timely warnings are not accepted, social upsurges are bound to develop in a mild or a violent form.

J.S. Neki has rightly said that "to help, to heal, to reconstruct, to comfort—and all along the line to act with compassion—all these bear testimony to the moral consciousness of the doctor. Whatever the new strains imposed upon medical ethics this structure will survive and continue to guide doctors in their professional conduct . . . Legal and juridical obligations they have, of necessity to fulfil. But these are not genuine ethics. Genuine ethics has to be integrated into character and does not have to depend upon external controls."[37]

R.S. Pathak, former Chief Justice of India rightly mentions that the vitality of an ethical dimensions in the discharge of public responsibilities is essential to a developing nation. In a developing nation, the release of nascent national energy is a great moment. It provides the power necessary for building of a nation.[38]

We suggest here some points to make ethical standards practicable and feasible:

(i) Top leadership should follow ethical standards to serve as bacon light for the health functionaries at the lower level.
(ii) We should encourage professional standards to inject in the medical team the spirit of service.
(iii) New entrants need be supervised properly so that wrong behaviours may be corrected in the initial stages.
(iv) There should be code of ethics which should be followed by all.
(v) Environment of the hospital should be such which can inspire confidence and loyalty.
(vi) Medical team should be respected and given due status.

3. ABSENCE OF REFERRAL SYSTEM CAUSING MISUSE OF RESOURCES

We may mention here that we cannot afford the scarce resources for health services being wasted in duplication, overlapping and mismanagement. There is at present no proper referral system in place. Once a patient is received at particular institution, the doctor examines the patient and decides whether he/she can be managed there itself, or needs a referral to a higher level facility. There is complete lack of co-ordination among the peripheral institutions, on the one hand, and between the institutions and district hospitals, on the other. There are no guidelines or procedures that govern the peripheral institutions and the higher-level hospitals in a referral chain. No written or unwritten conventions exist as to what types of conditions are to be treated, from where and when. There is also no prioritization of referred cases, either from private or government institutions. Lower-level facilities lack even basic facilities, equipment and major specialists, leading to a large number of self-referrals and overcrowding in the higher level facilities.

In the new millennium, we must promote forward and backward linkages among all levels and institutions of all systems of medicine to provide decent health services in new millennium. At present, our hospitals are working in isolation causing misuse of services. In the new millennium, we must define the clear-cut referral system to provide integrated health services and pooled wisdom of health experts.

Conceptually a multi-tier system which combines preventive, curative and specialized care is efficient when it provides patients access to levels of care that are appropriate to their health needs with a minimum of inconvenience and delay. It works best when the lowest tier is easily accessible to the community and provides the bulk of the preventive care as well as curative care services for common illnesses. Patients with more complex problems are identified in a timely and systematic manner and referred to the appropriate higher level. Each successive level provides services that are more complex and therefore more expensive. In such a system, the higher tier provides technical leadership and support for the lower tiers, and the community has confidence in the quality of care provided at each tier and the patients understand they will be in accordance with patient needs.[39]

4. HOSPITAL WASTE CAUSING ENVIRONMENTAL POLLUTION AND LEADING TO NEGATIVE RECYCLING WITH SERIOUS MEDICAL AND HEALTH CONSEQUENCES—NEED OF SERIOUS THINKING AND ACTION

Hospital waste is causing great health hazards especially in metropolitan and big cities where large number of hospitals are located. Hospital wastes include both infectious and non-infectious substances coming out of different wards, OTS, OPD, Emergency services, etc. Such wastes can create hospital infection as well pose major cause of environmental pollution.

Hospital waste will contain injurious items such as: infective exudates, tissues, or dressings; radioactive materials; and contaminated syringes and needles. Special care must be exercised in disposing of these items by incineration, burial, or other means. In particular, disposable syringes and needles may be sought by drug abusers, and should be rendered unusable. The channels for disposing of hospital waste will depend on local circumstances and legislation.

There is a need for every hospital to set-up hospital waste system. The hospital waste can cause infectious problems to:

(a) Patients and their relatives who come to the hospital.
(b) Personnel providing hospital services from doctors to sweepers.
(c) Impact on environment causing many health problems—Where hospital wastes are dumped, it becomes an ideal breeding ground for rodents, mosquitoes, bacteria, virus, flies, leading to many complex diseases. These can contaminate the water and air and can cause serious health problems for the residents.

The quantity of hospital wastes is on the increases as more and more disposal items are being used. In the new millennium, it may be very high. So, there is a need of scientific management of hospital wastes. It means removal and disposal of waste economically and hygienically on a scientific basis.

Generally two methods of waste treatment are in existence:

(i) Incineration.
(ii) Steam Sterilization.

Incineration is a process which converts solid wastes into harmless gases at 1400 degree Fahrenheit. While steam sterilization uses steam penetration.

Hospitals in India both Government and Private are not using scientific methods. They are dumping the wastes nearby or throw them at some distance of the hospital. In this way hospitals are becoming the cause of environmental degradation and causing many health hazards than providing good health care. Even, where incinerators are provided, these are non-functional.

In the new millennium, we suggest that hospital waste management must be given top priority, otherwise we would be creating our own health problems. We suggest the following to be done in new millennium:

(a) All hospitals with 30 beds and above should instal incinerators.
(b) All health centres must dispose of the wastes carefully.
(c) All health institutions should have a manual on waste handling procedure and those made responsible for it should be provided a training for it.
(d) Strict supervision must be done by directors/medical superintendents and local administration over the waste disposal.
(e) No private health establishment should be allowed to function until and unless they have developed proper waste disposal system.
(f) Care should be taken that unscrupulous element may not recycle the waste.

Tribune, May 19, 2000 has nicely reported the situation of waste disposal in Rohtak and Jhajjar districts. The Drug Control Department, Haryana has reportedly taken strict measures to check the sale and storage of medical waste in the state in view of the reports regarding the development of a "nexus" leading to the supply of used disposable syringes and intravenous (IV) sets for recycling and resale in market.

According to sources the Drug Control Department has alerted its officials and directed them to conduct raids at clinics and hospitals in rural and urban areas in the state. While the focus area remains the districts lying in proximity of the national capital, 'raids' can be conducted at any clinic anywhere in the state.

Officials of the department have conducted several "raids" in Rohtak and Jhajjar districts. According to reports the authorities had "recovered" used disposable syringes and Intravenous (IV) sets weighing about four kg from a clinic run by a registered medical practitioner (RMP) at Barahi village in Bahadurgarh sub-division, about 40 kms from Jhajjar. However, some of RMP's working in the same village fled before the officials reached their clinics. The "accused" medical practitioner is charged with storing used syringes and intravenous (IV) sets instead of destroying these immediately after use.

The authorities produced the samples of seized material in the court. The officials also recovered some expired medicines from a chemist's shop at Badli village in Jhajjar district. The shop is run by Ramesh Kumar.

Meanwhile, according to sources raids had also been conducted in Bahadurgarh and Rohtak towns, but with no major success. A senior official, however, said raids would continue.

The officials reportedly became alert after reports in the media regarding the recovery of two truck loads of medical waste (used syringes and IV sets) from Delhi. The matter became serious when the issue was raised in parliament and the government assured that proper action would be initiated to check the "entry" of recycled medical waste into market. The recycled hospital waste poses a risk of the spread of AIDS and Hepatitis-B.

The Drug Controller, Haryana, has issued instructions to the district drug inspectors and officials of the Health Department to step up the campaign and identify the persons engaged in storing, selling and recycling of medical waste.[40]

However, the shortage of staff and inadequate infrastructure in the department could hamper the campaign against recycling of medical waste.

Hospital waste poses a great hazard as it can spread infection, but most hospitals don't follow any standard waste disposal method. Government hospitals as well as the private nursing homes dump their waste just like ordinary garbage. Needless, syringes, dressings, swabs immersed with blood, pus or other body fluids, culture stocks, infected or unused blood are all disposed of in the same way. Only placenta and body parts are buried or burnt. Advent of new technologies has revolutionised the diagnosis and treatment methods, but at the same time it has also added to the quantum of hazardous waste.

The Ministry of Environment and Forests formulated certain rules called the Biomedical Waste (Management and Handling) Rules, 1998, to be followed throughout the country, but these are being flouted-everywhere.

For evolving national guidelines on hospital waste management, the All India Institute of Medical Sciences (AIIMS) organised a two-day expert committee meeting in November, 1998, where medical officers and health administrators evolved guidelines, which were published and circulated to all states. But they have hardly been followed.

The Ministry of Environment and Forest has categorised and notified two types of medical waste in the bio-medical handling and management rules. Each category needs a separate disposal treatment. But this is not done in most hospitals. The whole lot is dumped with waste from other sources infecting the latter also. Scavengers are the potential carriers of infections.

Rajan Kashyap in his article "Dangers from Medical Wastes — Need for multi-disciplinary approach" in *The Tribune,* dated July 13, 2000 stated that even as hospitals provide solace and relief from disease, the dangerous wastes generated by them have become a serious hazard which threatens public health. Indiscriminate disposal of hospital wastes is indeed a major source of pollution and infection. Bio-medical wastes from hospitals, nursing homes and clinics include hypodermic needles, scalpel blades, surgical gloves, cotton, bandages, clothes, medicines, blood and body fluid, human tissues and organ, body parts, radio-active substances and chemicals. Some of these contain harmful organisms. Reuse of discarded syringes/needles can transmit lethal disease like AIDS and hepatitis. Similarly, indiscriminate recycling of used cotton, clothes and medicines poses a host of health hazards.

For a solution, it is necessary to appraise both visible and invisible factors. A multi-disciplinary approach would have to be adopted for the management of bio-medical wastes. This must incorporate the following:

- *Legal measures*: The ministry of Environment and Forests, Government of India, has framed Bio-Medical Wastes (Management and Handling) Rules, 1995. The Central Pollution Control Board has formulated guidelines for safe handling of hospital wastes. Compliance must be enforced.
- Allocation of resources of the Central Government and the state government for an integrated programme of bio-medical waste management.
- Closer coordination between the Department of Health of the state government and municipal administration.
- The establishment of a commonly managed and integrated system of final disposal of medical wastes, linked to a fair debiting of costs to the generators of the hazardous wastes.
- Drastic reform measures in municipal administration for raising adequate financial resources for optimal utilisation for the management of hazardous wastes.
- Involvement of non-governmental agencies which are closely linked to the people who suffer the adverse impact of

mishandled hazardous wastes.

- A well-directed public awareness campaign.
- Harnessing technology for achieving clearly developed objectives.
- Structured training programmes for all staff members engaged in the handling of the wastes. These could include the introduction of specific diploma or even degree level courses in medical or engineering institutions, as also some practically-oriented courses for workers.
- A strong monitoring system, which determines accountability of the polluter and of the handler of the hazardous wastes.
- Enforcement of the polluter pays principle.

5. MUSHROOM GROWTH OF PRIVATE HOSPITALS WITH NO NORMS—NEED OF DEFINITIONS

Private hospitals are coming in a big way to make good the inefficiency of Government hospitals but with a heavy price. Ravinder Sood, reporting from Palampur (H.P.) said (*The Tribune*, May 22, 2000) that health services in this remote corner of the state has received a big boost with the setting up of a private hospital in the town. However, he cautioned that it is a sad state of affairs that despite spending crore of rupees every year, still, the government hospitals in the state has failed to meet the medical needs of the people. Every year the state government is spending over Rs. 120 crores on health services in the state but still the common man is deprived of health facilities.

In the new millennium hospitals would become big business exploiting both the doctors and the patients and benefiting the owners. Satya Prakash Singh in his article in *The Tribune* dated May 30, 2000 rightly observed that given the same environment and budget, hospitals in private sector provides better service, and can see the mushrooming of private nursing homes in a city like Chandigarh, which has the prestigious PGI and a modern government hospital. It would be tantamount to complacency if one thought that the growth of private nursing homes in the city was only due to the increased demand for medical service that government hospitals were not able to cope up with. There is a definite shift from government hospitals to the private sector. The future therefore, is that of private sector hospitals. Due to competition the quality of medical services is expected to improve to a satisfactory level for those who can afford to pay. The future of medical service for the teeming millions below the poverty line (and one should not believe that those above the poverty line are not poor) is indeed bleak. Even if the blissful world of perfect competition prevailed, in distant future, where the services would be produced and sold at a level of "prices equal to the marginal revenue equal to the minimum marginal cost", the poor would still not adequately be served. That level of minimum cost too would be too high for them to afford.

There is no harm in supplementing health services by private hospitals but with some state laws, norms and controls. State must help in providing various inputs in setting up private hospitals and also exercise its regulatory authority in respect of the following through medical council of India:

(a) Doctors engaged by private hospitals should be paid at least as per the government pay scales.
(b) Security of service must be ensured through service rules.
(c) Fees from patients need be approved by government for various services.
(d) Regular inspections need be done by experts to ensure quality of essential services.
(e) Hospital should not be located away from residential complexes.
(f) Mechanism of redressal of grievances of patients must be devised.
(g) Hospital must report on a pre-designed performa after a regular interval of time.
(h) Parameters for setting up private hospitals/nursing homes need be defined so that they may not become nuisance to people living nearby.
(i) Norms of services should be spelt out.

There is a need to make use of the private initiative in a big way and associate them as an equal partner in the provision of Health Care.

As the population is booming, with resultant increase in pressure on medical services, the inadequacies of Government managed hospital facilities are coming into focuss. While the Government cannnot wish away its role in providing some basic health and medical services to those, who can't afford it against cost, it is becoming increasingly evident that system failures can no longer be put under the carpet.

Now the time has come, when Government should restrict its role to providing primary health care and promote/support the private sector to establish and provide the remaining medical services. Let the private sector get pre-eminent role in management of health services, with administrtive and financial support coupled with some controls of the Government. This will save the public exchequer from unnecessary and wasteful expenditure and available costs of Governance in health and medical sector.

We can thus say that the government should come forward with a legislation defining parameters for setting up private hospitals/nursing homes, otherwise, the government would have to face greater challenges. However, there are many health institutions or private practitioners who are doing good work. The Government should encourage them and associate them in the total process of health care.[41]

6. LACK OF ARRANGEMENTS FOR KEEPING THE HOSPITAL STAFF EQUIPPED WITH LATEST KNOWLEDGE IN NEW MILLENNIUM IN CLINICAL, TECHNICAL AND MANAGERIAL COMPETENCE—NEED OF DESIGNING NEW METHODS

There is no doubt that the efficiency of the hospital services depends to a substantial extent on the clinical, technical and managerial competence of the hospital staff. However, it has been seen that doctors/ technicians, supporting staff, hospital administrators, once appointed, go on working in their narrow grooves. New millennium is unfolding many new skills in every area to make hospital system efficient and effective. A lot of research is being undertaken at various places in new methods but these do not reach to most of the hospital personnel and thus the benefits of new knowledge are never translated in practice. What can be done to overcome this? How can we keep hospital staff in tune with new millennium? How can we make them think tank of the hospitals? We suggest here some points which can keep the hospital staff effective and efficient.[42]

(i) There is a constant need of in-service training both for the government and private practitioners.
(ii) Teaching-*cum*-research institutions like PGI, AIIMS, etc. should start some evening classes or a fortnight course where doctors can undergo training in latest techniques. Medical associations, speciality associations and alumni associations of medical colleges can also play a significant role on this behalf.
(iii) Teaching-*cum*-research institutions can send the specialists in the concerned field to make doctors in the field aware of the latest development as well as distribute literature in the area concerned.
(iv) An Open Medical University may be set-up where courses in all areas are available. This can benefit in a big way. Modern techniques like tele-conferencing, computers may be used to reach the health and medical personnel in the remotest area.
(v) Telemedicine, a new technique can help the doctors to be in touch with the latest developments in the institutions in the entire world benefiting both the doctors and the patients.

Health Telematics is defined as a composite term for health-related activities, services and systems carried out over a distance by means of information and communications technologies for the purpose of global health promotion, disease control and health care, as well as education, management and research for health.[43]

Dr. Prakron Vuthipongse, permanent Secretary, Ministry of Public Health, Thailand, in Inter-country Workshop on Tele-Medicine for Health Development in 21st century from 30th March-3 April, 1998 at Bangkok said that as a decision-maker he was aware of the advancement in today's technology, especially in its applications which will help to bring better quality of health care to people in remote and rural areas in a cost-effective manner. He also said that the initiation of Tele-Medicine in the Ministry of Public Health has emerged from the fact that, in remote and rural areas, there has been maldistribution of medical specialities, resulting in poor health care services. He expected the workshop to come up with fruitful recommendations on regional and national plans of action as well as on inter-country cooperation.[44]

However, this very conference cautioned about the use of Tele-medicine: Health Telematics raises certain ethical issues, such as the acceptability of transmitting personal information across cultural boundaries; young doctors getting professionally affected, and the confidentiality of the relationship between the patient and the treating doctor. Full cooperation of the medical and paramedical staff involved, as well as patients is essential. Even in the most advanced form, Health Telematics might not provide a blanket solution for each situation. There would be cases where human intervention is needed. It also raises concern on widening the gap between the poor and the privileged.[45]

Thus, in the new millennium the use of tele-medicine offers a potential source of latest knowledge, however, we must use it with great caution and thought.

Dr. R.A. Mashelkar, Director General, Council of Scientific and Industrial Research, delivered the convocation address at the 30th Convocation of Indian Institute of Technology, New Delhi. He said, "Knowledge without innovation is of no value. It is through the process of innovation that knowledge is converted into wealth and social good. Innovative nations lead the world today. When one looks at India, one feels that centuries of subjugation have perhaps undermined our capacity for innovation and creativity, which has got to be revived. We cannot allow the 'I' in India to stand for imitation and inhibition, it must stand for innovation. This requires an all pervasive attitudinal change towards life and work—a shift from a culture of drift to a culture of dynamism, from a culture of idle prattle to a culture of thought and work, from diffidence to confidence, from despair to hope. Revival of creativity and the innovative spirit needs to be made into a national movement today, in the same spirit and on the same scale as marked our freedom struggle.[46]

Dr. R. Chidambaram, Chairman, Atomic Energy Commission and Secretary to the Government of India, Department of Atomic Energy, delivered the Convocation Address at the Third Annual Convocation of Shivaji University, Kolhapur, he said, "For a nation to grow and advance rapidly, it has to strive for excellence in all its spheres of activity.[47]

Dr. Shivayogi P. Hiremath, Vice-Chancellor, Kuvempu University, Shimoga (Karnataka) delivered the Convocation Address at the Graduation Day-1999 of JJM Medical College, Davanagere. He said,

"Doctors on the net is a common caption in most of the Western Countries. Why are so many people turning online for medical information? Experts suggest that there is something inherent in the quick turnover medical office visits that it leaves patients wanting more and more connection, more personal interest, more explanation and more help."

A doctor has to be a constant student and should always work hard to keep abreast of the field by regularly attending the Continuing Medical Education (CME) programmes.[48]

7. INCREASING COST OF HEALTH SERVICES: NEED OF RESOURCES MOBILISATION AND COST CONSCIOUSNESS

In the new Millennium, the cost of hospital services would increase beyond the capacity of the hospital resources. The expenditures on salary, equipment and drugs would be an ever increasing pressure on the capacity of the hospitals. The result would be either dilution of quality of services or limiting the hospital services. In both situations, hospital services and prestige would be affected. Let us explains with the help of Indira Gandhi Medical College, Shimla — As reported in *The Tribune* (June, 2000) out of even sanctioned strength of 186 posts comprising of 55 Class I, 70 Class II and 70 Class III are lying vacant while the number of OPD patients increased from one lakh in 1993 to 2.30 lakhs in 1999, and indoor patients increased from 11,295 to over 16,000 during the same period. Because of financial shortage, these posts instead of increase, have not been filled. Patient care has deteriorated. Patient care has been far from satisfactory as there are not enough nurses in the 661-bed hospital as against a requirement of 600 only about 200 were in position.

Even all the existing posts have not been filled and at present 186 posts, including 55 Class I, nine Class II and 70 Class III posts were vacant. While CT scan, ultrasound and other facilities were introduced, no new posts were created.

What can be done to keep the hospital services in operation in the new millennium? We suggest here some facts and suggestions:

(i) Hospitals should set-up an economy committee which should scrutinise the current activities, their mode of financing and their utility. An examination would indicate a great scope for curtailment of unwanted expenditure.

(ii) the Director/Medical Superintendent through financial experts apply the modern management techniques like performance budgeting, zero-base budgeting, cost accounting, etc. to ascertain the genuineness for expenditure and its utility, e.g. what is the cost per patient admitted to an emergency? What is the cost per operation? In this way, we can locate where expenditure can be controlled without affecting the delivery of quality health services.

(iii) Hospital staff should be made cost-conscious so that they should use hospital resources judiciously and economically. They should use only those services which are essential.

(iv) Since a large part of the hospital expenditure is on the salary of medical and supporting personnel there is a need to ensure optimisation of their services. It has been seen that a lot of time is wasted by the hospital staff in non-medical activities. By making use of method study, work measurement, activity analysis we can improve upon the utilisation time of hospital staff. Hospital authorities have to be strict on punctuality and availability of hospital staff to justify their salaries. In India, most of the hospital staff remain busy with private practice and work in private hospitals, therefore, they cannot justify their work in hospitals. Strict action is required on this account as doctors are already paid NPA.

(v) For resource mobilisation, there can be users' charges. The appropriateness of adopting cost sharing principles depends on the type of service provided. Hospital services are mostly patient-related curative services. There is a scope to charge on curative services provided, a mechanism exists to adjust fees depending on the patient's ability to pay. However, the additional revenues generated by cost sharing may not be adequate to cover fully the expenditure in improving quality through better facilities in terms of equipment and drugs. The argument for cost sharing is based on efficiency. If no fee is charged there will be an "excess demand" for services especially hospital beds. Government hospitals are crowded and often the resourceful but the undeserving people get free access, whereas the poor have to incur "transaction costs" to get treatment or a hospital bed. Graded cost recovery from the non-poor is expected to restrict demand for beds thereby releasing beds for the poor. Thus, cost sharing may be a step in restoring equity; the poor may benefit proportionately more than the non-poor.

Charging fees for services may only slightly affect the demand negatively for health services because demand for in-patient and out-patient care is highly inelastic. However, consumers will be more responsive to the quality of care, time costs and the relative prices of alternative types of care givers. Cost sharing will augment resources for the health sector and should, therefore, lead to improvements in supply both in qualitative and quantitative terms. Sustainability would also be promoted to a large extent because the revenue realized would finance a portion of the operational costs thereby, relieving the budgetary constraint. Cost sharing would result in improvements in the quality of care if the resources generated internally by a hospital are ploughed back for improving the availability of drugs and equipment in that hospital.

Introduction of measures to augment resources will not automatically raise the level of infrastructure unless the concerned institution is in a position to reinvest a substantial portion on the hospital. Ideally, each secondary and tertiary level hospital should establish a "Development Fund" and open a Bank account where the collections from Cost Sharing would be remitted.

All hospitals should also be entitled to receive donations from philanthropic organisations and individuals, undertakings in the private and public sector, etc. and credit to its "Development Fund" the money which can then be used for undertaking civil works, purchase of equipment, drugs, hospital supplies, etc.

Mobilisation of resources and injecting economy are the two important areas which can ensure the quality of hospital services in new millennium.

8. DETERIORATING QUALITY OF HOSPITAL SERVICES—NEED OF INTRODUCING HOSPITAL ACCREDITATION—QUALITY OF HEALTH CARE IN HOSPITALS IS DETERIORATING

The hospital system suffers from major handicaps. It was reported in *The Tribune* (June 2, 2000) that Doctors prescribes medicines of non-standard companies. To quote: "The Government Zonal Hospital has not been supplied stationery for a long time and various things like the OPD slips, in-door patient charts, X-ray prescriptions are being sought on donations. The hospital laboratories too are in a sorry state.

The ambulance service is also reported to be miserable. The three drivers have been posted on shift duties, but usually two of them remain on furlough. The only driver on duty takes his own time for attending emergency calls.

There is no casualty ward service available. The laboratory and X-ray technicians do not attend the emergency duties in protest against the failure of the government to pay them 10 percent house rent or emergency allowance. The ECG technician has not been posted for the past two years. A Class IV employee has been deputed for taking the ECG.

Budgets meant for maintaining equipment and building need to be stepped up. The hospital system in the State suffers from major handicaps. Budgets meant for maintaining equipment and building need to be steped up. Diagnostic facilities, equipment, ambulance and trained personnel require strengthening. Existing norms for staffing at various levels have to be reviewed, given the heavy pressure on the hospital system which currently results in poor quality of services. Similarly, norms for equipment and the range of clinical services at each level need to be worked out on a rational basis. The infrastructure needs thorough overhauling as well as expansion to meet the needs of the over strained hospital system. Management skills at the hospital level need to be continually upgraded. The overall environment in which the hospitals function need improvement.

Quality of health care is defined as "the degree to which health services for individuals and populations increase the likelihood of desired health outcomes and are consistent with current professional knowledge" (National Academy of Sciences, USA, 1997).

Quality of health care can be assured if the government introduces accreditation of hospitals in 21st century.

WHO, South Asia Regional Office organised a workshop in "Hospital Accreditation" at Bangkok, Thailand from 7-11 Dec. 1998. The group found the following advantages of accreditation:[49]

- Stimulates improvement of care.
- Strengthens community confidence.
- Reduces unnecessary costs.
- Increases efficiency.
- Promotes personnel training.
- Provides credentials for education.
- Can protect against lawsuits.
- Provides comparative data.

The Indian government proposed to take the following measures to introduce accreditation:

(1) Initiate the process for setting up a core group in the Ministry of Health.
(2) Sensitization of policy-makers by organizing national-level workshop by January 1999 for generating awareness about the need for hospital accreditation.
(3) Sensitization of professional bodies, service providers, and consumer groups by organizing regional workshops.
(4) Organize discussions on proposed legislation for compulsory registration of hospitals.
(5) Set-up expert groups to suggest minimum conditions for hospital registration.
(6) Set-up expert groups to suggest standards for hospital accreditation.[50]

Accrediation is going to be beneficial to both the providers and receivers of the services. Providers would be clear as to what standards are to be maintained and the receivers would know what to expect from the particular hospital. In this way, there can be a race among hospitals to get accreditation for better marketing of their services. Even in universities and colleges accreditation is being done in a big way by National Assessment and Acreditation Council (NAAC), an Inter-University Centre of University Grants Commission. Health Departments of the Union and State governments can set-up such accreditation councils for hospitals under the auspices of Medical Council of India. We have to take care that this work should be done in association with professional associations, research institutes, so that there may be less resistance at the implementation level.

9. NO HOSPITAL REVIEW: NEED OF STUDY AND RESEARCH IN DIFFERENT AREAS OF HOSPITAL ADMINISTRATION

Hospital administration is being run by hit and trial methods without undertaking in-depth studies in various areas of administration affecting hospital services.

In the new millennium, the hospitals should be run on scientific lines. This would require research and in-depth study of various administrative issues impinging on the medical services. Some of these areas may be mentioned here:

- the effective use of hospital services, e.g. X-rays, beds and of imaging and other services.
- staff issues such as job satisfaction and the retention of staff members, particularly nurses and other highly trained personnel;
- patient satisfaction;
- clinical data, such as readmission rate, length of stay for various illnesses, and the effectiveness and efficiency of referral to and from the hospital and health centres;
- cost-benefit analysis of different programmes;
- the incidence, etiology, and prevention of infection;
- design of new aids and gadgets for the care and comfort of patients, especially the disabled;
- management of human, financial, and material resources;
- quality assurance in hospitals;
- cost accounting of various services;
- utilization time of different categories of persons; and
- transport efficiency.

10. NEGLECT OF HOSPITAL MAINTENANCE: NEED OF MAINTENANCE AND BEAUTIFICATION

The first impression of the visitors to the hospital depends upon the proper upkeep of buildings, equipment, water-supply, electricity supply, etc. A visit to a number of hospitals revealed the following which should be taken care of in the new millennium:

(i) The surroundings of the hospital are covered with congress grass and is full of dirt. Even in many hospitals there are no boundary walls. It is suggested that green grass and plants should be grown to make the hospitals clean and greener.

(ii) Buildings of the hospitals are in bad shape. Because of the shortage of funds, these are not maintained properly. These become the breeding ground of insects and cause infection. In the hospitals, buildings must be maintained properly at regular intervals of time to avoid deterioration.

(iii) Sweepers and ward boys must be encouraged to keep the hospital clean. They must be told that cleanliness is very important for the recovery of patients.

(iv) Lavotaries are in bad shape and even stinking. Hospital authorities must attend to it seriously otherwise the foul smell make the whole environment of the hospital unpleasant.

11. NEED OF HARNESSING POTENTIALITIES BEING OFFERED BY NEW DEVELOPMENTS IN THE FIELD OF REGENERATIVE MEDICINE AND INFORMATION TECHNOLOGY

At the dawn of 21st century, we find the most important development in medicine is devėlopment of the science of Human Genome, involving human genetic engineering which will change the contours and contents of medical science.

William Haseltine in his article, "What the genome map means to your health." Enormous potential for both good and bad in *The Tribune,* dated July 2, 2000 clearly says that:

- **Molecular medicine** leads to improved diagnosis of disease; earlier detection of genetic predispositions to disease, rational drug design; gene therapy and control systems for drugs; and pharmacogennomics "custom drugs."
- **Microbial genomics** explores new energy sources (biofuels); environment monitoring to detect pollutants; protection from biological and chemical warfare; and safe, efficient toxic-waste clean-up.
- **Risk assessment** assesses health damage and risks caused by radiation exposure, including low-dose exposures; assess health damage and risks caused by exposure to mutagenic chemicals and cancer-causing toxins; and reduce the likelihood of heritable mutations.

Though less than a decade in the works, it is already clear that the combination of the genetic and information revolution will change medicine within the next 50 years more than in the past serveral centuries.

Current Medical Scene, Vol. 15, No. 1 (January-March 2000), in the Article "Medicine in the 21st Century has mentioned about the advancement of drug delivery system specially in relation to chronic diseases. To quote:

> "Scientists are working on a miniaturised sensor for diabetics that mimics the glucose detection systems in a healthy body. The device, possibly transdermal, would monitor blood sugar levels, then release insulin as necessary. Researchers at the Massachusetts Institute of Technology (USA) have made a proto-type for an entire mini pharmacy. It is a microchip (implanted or swallowed) with as many as 1,000 tiny reservoirs—each is the size of a pinprick and can hold anything from painkillers to antibiotics. The researchers claim the chip can be made even smaller and "smarter" by adding a sensor that will know when to release a drug and what the dose should be. Computerised diagnostic tools will read the patient's genetic profile, recorded on a computer chip. This will help physicians determine the exact levels of risk faced by a patient and the missing proteins and enzymes. In the not too distant future, we could expect genetically-based drugs for almost every serious ailment. These drugs would use the human gene, the human protein, the human cell and not a chemical as the medicine. Besides, this would help in prolonging healthy life."

Recently scientists have discovered a mutant fruit fly that lives for more than hundred days—about a third longer than the rest of its species. What makes the difference is a single gene, which scientists call Methuselah. Researchers are excited by the fact that if one gene can do that much for flies, then maybe something similar can be attempted in human genes. May be we can then swallow Methuselah pills or inject Methuselah genes and fool the body into thinking that it is forever young.

In addition, this science can help in curing age-related diseases which are incurable and thus can pave the way for healthier older life which would contribute to social and economic development of the society. To quote William Hastline in his article, "What the genome map means to your health" in *The Tribune,* dated July 2, 2000 that "the current medical practice of bone-marrow transplants shows that this idea is not at all farfetched. In that process, an older person with cancer, whose ability to form new blood cells has been damaged by chemotherapy, often receives marrow donated from someone younger. In effect, that person is an age-hybrid, with a 50 or 60 years old body, but with blood-derived tissues that are only 20 or 25 years old.

In short, rather than continually regenerate our body with aging stem cells, in the future we can regenerate them with our own younger cells. I expect this third wave of regenerative medicine to come into being sooner than the year 2050."

Prof. S.K. Brahmachari has stated (*Economic Times*, July 4, 2000) that the development of predictive medicine based on genomic information will allow better management of disease by early diagnosis and therapeutic or surgical intervention or through lifestyle change.

Professor G.P. Talwar in his article in (*Economic Times*, July 4, 2000) has said that "an advance of great importance is using stem cells for therapeutic purposes. Cells go through a stage where they have the ability to differentiate into various types of specialised cells depending on the environment in which the stem cells are placed. This has opened out new possibilities of populating such cells in different tissues. For example, inserted in the pancreas of a diabetic patient, these cells would differentiate to make insulin. Implanted in a discrete area of the brain, they would bring cure to a patient with Parkinson's disease by making the missing dopamine. Though at a nascent stage, this heralds a new era of Regenerative Medicine."

Kalpanan Jain in *The Economic Times* has rightly concluded that the human genome is in hand, holding answers not just to several diseases, but also to human origins. While there is a new promise to provide novel solutions to unmet health needs, the challenge at the same time is to use this gene power wisely, humanely and equitably.

Rick Weiss in his article "Human Health: Genomics and Beyond", *The Tribune*, July 5, 2000 stated that "the new science seeks to solve a simple but long-standing problem: Medicines are made and sold on a "one size fits all" basis, even though people vary substantially in how they respond to those compounds. As a result of this variability, more than 100,000 Americans die every year from side effects of prescribed medicines and another two million are made seriously ill.

Elbert Branscomb in his article, "It's genome, not a cure all" (*The Tribune*, dated July 5, 2000) has clearly said, "those far-reaching expectations should be tempered with realism: Mapping the genome will vastly increase the amount of our knowledge, but most will be knowledge we can't put into practice quickly. When it comes to medical treatment, far from offering new certainties, the genetic information will raise new questions and present difficult choices."

Machiavelli said in a famous work that there is nothing more difficult to take in hand more perilous to conduct, more uncertain in its success than to take the lead in the introduction of a new order of things.

12. NEED OF STREAMLINING THE UP-KEEP OF HOSPITALS THROUGH METICULOUS PLANNING OF HOSPITAL SERVICES

It has been seen that specialists and other staff are handicapped because of Non-availability of minor facilities which indicate callousness on the part of hospital authorities. For example, many a times, it has been found, trolleys are either not available or out of order, services of barber, bearers, communication facilities, transport facilities are not available. There is a need of planning in toto and not for some services only, as the absence of small services can lead to the death of a patient. Poonam Bath reporting about the death of a girl in (Chandigarh, *The Tribune,* dated July 2, 2000), mentioned the following factors responsible for it:

- ❑ Ambulance not available,
- ❑ CT scan machine out of order, and
- ❑ No barber to shave patient's head.

Besides the mother of the deceased complained of rude behaviour of the hospital staff, "The rude and callous behaviour of nurses and security staff also added to our woes. Nurses were busy chatting even as we kept requesting them to suck out blood from her lungs as she was finding it difficult to breathe."

Thus, the medical Superintendent must ensure the availability of these facilities or get these arranged from outside and not leave all these to be arranged by the patient's family as they are in a state of psychological trauma and shock.

Director of PGI, Chandigarh, where the death of the girl took place, instituted an enquiry into the incident and confirmed that the CAT Scan remains out of order till today (Chandigarh, *Newsline,* July 4, 2000).

In a government hospital in Cuttak (Orissa), three women died because of the infectious saline water. These cases are a daily occurence and can be avoided with careful hospital management.

13. CONSTRAINTS WITH WHICH MEDICAL PERSONNEL WORK AND LIMITATION IN SUCCESS OF TREATMENT

While endorsment of inefficiency or sheer neglect on the part of a hospital or its staff is uncalled for, it would be prudent to understand the constraints under which the hospitals and the medical personnel have to serve the ever increasing number of critical patients, some of which may not respond to a well proven treatment or the nature of affiction may be incurable or the delays in administration of treatment may occur despite the best efforts of the doctors on duty—due to multifarous pressures and bottlenecks, while judging their performance it is imperative to examine, whether the person was adequately skilled to handle the situation, whether there was intention to help to the best of his capability, whether an all out effort was made to render the service promptly and properly. If the answer to the above questions is 'Yes' no charge of negligence can be made out. It goes without saying that the staff has been accessible, humane, commitment . . . sympathetic in the hand of stren and grief, which patients and their attendants face in the hospital situation.

It is to be brought home loud and clear that medical treatment/ hospitalization does not gaurantee cure/amelioration in all cases. Things often go wrong, inspite of earnest care, concerted effort, advanced investigation, skillful surgical/medical treatment.

The adverse outcome of cases involved in serious injuries, often leads to sudden grief, manhandled of the medical and paramedical personnel and eventual media headlines, showing the medical profession/hospital in bad light. This require education to public on a continuing basis, besides providing security/insurance against outbursts of violent/anger leading to danger and risk to the life and property at the hospital.

It is suggested that local NGO/Red Cross play an important role in planning of utilization of services available and provide personnel services like transport, wheel chairs, drug, stores, barbers, bearers, etc. This can cut down an un-necessary delays, thus savings vital time between the onset of emergency situation and active intervention.

Any undue adverse publicity in the media against premier hospitals, will lead to greater stress on the minds of treating physicians/ surgeons and prove counter productive. However, the hospital administration should take seriously to healthy criticism and effect efficiency and improvement, whenever possible.

CONCLUSION

Besides, in the new millennium, the hospitals should attend to maintenance of buildings, equipment, dietry services, security services, registration services, etc. to maintain the prestige and dignity of the hospital as well as ensure quality health care in new millennium. In this great venture, hospital authorities may seek the involvement and co-operation of the people to make the medical services, patient-oriented. Hospitals in the new millennium should provide an environment of extended family where the patients can get professional and expert medical care and homely environment. Patients should be welcomed in this extended family type hospital services.

A spirit of service and dedication must pervade among the providers of the health care as they are considered second God on earth by the receivers of health care. In the new millennium, we must empower the patients by looking after them carefully and making them feel important.

The progress and achievements of the past 50 years are solid foundations for a healthier and better world. It is already time to build on them. Life in the 21st century could and should be better for all. We can pass no greater gift to the next generation than a healthier future. That is our vision. Together, the people of the world can make it a reality.

Notes and References

1. UN, 1974 Report on the World Social Situation, New York, 1975, p. 218.
2. WHO, *WHO Office Records*, No. 226, 1975, p. 113.
3. WHO, World Health *Papers*, 55, p. 83.
4. R.M. Findlay, Art of Administration, Edinburgh, Oliver, 1952, p. 48.
5. WHO, *Public Health Papers*, 55, p. 61.
6. Based on personal discussion.
7. L.D. White, Introduction to the Study of Public Administration, Macmillan, pp. 213-14.
8. For details refer to the respective Chapters.
9. L.D. White, *op. cit.*, p. 214.
10. V.O. Key, Politics and Administration in White (Ed.), *The Future of Government in the United States*, p. 155.
11. S.E. Finer, Primer of Public Administration, London, 1950, p. 68.
12. Granville Austin, The Indian Constitution: Cornerstone of a Nation, Clarendon Press, Oxford 1966, p. 50.
13. Christian Medical Commission: "An Exercise in the Development of Health Care Priorities", Geneva, 1974 (unpublished document—CMC/47/6), p. 1.
14. *The Tribune*, Chandigarh, August 1979.
15. UN, 1974 Report on the World Social Situation, New York, 1975, p. 219.
16. L.D. White: Introduction to the Study of Public Administration, Macmillan, N.Y., p. 201.
17. Gyan Chand, The Financial System of India, p. 1.
18. WHO, *Technical Report Series*, 925, p. 18.
19. Refer to the Chapter on 'Health Policy'.
20. Refer to J.H. Bryant, Health and the Developing World, Ithaca, N.Y., Cornell University Press, 1969.
21. WHO, Modern Management Methods and the Organisation of Services, Geneva, WHO, 1974 (*Public Health Papers*, No. 55).
22. P.K. Wattat, Parliamentary Financial Control in India.
23. UN (ESCAP), Economic and Social Survey of Asia and the Pacific, 1976, Bangkok, April 1977, p. 18.
24. Raymond J. Coleman and M.J. Rilley (Ed.), Management Dimensions, Holden-Day, INC, San Francisco, California, p. 5.
25. Morton F. Meltzer, The Information Centre: Management Hidden Asset, American Management Association, New York, 1967, pp. 136-37.
26. UNICEF, Health and Basic Services: Keys to Development, p. 50.
27. For details, refer to the Chapter on 'Health Planning'.
28. For details, see the Chapter on Health Manpower Planning and Development.
29. *WHO Chronicle*, 31:123-126 (1977), "Health Challenges for 1978-83."
30. Merle Fainsod, "The Structure of Development Administration" in Irving Swerdlow (ed.), *Development Administration: Concepts and Problems*, (Syracuse, N.Y., Syracuse University Press, 1963, p. 1).
31. *WHO Chronicle*, 30 (1976), pp. 177-78.
32. For details, refer to the Chapter on Primary Health Care Administration.
33. R.N. Rao, "Some Challenges in Health Administration", Background document to Xth Staff College Course at NIHFW, Mimeographed.
34. U.N.: ST/TAO/M/52/Add. I, p. 53
35. Erich Fromm: "Thoughts on Bureaucracy" (guest editorial), *Management Science* (Providence, R.I.), August, 1970.
36. U.N. Inter-Regional Seminar on Administration of Management Improvement

Services (Vol. I), Copenhagen, Denmark, 28 September-6 October, 1970, pp. 6-7 (ST/TAO/M/56).

37. J.S. Neki, "Medical Ethics: A View Point from the Developing World", *World Health,* July 1979, p. 15.
38. R.S. Pathak, Ethics in Public Life, Some Observations, in *IJPA,* July to Sept. 1995, p. 265.
39. Government of Karnataka, Karnataka Health System Development Project, Bangalore, 1996, p. 102.
40. *The Daily Tribune,* May 19, 2000.
41. *The Daily Tribune,* May 28, 2000.
42. *The Daily Tribune,* May 30, 2000.
43. WHO: SEARO, Health Telematics, Report of a WHO Intercountry Workshop on Tele-medicine for Health Development in the 21st Century, Bangkok, Thailand, 30th March-3rd April, 1998, p. 4.
44. *Ibid.,* p. 2.
45. *Ibid.,* p. 5.
46. AIU, *Unviersity News,* Sept. 20, 1999.
47. AIU, *University News,* April 21, 1997.
48. AIU, *University News,* Aug. 19, 1999.
49. WHO: SEARO, Hospital Accreditation Report of an Inter-country meeting, Bangkok, Thailand, 7-11, December, 1998.
50. *Ibid.,* pp. 41-42.

CHAPTER 4

ADMINISTRATION OF ENVIRONMENTAL HEALTH PROGRAMMES

O, mother earth, you are the world for us and we are your children. Let us speak in one accord, let us come together so that we live in peace and harmony.

—Atharva Veda

Administration of Environmental Health Programmes

A GOOD ENVIRONMENT IS THE KEY TO HEALTH AND DEVELOPMENT

Environment has been defined by Webster's New Collegiate Dictionary as "the aggregate of all the external conditions and influences affecting the life and development of an organism."

Shri T.N. Chaturvedi in his Editorial to *IJPA*, July-Sept. 1989 (Special Number on Environment and Administration) rightly sees the intimate relationship between human beings and nature since times immemorial. To quote, "Man, since his origin, has lived in harmony with Nature through the ages, holding Nature in awe and reverence. The Vedas, folklore and scriptures of different religions, faiths and beliefs also speak of the need for harmony with the universe, which is the habitat not only of man but also of all animals, bird, insects, plants and vegetation. The mutually supportive role of all living things is often mentioned as a crucial factor for a balanced social and harmonious existence. The ecological balance is inherent in the very process of creation. Everywhere, the seers, poets and thinkers, through the ages, have referred to the need for living in harmony with environment. In fact, the Taitariyopanishad looks at the relationship between man and his environment in its totality and stresses complete harmony and interdependence between them in order to attain real prosperity."

Dr. Hiroshi Nakajima, Director-General of World Health Organization, sounded a warning alarm about degradation of this planet in his Article, "A Wounded Planet." He rightly visualises that it is now increasingly evident that more and more diseases stem from the degradation caused by man to his own environment. The potential harmful effects of industrial development on our global ecosystem are now better known. Ozone layer depletion, acid rain, climate change, chemical pollution are some examples of the man-made wounds to our planet.[1]

We are at a turning point; warnings of the damage to our health and quality of life are growing louder. An increasing number of people are acting to stop the degradation of our environment. Lt. Gen. Jacob, PVSM (Retd.) former Governor, Punjab in his message "Fifty years of Indian Republic" in the *Daily Tribune* (26th January, 2000), remarked that with our rising population the civil services and environment, especially in the urban areas, are under great stress and strain. The degradation of our environment has to be arrested immediately otherwise it would have long-term impact on the quality of life of future generations . . . . We should also take this opportunity to educate our children regarding the importance of the preservation of our environment. Dr. Wilfried Kreisel also elaborates the aspects of environment which affect health of mankind.[2]

How can we make environmental health a more potent force to serve people faced with growing threats to their health? How can our improving environmental health technology be better used to foster positive health? I know of no country-developing or industrialised in which this issue is not urgent and important. I know of many countries in which it is critical.

The remarkably wide range of environmental concerns include the international problems of acid rain, the greenhouse effect, and depletion of the planet's ozone layer. It includes national concerns with medical wastes disposal, radioactive and toxic wastes control, transportation accidents, health aspects of urbanisation and traffic, occupational health and safety, and air and water pollution. It also includes local concerns over inadequate water supplies and sanitation facilities, water quality, clean air, solid wastes management, and finding a balance between the economic incentives of development and a decent quality of life. In the report on Our Common Future, the World Commission on Environment and Development (sometimes called the Brundtland Commission) pointed out that the situation is getting increasingly critical.

WHO, South-East Asia Regional Office Declaration on Health and Development in the South-East Asia Region in the 21st Century mentions that significant differences exist between the environmental problems of rural and urban areas.[3] In rural areas, poverty, unsafe drinking water, inadequate excreta disposal, combined with contaminated food and illiteracy, are responsible for a majority of illnesses. Poor ventilation, coupled with the use of poorly-designed cooking stoves, cause severe indoor air pollution and health problems, particularly in children and infants. With the intensification of agricultural activities large quantities of pesticides and herbicides are being applied without taking adequate precautionary measures.

In urban areas, on the other hand, environmental problems are the result of rapid and massive population migration from rural to urban areas and of uncontrolled industrialization. Municipal services are unable to keep pace with the urban growth, like providing adequate water supplies, sewerage and sanitation. Overcrowding, inadequate housing with poor ventilation and absence of protection against rain, heat and cold add to the stresses and dangers of urban living. Industries are often located in and around urban areas with uncontrolled disposal of wastes. The Bhopal gas tragedy in India over a decade ago is an example.

Of course, there are other major environmental concerns such as deforestation, global warming, ozone depletion, cross-border movements of hazardous products and other forms of environmental degradation. Protection of the environment and of health endangered by environmental hazards comprise a very large and important international public policy agenda. In developing countries the problems are doubly difficult because of the immediacy of local environmental threats as well as the larger regional and global issues.

ENVIRONMENTAL ADMINISTRATION IN INDIA: GENESIS, GROWTH AND LEGAL FRAMEWORK

As stated in India 1999—A Reference Manual published by Ministry of Information and Broadcasting, in the beginning of the Fourth Five Year Plan, problems and issues centred around environment. This resulted in the establishment of the National Council of Environmental Planning and Coordination in 1972 at the Department of Science and Technology. Another empowered Committee was set-up in 1980 for reviewing the existing legislative measures and administrative machinery, for ensuring environmental protection and for recommending ways to strengthen them. On the recommendations of this empowered Committee, a separate Department of Environment was set-up in 1980 which was subsequently upgraded in a full-fledged Ministry of Environment and Forests in 1985 to serve as the focal point in the administrative structure of the Government of India for the planning, promotion and coordination of environmental and forestry programmes. The state department of environment, Central and state pollution control boards, the Botanical and Zoological Survey of India, the Forest Survey of India, the National River Conservation Authority (formerly Central Ganga Authority), the National Afforestation and Eco-development Board, the Indian Council for Forestry Research and Education, the Wildlife Institute of India, the National Museum for Natural History, etc., are the Ministry's partners in carrying out environmental protection activities.

Prevention and Control of Pollution

The policy statement on Abatement of Pollution, adopted in 1992, provides instruments in the form of legislation and regulation, fiscal incentives, voluntary agreements, educational programmes and information campaigns to prevent and control pollution of water, air and land. Since the adoption of the policy statement, the focus of activities has been on issues such as promotion of clean and low waste technologies, waste minimisation, reuse/recycling, improvement of water quality, environment audit, natural resource accounting, development of mass-based standards, institutional and human resource development, etc. The whole issue of pollution prevention and control is dealt with by a combination of command and control methods as well as voluntary and regulatory, fiscal measures, promotion of awareness and involvement of public.

Central Pollution Control Board

The Central Pollution Control Board (CPCB) is the national apex body for assessment, monitoring and control of water and air pollution. The executive responsibilities for enforcement of the Acts for Prevention and Control of Pollution of Water (1974) and Air (1981) and also of the Water (Cess) Act, 1977 are carried out through the Board. The CPCB advises the Central Government on all matters concerning the prevention and control of air, water and noise pollution and provides technical services to the Ministry for implementing the provisions of the Environment (Protection) Act, 1986. Under the Act, effluent and emission standards in respect of 61 categories of industries have been notified.

Education, Awareness and Information

Priority is accorded by the Ministry of Environment and Forests to promote environmental education, create environmental awareness among various age-groups and to disseminate information through Environmental Information System (ENVIS) network to all concerned. Special emphasis is given to non-formal environmental education through seminars/symposia/workshops, training programmes, eco-camps, audio-visual shows, etc. The Ministry has been organising a National Environment Awareness Campaign (NEAC) since July 1980. As a part of this campaign, 19 November to 18 December every year is observed as the National Environment Month. The main themes for the 1997-98 campaign were Pollution Prevention and Control, and Conservation and Plantation of Trees for Environmental Protection. A large number of organisations have been granted financial assistance by the Ministry to organise various activities for creating environmental awareness. The Ministry also provides financial support for setting up eco-clubs at schools and for production of films on environment.

A new scheme, Paryavaran Vahini, was launched in 1992-93 to create environmental awareness and to ensure active public participation by involving the local people in activities relating to environmental protection. Paryavaran Vahinis are proposed to be constituted in 194 selected districts all over the country which have a high incidence of pollution and density of tribal and forest population. The Vahinis also play a watch-dog role by reporting instance of environmental pollution, deforestation, poaching, etc. They function under the charge of District Collectors, with the active cooperation of the State/Union Territory governments. This scheme is entirely financed by the Ministry of Environment and Forests.

International Cooperation

The Ministry of Environment and Forests functions as a nodal agency for United Nations Environment Programme (UNEP), South Asia Cooperation Environment Programme (SACEP) and International Centre for Integrated Mountain and Development (ICIMOD), International Union for Conservation of Nature and Natural Resources ((IUCN) and various international agencies, regional bodies and multilateral institutions.

India is signatory to the following important international treaties/ agreements in the field of environment: (i) International Convention for the regulation of Whaling; (ii) International Plant Protection Convention; (iii) The Antarctic Treaty; (iv) Convention on Wetlands of international importance; (v) International Convention on International trade in endangered species of wild flora and fauna; (vi) Protocol of 1978 relating to the international convention for the prevention of pollution from ships; (vii) Vienna Convention for the protection of the ozone layer; (viii) Convention on Migratory Species; (ix) Basel Convention on trans-boundary movement of hazardous substances; (x) Framework convention of climate change; (xi) Convention on conservation of biodiversity; (xii) Montreal protocol on the substances that deplete the ozone layer; and (xiii) International Convention for Combating Desertification.

Environmental Legislation

Major legislations directly dealing with the protection of environment are the Wildlife (Protection) Act, 1972, the Forest (Conservation) Act, 1980, the Water (Prevention and Control of Pollution) Act, 1974, the Water (Cess) Act, 1977, the National Environment Appellate Authority Act, 1977, the Air (Prevention and Control of Pollution) Act, 1981, the Environment (Protection) Act, 1986, the Public Liability Insurance Act, 1991 and the National Environment Tribunal Act, 1995.

The Constitution (Forty-second Amendment Act of 1976) gave Parliament the power to enact laws on virtually any entry in the State list, and through Article 253 brought environmental regulation under the Concurrent List.

India has increasingly institutionalized its environment concern after the United Nations Conference on Human Environment at Stockholm in 1972, to serve as a guideline to the governments, both Central and State, Article 148A was added to the Directive Principles of

State Policy in 1976, which said, "The state shall endeavour to protect and improve environment and safeguard the forests and wildlife of the country." In a new chapter entitled 'Fundamental Duties', Article (51 Ag) imposed a similar responsibility on every citizen to protect and improve the natural environment including forests lakes, rivers and wildlife and to have compassion for living creatures. Supreme Court of India has held whenever a problem of ecology is brought before the Court, the Court is bound to bear in mind Art. 48A of the Constitution.

ENVIRONMENT VIS-A-VIS DEVELOPMENT

Nature and Scope of Environmental Health Programme

Meaning

Environmental health refers to the ecological balance that must exist between man and his environment in order to ensure his well-being. The deterioration of the human environment through the population explosion, pollution of air and water, and other disruptions of the ecological balance pose a major international health hazard and a serious challenge. Professor J. Logan, in a paper published in *American Journal of Tropical Medicine* in 1960, was able to show that environmentally transmitted diseases were responsible for the sufferings of 500 million people every year particularly among infants and children.[4] The UN Secretary-General's report on problem of the human environment sounds a similar ominous note: "If current trends continue, the failure of life on earth could be engendered and thus, it is urgent to focus world attention on these problems which threaten humanity in an environment that permits the realisation of the highest human aspirations."[5]

The close relationship that exists between an unhealthy environment and the economic condition of a community was pinpointed by a panel of experts which met in 1971 to discuss the environmental problems of the developing countries. "Poverty and the very lack of development", these experts said, "constitute an essential environmental problem in the developing countries. They recommended an attack on the problems of inadequate water supply, poor housing, sanitation, nutrition and widespread disease as prime targets in an effort to improve the environment of millions of people, and to lay the groundwork for their economic betterment."[6]

Ninth Five Year Plan (Draft) also warns about the bad consequences of poor environment on Health. Environment can affect human health in many ways. Deficiency of iodine in soil, water and foodstuffs is the cause of iodine deficiency disorders. Excessive fluoride content in the water is the cause of fluorosis. Environmental degradation may affect air, land and water. Pollutants may enter the food chain. All these may enter human body through various portals and affect the health status.

Rapidly growing population, urbanisation, changing agricultural, industrial and water resource management, increasing use of pesticides and fossil fuels have all resulted in a perceptible deterioration in the quality of environment and attendant adverse health consequences. Environment pollution due to developmental activities are increasingly becoming the focus of concern. The interactive interdependence of health, environment and sustainable development was accepted as the fulcrum of action under Agenda 21 at the Earth Summit in Brazil in 1992. Environmental health in its broader perspective would have to address the detection, prevention and management of:

(i) existing deficiencies or excesses of certain elements in natural environment;
(ii) macro-environmental contamination of air, land, water and food; and
(iii) disaster management.

Aspects of Environmental Health

The environment can be defined as an aggregate of all the external conditions and influences affecting the life and development of an organism. Human environment means everything that is experienced by man and it is the total nature of this experience that determines the quality of life. According to Roggers, "the environment appears to possess two main avenues by which it may reach man and affect man's health; it may act upon his body as a material agent or it may act upon his mind and emotions as non-material agent, although sooner or later this may very well produce a material effect."[7] The effect of both is the pollution of environment. Prof. Samuel Halter, Professor of Public Health at the University of Brussels defines pollution as the "presence in the ambient environment of chemical, physical or biological factors capable of inducing disturbances in the normal physiology and functioning of human organs."[8]

We can classify the environmental factors impinging on the health of the people as follows:

(a) Physical, Chemical and Biological factors.
(b) Social, Economic and Cultural factors.
(c) Ecological, Economic and Aesthetic factors.
(d) Individual human system.

All these agents in the environment interact with one another and produce the favourable or unfavourable impact on the health of the people.

MEANING AND ROLE OF ENVIRONMENTAL HEALTH ADMINISTRATION (Refer Table 4.1)

Environmental Sanitation Administration is an activity of diagnosing and controlling the environmental factors which exercise or may exercise a deleterious and unhealthy effect on the physical, social, and mental life of the people. The Draft Five-Year Plan (1978-83) has rightly mentioned: "The essence of sound environmental growth lies in a happy blend of the realisation of the physical out limits to the exploitation of environmental resources and the inner limits to human needs and aspiration."[9] Environmental health administration is quite complex and complicated owing to the complexity and diversity of the socio-political and institutional arrangements in which the programmes are implemented and the complexity, multiplicity of the physical, biological, social and economic factors that they must take into account. The objective of the environmental sanitation administration is to plan thoroughly to change favourably the environment itself and modify the interaction of human beings with the environment so that the people can enjoy a good quality of life. The administration of environmental programme is not within the purview of any single discipline but presents a challenge to many disciplines. The administrators responsible for such programmes must plan to attack the unfavourable factors in concert with one another. We may mention some of the important areas which need the immediate attention of the planners, policy-makers and administrators to solve these impending problems—potable safe water supply and water pollution, solid wastes management, air pollution control, occupational health, food sanitation, urban planning and housing, slum clearance, soil erosion, noise pollution, etc. The administration must define in the geographical context the magnitude of each problem, its relationship with others and the benefits expected, direct outputs, intermediate effects or impacts and the ultimate effects or benefits. Some of these have been indicated in the form of a table (see Table 4.1). The administration of environmental health programmes are very expensive and complicated. In order to translate the benefits of such programmes to the society, the administrators must ensure that the programme:

(a) receives acceptance and support;
(b) achieves the desired objectives and results;
(c) links its efforts with those of other health and socio-economic development programmes; and
(d) accomplishes its work economically, with a minimum waste of money and other scarce resources.[10]

We may now take up two important aspects of environment, i.e. water supply and sanitation which affect health development in a big way.

TABLE 4.1

Types of Output in Illustrative Environmental Health Programmes

Programmes	*Direct Outputs*	*Intermediate Effects or Impacts*	*Ultimate Effects or Benefits*
Water Supply	State water provided to households in adequate amounts and used efficiently.	Reduced disease from water borne pathogens; support to hygiene, nutrition and economic activity	Longer survival
Water Pollution Control	Reduced contamination of (used water returned to) watercourses, seas, soil and food	Improved water resources for human use; reduced damage to marine life; improved aesthetics	Less disability, suffering impairment and pain
Solid Wastes Management	Wastes confined, removed and disposed of (treated recycled)	Reduced disease from vectorborne pathogens and from pathogens and chemicals transferred to air, water and land; economic gains; improved aesthetics	More efficient personal and social perforamnce
Air Pollution Control	Reduced introduction of toxic, irritant and nuisance elements into ambient air	Reduced death, disease and discomfort; reduced economic losses; improved aesthetics	Improved quality of life
Occupational Health	Reduced physical/chemical hazards in work environment, through primary and secondary disease prevention services	Reduced illness, trauma and poisoning; safer work environment; improved working conditions and productivity	Socio-economic development
Food Sanitation	Food safeguards against contamination in production, processing, delivery, preparation and consumption	Reduced disease and death from pathogens and toxins in food; enlarged markets; improved aesthetics	

Source: WHO, Public Heath Paper No. 59, p. 111.

Water Supply and Sanitation

Safe water and improved sanitation are a necessary condition for better health, and there can be no lasting improvement of public health without them. There is no denying the fact that inadequacy of safe drinking water, improper disposal of human excreta, solid and liquid wastes leading to unfavourable environmental condition have been the causes of many killer diseases.

M. Aktar has stated that inadequacy in the availability of safe drinking water, unfavourable environmental conditions and lack of personal hygiene have been the major causes of disease and disability among people. As per WHO statistics, 80 per cent of diseases in the developing countries are related to unsafe water supply and inadequate sanitation causing high child mortality, low life expectancy and poor quality of life. In India, more than one million children below 5 years died from dehydration caused by diarrhoea annually, while another 250 thousand are victims of tetanus. Poliomyelitis has been a cause of lameness among 170 thousand children per year. There is also a very high rate of occurrence of intestinal worms, particularly in West Bengal, Bihar, Orissa, Andhra Pradesh, Tamil Nadu, Kerala and Maharashtra. The national goal to reduce child mortality from 146 per thousand to 125 by 1995 and 70 per thousand by 2000 cannot possibly be achieved without a significant change in the existing mortality-morbidity related to water and sanitation. Also important is to change the peoples' perception about the link between sanitation and health. According to a recent KAP survey in the country, 37 per cent people do not know/do not believe that exposed excreta can harm health. Outdoor defecation is not generally seen as a problem except in terms of inconvenience during rain, night or winter and to women.

Y.N. Nanjudiah has stated that majority of the rural people practice open air defecation as the coverage of sanitation facilities has reached only a negligible population. For want of awareness on health on the part of users quite a large number of latrines are out of use or misused. Further, open air defecation generally enjoys social acceptability. It is considered hygienic and wholesome and in tune with the nature and fresh air. At the same time toilet has a poor image. It is believed to be dirty and a breeding place for flies and mosquitoes. Social surveys carried out so far have highlighted that there is lack of knowledge regarding latrine, which can be summarised as under:

(a) Faecal-borne diseases can be prevented by using a latrine.
(b) Pathogenic microbes survive from days to years in the moist soil and may become wind borne.
(c) Social status and prestige can be attained by having a latrine.
(d) Constipation, particularly among rural women, can be eliminated.
(e) Privacy can be achieved.

(f) Low cost sanitation options are available, and these can be maintained in an eco-friendly way.

Dr. H. Mahler, former WHO Director-General, has rightly said that he is utterly convinced that the number of water taps per 1,000 population will be an infinitely more meaningful health indicator than the number of hospital beds per 1,000 population. Mr. Kurt Waldheim, former UN Secretary-General also stressed that, the provision of safe water and sanitation does not merely mean happier, healthier citizens; it also means increased economic productivity.

Nikolas P. Napulbow in his editorial, "Water For All, a Human Right" has rightly said that, "water is a basic human need for health—indeed, for survival—and therefore it is not an exaggeration to call it one of the basic human rights. Without safe water and sanitation, there is no real development. A community ravaged by diarrheal diseases, dracunculiasis or schistosomiasis cannot look beyond its immediate problems towards social and economic welfare. Safe water is the doorway to health and health is the prerequisite for progress, social equity and human divinity."[11]

Infectious diseases resulting from water pollution can be classified into four groups, depending upon the ways in which their incidence can be lessened by improvements in water supply. (See Chart 4.1)

(1) "Water-borne" diseases are those in which infectious agent remains alive in drinking water e.g., typhoid, paratyphoid, gastroenterities, etc. The incidence of these disease can be reduced by the purification of water.
(2) "Water-washed" diseases include infection of the outer body surface, e.g., trachoma, skin ulcers, scabies and typhus, bacillary and amoebic dysentery and gastro enterities. The incidence can be reduced by augmenting water quantity.
(3) "Water-based" infections, i.e., schistosomiasis, guinea worms. The infection occurs when the skin is in contact with water or through drinking water.
(4) "Water breeding" or water proximity diseases are caused by mosquitoes or flies living near aquatic conditions.

There is probably no single factor that has a greater effect on the health, well-being and development of a community than the provision of ample and convenient supply of wholesome and good quality water. In towns and cities water supply is recognised as a basic necessity for industrial and commercial purposes; it is vital for the maintenance of public health and the prevention of epidemics. Dame Barbara Ward, President of the International Institute for Environment and Development, rightly observes that, "Water is everywhere, the key to human health . . . clean water is a key to human comfort, health and

CHART 4.1

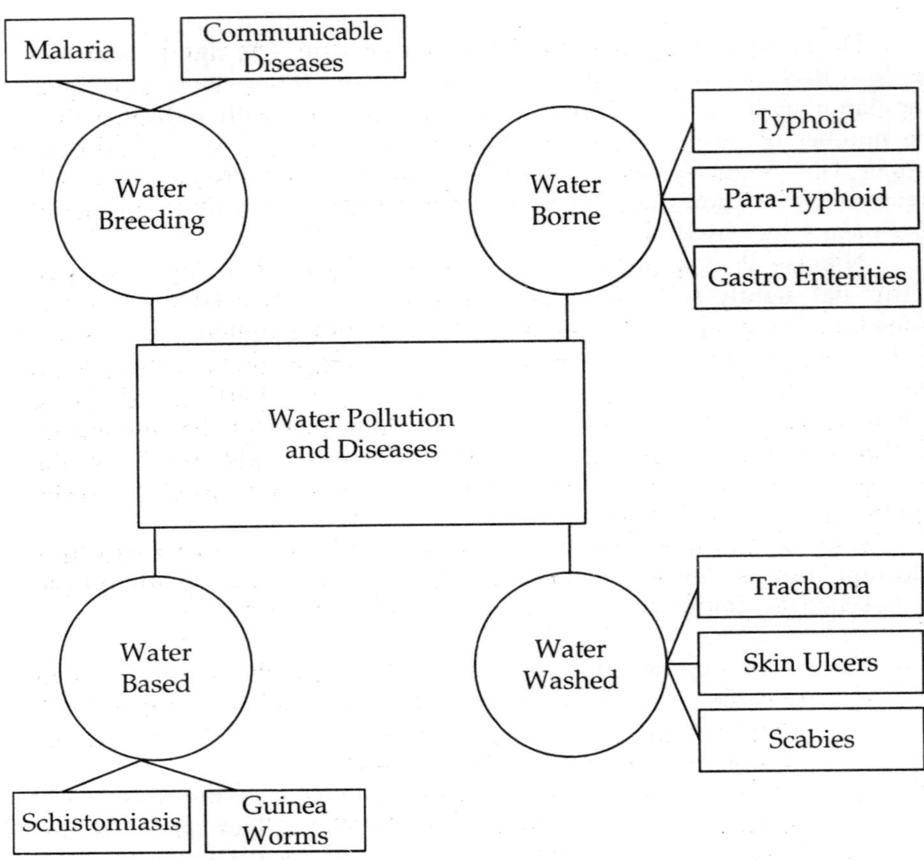

even survival.[12] Martin Boyer, Adviser, Drinking Water Programme, UNICEF has observed that, "The provision of ample supplies of safe water and the sanitary disposal of excreta have a direct and far-reaching effect upon the health and well-being of rural populations. Indeed, it is believed that no other single measure can make a comparable contribution to the improvement of their health and standard of living. The choice of an appropriate technology depends on local conditions."[13] To quote WHO: "One hospital bed out of four in the world is occupied by a patient who is ill because of polluted water. . . . Provisions of a safe and convenient water supply is the single most important activity that could be undertaken to improve the health of people living in rural areas of the developing world."

WHO estimates that as much as 80 percent of all diseases in the world are associated with water. Iain Guest (Geneva), a specialist in development topics submits that an astonishing number of people suffer from these water-related diseases at any time, 400 million with gastro enterities, 160 million with malaria, 30 million with river blindness, 200 million with Schistosomiasis.[14] At the 1969 World Health Assembly, a delegate from the region (SEA) estimated that water-borne diseases accounted for 40 percent of all morality, and 60 percent of all morbidity in his country.[15]

I.V. Rajeshwar, ex-Governor of West Bengal in his article, "Endemic Problems defying solution" in the *Daily Tribune*, dated January 16, 2000 rightly says that fifty-two years after independence even basic amenities like drinking water supply and unpolluted air are not available to most citizens. At present, water supply is available to 84.33% of urban population and 76.68% to rural population. However, sanitation coverage is 49.91 to urban areas and 14.02 to rural areas.

Ninth Plan finds that the existing norms for rural water supply is 40 liters of drinking water per capita per day (LPCD) and a public stand post or a hand pump for 250 persons. Further, the sources of water supply should be within 1.6 km. horizontal distance in plains or 100 metres elevation distance in hills. For cattle in Desert and Drought Prone (DDP) areas, an additional 30 LPCD is recommended. Against this, the norm for urban water supply is 125 LPCD piped water supply with sewerage system, 70 LPCD without sewerage system and 40 LPCD in towns with spot sources. At least one source for 20 families within a maximum distance of 100 metres has been laid down.

As against these norms, the studies as on 1.4.1997 revealed that there were 61,724 habitations without any safe source of drinking water (called not covered habitation), 3.78 lakh habitations which were partially covered and 1.51 lakh habitations which had quality problems like excess fluoride, salinity, iron and arsenic, etc. Apart from the provision in the state plans for water supply, there are major Centrally Sponsored Schemes called the Accelerated Rural Water Supply Programme and the Urban Water Supply Programme for small towns with population of less than 20,000. In order to cover this backlog in rural drinking water supply, it has been estimated that approximately Rs. 40,000 crore will be required including the funds required for operations and maintenance and funds to tackle quality problems. Similarly, the estimates of investment required for full coverage of urban water supply is Rs. 30,734 crore.

Drinking water and sanitation improvements could reduce the overall incidence of infant and child diarrhoea by one quarter and cut total infant and child mortality by more than one-half. Country programmes are increasingly taking measures to improve water supply and sanitation within their primary health care programmes.

Guinea worm disease can be effectively prevented by providing safe drinking water and its global eradication is clearly possible within the next few years. As for schistosomiasis, some 60% reduction could be achieved by improving water supplies. Building latrines, giving health

CHART 4.2

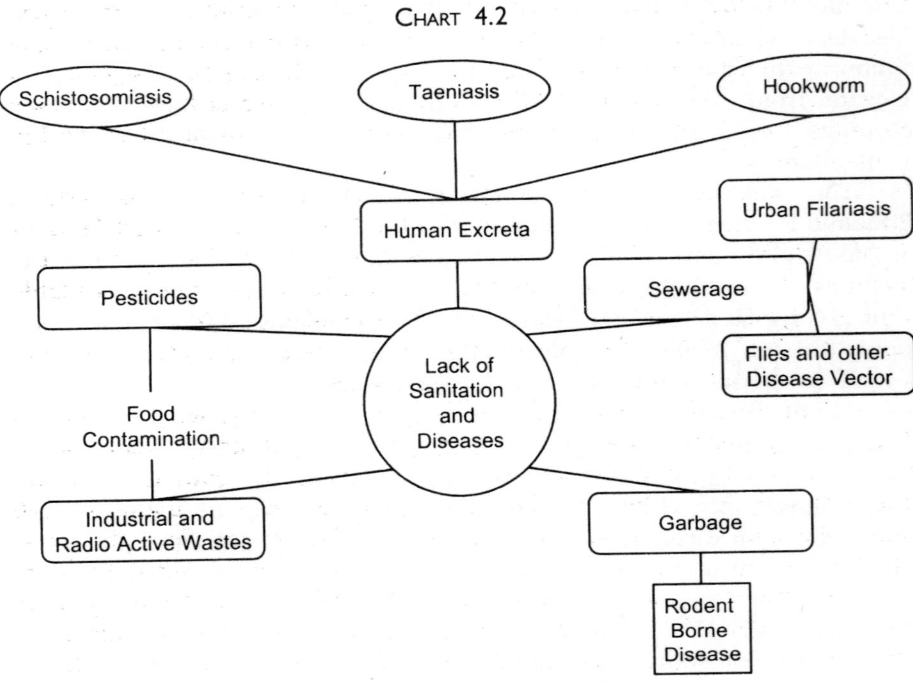

education and introducing selected drug therapy could reduce the prevalence even more.[16]

A great surge in the population of India's big cities, poses huge problems for safeguarding water supplied.

We suggest here the methods of conserving water supply:

- Integration of water and waste water management, coupled with health education for cost-effectiveness and promotion of preventive measures for health;
- Prospecting for water resources through state of the art techniques of remote sensing and geophysical surveys;
- Protection of water sources against pollution;
- Decentralization of water supply matching the required quality and quantity through waste recycle and reuse;
- Maintenance of the water distribution system, which can prevent up to 50% of the purified waste water from being lost; and
- Application of mathematical programming techniques with exact fluid flow relationships in the design of water and waste water systems, so as to ensure functionality and to conserve material and financial resources.

Lack of sanitation causes many diseases related to human excreta, sewerage disposal, Garbage and the use of pesticides and the industrial and radio active wastes, (See Chart 4.2 on previous page). Following the suspected plague outbreak in the country during 1994 the Planning Commission constituted a High Power Committee on Urban Solid Waste Management in India under the Chairmanship of Member (Health). This committee undertook a comprehensive review of current situation of urban solid waste management, specially in cities with one million or more inhabitants and made recommendations for safe methods for collection, transportation of waste and suitable cost-effective, environmentally friendly methods for disposal of these wastes. Pilot projects exploring the dimensions of the problem and aimed at seeking realistic solutions were initiated during the Eighth Plan period. During the Ninth Plan period it is expected that many more cities will initiate programmes for the efficient methods of management of wastes generated and improve environmental sanitation.

So far, the major focus has been on communicable disease burden due to poor environmental sanitation in urban areas and due to improper disposal of human excreta, garbage and waste water in rural areas and methods to tackle these. These efforts will be intensified during the Tenth Plan. In addition, efforts to reduce pollution and related non-communicable disease burden will also be strengthened. Efforts will be made to document the extent of the problem of environmental pollution and its impact on health status of the population through linkages between existing environmental monitoring data and data on health status of population living in these areas. Prevention and management of health consequences of environmental deterioration will receive increasing attention.

The Expert Committee on Public Health System had noted that major developmental activities in any field such as agriculture, industries, urban and rural development may result in environment changes which could have adverse health implications and recommended that health impact assessment may become a part of environmental impact assessment of all large developmental projects. The feasibility of making appropriate provision for health care of people involved in developmental activities and prevention and management of health consequences of developmental activities on the population living in vicinity of the project as a part of the project budget will be explored.[17]

CRITICAL ASSESSMENT AND SUGGESTIONS TO IMPROVE THE PROGRAMMES

The situation pertaining to environmental sanitation is horrifying at the global, regional and national levels. It has been admitted by various agencies responsible for it at all levels. Attainment of the global target of the UN Second Development Decade (DD2) had not been feasible in most countries of the region. The Regional Director of the WHO in his

Annual Report has warned the member-states:

> "In spite of the continuing efforts of governments and international and bilateral agencies, only the fringe of the problem has been tackled. . . . there is an urgent need to mobilise further support from all available sources to solve this difficult problem. Investment in this field will be amply rewarded not only in terms of reduction in the incidence of communicable diseases, but also by substantially contributing towards an improvement in the standard of living."[18]

Dr. Abel Wolman, one of the "father-figure" of environmental health and Professor Emeritus of Sanitary Engineering at the Johns Hopkins School of Engineering, Baltimore, USA says while talking of the World Health situation, "It always leads great conferences to pass resolutions to do something about providing water to impoverished people. Resolutions become opiates because they are gratifying substitutes for action."[19] He warns the policy-makers and administrators against complacence and says, "Viewed on a global basis, we have little to be sanguine about. The disease-consequences of poor and insufficient water, of living with human excreta, and of unhygienic personal habits, are disastrous—they have been familiar for so long a time that they no longer excite even the statistician or epidemiologist. People accept their devastation, as they so often abjectly bear their real and spiritual poverty. We speak of the toll of deaths, due to environmental deficiencies in a casual way, even though the figures mount to hundreds of millions. The communicable diseases, often the sequels of poor sanitation are maiming and killing men, women and children—not computer data."[20] It is beyond doubt that a lasting solution to many of the existing and future problems of public health require control on environment. The question arises as how to provide sanitary facilities to hundreds of millions of people still without even minimum sanitary facilities? How to tackle such programmes? How to find the resources required for these programmes? What should be the administrative set-up to ensure speedy implementation? What are the responsibilities of planners and policy-makers to ensure integrated approach? We shall discuss the facts and suggestions to provide good environment for the healthy growth of the people.

(I) Need of Cooperation and Coordination among Allied Programmes

There is a close relationship between the environmental programmes and other programmes. In practice, this relationship is ignored by the planners and administrators of these programmes, e.g., a dam has to be constructed for irrigation and power purposes; its consequences on human health or soil salinity are ignored or underestimated. To remedy such unfortunate situations it is suggested that an 'integrated' approach may be adopted. It presumes an unprecedented, ungrudging cooperation between different services, as well as between various brands of natural scientists on the one hand and of social and human scientists on the other. We have to encourage such integrated approach to have full impact rather than piecemeal goals and approaches. It was mentioned in a WHO document that, "more effective administration requires that planners and managers take account of the full range of implications of their own programme goals and further, that they actively seek to participate as consultants and collaborators in the planning and execution of other community programmes that demonstratively or potentially interact with environmental health."[21]

UNESCO's MAB Programme (Man and the Biosphere Programme) coordinates various disciplines by mobilising applied research efforts all over the world on major man environment resources interactions. It relies on international cooperation among governments and the participation of all specialists. A major UNESCO research programme is closely studying the effects of human interventions in the environment and man himself in all the major socio-economic systems. We can get benefit out of such programmes.[22]

(2) Improve Administrative Capability and Competence

Environmental health programmes are administered by technically qualified people but such people lack administrative capability and capacity, i.e., the ability to achieve results. We have doctors, engineers, town planners, inspectors, nutritionists, geologists who are responsible for improving the environment. Every programme has its administrative component which is the heart and soul of that programme. It is suggested that the persons engaged on these programmes may be given suitable training in administration to enhance their competence.

(3) Deploy more Resources

The Environmental Health Improvement programmes require considerable financial investment. The World Bank and WHO reported to the Mar Del Plata Conference that $ 140,000 million would be needed to reach the target of clean water for all by 1990. Today, we need double this amount to cater to increased population. Where will it come from? External aid is limited. So, there is a need to exploit the resources available within each country. It is only a question of proper allocation of resources. Voluntary effort can be encouraged to accelerate the pace of development. With exploitation of local self-help, money can be generated. It is also a question of political will. This programme must be made an integral part of the community development programme. It should take the form of self-aided programme. The funds allocated should be used to achieve the aims of the policy and care should be taken that the funds are not diverted for other purposes. It was mentioned by Dr. B.H. Dieterich, Director, Division of Environmental

Health, WHO that Development planners confronted with meagre budgets are often forced to keep some projects in abeyance and give priority to others that may bring immediate economic benefit. It is now being increasingly realised that it is not a practicable or economically sound idea to defer environmental health projects. Planners are beginning to look at environmental health projects in the context of the ultimate socio-economic objectives of the development process."[23]

(4) Need of Action Research to Meet the Requirements of Different Geographical Areas

There are many potential health hazards. We know much about some of these hazards and little about many of them. We must encourage research in the experimental laboratory and epidemiology to pin-point the areas of ignorance. Secondly, national institutes should carry out research to develop models for adapting measures to reduce costs. They may also find simple disinfection devices suited to rural needs. We may not adopt costly western models to supply safe water and sewerage disposal, e.g., the British Development Agency, Oxford has made a latrine which turns the human excreta into organic manure producing some 6,000,000 tons a year. In the Republic of Korea, human excreta is being exploited to produce methane gas. There is need to change the attitudes of experts so that they can design the machinery and equipment suitable and feasible in our country.

(5) Encouraging Local Participation

Public Health administration is manned by and meant for human beings. It is therefore necessary to associate the people with the programmes of water supply and rural sanitary latrines. Sociologists, behavioural scientists and public relation experts should be associated with programmes to make the local involvement more effective.

Social mobilisation, People's participation and health and sanitation education are essential inputs into water supply and sanitation programmes. These help to make sure that the proposed activities fit into the targeted population's habits and socio-cultural environment. Where they do not suggest changes, it intends to ensure that the proposed water supply and sanitation technologies and activities are appropriate to men, women and children.

(6) Strong Political Will and Determination

It has been mentioned that the programmes of environmental health are deferred because of the lack of resources or the apathy on the part of the politicians. This assumption is totally wrong and baseless. "The major cause for delinquent action lies in the motivation of governments. Do they really mean what their resolutions say—militantly enough to go into action? Is only lip service the main response of Presidents, Prime Ministers, kings and ministers? The task for the future is difficult but possible. People should not be consigned to premature death simply because we are less than courageous and diligent. The pace must be accelerated."[24]

(7) Effective Maintenance

It is not only important to build the infrastructure for the environmental sanitation programmes but also to see that these projects function efficiently and regularly. We must ensure their efficient construction, effective and fool-proof operation and maintenance of completed supplies and effective surveillance on quality of drinking water. The maintenance is very poor in the developing countries. Even in the planned cities like Chandigarh—the headquarters of three governments—we are shocked to find germs, mosquitoes and flies coming in the tap water. Besides, the dirt is scattered in the whole of the city. Thus, there is a need to maintain the services once provided to the people through efficient and economical administration, involving the people.

(8) Guidance and Assistance from Bilateral and Multilateral Agencies

The capacity of the developing countries to solve the problem pertaining to environmental sanitation programmes are limited. International and bilateral agencies should be encouraged to increase their direct technical assistance to member-countries in the following ways:

(a) In making assessment studies;
(b) In the establishment of information systems and programme formulation, implementation and evaluation;
(c) In identifying and helping to meet specific needs for multilateral or bilateral assistance by way of expertise, equipment, materials and soft loans;
(d) In setting up research and training centers and collaborating laboratories;
(e) In assisting training programmes, including programmes for the production of manuals and training guides;
(f) In establishing health criteria and codes of practice; and
(g) In the local production of materials.

In addition to providing assistance itself, WHO should act in a coordinating capacity in respect of assistance received from these and other sources."[25]

(9) Civic Consciousness

Environmental sanitation cannot be achieved by the effort of the Government alone. It requires the active support and cooperation of the people. It was indicated to the writer by the authorities responsible for water supply that 25 per cent of the resources are being wasted because the people do not care to use the services only when in need. Most of the public and private taps remain working without any utility. Besides, the people lack civic consciousness and they do not cooperate in the maintenance of hygienic conditions. One is shocked to see the beautiful city of Chandigarh with heaps of debris all around. The difficult task of improving environmental sanitation is possible only if the people develop civic consciousness.

(10) Environmental Education

Dr. T. Sundaran in his Article from literacy to health in *Kurukshetra* (Oct. 1992), suggests Health education and personal hygiene are necessary components of all such plans. Such education inputs may relate to:

(a) washing hands before collecting and carrying water, and pouring out water from a storage container without touching it or using a clean long handled dipper to take the water out;
(b) making sure that the water container, the cups and mugs used for drawing water are clean and that the water is kept covered at all times; and
(c) washing hands after defecation, before preparing and eating food, cutting of nails and other such basic measures.

Special care to ensure implementation of these measures in hotels and other public eating places is more difficult but essential to really checking diseases like typhoid.

The Stockholm Conference held in 1972 drew the urgency of tackling environmental problems through various efforts. One recommendation of this conference called for development of 'environmental education' as one of the most important steps to attack world's environmental crisis. The conference pleaded that "new environmental education must be broad-based and strongly related to the basic principles outlined in the United Nations Declaration on the New International Economic Order." Environmental education has been defined as an educational process dealing with men's relationship with his natural and man-made surroundings, and encompass the relation of population, health, pollution, technology, urban and rural planning, housing, proper nutrition to the total human environment. The scope of environmental education is vast, touching every aspect of man and environment. The purpose of environmental education is to provide knowledge to the people so that they can adjust with the environment and enjoy decent environment The goals of environmental education as discussed in the Inter-Governmental Conference on Environmental Education, organised by the UNESCO in cooperation with UNEP, at Tbilisi (USSR), from October 14-26, 1977, are mentioned below:

(a) To foster clear awareness of and concern about economic, social, political and ecological interdependence in urban and rural areas;
(b) To provide every person with opportunity tc acquire the knowledge, value, attitudes, commitment and skills needed to protect and improve the environment; and
(c) To create new patterns of individuals, groups and society as a whole towards the environment.

The Secretary-General of the UN in his report on Population, Resources and Environment sums up the benefits of environmental improvement programmes. He mentions four social and economic benefits that would result from government action for environmental betterment in the poor countries besides the improvements in the people's health from control of infectious diseases.

(a) Employment of large number of poor people in public works projects;
(b) Reduction of food requirements and costs by lessening the mal-absorption caused by intestinal parasites. This might ultimately save $ 2,000 million per annum in India alone. This annual saving would be equal to the entire capital cost of needed water supply improvements in the whole of rural India;
(c) Increases in potential economic productivity through improved health of adults; and
(d) Greater receptivity of children at the early ages by improvements in health."[26]

(11) Appropriate Technology

A.S. Bal, A.N. Khan and P.R. Sarode in their Article, "Technological Options for Rural Sanitation" in *Kurukshetra* (October 1992), rightly suggest that high incidence of excreta-related diseases in the developing countries warrants that the sanitation programmes be designed with the primary objective of bringing about improvement in public health. This objective can be achieved through alternate sanitation technologies which are simpler and cheaper as also socially acceptable. An inter-disciplinary sanitation programme could prove to be more successful not only from the sanitation point of view but also from the point of view of problems faced by the local bodies by way of poor financial returns from provision of sewerage facilities in the low income areas. Selection of appropriate sanitation technology for a given community and its proper operation and maintenance after installation is ensured only when socio-cultural aspects are considered along with economic, financial, ecological and technical features in the planning process.

The task of providing water and sanitation to the unserved population is so immense that it would be almost impossible to accomplish it without the development and application of low-cost technologies. Low-cost technologies are generally applied at the peripheral level, where construction, operation, maintenance and surveillance may vary greatly from one location to another, affected by the level of community motivation and participation.

Non-sewerage onsite sanitation facilities may be all that are needed when water supplies are limited, but if improvements result in greater water usage then eventually the need will escalate for sewers and offside disposal. In this case it can create a need for concentrated population to be controlled by treatment.

(12) Holistic Approach

Nirmal Deshpande, an eminent Gandhian has stressed the need to adopt holistic approach to sanitation, it is necessary to approach the problem in a holistic manner by linking sanitation with religion, culture, health, agriculture, environment and production of energy. The basic attitude that needs to be formed is to link it with Bhakti. It has to be stressed that cleanliness is godliness and unless cleanliness becomes a part of our lives, we cannot be true devotees of God. Construction of toilets, their proper use, maintenance and clean habits should form part of the psyche. The wrong notion that night soil is not to be touched has to go. Cleaning should become a part of daily practice. The linkage of cleanliness with health is also very important. It has to be impressed upon the minds of the people that this programme is essential for keeping good health and protecting the family and village from various diseases. With charts, slides, films, songs, cultural shows, this knowledge can be imparted. Imaginative and innovative methods have to be adopted to make people aware of health.

CONCLUSION

Dr. Zbigniew Bankowski,[27] spells out the code of ethics to protect the environment. It would be unrealistic, however, to suppose that the damage that has been done, and still continues to be done, can be arrested and undone in the short-term. Rather, long-term global policies must be envisaged and, if they are to be successful, they will require changes in our perceptions of man in nature. If our global physical environment is not to be further degraded, we must change our conceptual environment, our ways of thinking and behaving. Perhaps the worst environmental pollution is pollution of the mind, and the greatest need is for well thought out principles of environmental ethics.

All spheres of human conduct—private and public, are subject to ethical principles or rules. When governments or other corporate bodies despoil the environment in the name of development or political dominance or national security, when government adopt *laissez faire* policies that permit the exploitation of nature for narrow, short-term gains, they contravene the basic ethical principle of the greatest good for the greatest number of people.

Sh. M. Akhtar, Chief WESS/ICO UNICEF, New Delhi in his Article, "Strategies for Rural Sanitation (UNICEF Experience)" suggested the following based upon UNICEF experience to ensure fruitful application of strategies for safer water supply and sanitation. (*Kurukshetra*, October 1992).

1. If sanitation has to be a 'way of life' it should be treated as a package of facilities/services and not identified with latrines. All the low-cost sanitary facilities, both at domestic and community level, such as latrine, soak pit, garbage pit, smokeless chulha, bathing cubicle, drainage improvement, ground water sources and other community-based facilities should form a part of the package. A distinction may have to be made among 7 components of sanitation. These are: (i) Handling of drinking water; (ii) Disposal of waste water, (iii) Disposal of human excreta; (iv) Garbage disposal; (v) Home sanitation and food hygiene; (vi) Personal hygiene; and (vii) Sanitation in the community. This should be supported by a strong IEC back up to create awareness with regard to various sanitary practices including personal hygiene. It is necessary to modify the guidelines both at the Government of India and State Government levels to reflect the package deal and how to achieve the same.
2. In order that sanitation becomes a "peoples' movement", it is essential that their active involvement and participation receive due importance. In this regard subsidy can play only a limited role. Alternate financing mechanisms have to be developed to facilitate greater adaptability.
3. The low-cost sanitary facilities should have different technological options to suit different geohydrological conditions and also the varying socio-economic segments of the population. Such technologies should be affordable, acceptable and replicable. Identification and use of alternate materials should be a continuous process so as to keep the cost escalation under check.
4. Demand generation for sanitary facilities should get a high priority in Rural Sanitation Programme. For this purpose, a comprehensive and systematic communication strategy has to be developed and all possible methods and channels should be used to motivate people. In this regard inter-personal communication through village level motivators seems to be quite promising. Willing village level functionaries like

Anganwadi workers, DWCRA group organisers, Traditional Birth Attendants, primary school teachers, Youth Club/Mahila Mandal office-bearers, etc. could be the core group of motivators. The panchayat members can also play an active role in this regard.

5. The demand generation strategy should be backed up by an efficient delivery system which need not be a part of the subsidy-oriented programme. At present, even if a person wants to have his/her own latrine in rural areas, it is not easy to find the required pan/trap/pit cover, etc. as adequate infrastructure has not developed as yet. Only in an area where government programme is under implementation, things are more readily available. It is, therefore, necessary to create alternate delivery channels/mechanism to have improved sanitation coverage.
6. Private initiative is a must to make the sanitation programme a success. The government-supported activity could at least be a stimulant. The results of the 44th Round on Sanitation Coverage is a pointer to this assumption. While figures from the government sources show a 3 percent coverage, the NSS survey reveals that more than one-tenth of the households were using latrines. The difference could be accounted for by the spread effect of the government programme. It is high time that a clear-cut policy on how to encourage private initiative outside the subsidy-oriented approach is laid down. The policy should keep a flexible approach and suggest alternate social marketing strategies to promote sanitation through private initiative. Involvement of industrial houses/ public sector units including the manufacturers of sanitary goods could form a part of it.
7. NGOs can play a very crucial role in promoting rural sanitation. They can very effectively be used to encourage private initiative because of their rapport with the community and can serve as an efficient channel for information dissemination, awareness creation and motivation. Only those NGOs who have the required capacity to take up activities at a district level or at least for a group of blocks should be encouraged. The Government should come out with separate guidelines for involving NGO's in the Rural Sanitation Programme. The State Government should be well aware of such guidelines.

Dr. Martin Kaplan[28] has desired to look positively and is hopeful of solutions by mankind. He stated, "hazards to human health arising from environment factors are many and varied. We know much about some and little about many of them. We must therefore depend on future research both by the experimental laboratory and by epidemiology to clarify many of our areas of ignorance. The development of surveillance and monitoring mechanisms for changes in health status correlated with environmental components should provide the warnings necessary to avoid serious harm to present and future generations of the human race.

In reviewing all these environmental effects and their possible dangers, we should not however reach too gloomy a conclusion. A comforting finding, which may be extended to many other aspects, is the recent discovery that fish caught in the last century and preserved in museums have been found to have similar mercury levels as those found in fish today. And after all, the human race with its great adaptability has survived the innumerable disasters and environmental hazards it has encountered for several million years. Modern life and times represent for man merely a new set of problems replacing old ones, and there is no reason to doubt that man's ingenuity and intelligence will prevail as far as environment problems are concerned."

Notes and References

1. Hiroshi Nakajima, "A Wounded Planet", in *World Health*, January-February 1990, p. 3.
2. Dr. Wilfried Kreisel, "Environmental Health in the 1990s" in *World Health*, January-February 1990, p. 5.
3. WHO: SEARO, Declaration on Health Development in the South-East Asia Region in the 21st Century, New Delhi, 1997, pp. 17-18.
4. WHO, *World Health*, May 1972, p. 28.
5. U. Thant quoted in Clellan, M.C. and S. Grant (ed.), Protecting our Environments (New York., 1970), p. 206.
6. WHO, *World Health*, May 1972, p. 29.
7. Edwards S. Roggers, Human Ecology and Health Environment, *Administrator*, New York, 1960.
8. WHO Samuel Halter; "Man and his Environment", in *World Health*, July, 1975, p. 18.
9. GOI, Planning Commission, Draft Five Year Plan (1978-83), p. 117.
10. WHO, *World Health Paper*, 59, p. 12.
11. Nikolas P. Napulbow, Water For All: A human right, in *World Health*, July-Aug., 1992, p. 3.
12. Barbara Ward, "The Key to Health" in *World Health*, January 1977, p. 3.
13. UNICEF, Assignment Children, 34, April-June 1976, p. 11.
14. WHO, *World Health*, January 1979, p. 3.
15. UN, 1970, Report on the World Social Situation, New York, 1971, pp. 167-68.
16. *World Health*, July-August 1992, p. 7
17. Purshotam Khanna and Bindo Koshy, "When City Growth Exceeds Supply" in *World Health*, July-August, 1992, p. 11.
18. WHO, SEARO: Annual Report of the Regional Director, 1976-77, pp. xii-xiii.
19. WHO, *World Health*, January 1977, p. 17.
20. *Ibid.*
21. WHO, *Public Health Papers*, 59, p. 116.

22. Batisse Michel, "Man and Biosphere" in *World Health,* June 1978, p. 4.
23. WHO, *World Health,* May 1972, p. 29.
24. WHO, *World Health,* January 1977, p. 17.
25. WHO, SEA/RC27, p. 41.
26. UN, ST/ESA/SERA/57, New York, 1975, p. 101.
27. Zbigniew Bankowski, "A Code of Ethics" in *World Health,* January-February 1990, p. 18.
28. Dr. Martin Kaplan, "Environmental Hazards for Human Health" in *World Health,* May 1972, p. 11.

PART II

POPULATION POLICY, CONTROL AND HEALTH DEVELOPMENT

CHAPTER 5

ADMINISTRATION OF FAMILY PLANNING PROGRAMME

The ultimate goal of the world's population policy must be to achieve an equilibrium based on low birth and death rates that can be sustained throughout a distant future for the world and its several parts.

—*F.W. Notestein*

The programme of family welfare and family planning is in the interest of peace and humanity in order to improve the quality of life for families in developing countries particularly in rural areas and in urban disadvantaged poor.

—Tokyo Declaration of Parliamentarians issued in March, 1978.

Administration of Family Planning Programme

The growth rate in population absorbs the national income and lowers the standard of living. The world population conference indicated in the population plan of action that population growth and population policy must be viewed not in isolation, but in the context of development. It was mentioned by the Secretary-General that "Current and potential world-wide population trends evidently cannot continue for as long as even one century without causing serious dislocations and crises in many areas.[1]

Myrdal in his book "Asian Drama" gave a stern warning to the world in regard to population explosion when he said, "Demographers are of the view that if fertility does not decrease, a time will come when mortality will lose its relative independence of levels of living and begin to rise again."[2]

Alexander Kessler[3] in his article, "Family Planning and the role of WHO" in *World Health,* May-June 1994 stated that the success of family planning programmes has led to a considerable decrease in average family size in developing countries, yet actual numbers continue to increase. This poses enormous challenges in terms of providing food, water, energy and services, let alone improving the quality of life. Far more emphasis must be placed on the importance of family planning services.

Family planning and health are intimately related. Family planning can promote women's health through the prevention of unwanted pregnancies, limiting number of births, and proper spacing, timing of births and foetal health. Family planning also promotes the health of the child through the reduction of child mortality, and promotion of the child development. Maryellen Fullam stresses the importance of family planning as instrument for the promotion of health. He says:

> "Uncontrolled fertility directly threatens the health of mothers and infants and may undermine the health of other family members. Today, no health programme can be considered complete unless it offers ready access to the appropriate family planning measures for all potential parents."[4]

Rapid population growth leads to social and psychological tensions, and breakdown of a distribution system. Civil amenities such as water and power supply, housing, transport and social utilities like schooling, educational, health and medical services fall much short of demand in spite of their constant expansion. Besides, it leads to political and social corruption and accentuates economic disparities.

The experiences and lessons gained from Indian Planning suggests that effective population control, designed to restore the balance between vital rates by reducing the level of fertility, has a positive influence on the process of economic development and modernization. An eminent scholar has rightly mentioned that "A reduction in fertility would make the process of modernization more rapid and more certain. It would accelerate the growth of income, provide more rapidly the possibility of productive employment of all adults who need jobs, make the attainment of universal education easier and it would have the obvious and immediate effect of providing the women of low income countries some relief from constant pregnancy, prostitution and infant care.[5]

Thus, we can say that the problem of growing population has reached such menacing proportions that it has become a real threat to the socio-economic stability of the country. The excessive growth in population does not affect the stability of the national economy alone, it disturbs the stability of the entire body politic. It poses a colossal threat to our social structure. In our fight against poverty, disease, hunger, malnutrition and unemployment, checking the rapid growth of population is as important as raising production in the farms and factories and provision of social services. Population control is one of the chief issues which the country has to resolve and accord top priority in its march towards social and economic development. The programme of family planning is of vital importance for our country. It is a positive and constructive approach to the betterment of the quality of life of the community. Thus, it is evident that the key to India's economic future based on social justice lies in the immediate and effective implementation of a nation-wide population programme.

MEANING

Family Planning Programme makes a planned and scientific approach to the issues and problems of family life and attemps to solve them to make the family life happier, harmonious and fruitful. Family planning was thought of as a public health problem. It was stated in the First Five Year Plan:

> It is apparent that population at a level consistent with the requirement of national economy should be stabilised. This can be secured only by the realisation of the need for family limitation on a wide scale by the people. The main appeal for planning is based on considerations of health and welfare of the family. Family limitation or spacing of the children is necessary and desirbale in order to secure better health of the mothers, and better care and upbringing of children. The measures described to this end should, therefore, form part of the public health programme.

A distinction must be made between population control and family planning. Population control is influenced and determined by a government policy motivated by socio-economic considerations. Family planning, on the other hand, is a responsibility of the family. Who has given various definitions of family planning.

An Expert Committee (1991) of the WHO defined family planning as: "a way of thinking and living that is adopted voluntarily upon the basis of knowledge, attitudes and responsible decisions by individuals and couples, in order to promote the health and welfare of the family group and thus contribute effectively to the social development of the country."[6]

Mr. Ramakrishna Mukherjee has defined family planning in broader and narrower context. In broader context, he says that:

(i) It is not matter of mere biological arrangement between a man and a woman, albeit in the "social" setting of a family.
(ii) It is not exclusively a "cultural" issue: culture defined as an aggregate of what a person or group of persons desires and detests in every-day-life, the aggregate being formed, from the past upto date in the course of socialisation and, thus, provides the person or the group with a matrix of perception of life itself.
(iii) It is a matter of systematic understanding of the human kind with reference to the world as a whole and not merely one of its sectors: The Third World.

In the narrower sense, he says, that family planning is, regarded as a managerial issues particularly relevant to the Third World. It involves the following measures:

(a) Propogation of appropriate slogans for a "small family."
(b) Running family planning centres for sterlisation; and

(c) Distribution of contraceptives and education of the people to use them for their own good.

Another Expert Committee (1971)[7] defined and described family planning as follows: "Family Planning refers to practices that help individuals or couples to attain certain objectives:

(a) to avoid unwanted births;
(b) to bring about wanted births;
(c) to regulate the intervals between pregnancies;
(d) to control the time at which births occur in relation to the age of the parents; and
(e) to determine the number of children in the family."

Dr. H. Mahler, ex-Director General of WHO has rightly said in *World Health* (June, 1984) that in all societies, the family in one form or another is the Central nucleus for people, for their lives, their loves, their dreams and their health. So the people must be helped to understand that it is in their own interest to plan their families. And when they want to plan their family, appropriate information and services must be available in a context that provides confidence and security. Clearly what most parents want are healthy children who will grow upto become healthy adults. Today, it is possible for families through the use of technically and culturally appropriate contraceptive means to choose the timing and spacing of their children, and thus to complement other traditionally accepted means of child spacing such as breast-feeding. And quite apart from the positive health effects of family planning, the ability of couples to control their own fertility has opened the way for women to achieve the full and equitable participation in social and economic development that is their due.

In *World Health* (June 1984), it is correctly stated that healthy families do not just happen, they are planned. The birth of a healthy wanted child is a joyous occasion. A child has chance of being born healthy, of surviving the first few years of life and growing well are enchanced if parents plan their children, so that they are born not before the mother is 18 or after she is 35—at least 2 years apart. Family Planning improves the health of women by helping them avoid high-risk pregnancies.

A WHO Expert Committee (1970)[8] has stated that family planning includes in its purview: (1) the proper spacing and limitation of births, (2) advice on sterility, (3) education for parenthood including pre-natal and post-natal care, (4) sex education, (5) screening for pathological conditions related to the reproductive system (e.g. cervical cancer), (6) genetic counselling, (7) pre-marital consultation and examination, (8) carrying out pregnancy tests, (9) marriage counselling, (10) the preparation of couples for the arrival of their first child, (11) providing services for unmarried mothers,

(12) teaching home economics and nutrition, and (13) providing adoption services. These activities vary from country to country according to national objectives and policies with regard to family planning. This is the modern concept of family planning.

STATUS IN INDIA

Population of the country has multiplied by more than four times during the century. It became 84.6 crore in the 1991 census and is 1,027 million as on March 1, 2001 (531 million males and 496 million females from 361 million at the time of independence. The India's population now is thrice that of USA (For details see Table 5.1). According to United Nations Fund Population Activities (UNFPA) estimates, world population is currently increasing at the rate of about 80 million per year. India alone is contributing to a fifth of the total increase in world population, every year. This is excessive as can also be seen from the fact that India has only 2.4% of the world land area, while its population constitutes 16% of the present world population. The already unusually large pressure of population on land in India, coupled with still continuing large annual increase indicates that the population situation in India is already critical.

TABLE 5.1

Decadal Variations in Population Growth in India, 1901-2001

*Census year**	*Total population in million*	*Average annual exponential growth rate*	*Progressive growth rate over 1901 in per cent*
1901	238.4	—	—
1911	252.1	0.56	5.8
1921	251.3	-0.03	5.4
1931	279.0	1.04	17.0
1941	318.7	1.33	33.7
1951	361.1	1.25	51.5
1961	439.2	1.96	84.3
1971	548.2	2.20	129.9
1981	683.3	2.22	186.6
1991	846.3	2.14	255.0
2001	1027.0	1.93	330.8

* Including Assam and Jammu & Kashmir. The 1981 Census was not held in Assam and the 1991 Census was not held in Jammu & Kashmir due to disturbances. The 1981 and 1991 census data include estimated figures for these two states.

Sources: Census of India, 1981, General Population Tables, Series 1, India, Part II-A (i), pp. 35-50, 536-37; *Census of India, 1991, Final Population Totals: Brief Anaysis of Primary Census Abstract*, Series 1, India, Part 2 of 1992, p. 86; *Census of India, 2001, Provisional Population Totals*, Series 1, India, Paper 1 of 2001, p. 34.

Such large and still increasing population has big implications for availability and incidence of unemployment in the society. The pressure of population is also very relevant for the state of enviornment. The high levels of population on land, in air and in water in large parts of the country indicate that the carrying capacity of land and environment is being exceeded.

NATIONAL POPULATION POLICY

India adopted a comprehensive and holistic National Population Policy (NPP)—2000 with clearly articulated objectives, strategic themes and operational strategies. The Policy enumerates certain socio-demographic goals to be achieved by 2010, which will lead to achieving population stabilization by 2045. The Policy also prescribes an Action Plan for implementing the strategic themes listed in the Policy.

The National Population Policy, 2000 has identified the immediate objectives as meeting the unmet needs for contraception, health care infrastructure and trained health personnel and to provide integrated service delivery, with the following interventions: (i) Strengthen community health centres, primary health centres and sub-centres; (ii) Augment skills of health personnel and health care providers; (iii) Bring about convergence in the implementation of related social sector programme so that the Family Welfare Programme becomes a peoples' programme; (iv) Integrate package of essential services at village and household level through mobile clinics and counselling services; and (v) Explore the possibility of accrediting private medical practitioners and revive the system of licensed medical practitioners, who could provide specified clinical services.

S.P. Singh in his Article, "Problems of Population and Sustainable Development in India" in *IJPA*, January-March 2003, observed that, With a population of about one billion, India has achieved many dubious distinctions. Now India is a country with largest number of unemployed youth, handicapped people, beggars, slum-dweller and illiterates in the world. The population of illiterates in India is larger than the total population of any country in the world except for People's Republic of China. Every third illiterate in the world is an Indian. It is irony that in all these areas India, come what may, will lead the world for many more years to come. It is pity indeed that in near future we will be able to achieve a few more dubious demographic distinction.

GENSIS AND GROWTH

Policy-making and Planning for Family Welfare

Family planning as an official programme was adopted in India in 1952. Before this, the Family Planning Association of India was formed in 1949 in Bombay. On 11 April 1951 the Advisory Panel on Health

Programmes appointed a sub-committee on Family Planning. The sub-committee strongly recommended that family planning should be recognised as an official programme to protect the health and welfare of mothers and children and to aid the national economy by reducing the birth rate concurrently with the death rate in order to stabilise the population. During the first two Five Year Plans (1951-61) the programme was taken up in a modest way with a clinical approach. During the Second Plan period, 549 urban and 1,100 rural clinics were set-up.

The programme was reorganized in the Third Plan after the publication of the 1961 census result which showed a higher growth rate than anticipated. It was towards the middle of the Third Plan that the emphasis was shifted from the clinical approach to the more vigorous extension educational approach for motivating the people for acceptance of the small family norm and for provision of services.

A full-fledged Department of Family Planning was created in the Ministry of Health and Family Welfare. During the three annual plans (1966-69), the programme which was described as the 'kingpin' of the plan was made time-bound and target-oriented with vastly increased funds. In the Fourth Plan, the programme was accorded the highest priority. More emphasis was given to training, research, publicity, organisation, supplies and evaluation. Medical Termination of Pregnancy Act, 1971, was passed which came into force from 1 April 1972. With this Act, State Governments were empowered to constitute relevant boards to certify the registered doctors who were willing to perform the operations causing termination of pregnancy. Though the MTP Act is mainly a health measure, it also supplements the family welfare programme because a large percentage of women undergoing medical termination of pregnancy readily accept family planning measures to avoid future conceptions.

The experiences gained within the country and outside had amply established that health of women in the reproductive age group and of small children (up to 5 years of age), is of crucial importance for effectively tackling the problem of the growth of population. This perception has led to change in the approach from Family Planning to Family Welfare. Since the Seventh Plan implemented during 1984-89, the FW programmes have evolved with the focus on the health needs of the women in the reproductive age group and of children below the age of 5 years on one hand and on the other hand, to provide contraceptives and spacing services to the desirous people. Thus, the family welfare programme has objectives of stabilising population of the country early and to ensure good reproductive and child health status of the existing population. These objectives are pursued by addressing contraception issues, maternal health issues, child survival issues and by encouraging citizens through IEC to use these services.

Various programmes have led to very substantial improvement in health indicators. The achievements with regard to some prominent health and population indicators is depicted in the Table 5.2.

TABLE 5.2

Achievements of the National Family Welfare Programme

Indicator	*Past Level*	*Current Level*
Crude Birth Rate	41.7 (1951-61)	25.4 (2001)
Crude Death Rate	22.8 (1951-61)	8.4 (2001)
Infant Mortality Rate	146 (1951-61)	6.6 (2001)
Maternal Morality Rate	437 (1992-93)	4.07 (1998)
Life Expectancy at Birth		
(years) Est. Male	37.1 (1951)	63.87 (2001)
Female	36.1 (1951)	66.9 (2001)
Effective Couple Protection Rate	10.4 (1970-71)	48.2 (1998-99)
Total Fertility Rate	6 (1951)	3.2 (1999)

(Relevant year in parentheses)
* Universal Immunisation was started in 1985-86.

The Approach Paper to the Ninth Plan brought out by the Planning Commission has shown the inadequacy of the investment made for family welfare. This is a severe handicap, particularly when it is noted that in almost all respects, the health care system needs up-gradation and it needs to reach out to many more people for the national goals to be achieved. While there is a steady improvement due to economic development, spread of education/literacy and empowerment of citizens, substantial problems in regard to education/literacy, particularly among the weak performing states and in regard to empowerment particularly of women, remain. It has been now renamed as Reproductive and Child Health (RCH).

Containing population growth was one of the six major objectives of the Eighth Plan Recognizing the fact that reduction in infant and child mortality is an essential pre-requisite for acceptance of small family norm, Governmnt of India has attempted to integrate MCH and Family Planning as part of Family Welfare services at all levels, NDC approved modified Gadgil Mukherjee Formula which for the first time gave equal weigtage to performance in MCH Sector (IMR reduction) and FP sector (CBR reduction) as a part basis for computing central assistance to non-special category States. This initiative ensured that the inter-linkages between Family Welfare Programme and Development was kept in focus in State Plans.

In order to give a new thrust and dynamism to the ongoing Family Welfare Programme the National Development Council set-up a Sub-committee on Populatiion to consider the problem of population stabilisation and come up with recommendations to improve performance. The report of the sub-committee was considered and the recommendations were endorsed by the NDC in its meeting in September 1993. The NDC Committee on Population had recommended that Family Welfare Programme should take cognizance of the area specific socio-economic, demographic and health care availability differentials and allow requisite flexibility in programme planning and implementation. For this purpose the NDC Committee recommended that there should be:

(a) Decentralised area specific planning based on the need assessment.
(b) Emphasis on improved access and quality of services to women and children.
(c) Providing special assistance to poorly performing states/ districts to minimise the inter and intra-state differences in performance.
(d) Creation of district level database on quality and coverage and impact indicators for monitoring the programme.

ORGANISATION

The apex body at the centre is a cabinet committee which is presided over by the Union Minister of Health and Family Welfare. It includes Ministers of States for Finance, Human Resource Development, Home Affairs. It also includes a member from the Department of Electronics and Scientific and Industrial Research. This body has the overall responsibility for the formulation of national policies on the family planning and for reviewing the progress in their implementation. (See Chart 5.1).

To Co-ordinate the family planning activities among the different States, the Central Family Planning Council has been set-up as an advisory body for policy-making. It includes Health Ministers from all the States and is presided over by the Union Minister of Health and Family Welfare, Vice-President in Union Minister of State. The Union Deputy Minister in the Ministry of Health. Other members are from the Planning Commission, representatives of the Union Territories, representatives of major voluntary organizations, labour organizations, selected members of Parliament, Eminent individuals in their personal capacity and officials from the various ministries. It has representatives from a wider section of interests in family planning, including those that are directly charged with the implementation of the programme.

The Department of Family Welfare (earlier Family Planning) within the ministry is responsible for the implementation of policies. The Secretary to the Government of India in the Ministry of Health and Family Planning is overall in-charge of the Department of Family

Welfare. An Additional Secretary assists the Secretary and provides overall direction to programme implementation. He is known as Additional Secretary and Commissioner for Family Welfare. There is a Joint-Secretary who supervises the working of the Technical Wing of the Department which provides technical guidance to the various programme activities, i.e., Sterilisation, IUD, Post-Partum, M.C.H., Training, Mass Education, besides Evaluation and Research. The Additional Secretary's duties include policy formulation, programme planning, supervising the programme implementation and co-ordination of activities of the department with other related ministries and departments of the Government of India.

There are two wings of the department: (A) Administrative Wing (the Secretariat), and (B) Technical Wing with many divisions.

On the secretariat side, there is: (i) Policy Division, (ii) an Aided Programme Division, (iii) an organised sector, (iv) Voluntary Organisations Division, and (v) a Plan Budget Division.

(i) The Policy Division looks after formulation of policies concerning family welfare.
(ii) The Aided Programme Division looks after the activities of organizations which receive extra government assistance and aims at improving upon the scope and quantum of medical and health care services.
(iii) The Organised Sector Division Co-ordinates Departmental Policies and Measures affecting the family planning activities of public bodies and private organisations which are collectively called institutions in the organised Sector.
(iv) The Voluntary Organisations Division assigns programmes to voluntary agencies and aims at assessing the efficiency and effectiveness of these agencies.
(v) A Plan Budget Division looks after the finances of the Programme.

On the technical side, the following divisions are functioning. The functions are clear from the names of the divisions:

(i) Programme Appraisal, Co-ordination and Training and Sterilisation (including Research) Division.
(ii) Technical Operations Division.
(iii) Maternal and Child Health Division.
(iv) Evaluation and Intelligence Division.
(v) Mass Education and Media (including population education) Division.
(vi) Nirodh Marketing Division.
(vii) Transport Division.
(viii) Projects Division (Area Projects).

Chart 5.1

Organisation Chart: Department of Family Planning*

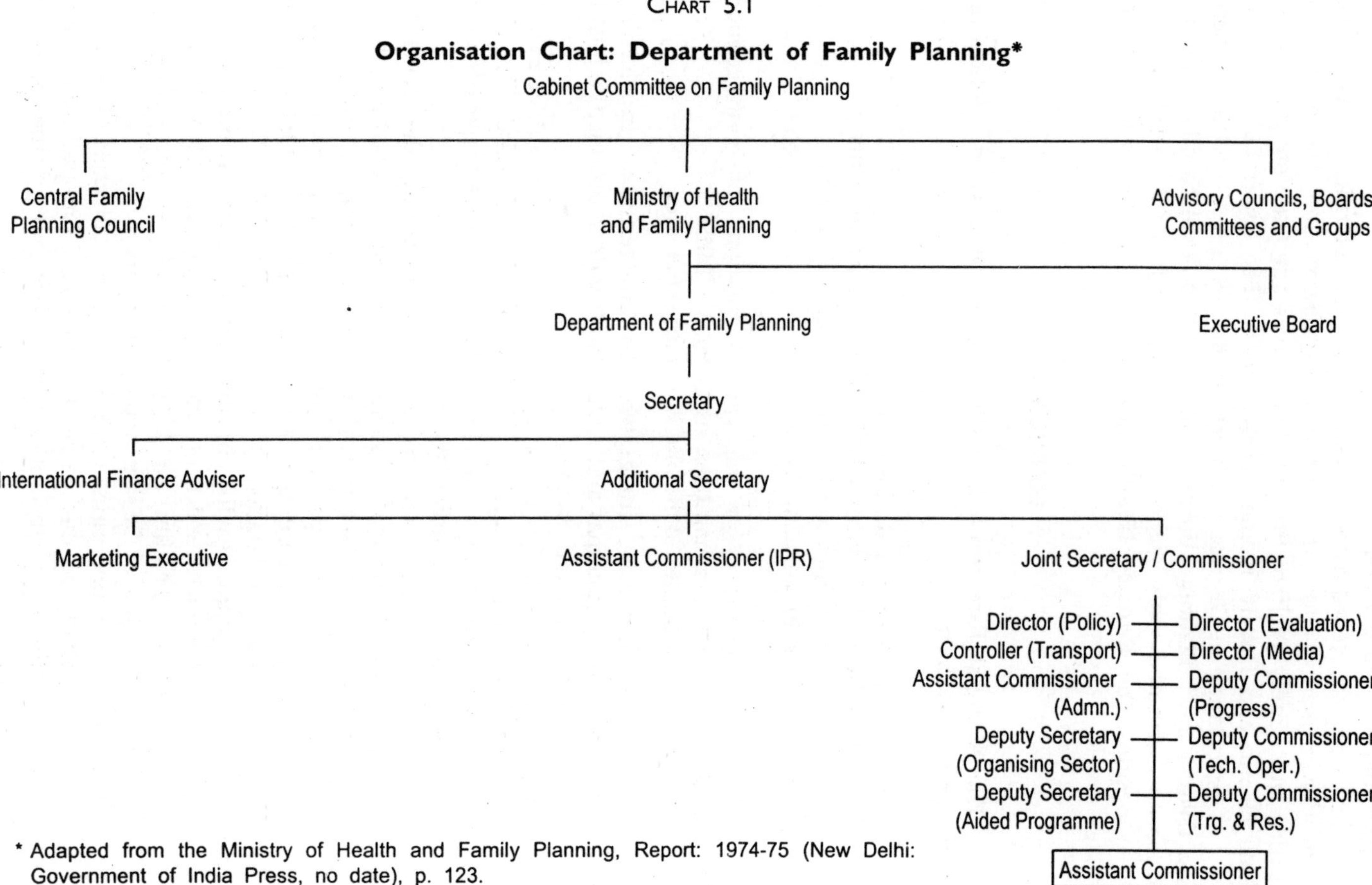

* Adapted from the Ministry of Health and Family Planning, Report: 1974-75 (New Delhi: Government of India Press, no date), p. 123.

Organisation at State Level

In order to co-ordinate the family welfare activities between the State Governments and the Central Government, the Directorate of Health and Family Welfare for each State gives adequate support to the State Health and Family Welfare Departments. (See Chart 5.2)

Organisation at District and block levels—At the district level there is a Distt. Family Planning Bureau while at block level Family Planning has been integrated with health services (Refer Charts 5.3 and 5.4).

Besides, the Primary Health Care complex is responsible at the village level.

SERVICES

The National Family Welfare Programme provides the following contraceptive services:

- Sterilization as a terminal method.
- Intra-Uterine Devices (IUD) for the spacing births.
- Daily Oral Contraceptive Pill for spacing births.
- Condoms for spacing births.

The acceptance level of the various methods of contraception during the last four years has been as given in Table 5.3.

The main Highlights of the RCH Programme are:

(i) The Programme integrates all interventions of fertility regulation, maternal and child health with reproductive health of both men and women.

(ii) The services to be provided will be client-centred, demand-driven, high quality and based on the needs of the community arrived at, through decentralised participatory planning and a target free approach.

(iii) The programme envisages up-gradation of the level of facilities for providing various interventions and quality of care. The First Referral Units (FRUs) being set-up at sub-district level will provide comprehensive emergency obstetric and new born care. Similarly, RCH facilities in PHCs will be substantially upgraded.

(iv) The Programme will improve access of the community to various services which are commonly required. It is proposed to provide facilities for MTP at the PHCs, counselling and IUD insertion at SCs in a phased manner.

(v) The Programme aims at improving the outreach of services, particularly for the vulnerable groups of population which have till now substantially been left out of the planning process:

CHART 5.2

Organisation for Family Planning in a State

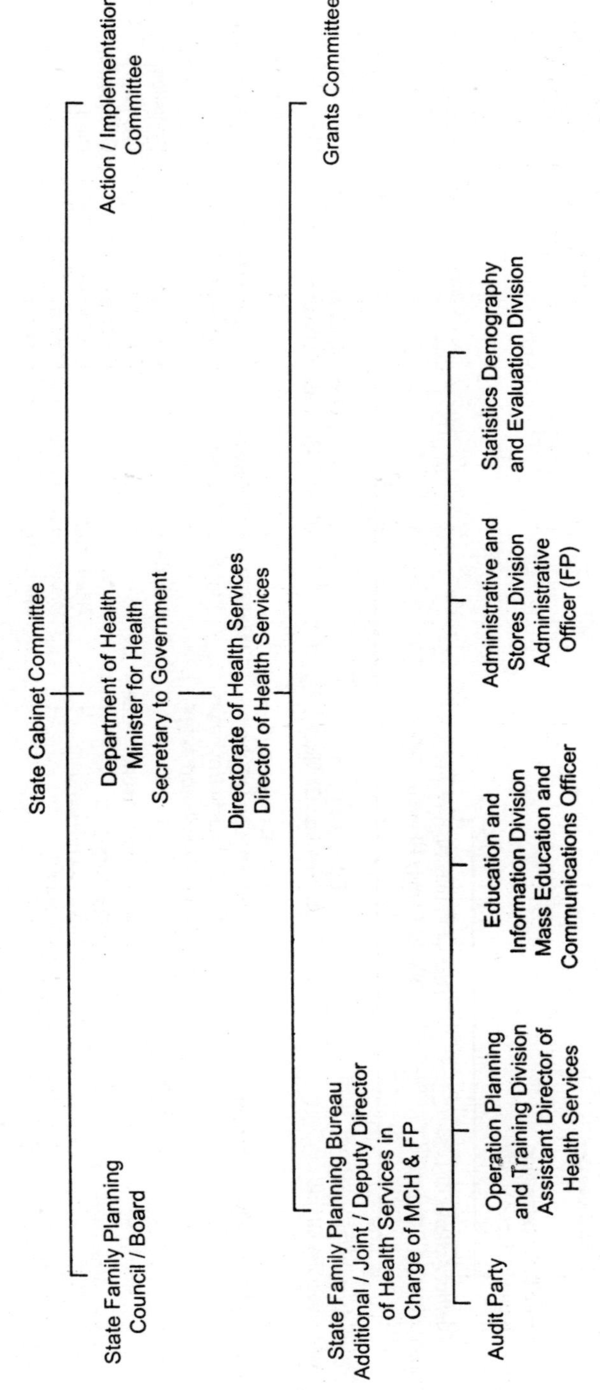

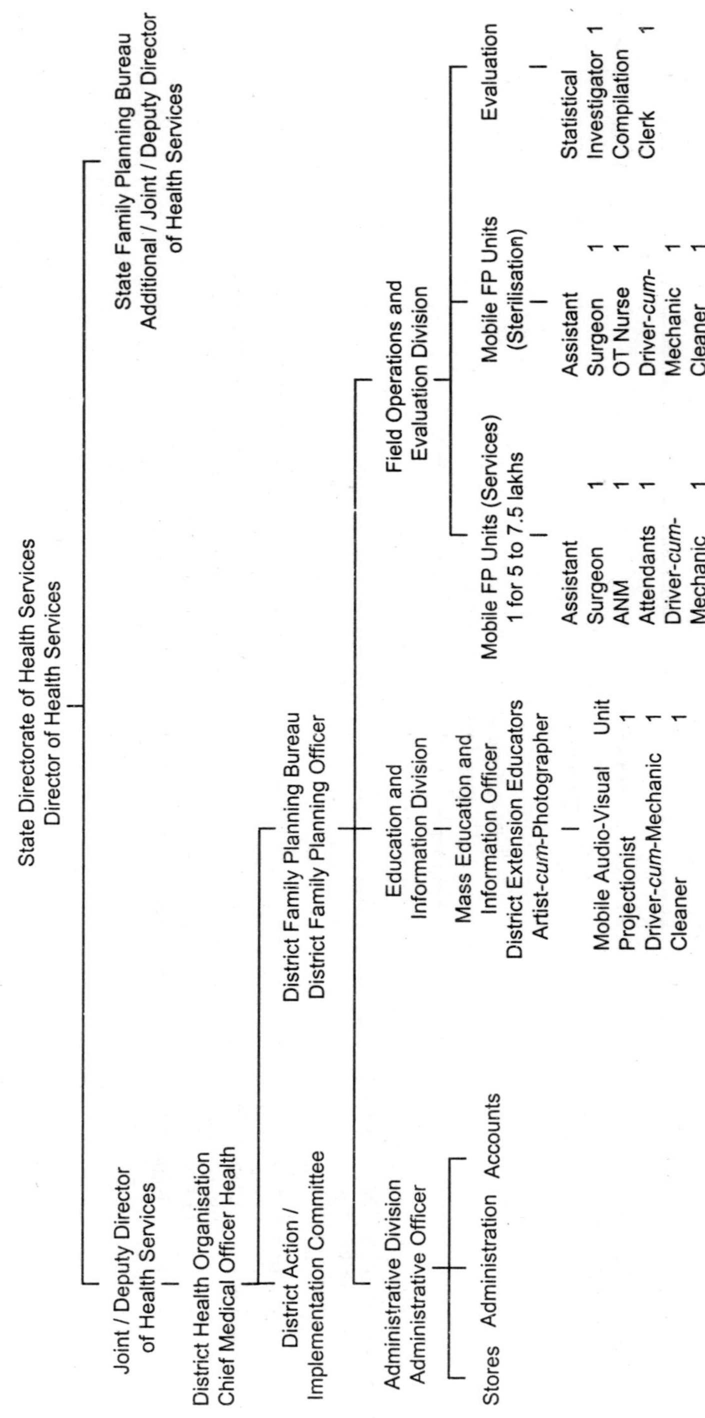
CHART 5.3
Organisation for Family Planning in a District
State Directorate of Health Services
Director of Health Services
Joint / Deputy Director
of Health Services
State Family Planning Bureau
Additional / Joint / Deputy Director
of Health Services
District Health Organisation
Chief Medical Officer Health
District Action /
Implementation Committee
District Family Planning Bureau
District Family Planning Officer
Administrative Division
Administrative Officer
Stores
Administration
Accounts
Education and
Information Division
Mass Education and
Information Officer
District Extension Educators
Artist-cum-Photographer
Mobile Audio-Visual Unit
Projectionist 1
Driver-cum-Mechanic 1
Cleaner 1
Field Operations and
Evaluation Division
Mobile FP Units (Services)
1 for 5 to 7.5 lakhs
Assistant
Surgeon 1
ANM 1
Attendants 1
Driver-cum-
Mechanic 1
Mobile FP Units
(Sterilisation)
Assistant
Surgeon 1
OT Nurse 1
Driver-cum-
Mechanic 1
Cleaner 1
Evaluation
Statistical
Investigator 1
Compilation
Clerk 1

Chart 5.4

Organisation for Family Planning in a Block

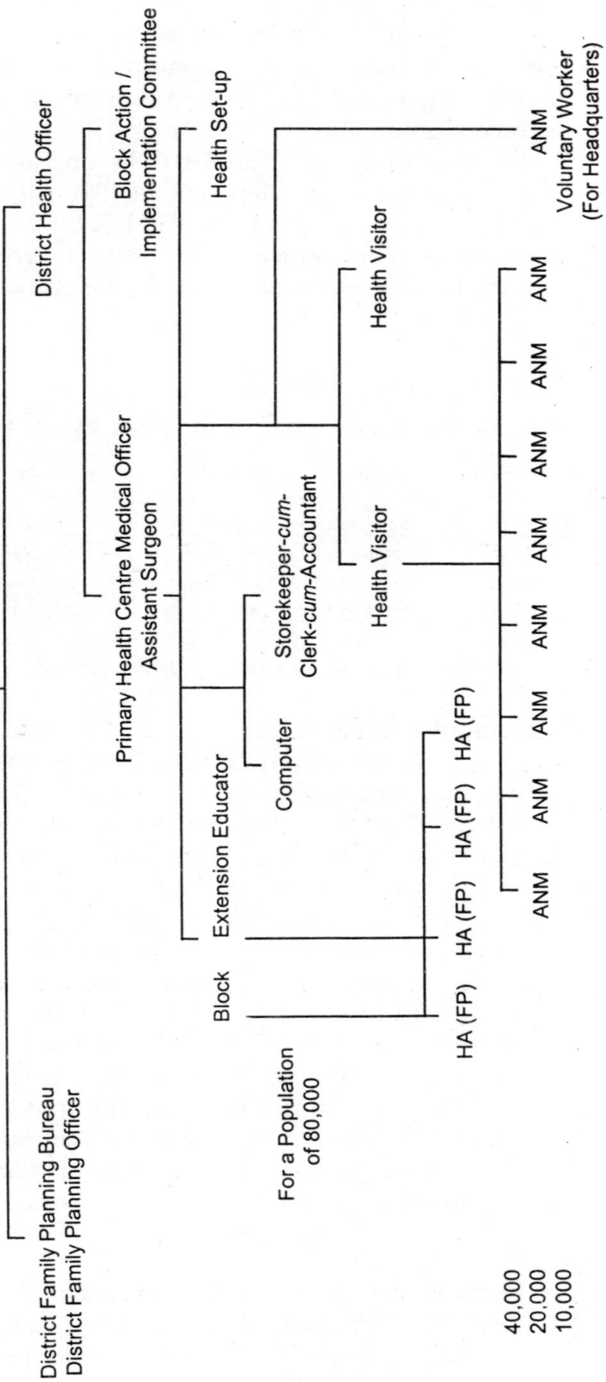

District Health Organisation
Chief Medical Officer of Health

District Family Planning Bureau
District Family Planning Officer

District Health Officer

Primary Health Centre Medical Officer
Assistant Surgeon

Block Action /
Implementation Committee

Block

Extension Educator

Health Set-up

For a Population
of 80,000

Computer

Storekeeper-*cum*-
Clerk-*cum*-Accountant

Health Visitor

Health Visitor

HA (FP) HA (FP) HA (FP) HA (FP)

40,000
20,000
10,000

ANM ANM ANM ANM ANM ANM ANM ANM

ANM
Voluntary Worker
(For Headquarters)

- Special programmes will be taken up for urban slums, tribal population and adolescents.
- Non-Government Organisations will be involved in a much larger way to improve out-reach and make it people's programme.
- Skills of practitioners of ISM will be upgraded by training and research and development in ISM will be supported to improve the range of the RCH Services.
- Panchayati Raj system will have a greater role in planning, implementation and assessment of client satisfaction.

TABLE 5.3

Acceptance of Various Services from 1995-96 to 1998-99

	1995-96	*1996-97*	*1997-98*	*1998-99*	*2002-2003*
Sterilisation	4422319	3870226	4127065	1283402	4731000
IUDs	6857882	5680671	6085744	263463	6108000
Oral Pills	5090850	5250179	6249222	5081306	16537000
Condom	172974291	17214327	16730468	12984061	8243000

Source: Annual Report, Ministry of Health and Welfare Work, 1998-99.

Prevention of Unwanted Pregnancy

The data from National Family Health Survey has shown that awareness regarding contraception is nearly universal. But there is an unmet for contraception. The Family Welfare Programmes will gear itself to meet the unmet need during the Ninth Plan period. Vasectomy is safer than tubectomy and efforts will be made to increase acceptance of vasectomy, so that there is substantial reduction in the morbidity associated with terminal methods of contraception. Quality of contraceptive care will be improved. Couples will be provided with balanced information on all available methods of contraception and the advantage and disadvantage of each of these methods so that they choose the method best suited to their needs. Such a balanced presentation and counselling will in the long-run not only improve acceptance of contraceptive care, but also improve continuation rates of temporary methods of contraception. The quality of services will be improved through appropriate training of service providers at all levels.

MTP Services

Over two decades have elapsed after the enactment of legislation for Medical Termination of Pregnancy (MTP) Act. Over the last two decades the Government of India has taken steps to provide trained manpower and equipment at secondary and primary health care level for safe legal abortion services.

It is obvious that after the initial rise, the reported number of MTPs has remained below 0.6 million for the last 15 years. In 2001, it was 7,66,762. In spite of efforts to improve the availability of, and access to, induced abortions services in the primary health care set-up, safe abortion services are not available to majority of rural population in India. Even today majority of the estimated 7.6 million induced abortions are not carried out in settings recognised for legal abortion and about 8.9% maternal deaths in India are due to septic abortion.

Efforts to improve access to family planning services to reduce the number of unwanted pregnancies and cater to the request for induced abortion will continue to receive intensified attention during the Ninth Plan. In addition, efforts will be made to improve access to safe abortion services by training physicians in MTP and recognising and strengthening institutions which are capable of providing safe abortion services for the first trimester. IEC efforts through appropriate channels of communications to improve awareness among women about availability of safe abortion services at affordable cost through appropriate channels of communication will be intensified. Provision for first trimester abortion will be coupled with appropriate contraceptive care so that these women do not incur the risk of yet another unwanted pregnancy and induced abortion.

RESEARCH AND DEVELOPMENT

The ICMR is the nodal research agency for funding basic, clinical and operational research in contraception and MCH. In addition to ICMR, CSIR, DBT and DST are some of the major agencies funding research pertaining to Family Welfare Programme. The National Committee for Research in Human Reproduction assists the Department of Family Welfare in drawing up priority areas of research and ensuring that there is no unnecessary duplication of research activities. Some of the major institutions carrying out research in this area include the Institute for Research in Reproduction, Bombay, National Institute of Nutrition, Hyderabad, National Institute of Health and Family Welfare, New Delhi, Central Drug Research Institute, Lucknow and the Central Council for Research in Ayurveda and Siddha, Delhi. A network of 18 Population Research Centres conduct studies on different aspects of the Family Welfare Programme and undertake demographic surveys.

Basic and Clinical Research

Development and testing of new contraceptives including contraceptives which are considered to be effective in Indian Systems of Medicine.

Research on methods for male fertility regulation,
Clinical trials on newer non-surgical methods of MTP, and
Post-marketing surveillance of Centchroman.

Operational Research

- Studies on the ongoing demographic transition and its consequences.
- Studies on continuation rates and use of effectiveness of contraceptives.
- Research on operationalising integrated delivery of RCH services nutrition, education, women and child development, rural development and family welfare services at village level.

MONITORING OF FAMILY WELFARE SERVICES

Monitoring and evaluation form an essential component of FW Programme. Indicators used for monitoring and evaluation include process indicators and impact indicators. Process indicators are used to monitor the progress of implementation of the programme through monthly progress reports as compared to the annual targets/expected Level of Achievements (ELAs).

Training

Training to medical and paramedical health professional is imparted in various training institutes, centres and school. Basic training is imparted in ANM training schools, LHV training schools and MPW (M) training schools and selected Health and Family Welfare Training Centres. In-service training is imparted in National Institutes; State Regional Health and Family Welfare Training Centres, HFWTC's and by District Training Teams.

CRITICAL APPRAISAL

To quote S.P. Singh again, What has happened elsewhere can happen in India too provided there is a massive campaign to educate eligible couples, particularly in villages, about the benefits of limiting the size of the family. This point has of course been emphasised innumerable times and at different places but it has never been sincerely implemented. Rural people, steeped in ignorance and obsolete religious belief, still do not know the harm that big family size brings to them and consider every child as a gift of God. This notion must be altered if family planning is to succeed. However, the education campaign must always be backed by easy availability of modern contraceptive measures that can enable people to plan their families. One of the reasons why family planning measures have not yielded the desired results is that it has not been honestly implemented. The unmet need for family planning has been reported to be quite high. According to the National Family Health Survey 2, the current unmet need for family planing is 16 per cent and it is higher in rural areas than in urban areas.

Inspite of the existence of infrastructure and availability of technology to control the growth of population, we have not been achieving the desired results. K.B. Sahay[9] in his article, "Population: Time for Tough Measures", in the *Daily Tribune* (January 28, 2000) has rightly portrayed the present population scene which present a depressing picture. To quote him: "It is very well known that we are adding at least about 1.5 crore "additional" children every year to our population. Thus, the reality is that hardly 10 percent of the "additional" children accruing every year in India are getting (even) enrolment in primary schools and the rest 1.35 crore per year are being left to grow up without any school education. Thus, we need to open at least 60,000 new primary schools per year to meet the constitutional requirement whereas we have been opening only 6000 new primary schools per year. Thus, our "educational rate" is, in fact, declining about 1.4 per cent per year. It is feasible now for the country to open 60,000 new primary schools per year and provide free and compulsory primary education to all the children as required in the constitution without first controlling our population growth? And, again, it is possible to empower women without even primary school education?

It might be recalled that in 1970 Dr. Norman Borlaug, in his speech that he gave on the occasion of receiving the Nobel Prize cautioned that whatever was being done by way of increasing food production would give us a breathing time of not more than 30 years which should be used to tame the population monster. We have now come to the end of that grace period but our population is still increasing by about 1.6 crore per year. Also, according to a recent study report, "Population, Food Production and Nutrition in India", published by UNFPA, India (Oct. 1999), "there is an urgent need to reduce population growth so that the demand for foodgrains can be reduced and effectively met."

The question arises as to what is the major problem? It may be mentioned that the main problem in the less developed world including India is that of inadequate and inefficient administration which directly or indirectly impinge on the implementation of family planning programmes. The success of family planning programmes can be ensured only through innovative, impartial, honest and efficient administration.

There is a need that Family Planning Administration must be modernized, i.e., recreated, renewed and revitalized to achieve the predesigned changes and output. This needs a different trend and magnitude of Administrative Management, culture and capability especially in a challenging area of Family Planning.

Let us analyse some of the problems in detail which affect the functioning of family planning programme:

1. Ineffective Environmental Linkages

It is understood that the implication of family planning programme is a quite complex process in which medical, cultural, psychological, social, economic, administrative and even political factors are involved and intermingled. The existing family planning organisations are operating like other government departments and thus their performance is not adequate. A good organisation must respond to and react to the changes in the environment and establish environmental linkages. Linkages are points of interactions with the environment. They can be classified into four categories: (a) enabling, (b) functional, (c) diffused, and (d) normative linkages.

(a) Enabling Linkage

It ensures and protects the organisational authority to operate its access to resource and its power to achieve results. One of the most important factors which impinges on the programmes from its formulation to execution is political and its impingement on both the programme and its executors occur at al levels (national, regional, provincial, district) and at the programme input levels (financial allocations, personnel, material resources). The impact of policies and the political processes on the programme is both positive and negative and this insight provides the directions and options available to ensure greater success in programme implementations. Since political constraints are neither permanent nor inseparable there is urgency in adopting measures designed to optimise the positive contributions of political support as well as minimise and mitigate the harmful effects of partisan interferences. To make Family Planning Programme effective and stronger there is a need of more visible political commitment and commitment for demographic rather than health or welfare reasons.

For Family Planning administrators to operate successfully in this political environment they must acquire not only a deeper insight of the 'political games' as well as the 'political skills' needed to serve and thrive in that environment. An important asset is the capability of programme leaders to seek and maintain support from key political elites both at the national and local levels.

The Family Planning Workers at all levels must keep in touch with political elite to generate favourable public opinion. In this context, there is a great need at the local level where the family planning programmes are being implemented. Here, they must involve the members of Panchayat and other local leaders so that they can help the family planning workers in developing momentum.

(b) Functional Linkage

It is to link the programme with the task environment, i.e., university, research institutes, hospitals, etc. The Family Planning workers must analyse the agencies interested in the developmental activities and then get their support and guidance in their work. Such agencies are existing from national to local levels. For examples, at the grass-root level, we have teaching institutions, extension offices of many development departments. The need is to develop effective linkages in order to get the benefit of their existing structures and mechanisms. Let us discuss some of them.

(i) Collaboration with the Elites

In this connection, it is suggested that there should be effective collaboration between the universities and the family planning programme as the universities can be a sources of strength to the programme from the policy formulation to evaluation. To quote K.P. Bahadur:

> "The involvement of intellectuals in the programme has distinct advantages. This was done in Turkey with excellent results. They have the ability and the social position to carry its message to the lower classes and to convince those who are hovering on the fringe of doubt."[10]

At the moment there is a dichotomy between the social scientists and the medical specialists which must fade away as early as possible. In South Korea, one of the reasons ascribed for the success of the programme is the association of the university with the family planning programme.

(ii) Collaboration with the Hospital

The success of family planning programme depends to a great extent on the way the programme can operated through the health services network in the country. The hospital provides a good platform from the educational and motivational point of view. About 200 million people approach the hospitals every year in the country and there the people are most amenable to advice upon any aspect of their personal behaviour including family planning. Maternity wards are special places for such work. Moreover, the hospital is the best place for family planning as it can provide all the services to deal with after effects. Conventional contraceptives are not being used by the people in India because it requires high motivation and good standard of living, e.g., the sale of Nirodh has touched 50 million mark in India while in USA with half the population, sale is about 600 million per year, in Japan with one-fifth of India's population, the sale is 250 million per year. Therefore, the country should rely on sterilization, IUD, etc. Both of these require supervision of a high order. Hence, we must streamline the administration of the hospitals so that the hospital staff can also take up Family Planning Programme work with more earnestness and seriousness.

(iii) Co-ordination with Voluntary Agencies

Voluntary agencies can play an effective role in mobilizing the public opinion in support of the programme. The Family Planning Association of India and its branches in the States are rendering useful service. In this connection, it may be suggested that to revolutionise the programme, FPAI may take initiative in setting up the "Women's Club" in every village as in South Korea. At present, the 'Mother's Club' having a membership of 20-40 women in each of 19,000 villages has become a multi-purpose basic organ for the nation-wide 'New community movement' since 1971, in Korea. It is significant to note that the family planning programme became integrated into a broader community movement by the Mother's Club at the village level.[11] This experiment has been a great success in South Korea. We can bring these members in the communication network with the help of a four-step strategy mentioned below:

(a) Provide the opinion leaders with the information necessary for a full understanding of the reasons for family planning including its relationships to national and particularly local development,
(b) Invite their suggestions for local activities,
(c) Involve them in the purview of radio and television programmes, and
(d) Invite them to open discussion about family planning in the community whether formally or informally.[12]

Mrs. Helvi Sipila has also stressed that the associations of women organisations will surely help in checking the menace of population explosion.[13] A study of the inter-relationship of the status of women and family planning was conducted in accordance with economic and social council resolution.[14] The report affirmed:

(a) The right to decide freely and responsibly on the number and spacing of their children is a fundamental right of individuals which facilitates the exercise of other human rights especially by women.
(b) Adequate information, education and services enabling individuals to exercise this right are essential prerequisites for ensuring their complete integration in social and economic development at all levels.
(c) Family Planning which should constitute an integrated and essential part of development plan and programme in countries suffering from over-population can only succeed in concert with other measures which also improve the status of women.[15]

It can be said that the best contraceptive in the world is the involvement and the overall improvement of the status of women. Meher

C. Nanavatty in his Article, "Organising Communities" has rightly stated that the process of Community Organisation, which is necessary for shouldering this work, has to be generated in developing community education for population control. The development of the nucleus of local leadership, involving the community in the study of the needs and requirements of the programme, the association of existing groups and their leader in the promotion of the programme, the effective use of educational and audio-visual aids with emphasis on creating the climate of change for and acceptance of programme. Their inclusion needs to be ensured by the non-official Organisations which would take upon themselves the responsibility of promoting community education for population control.[16]

(c) Diffused Linkage

"Life enlighten movement" means to reach the clients through mass-media. Organized family planning programme requires a high level of user participation. Any successful family planning effort must be understood and accepted by the people and be based on public trust and confidence. It cannot be solely dictated or legislated. Family planning is such a multifaceted personal and intimate subject that its practice can only occur on an individual, voluntary basis.[17]

The art of developing common understanding among people is vital to bring about change of attitudes and behaviour. Sociologists have classified the diffusion process which leads to a widespread acceptance of the programme into five stages:

Awareness (the individual's first introduction to a new idea or practice).
Interest (the stage at which he actually seeks further information and background data).
Evaluation (the stage of assessment on theoretical grounds).
Trial (a limited phase of experiment), and finally acceptance or adoption.

Naturally, the duration of the process depends upon personality factors which differs with individuals. Mass-media helps in creating awareness, in providing stimulation and motivation and in giving ready access to information. But at the specific stage of evaluation, trial and adoption, inter-personal, face to face, communication counts for much more and the inability of the mass-media to maintain a two-way dialogue with regular feedback restricts their utility.[18] Therefore, no medium of communication is as effective as one human being talking to another. The UNESCO has rightly stated:

> The process of social and economic development is a process of human development for people are the targets as well as the

essential variable in development. Communication being a two-way process, provides for participation at whatever stage of enlightenment of the individuals composing a society find themselves. Change agents are key factors in both the communication development processes since they are instruments for getting facts to the people upon which decisions can be based.[19]

The function is to be performed mostly by the field workers. At present, the field workers are not fully equipped to do this interpersonal communication resulting into much mis-informed criticism of the programme. For example, on the personal discussion of the writer with a group of rickshaw-pullers, it was revealed that they were not undergoing family planning operations as they thought that they would not be able to ply their rickshaws afterwards. Similarly, in a discussion with educated people one finds that the adoption of family planning programme would lead to many social and psychological maladjustments. It was found in a survey that multi-purpose workers felt a need for more training to develop skills and techniques to contact, communicate and persuade their clients in their own particular setting and identity of personality. Even the Haryana Government has admitted that training of the workers in the field needs re-orientation and pre-service training of multi-purpose workers is absolutely necessary. [20]

The ultimate test of establishing diffused linkage can be ascertained from the following:

(a) Awareness of the needs and problems of population control;
(b) Knowledge of schemes in operation, their objectives, service, eligibility criteria, agencies and functionaries for the delivery of services;
(c) Community's conviction about the efficacy and usefulness of the services;
(d) Community's clear understanding of its participation and contribution; and
(e) Active involvement of the people, their leaders, institutions, organisations.

(d) Normative Linkage

There has been little attempt to incorporate the family planning behaviour into the existing value system of the society. Social values act as a hindrance to ready adoption. For example, if people talk about birth control behaviour naturally related to sex, it is traditionally regarded as impolite. Besides, the demand for sons to carry on the family line has been predominant in the Indian society. Not only social values but also religious values often act as a hindrance.[21] Therefore, the mass-media and communication officers and family planning workers must dispel all these false impressions and taboos after a careful survey and research in demography. Mass-media and communication officers may intensify their efforts by organising public meetings of different groups—labourers, farmers, workers, union leaders and extensive use of various media like, cinema, exhibition, radio, TV, etc. may be made. At present, the full use of mass-media is not being made in the real sense inspite of the availability of the arrangements. More attention is to be paid to uneducated rural people and economically depressed classes. Family planning and fertility control behaviour of the client group especially eligible women have been affected by their socio-economic background. It is found that the higher educated women tend to have a small number of children and the use of contraceptives and induced abortion is more prevalent among them. The socio-economic status as well as the urban-rural diffusion of client groups are clearly pronounced in their family planning behaviour. The Government of India, Ministry of Health, has also admitted that "high fertility rates have been identified as more a function of poverty than of anything else." Therefore, more attention must be paid to groups living under conditions of poverty.

2. Limited Financial Resources and Absence of Cost Consciousness Among Family Planning Personnel

The most important aspect about the finances for the Family Planning Welfare is its effective utilisation, i.e., to ensure optimization. This can be ascertained from the physical results achieved. V.M. Dandekar in his Article, "Population Front of India's Economic Development" in *Economic and Political Weekly*, April 23, 1988 has analysed the Family Planning Programmes. He states that the expenditure on family planning increased from Rs. 12.14 per eligible couple in 1980-81 to Rs. 37.7 in 1985-86. There is a great variation in States, the expenditure per eligible couple varied from Rs. 59.59 in Kerala to Rs. 23.47 in Bihar. The cost per birth averted has increased from Rs. 285.63 in 1980-81 to Rs. 590.87 in 1985-86. Study the Deptt. of Family Welfare also found this. Expenditure on Family Welfare per eligible couple is the highest in Punjab.

This analysis clearly indicates that the resources allocated to Family Planning are not being fully utilized. Though, there are no two opinions regarding the urgency of averting birth. To quote Mr. V.M. Dandekar, "Whatever the cost, the Family Planning Programme must be pursued steadily. But, it must perform."

"It has been a matter for concern that there are considerable shortfalls in expenditure and disturbing increase in the cost per acceptor . . . Although expenditure has been mounting since the beginning of the Fourth Five Year Plan, Physical Performance has not been keeping pace with it. Capital expenditure on construction activities and vehicles has grown since 1969-70, but the number of equivalent sterilizations has been going down."[22]

3. Not Enough Use of Modern Management Techniques

In a developing country, such as ours, there is a great urgency to control population growth in the shortest time possible before it becomes too late. It is felt that the scope of experimentation is a costly and slow process. As such, we need to apply the new management technique to accelerate the process of population control.

Family Planning functions are so pervasive, diverse and vast, in terms of the range of functions, the number of functionaries, and the areas of operation, that it would be risky to fail to appreciate the need for rationalization of the processes of management.

To quote Dr. Chi-Yuen Wu of the UNDP:

> "To create administrative capabilities, commensurate with requirements, developing countries must be able among other things, to use modern management techniques more effectively than in the case of the industrially advanced countries."

Family Planning and Population Programme involve large, complete and inter-related activities which need to be managed consistently to include the desired social change. Though there are a large number of these techniques like PERT/CPM, Operational Research, Organisational Development, Cost-Benefit Analysis, Management Information System, Work Study, Method Study, Performance Budgeting, etc. which can be used profitably to optimise the family planning activities. But, the management techniques suitable for industrial and commercial enterprises may not help in their pure forms. There is a need to modify and develop these techniques to make them applicable to family planning activities. We generally forget it and the result is frustration.

4. Less Emphasis on Relevant Research

Mr. Prodipto Roy in his Article, "The Uses of a Rapid Survey and Feedback to Accurately Assess Demographic Trends" has emphasized the need of co-ordination between researchers and policy-makers, planners and decision-makers. He states that the dialogue between the research workers, decision-makers and action workers must be maintained. The latter must feel free to ask foolish but sometimes difficult research questions and the research machinery must be geared to answer these questions. A continual feeding of problems from high political places or low action places to simple or complex research design and execution must maintain a steady cycling and recycling. It is only when this level of research capability is built flexible, fast and with the capacity to save the entire range of problems that arise, will the population problem be put on an intelligent footing so that the policy can be based squarely on scientific facts.[23]

The researches so far conducted have not devoted sufficient

attention to fields of organistional structure and functioning of family planning progrmme and modern methods of administrative management. Evaluation machinery needs strengthening at all levels. Independent evaluation may be undertaken to ensure that qualitative aspects of the programme have not been ignored by the states.

Research is not an end in itself, it is only a means to an end. There has been a lack of co-operation and co-ordination among the institutions engaged in teaching and research. This resulted in disjointed, isolated and rank duplication of scientific research in the institutions engaged in population/Family Planning Research resulting in waste of scarce resources. Thus, there is a need that energetic steps may be taken to enlarge the scope of collaboration to avoid repetitive research.

Besides, over the years, for a variety of reasons, the medical and family planning programme in the country could not follow the path of problem-oriented research in priority areas. The Sixth Draft Plan (1978-83) was also critical of the research policy pursued so far. It was stated that medical research in the past had by and large failed to lay emphasis on problems of immediate practical importance. The Estimate Committee in its 102 Report pointed out that it is unfortunate that resources, time and talent of the medical community of the country have not been meaningfully utilized over the years according to well thought out priorities. [24]

5. Lack of Area Development Profiles and Programmes

The policy of the Family Planning Programme Organisation in terms of targets are made only for the state or country as a whole. No attempt has been made so far to prepare action plans for each sub-centre/primary health centre or urban centre in terms of money, equipment, personnel, time, physical targets, etc. Such action programme if designed would help in effective implementation and monitoring. Here, we can make use of the new techniques of management—PERT/CPM for proper programme planning and resource deployment.

It is understood that planning covers not only the determination of programme objectives and overall targets but also the detailed specification of activities and projects as well as resources allocation for the achievement of specific project targets during a given period of time. In the case of most Asian countries, planning of FP programmes covers only the official statement of programme objectives in terms of national demographic goals and the determination of the overall targets of FP acceptance. There is no such management planning that is conducive to programme implementation through the provision of guidelines for managers and administrators of FP programmes at every level regarding specific actions to be undertaken in terms of what to do (specification of activity design), how much to do (individual activity targets and budgeting), what is required (standard of performance), how to secure the desired performance (monitoring), how to co-operate (organisation), etc. In most Asian countries, FP programmes are conceptually specified into primary functional categories such as: (1) contraceptive services and supplies (FP delivery), (2) information, education and communication (IEC) for mass education, (3) training of FP personnels, (4) research and training, (5) administration, etc. According to information revealed in the plan documents of programmes, however, the elaboration of these activities into further specific sub-functional categories is not made and thus managerial strategies for achieving the programme targets are hardly demonstrated. The lack of specification of FP programmes in the planning stage does not help in guiding adequately the administrators' role in management planning, monitoring and evaluation.

6. Lack of Team Work in Family Planning

Besides Planning and Training, we may keep in mind that team-work among different categories of personnel engaged in family planning activities is of vital significance.

Most of the Family Planning workers are working in isolation, i.e, their activities are not co-ordinated properly resulting into lower output of services. According to Antonia Ordonex-Plaja":

> "Team work requires, among other things, that the members have an image of their team-mates, which coincides as precisely as possible with reality. In addition, each member must have a self-image which adjusts to reality as much as possible and thus coincides with the image the other membrs have of him."[25]

The team work would develop common practices and shared practices. This would also raise the morale of the personnel working at the grass-root level.

Another important area is of Organisational Communication which can bind and keep united all the Family Planning workers. Effective communication in the Family Planning organisation is very important because:

(i) Unless employees know the organisational objectives, they cannot associate them with their own;

(ii) It is essential to the management of change in the organisation. Without facts, understanding, and acceptance, efforts to change are doomed to failure, without well directed communication, there is not a chance; and

(iii) Without a communication, sharing of ideas with others will take place.

Let us now mention some other problems:

1. No reliable criteria for evaluation of the impact of family planning programme.

2. Inadequate Management Information System to Monitor Family Planning Programmes to ensure effective policy-making, implementation and evaluation.
3. Lack of dedicated and committed leadership.
4. Inadequacy of personnel planning and development.
5. Lack of effective public responsibility and accountability.
6. Lack of adequate administrative machinery for implementation.
7. Increasing women's status through women empowerment.

CONCLUSION

Joung Wahang has identified some potential areas where administrative reforms and improvements can help in increasing operational efficiency, i.e.,

(a) To get F.P. methods (including instruments and services) identified and defined;
(b) To get sufficient amount and reliable quality of F.P. instruments and services available to the clients;
(c) To get F.P. instruments and services available to clients in the most appropriate places;
(d) To get F.P. instruments and services available to clients at the most reasonable prices and costs; and
(e) To get F.P. instruments and services available without any psychological embarrassment and disturbance to the privacy of clients.

We should not be pessimistic. We should hope that the present momentum built-up since the Sixth Plan would continue. We should not hesitate to bring about innovative changes to make the programme realistic. We cannot afford to allow the programme to go slow as the programme is a source of strength to all other schemes of socio-economic development, whatever may be their immediate goal. Prime Minister Indira Gandhi, has rightly said on September 30, 1983, at New York, while receiving the United Nations Population Award.

The enabling objectives during the Ninth Plan period, therefore, will be to reduce the population growth rate by:

(a) meeting all the felt-needs for contraception, and
(b) reducing the infant and maternal morbidity and mortality so that there is a reduction in the desired level of fertility.

The strategies during the Ninth Plan will be:

(a) To assess the needs for reproductive and child health at PHC level and undertake area specific micro-planning, and

(b) To provide need-based, demand-driven high quality, integrated reproductive and child health care.

The programmes will be directed towards:

(a) Bridging the gaps in essential infrastructure and manpower through a flexible approach and improving operational efficiency through investment in social, behaviour and operational research.
(b) Providing additional assitance to poorly performing districts identified on the basis of the 1991 census to fill existing gaps in infrastructure and manpower.
(c) Ensuring uninterrrupted supply of essential drugs, vaccines and contraceptives, adequate in quantity and appropriate in quality.
(d) Promoting male participation in the Planned Parenthood movement and increasing the level of acceptance of vasectomy.

Efforts will be intensified to enhance the quality and coverage of family welfare services through:

(a) Increasing participation of general medical practitioners working in voluntary, private, joint sectors and the active cooperation of practitioners of ISM and H.
(b) Involvement of the Panchayat Raj Institutions for ensuring inter-sectoral coordination and community participation in planning, monitoring and management.
(c) Involvement of the industries, organised and unorganised sectors, agriculture workers and labour representatives.

It is said that prosperity is a good contraceptive. But the effects of development are submerged unless we bring about a low birth rate. Family Planning is an input for development, an indispensable exercise in human capital formation. Education, better capacity for producing and earning a higher rise in per capita income are possible only when population growth is curbed.

Government of India has enunciated the new Population Policy in February, 2000. Commenting on the New Population Policy *Business Standard* Editorial, "Sense on Popuplation" dated February 17, 2000, remarked, The new national population policy, 2000, however may have a greater chance of acceptances it incorporates some of the lessons learnt from recent successes in curbing population growth. While the earlier attempts merely emphasised physical targets and ignored the vital aspects of health and education, especially that of the girl child, which are vitally linked to birth rates, the latest policy seeks to squarely address these issues. Besides, it also makes the right kind of noises about investment in social infrastructure as an essential prerequisite for promoting small family norms.

Success of the new policy will depend largely on the way it is implemented by the laggard states and the pace of socio-economic development (including in the field of health and education) that accompanies it. Measures like freezing the number of seats in the Lok Sabha at the current level are essentially facilitators, dispelling states' fears that population control will reduce their quota of MPs. There has to be an adequate political will to achieve the twin, vertiably inseparable, objectives of reducing family size and improving the quality of life.

However, *The Tribune* Editorial "Gaps in Population Policy" dated February 17, 2000, suggested the gaps in new policy and stressed the need to make up these gaps. Increasing population packs a greater destructive power than what Pakistan can cause by hurling a few nuclear bomblasts. That is because it is concentrated at the bottom of the social and economic pyramid covering three-fourth of the population. The failure to control the exploding numbers is the most damaging of all failures. What the country needed was a radical review of the old policies, alertness to deploy all available instruments and establish enduring contacts with the target segment in rural India. Sadly these are missing in the New National Population Policy unveiled. The document still pins its hopes on a few tired incentives and shapeless promises to rein in population growth. Such sops will be available only after the event — that is, after individuals or couples take themselves out of the reproduction cycle. Actually, the concentration should have been on goading people to enter the charmed circle.

To quote S.P. Singh again, According to the provisional results of the 2001 Census, India's population stood 1,027 million on March 1, 2001, comprising 531 million males and 496 million females. From 361 million at the time of Independence the population reached one billion in 2001, registering an increase of nearly three times. All this had happened when the country is not in a position to guarantee adequate nutrition, health-care and education to the burgeoning population. At the same time, it is also true that all this has happened because of mass poverty in the country. Indifferent governance is also partly responsible for the current demographic and health scenario. Every year about 18 million people were added to India's population during 1991-2001 as against 16 million annually during 1981-91 (see Table 5.1). In other words, each year India's population increases by the equivalents of the number of inhabitants of Ghana, Australia, Mozambique or Saudi Arabia.

Notes and References

1. UN: E.F.S. 75, XIII. 4, p. 76.
2. Gunnar Myrdal, "Asian Drama: An Inquiry Into the Poverty of Nations", Vol. III, London, 1968, p. 154.
3. Alexander Kessler, "Family Planning and the role of WHO" in *World Health*, May-June 1994, p. 30.
4. Maryellen Fullan, "People—A Journal of the International Planned Parenthood Federation", Vol. 5, Number 4, 1978, p. 27.
5. Ansley, J. Coale, "Population and Economic Development", in Phillip M. Hauser (ed.), The Population Dilemma, p. 69.
6. WHO, (1971) Technical Report Series, No. 483.
7. WHO, (1971), Technical Report Series, No. 473.
8. WHO, Technical Report Series No. 442.
9. The *Daily Tribune*, January 28, 2000.
10. K.P. Bahadur, Population Crisis in India, National, New Delhi, 1977, p. 37.
11. Joung, Whaff, Ph.D., Graduate School of Public Admn., Seoul, National University, Seoul, Korea, Seventh General Assembly and Conference on "Implementation — The Problem of Achieving Results", EROPA, 24-31, October, 1973, Tokyo, Japan, pp. 69-106.
12. U.N., F/F/S. 75, XIII, 5, p. 383.
13. Mrs. Hevli Sipila, Assistant Secretary General, "Social Development and Humanities Affairs", UN, June 17, 1975, *Weekly News Letter*, UN Information Centre, New Delhi, Vol. 25, No. 3.
14. UN, 1326, (XLIV).
15. UN, F/C/N/6/5755, Add 13, ECOSOC.
16. Council for Social Development, New Delhi, 1969.
17. UN, Public Administration Division of the Department of Economics and Social Affiars, "Organisation and Administration of Family Planning Programme", UN: F/E/75, XIII, 5, p. 494.
18. UNESCO, Communication Media, Family Planning and Development, No. 1, Paris, 1975.
19. UNESCO, Communication in Support of Population, Family Planning and Development, E/F/S.75, XIII, 5, p. 482.
20. State Family Planning Bureau, Haryana: National Population Conference (6th to 8th December, 1974), Population Statement of Haryana State.
21. S.S. Kamalai, and C. Parvathemma, "Family Planning and Social Values", *Family Planning News*, March 1970, Vol. XI, No. 3.
22. Fourth Five Year Plan, Mid-Term Appraisal, pp. 223-24.
23. Council for Social Development, Aspects of Population Policy in India, New Delhi, 1969, p. 56.
24. Lok Sabha Secretariate Estimates Committee, 102nd Report (5th Lok Sabha), New Delhi, 1975, pp. 92-94.
25. Antonio Ordonex-Plaja, Teamwork at Ministry level, in Teamwork for *World Health* (ed.), *op. cit.*, p. 170.

CHAPTER 6

REPRODUCTIVE AND CHILD HEALTH PROGRAMME

> It is the flagship programme of family welfare which combines the trinity of objectives, viz. reproductive health, child survival and fertility regulations with a policy and programme orientation markedly different from previous programmes.
>
> —India 2004

Reproductive and Child Health Programme

I. GENESIS

The Universal Immunisation Programme (UIP) aimed at reduction in mortality and morbidity among infants and younger children due to Vaccine Preventable Diseases, was started in 1985-86. The Oral Dehydration Therapy (ORT) was also started in view of the fact that diarrhoea was a leading cause of deaths among children. Various other programmes under Maternal and Child Health (MCH) were also implemented during the Seventh Plan. The objectives of all these programmes were convergent and aimed at improving the health of the mothers and young children and to provide them facilities for prevention and treatment of major disease conditions. While these programmes did have a beneficial impact, but the separate identity for each programme was causing problems in its effective management and this was also reducing somewhat the outcomes. Therefore, in the Eighth Plan, these programmes were integrated under Child Survival and Safe Motherhood (CSSM) Programme which was implemented from 1992-93.

The process of integration of related programmes initiated with the implementation of the CSSM Programme was taken a step further in 1994, when the International Conference on Population and Development in Cairo recommended that the participant countries should implement unified programmes for Reproductive and Child Health (RCH). The RCH approach has been defined as "People have the ability to reproduce and regulate their fertility, women are able to go through pregnancy and child birth safely, the outcome of pregnancies is successful in terms of maternal and infant survival and well-being and couples are able to have sexual relations free of fear of pregnancy and of contacting diseases."

This concept is in keeping with the evolution of an integrated approach to the programmes aimed at improving the health status of young women and children, which has been going on in the country. It is obviously sensible that the integrated RCH Programme would help in reducing the cost of inputs to some extent because overlapping of expenditure would no longer be necessary and integrated implementation would optimise outcomes at the field level. During the Ninth Plan, the RCH Programme, accordingly, has integrated all the related programmes of the Eighth Plan. The concept of RCH is to provide to the beneficiaries need-based, client-centred, demand driven, high quality and integrated RCH services. The RCH Programme is a composite programme incorporating the inputs of the Government of India as well as funding support from external donor agencies including the World Bank and the European Commission.

The RCH programme incorporates the components covered under the Child Survival and Safe Motherhood Programme and includes two additional components, one relating to sexually transmitted diseases (STD) and the other relating to reproductive tract infection (RTI). The main highlights of the RCH Programme are:

(i) The Programme integrates all interventions of fertility regulation, maternal and child health with reproductive health of both men and women.

(ii) The services to be provided will be client-centred, demand-driven, high quality and based on the needs of the community arrived at, through decentralised participatory planning and a target free approach.

(iii) The programme envisages upgradation of the level of facilities for providing various interventions and quality of care. The First Referral Units (FRUs) being set-up at sub-district level will provide comprehensive emergency obstetric and new born care. Similarly, RCH facilities in PHCs will be substantially upgraded.

(iv) The Programme will improve access of the community to various services which are commonly required. It is proposed to provide facilities for MTP at the PHCs, counselling and IUD insertion at SCs in a phased manner.

(v) The Programme aims at improving the outreach of services, particularly for the vulnerable groups of population who have till now substantially been let out of the planning process:

- Special programmes will be taken up for urban slums, tribal population and adolescents.
- Non-Governmental Organisations will be involved in a much larger way to improve out-reach and make it people's programme.
- Skills of practitioners of ISM will be upgraded by training

and research and development in ISM will be supported to improve the range of the RCH services.
- Panchayati Raj system will have a greater role in planning, implementation and assessment of client satisfaction.[1]

Ninth Five Year Plan (Draft) has mentioned the following features of RCH Programme:

- Effective maternal and child health care,
- Increased access to contraceptive care,
- Safe management of unwanted preganancies,
- Nutritional services to vulnerable groups,
- Prevention and treatment of RTI/STD,
- Reproductive health services for adolescents,
- Prevention and treatment of gynaecological problems, and
- Screening and treatment of cancers, especially that of uterine cervix and breast.

For over 30 years Family Welfare Programme was known for its rigid, target-based approach in contraceptives. The performance was measured by the reported numbers of the four contraceptive methods—Sterilisation, Intrauterine device, Oral pills and Condoms. This was widely criticised for being a coercive approach.

The 1994 Cairo International Conference on Population and Development (ICPD) formulated a growing International consensus that improving reproductive health and family planning is essential to human welfare and development.

A growing body of evidence and the Cairo consensus suggest "Numerical method specific contraceptive target and monetary incentives" for providers to be replaced by a broader system of "programme performance goals" and measures focussed on a range of reproductive health services.

We can say in brief that reproductive and Child Health Services which is equivalent to:

- Family Planning, to focus on fertility regulation,
- Child Survival and Safe Motherhood Programme, and
- Treatment of Reproductive Tract Infections and Sexually Transmitted Infections and prevention of AIDS,

Through

1. Client-Oriented/Mother-Friendly/user-specific, family welfare services, and
2. High quality services.

The specific programmes under Reproductive and Child Health Services are:

1. Prevention and management of unwanted pregnancies,
2. Maternal care:
   (a) Ante-natal services,
   (b) Natal services,
   (c) Post-natal services,
3. Child Survival, and
4. Treatment of Reproductive Tract Infections (RTI) and Sexually Transmitted Infections (STI).[2]

The following definition of reproductive health was approved in April 1994, by the WHO Global Policy Council, provides the basis for action in this field:

> "Reproductive health implies that people are able to have a responsible, satisfying and safe sex life and that they have the capability to reproduce and the freedom to decide if, when and how often to do so. Implicit in this last condition are the right of men and women to be informed of and to have access to safe, effective, affordable and acceptable methods of fertility regulation of their choice, and the right of access to appropriate health care services that will enable women to go safely through pregnancy and childbirth and provide couples with the best chance of having a healthy infant."

Reproductive health must address, as its basic elements, sexual behaviour, family planning, maternal care and safe motherhood, abortion, reproductive tract infections (including sexually transmitted diseases and HIV/AIDS, and certain reproductive tract malignancies such as cervical cancer.[3]

II. THE PACKAGE OF REPRODUCTIVE AND CHILD HEALTH SERVICES

The different services provided under RCH programme are:

I. For the Mothers

- TT Immunization,
- Prevention and treatment of anaemia,
- Ante-natal care and early-identification of maternal complications,
- Deliveries by trained personnel,
- Promotion of institutional deliveries,
- Management of Obstetric emergencies, and
- Birth spacing.

II. For the Children

- Essential newborn care,
- Exclusive breast feeding and weaning,
- Immunization,
- Appropriate management of diarrhoea,
- Appropriate management of ARI,
- Vitamin A prophylaxis, and
- Treatment of Anaemia.

III. For Eligible Couples

- Prevention of pregnancy, and
- Safe abortion.

IV. RTI/STD

- Prevention and treatment of reproductive tract and sexually transmitted diseases.[4]

Principles and Approach

The guiding principles and approach of reproductive health care are to a great extent different than those of the existing dominant approach of MCH and FP programme.[5] A glimpse of the shift in approach and principle can be studied from the Table 6.1.

The guiding principles of reproductive health care are those of human rights, ethics, equity, quality of care, universal access, participation, partnership, integration, optimal use of resources and sustainability. Partnerships and sharing of responsibilities between government, governmental organizations and the private sector are important in stimulating new ideas and approaches and ensuring service coverage and quality of care. These principles are the same as the principles of primary health care.

We must keep in mind that reproductive health is a crucial part of general health and is central to human development. It affects everybody; it involves intimate and highly valued aspects of life. Not only is it a reflection of health in infancy, childhood and adolescence, it also sets the stage for health beyond the reproductive years, for both men and women, and has effects from one generation to another. Reproductive health includes sexual health care, for maintaining and enhancing the functions of the reproductive system, and the prevention and management of RTIs, HIV/AIDS and infertility. Reproductive health care is an integral part of primary health care. The guiding principles and the approaches of reproductive health care are similar to the delivery of primary health care. These are:

TABLE 6.1

Principles and Approach of Existing MCH/FP Programme and of RHC Programme

Existing MCH/FP Programmes	*Reproductive Health Programmes*
Target population is primarily women	Target population is both women and men
Vertical programmes	Integrated and inter-sectoral programmes
Top-down planning and implementation	Bottom-up planning respoding to local reprodutive health needs within socio-cultural and economic milieu and decentralised implementation
Focus on individual cases	Public health approach with familiy and community focus
Pregnancy-based approach	Life cycle approach
Medical approach: health needs identified by providers; reliance on medical solutions	Community-based approach: respect women's knowledge and definition of their health needs; reliance on holistic solutions that take into account the social, biological and psychological factors determining health
Provider centred: prescribe fertility control methods	Client centred: provide inforamtion and enable women to choose the methods they wish to adopt
Method specific information provided	Apart from information on all methods of fertility regulation, provide knowledge on sexuality and reproduction
Emphasis on achieving output targets	Emphasis on coverage and quality of services
Services provided in a clinical atmosphere	Provide services in a humane and caring setting
Vague general health rights	Respect specific reproductive health rights

Source: WHO: SEARO, Managing Essential Reproductive Health Care, New Delhi, p. 5.

- education concerning prevailing health problems and the methods of preventing and controlling them;
- promotion of food supply and proper nutrition;
- an adequate supply of safe water and basic sanitation;
- maternal and child health care, including family planning;
- immunisation against the major infectious diseases;
- appropriate treatment of common diseases and injuries; and
- provision of essential drugs.

Let us new mention the health interventions required for different services at different levels. (See Table 6.2).

Advantages of the Scheme

RCH can avoid the problems prevalent in earlier family planning programme and can improve the coverage and quality of services provided the RCH programme is implemented as scheduled.

1. Target-free Approach can make the Programme Flexible

The achievements of family planning programmes were judged simply on the completion of targets fixed from above. It was found that the top down approach is not realistic and based on field situations. Thus, the users preference is not reflected in the targets. A major feature of the target-free approach in its emphasis on the promotion of modern spacing methods. The approach intends also to achieve a greater participation of males in the family welfare programme. Moreover, in the absence of method-specific targets, the grass-root level workers including the ANM and the Multi-purpose Health Workers (both male and female) are expected to work closely with the community and arrive at an estimate of the various family welfare activities required in the area/ population covered by them. The male health workers, in particular, are made responsible for motivation for vasectomy and condoms. These activities are expected to result in an improvement in the knowledge of modern temporary methods as well as male methods of contraception; and an improvement in the proportion of spacing as well as male methods in the contraceptive method-mix.

2. Target-free Approach can make the Reporting Honest and Reliable

Field Staff used to do false reporting in order to prove the progress to avoid disciplinary action. This approach has made the reporting realistic and thus can help in effective policy-making and planning.

Earlier, we had malpractices of performing sterilisation/ vasecotomy upon ineligible persons. All such cases and practices would be avoided.

3. New Programme can Infect Forward and Backward Linkages

The RCH programme can promote linkages to make it effective forwards positive health. Since it is not merely a family planning programme, it is a total package covering the total health of women and children, a very positive view.

4. Over-head Cost can be Reduced

Costs incurred in managing programmes in an integrated way can reduce a lot of cost as overhead cost can be reduced.

TABLE 6.2

Essential Reproductive and Child Health Services at Different Levels of the Health Services System

Health Intervention	*Community Level*	*Sub-centre Level*	*Primary Health Centre Level*	*First Referral Unit/ District Hospital Level*
1. Prevention and management of unwanted pregnancy	1. Sexuality and gender information education and counselling 2. Community mobilization and education for adolescents, newly married youth, men and women* 3. Community-based contraceptive distribution** (through panchayats, Village Health Guides, Mahila Swasthya Sanghas, etc. with follow-up) 4. Motivating referral for sterilization 5. Social marketing of condoms and oral pills through community sources and G.P. (Oral pills to be distributed through health personnel including GPS to women who are starting pills for the first time) 6. Free supplies to health services * to be piloted ** Panchayats to distribute only condoms	No. 1. as in community level 2. Providing* oral contraceptives (OCS) and condoms 3. Providing IUD after screening for contraindications 4. Counselling and early referral for medical termiantion of pregnancy 5. Counselling/ management/ referral for side effects, method-related problems, change of method where indicated 6. Add other methods to expand choice 7. Providing treatment for minor ailments and referral for problems * Social marketing of pills and condoms through HW (M & F) may be explored by permitting her to retain the money.	Nos. 1-6 and 7. Performing tubal ligation by minilap on fixed dates* 8. Performing vasectomy 9. Providing first trimester medical termination of pregnancy upto 8 weeks (includes MR) 10. Facilities for Copper 'T' insertion to post-natal cases 11. Treatment facilities for all types of referrals * PHCs should have facilities for tubal ligation and mini-lap including OTs and equip-ments	Nos. 1-11 and 12. Providing services for medical termination of pregnancy in the first and second trimester (upto 20 weeks) where indicated

TABLE 6.2 *(Contd.)*

Health Intervention	*Community Level*	*Sub-centre Level*	*Primary Health Centre Level*	*First Referral Unit/ District Hospital Level*
2. Maternity Care Prenatal Services	1. Early registration of all pregnant women 2. Awareness raising for importance of appropriate care during pregnancy and identification of danger signs 3. To mobilise community support for transport, referral and blood donation 4. Counselling education for breast feeding nutrition, family planning, rest, exercise and personal hygiene, etc. 5. Early detection and referral of high risk pregnancies 6. Observing five cleans or through social marketing of disposal delivery kits. Delivery planning as to where? when and from whom?	No. 1-4 and 5. Three antenatal contacts with women either at the sub-centre or at the outreach village sites during immunisation/ MCH sessions 6. Early detection of high risk factors and maternal complications and prompt referral 7. Referral of high risk women for institutional delivery 8. Treatment of malaria (facilities including drugs to be made available at sub-centres) 9. Treatment for TB and follow-up 10. Preventive measure against all communicable disease	Nos. 1-10 and 11. Treatment of TB 12. Testing of syphilis for high risk group and treatment where necessary including for RTI's	Nos. 1-12 and 13. Diagnosis and treatment of RTIs/STIs 14. Weekly clinics for High risk pregnancies
	* The need of IC support and establishment of first referral facilities.		* training of laboratory technicians, equipment and reagents required.	

TABLE 6.2 *(Contd.)*

Health Intervention	*Community Level*	*Sub-centre Level*	*Primary Health Centre Level*	*First Referral Unit/ District Hospital Level*
3. Delivery Services	1. Early recognition of pregnancy and its danger signals (rupture of membranes of more than 12 hours duration, prolapse of the cord, hemorrhage) 2. Conducting clean deliveries with delivery kits by trained personnel 3. Detection of complications referral for hospital delivery 4. Providing transport for referral 5. Referral of new born having difficulty in respiration 6. Management of Neonatal hypothermia	No. 1-4 and 5. Supervising home delivery 6. Prophylaxis and treatment for infection (except sepsis) 7. Routine prophylaxis for gonococi eye infection	Nos. 1-7 and 8. Modified partograph 9. Delivery services 10. Repair of episiotomy and perennial tears	Nos. 1-9 and 10. Treatment of severe sepsis 11. Delivery of referred cases 12. Treatment of high risk cases 13. Services for obstetrical emergencies anesthesia, cesarean section, blood transfusion through close relatives linkages with blood banks and mobile services
4. Post-partum Services	1. Breast-feeding support 2. Family Planning counselling 3. Nutrition counselling 4. Resuscitation for asphyxia of the newborn 5. Management of neonatal hypothermia 6. Early recognition of post-partum sepsis and referral	Nos. 1-6 and 7. Referral for complications 8. Giving inj. Ergometrine after delivery of placenta	Nos. 1-8 and 9. Referral of FRUs for complications after starting an I.V. line and giving initial dose of antibiotics and oxytocin when indicated 10. Management of asphyxiated new born (equipment to be provided)	Nos. 1-10 and 11. Management of referred cases PHCs and FRUs would require additional equipment and training for management of asphyxiated new borns and hypothermia. These include a resuscitation bag and mask and radiant warmers
5. Child Survival	1. Health education for breast feeding nutrition immunization, utilisation of services, etc.	Nos. 1-6 and 7. Treatment of dehydration and pneumonia and referral of severe cases	Nos. 1-9 and 10. Management of referred cases	Nos. 1-10 and 11. Handling of all paediatric cases including encephalopathy

TABLE 6.2 *(Contd.)*

Health Intervention	*Community Level*	*Sub-centre Level*	*Primary Health Centre Level*	*First Referral Unit/ District Hospital Level*
	2. Detection and referral of high risk cases such as low birth weight, premature babies, babies with asphyxis, infections, severe dehydration acute respiratory infections (ARI), etc. 3. Help during Immunization by ANM 4. Help during Vitamin 'A' supplementation by ANM 5. Detection of pneumonia and seeking early medical care by community and treatment by ANM 6. Treatment of diarrhoea cases and ARI cases	8. First aid for injuries, etc. 9. Closing watching on the development of child and creating awarness of cheap and nutritious food		12. Identification of certain FRU's to provide specialist services and training
6. Management of RTIs/STIs	1. IEC, counselling and awareness and prevention 2. Condom distribution 3. Creating awareness about usage of sanitary pads by women of reproductive period 4. Creating awareness of about RTI's and personal hygiene	Nos. 1-4 and 5. Identification and referral for vaginal discharge, lower abdominal pain, genital ulcers in women, and urethra discharge, genital ulcers, swelling in scrotum or groin in men 6. Diagnosis of RTI's and STI's by Syndrome approach 7. Referral of cases not responding to suavely treatment 8. Partner notification/ referral	Nos. 1-8 and 9. Treatment of RTIs/STIs 10. Syphilis testing in ante-natal women	Nos. 1-9 and 10. Laboratory diagnosis and treatment of RTIs/STIs 11. Syndromic approach to detect and treat STD in ante-natal, post-natal and at risk groups

Source: Department of Family Welfare, GOI, Reproductive and Child Health, Vol. I, March 1997, pp. 42-45.

5. *Effective Maternal and Child Health*

At the village level, the Auxiliary Nurse Midwife is responsible for rendering maternal and child health services alongwith family welfare services. She is supposed to register pregnant women as assess their health throughout pregnancy, by at least three visits. Regular height and weight checkup, blood pressure test, urine test as well as providing tetanus toxoid injections and iron and folic acid tablets constitute important aspects of any antenatal checkup. Another responsibility of the ANM is to refer pregnant women who have symptoms of abnormal pregnancy or labour, or who have gynaecological problems that are beyond her level of competence, to the Primary Health Centre.

At the instance of the Ministry of Health and Family Welfare, Government of India, New Delhi and as a part of monitoring and evaluation of the performance of the family welfare programme under the new target-free approach, the Population Research Centre, J.S.S. Institute of Economic Research, Dharwad, undertook a rapid survey in the rural areas of Belgaum District, Karnataka state during the last two weeks of December 1997 and first two weeks of January 1998. Using a simple and short questionnaire, the survey interviewed a total of 1,000 currently married women age 15-44, from 50 villages, at the rate of 20 women per village. Apart from several background characteristics of women, the survey collected information on utilization of ante-natal care, place of delivery, and assistance during delivery, child immunizations, knowledge and practice of family planning, visits by the ANM and services received from her; health problems of the women including side-effects of family planning methods, and respondents ratings on various aspects of quality of care provided by the nearest PHC, sub-centre or the ANM.

(a) While the provision of tetanus toxoid injections and iron/folic tablets is better, other components of ante-natal care such as monitoring the weight and blood pressure, and urine tests were not carried out for the majority of women during their pregnancy by multi-member females.

(b) Overall, 51 percent of the deliveries which occurred during the five years preceding the survey took place at home, 30 percent in private hospitals or nursing homes, and little less than one-fifth in government health facilities. Of the births that took place at home, the majority (62 percent) were attended by untrained persons including relatives, friends and neighbours.

(c) Little less than one-quarter of women in the rural areas of Belgaum District have an unmet need for family planning, that is, they are not using contraception even though they do not want any more children or want to wait at least two years before having their next child. The unmet need for spacing (11 percent) is almost the same as that for limiting births (12 percent). If all the women with an unmet need were to use family planning, the contraceptive prevalence rate would increase from 62 percent to 85 percent.

(d) Among the three registers (Eligible Couple register, ANC register, and immunization register) examined, the EB register was found to be relatively more complete and accurate than the other two registers.[6]

In another study a rapid research survey was conducted in rural areas of Dharwad district in Karnataka during February-April, 1997 to check the coverage, quality of services and client satisfaction under the new strategy of 'target-free' approach. The analysis of service statistics for the district showed that removal of targets appears to have made no significant impact on the total number of annual acceptors. However, it had a favourable impact on method mix as sterilizations have come down slightly while acceptors of IUD and Pill have gone up from that of the previous year.

The unmet need for contraception was estimated to be 10 percent, 6 percent for limiting and 4 percent for spacing.

It was found that immunization levels are yet to become universal. About 70 percent of pregnant women had two doses of Tetanus toxoid vaccination and only half of the children were fully immunized.

Measurement of weight and blood pressure, as well as urine tests were reported rarely. Only 40 percent of deliveries were attended by trained persons. On record maintenance, it was observed that EC register was better maintained than ANC and immunization registers. Some of the important policy recommendations emerging from the study are:

1. Improve ANM services, especially make them visit women with unmet need for contraception, and past acceptors of sterilization.
2. As a large number of sterilization acceptors complain about method side effects, a special health campaign for sterilized men and women should be launched by multi-purpose workers female. In order to safeguard future levels of acceptance, past acceptors should be made to feel that they are looked after well by programme functionaries.
3. It should be ensured that sub-centres have adequate supply of drugs, and attempts should be made to reduce waiting time and provide free services at primary health centres. The guilty should be punished.
4. A television set could be placed in PHC waiting room and also a VCP to disseminate information and messages on health and family welfare and facilities in sub-centres.

5. Concerted attempts should be made to raise immunization levels by workers as they appear to have reached a point of stagnation before acquiring universality.[7]

National Institute of Health and Family Welfare (Role in RCH)

History and Need

The National Institute of Health and Family Welfare came into being with effect from 9 March, 1977, by the amalgamation of the erstwhile institutes, namely, the National Institute of Family Planning and the National Institute of Health Administration and Education. It has been established as an autonomous body (registered under the Societies Registration Act, 1860) and its object is to act as an apex technical institute for promoting the Health and Family Welfare Planning Programme in the country through education, training, services, research and evaluation. The overall objective of the Institute has been to play a leading role in orienting training and research in health administration and education to the newer concepts of administration and education and thereby strengthen and accelerate India's health and family welfare programmes.

Organisation

The Institute is governed by a General Executive Council with the Union Minister for Health and Family Welfare as the President/ Chairman. The day-to-day activities are administered by the Director. The Institute is supported in its activities by International Agencies such as WHO/SEARO and UNICEF. Closer contacts and collaboration exist between the Institute and numerous other organisations in the country. The finances for the functioning of the Institute are provided by the Government of India through grants-in-aid.

Structure

As health administration is based on the concept of 'multi-disciplinary' approach, the Institute has departments embracing various disciplines. These are the departments of Public Health Administration, Hospital Administration, Family Welfare, Maternal and Child Health Programme Planning, Evaluation, Social Sciences, Epidemiology, Health Education, Public Administration, Biostatistics, Education and Training, Field Training, Public Health Nursing and Field Services. A field practice area in the Rohtak district of Haryana State exists for experimentation and field training exercises of the participants of the institute. Research in the field of Health Administration is reckoned to be a key factor for the development of the activities of the Institute and is therefore, an integral part of the functioning of all departments of the Institute. The new Institute has been renamed as the National Institute of Health and Family Welfare.

Activities

The main activities of the Institute are:

(a) Education and Training.
(b) Research.
(c) Evaluation of Health Programmes.
(d) Consultation Services.
(e) Clearing House Functions.
(f) Publications and Documents.

Objectives in the Context of RCH

(i) To organise, co-ordinate and monitor training in the country.
(ii) To upgrade the competence of family welfare personnel and managers to provide technically sound client centred and gender sensitive RCH services.
(iii) To create mass awareness of RCH and population stabilization issues by holding orientation training programme.
(iv) To involve other government departments in promotion of RCH programme by team training for convergence of services.

III. SPECIFIC OBJECTIVES

(a) *To coordinate*: (i) training financed by the Family Welfare Department in RCH management, clinical and interpersonal counselling skills and communications (IEC), and (ii) awareness generation and community mobilization (including convergence of related programmes such as ICDS) as requested by MOHFW.
(b) To coordinate the development and or adaptation, as necessary, of model training curricula, facilitators, guides, and prototype manuals/materials, and provide such materials to collaborating centres and training centres for local adaptation and use.
(c) To assist MOHFW in the development of clinical management protocols for safe motherhood, fertility regulation methods, reproductive tract infections and sexually transmitted diseases and child survival as specified in the essential package of RCH services and ensure that such protocols are integrated into training.
(d) To assist MOHFW and national procurement support agency for appointment of suitable collaborating institutions from Government, NGO and private/corporate sector in accordance with World Bank Guidelines and to organise training of trainers of these institutions.
(e) To review the work of the collaborative institutions annually

and to assist the MOHFW in determining suitability of the institution to continue as a collaborating institution.

(f) To assist states, districts through collaborating institutions, in formulation of integrated training plans at State and District levels so as to: (i) avoid unnecessary duplication; (ii) ensure here are no critical gaps in the training plans; and (iii) coordinate scheduling of training with other programme inputs such as equipment, civil works, IEC and NGO activities.

(g) To assist States in the establishment of system of proficiency certificate award to trainees and monitor and report on state specific achievements on the project performance.

The RCH programme should take care of following factors before formulation, implementation and evaluation strategy:

(a) according to the topography of the District,
(b) according to the priority needs of the people,
(c) linked properly with the objectives and goals of District planning,
(d) fitted into the overall economic and social development of the country,
(e) properly linked with projects in the allied area, and
(f) able to achieve useful and permanent results.

Let us now analysis the factors which impede the effective functioning of RCH programme. It is based on authors' study in Punjab and Karnataka. We have also given suggestions to improve RCH programme.

Let us mention the schedule of operation of RCH programme in Punjab and Karnataka (See Tables 6.3 and 6.4). We may also mention the facilities required in A, B and C categories of Districts. The project has not so far been implemented fully. However, we discuss our observations and findings on the basis of the experiments done so far.

Though it is desirable that the entire package of services indicated above is made available to all those who need it, it will not be possible to immediately implement such a comprehensive package on a nation-wide basis. Hence, it is envisaged that improvement in quality and coverage of services over and above the existing level will be attempted in all states in an incremental manner so that maternal and child health indices improve.

After consultation with experts a package of essential reproductive health services for nation-wide implementation at various levels of health care has been identified. Essential components recommended for nation-wide implementation include:

TABLE 6.3

Punjab—Year-wise Category of Districts

Category	*Year-I*	*Year-II*	*Year-III*
A			
B	Hoshiarpur	Jalandhar	Faridkot
	Patiala	Ludhiana	Rupnagar
	Moga	Kapurthala	Bathinda
		Gurdaspur	Muktsar
		Amritsar	Nawanshahar
		Sangrur	
C	Firozepur	Mansa	
	Fatehgarh Sahib		

TABLE 6.4

Karnataka—Year-wise Category of Districts

Category	*Year-I*	*Year-II*	*Year-III*
A	Dakshin Kannada Kadagu (Coorg)		
	Mandya		
B	Uttar Kannada	Hassan	Shimoga
	Chikmaglur	Bangalore (R)	Chitradurga
	Dharwad	Tumkur	
		Mysore	
		Belgaum	
C	Bijapur	Bellary	
	Bidar	Raichur	
	Gulbarga		
	Bangalore		

- Prevention and management of unwanted pregnancy.
- Services to promote safe motherhood.
- Services to promote child survival.
- Prevention and treatment of RTI/STD.

Most of the services are already included in the Family Welfare Programme. However, there are wide variations in the quality and coverage of services not only between states but also between various districts in the same state. The focus is therefore on the improvement in the quality and coverage of the services. A project preparation workshop held in September 1995 discussed the issues and problems in implementation of essential RCH package and recommended reproductive and child health services that should be made available at community, sub-centre, PHC and FRU/District Hospital.

Implementation schedule of Punjab and Karnataka is given in

Tables 6.3 and 6.4.

The Ministry of Health and Family Welfare has got the research conducted on the impact of RCH programme in the districts. Analysis of the reports indicate that:

(a) Infrastructure facilities non-existent.
(b) Personnel responsible for RCH lack motivation.
(c) Lack of effective supervision.
(d) Slackness in work.
(e) Non-availability of funds.
(f) Lack of team work.
(g) Not following the work as schedules.

The study in Punjab in some districts revealed not impact of the new RCH programme. The personnel responsible lack motivation and interest. Because of financial crisis, normal functioning of the health department is at a stand still. Besides, there is no supervision, resulting into a absentism and irregulately.

1. Lack of Adequate Facilities in the Institutions Responsible for the Provision of RCH Services

After the project is formulated, the project manager must ensure the availability of necessary inputs. It has been generally observed that the projects are delayed because of the absence of timely availability of all the inputs simultaneously. In one of the projects, the health personnel had no work to do because of the non-availability of vaccine. Obtaining resources is a process that takes place periodically throughout the life of the project. It was revealed that failure to obtain resources simultaneously in time is the most common cause of delay in implementation. The project manager must begin the process of procuring resources immediately after the formulation stage. Sometimes, the process may be started quite early if the resources are scarce and not easily available. The absence of one resource would inflate the cost of the project as the other resources would remain idle. The project manager must take the following steps:

(a) Working with the relative administrative units in preparing a time-table of administrative steps to be taken to obtain the planned resources.
(b) Monitoring this time-table to ensure that the administrative steps are being completed in time.
(c) Taking corrective action as and when necessary.

Inspite of all these precautions, there is a possibility of not reaching the resources in time. What can be done under such critical situation? Most of the experts indicated that the whole project staff remains idle for months together. This is very serious in big projects. It is suggested that project officers may be delegated powers to purchase the inputs locally or employ persons, if not available from the agency as planned. This would ensure that the project is one schedule.

2. Lack of Clarity among the Person Responsible for Implementation of RCH Programme

There is a dichotomy between the personnel responsible for the formulation and the personnel responsible for the implementation of the RCH project. The latter are not clear about the implications of the project. Because of lack of identity, they develop low morale resulting into the poor management. It was mentioned by a number of persons working on some projects that, "they are thrown into the fields to operate the RCH project without proper briefing about the project and its rationale in the total system. Besides, the supervisors, at the head-quarters, never guide them about their role in the projects."

3. Poor Linkages Among the Allied Projects

In a particular geographical or functional area, a number of projects are being implemented to improve the standard of living of the people. Most of the projects are complementary and supplementary. Because of the poor co-ordination among the various departments, at the state level, the projects are implemented in the area without developing linkages with each other. For example, a project for the agriculture development to grow more food can be beautifully linked with the health projects on nutrition. Population control has many dimensions and needs the co-operation of many agencies. Thus, there is a need of area planning and developing an integrated area approach where different projects may develop linkages to have optimum benefit.

4. Absence of the Full Involvement of the Beneficiaries in the Formulation and Implementation of Projects

The success or failure of the RCH project ultimately depends upon the acceptance of these projects by the people. If the people are not taken into confidence during the formulation and implementation of RCH projects, these would be less successful. People's participation would provide extra nuclear energy to the success of the RCH projects. Most of the beneficiaries contacted by the writer were of the view that they are not treated as equal partners in the process of formulation and implementation of projects. The failure of the scheme is because of the absence of identity of the people with the programmes. It is essential for the experts to motivate and encourage the people to participate in the formulation and implementation of projects. Although people's participation in affairs governing their lives dates back to the beginning of human society, the concept has taken a new dimension as societies have grown in size and complexity. This is partly because the management has become more and more a specialized enterprise, an area for technocrats and trained general administrators and political leaders. Although they officially advocate and preach people's involvement, in practice, they bring them into picture only after the major decisions have been made. Hence, they often leave the ordinary citizens to follow their pre-determined paths. Peter Druker agrees with this contention when he says that "the overwhelming majority of these people have little or no opportunity to influence policy, and their perspectives on the situation are systematically ignored by almost all theorists. For them the problem of development is one of the everyday life."

5. Local Communities are Treated as Passive Participants in Improvement and Bettering of their Lives

Most of the project personnel working in the villages return to the cities after their duty hours. The villagers cannot make their views known to them in cities. The result is lack of communication among them. When the project fails, it is intentionally ascribed to the obstinacy, fatalism, illiteracy or apparent irrationality of the poor people. The potential for community involvement has been seriously underestimated. We must encourage people's participation through all methods to promote development.

6. Absence of any Satisfactory Monitoring System to Measure the Regulated Performance during Implementation

Project control is the managerial function that helps the managers to keep the project functioning as scheduled. It is possible only if the realistic advance targets of output are fixed before implementation. This is not being done as is evident from the perusal of most of the projects studied. Monitoring if properly designed, projects can help the managers in keeping the process of implementation as scheduled. The project performance is compared at different intervals of time with the control indicators. Whenever deviations are located, causes of deviations are examined, solutions are found to correct the deviations. The following are the general causes of deviation:

(1) "Excessive optimism on the part of the project planners, resulting in unrealistic estimates in respect to:
- the time, funds, manpower or other resources required to do an activity, and
- the passability of achieving the expected results.

(2) Unfrozen resistance from or changes in the environment of the project (natural disaster, political changes, etc.).

(3) Decisions at higher, managerial levels to change the planned resources inputs of the project (change of a staff member).

(4) Inefficient administrative procedures.

If there is any unavoidable deviation beyond the control of the project authorities, we can think of alternative proposals immediately without wasting the future resources. If such timely action is taken, the developing countries can be sure of the success of the projects. More safely designing the control system means specifying who reports what to whom and when.

7. Unscientific Manpower Planning and Insufficient Utilisation of Project Personnel

The success of the project depends upon the quality and quantity of personnel associated with it. It was observed that in many projects, the projects personnel have their utilisation time as low as 20 per cent. This is highly serious as the resources are being consumed by the establishment rather than invested in the RCH programme. Because of the absence of manpower planning, personnel of the project utilize very little time. People in the area remarked about the workers appointed to motivate people to adopt family planning norm: "They are not available at all. They rarely devote any time for this work. They remain away from their work." It is essential to see through proper manpower planning that only needed persons are appointed and they are utilised to increase in the overall cost-productivity, efficiency and effectiveness. The projects should be so administered as to lead to overall improvement in its performance.

8. Lack of Clarification of Authority, Responsibility and Relationships

In the developing world, the persons responsible for implementation of the project do not work as a team as there is no clarification of authority, responsibility and relationships amongst them, i.e. the roles of the various participants are not often mutually understood. This result into friction among these persons. Most of the time of these persons are spent in their mutual disputes. It becomes very difficult for them to devote their whole attention to the project.

9. Private Sector Engaged in Merely Curative Services

Ninth Plan suggested the Private Sector participation in RCH. It is estimated that the private sector accounts for more than three quarters of all health care expenditure in India. Private sector provides MCH and family planning services also but to a lesser extent. It is increasingly recognised that the private sector represents an untapped potential for increasing the coverage and improving the quality of reproductive and child health services in the country. The challenge is to find ways and means to optimally utilise their potential. The major limitations in the private sector include the following:

(a) the focus has till now been mainly on curative services,
(b) the quality of services is often variable, and

(c) as the users have to pay for the services, the poorer sections of population cannot afford these services.

Some of the initiatives could be through collaboration between public and private sector in providing health care to the poorer segments of population who cannot afford to pay for health services. While organising the involvement of private medical practitioners in RCH care, it is essential to provide orientation training to all and ensure utilisation of their services is a cost-effective and sustainable basis.

Private/voluntary organisations providing health care to women are relatively small in number but they could play an effective role in the delivery of reproductive and child health care services at affordable cost, especially in certain specific locations such as urban slums. Giving the private sector and voluntary organisations appropriate incentives to broaden the range of activities and improve the quality of reproductive and child health-related services they offer are other avenues that require exploration. Continued collaboration, training and technical assistance by governmental agencies to private medical practitioners and private/ voluntary organisations may help in strengthening reproductive and child health services in remote or under-served areas.

10. Previous Implementation Experience of the Completed Project not Referred to

It was a great surprise to learn that there are no records of past experiences in relation to project implementation. One can always learn from the mistakes of others. Some of the project personnel remarks that "they do not know anything about the difficulties encountered by the project personnel and the causes of the failure of the project undertaken earlier." It is beneficial to examine how major projects have been managed in the past. It would also be better to identify those approaches which have been most successful. We can keep a record of good and bad points of the past project and this cumulative experience may be passed on to the present project managers. In this way, many of the difficulties likely to be encountered would vanish.

Frank A. Wilson in his article "Planning for Project Management" in the *Journal of Administration Overseas* (July 1979) has rightly mentioned that, "Disappointing and inefficient project performance is a fact of life. . . . . Ex-post evaluation of existing projects can be the means by which we can systematically seek to analyse the potential for improving project management. Evaluation studies give the opportunity for developing a greater understanding of the way projects are managed and implemented."

11. Faulty and Cumbersome Administrative Procedures

Whenever a project is formulated, we do not pay much attention to the problems of communication, co-ordination, headquarters field relationship, supervision, etc. The purpose of these procedures is to help in the smooth functioning of the project. Without proper procedures developed most of the project personnel remain engrossed in preparing unnecessary reports. These procedures should be clarified in the initial stages of project management, so that no confusion arises later on. If there are already set procedures in a particular organization, these may be adopted otherwise new procedures may be adopted and made known to the project personnel. It must be clear that administrative procedures are an aid to help the efficient functioning of the project. The meticulous applications of these procedures may result into red-tapism and inefficiency.

The Five Year Plan (1978-83) has also indicated the technical, administrative and managerial problems which affect project efficiency. They are mentioned below:

(a) Inadequate investigation and data collection as a result of which the project appraisal, even when it is sought to be done in a systematic way, has to be carried out on the basis of wholly inadequate information, thus leading to wrong investment decisions.
(b) Inadequate detailed planning of projects in terms of their time schedule, input resource requirements and skills needed for project implementation.
(c) Lack of delegation of authority to subordinate organization levels.
(d) Delays in issuing sanction, approvals, fund authorisations and releases.
(e) Organizational weaknesses in planning and implementation at various levels.
(f) Lack of specific assignment of responsibility and accountability for results.
(g) Problems of industrial relations and inadequate motivation of personnel, lack of proper career planning and incentives and commitment to results.
(h) Inadequate share of representation of the weaker sections in elected bodies in the village, district and block levels and agencies.

We can improve upon the management of projects if we keep these difficulties or problems or obstacles in mind and try to reduce them to negligible proportions. Besides, there is a need of training project personnel in the art of project management.

CONCLUSION

The new RCH programme has been designed scientifically keeping in view the minor details meticulously. The programme is certainly better than the earlier Family Planning maternal and child health programmes aimed at specific activity. The RCH programme is operative in the whole of the country.

However, with the overall policy made by the Ministry of Health and Family Welfare, each district should design its own programme keeping in view the needs, resources, topography, quality of the peoples, facilities and infrastructure available as well as plan implementation and evaluation to inject flexibility as situations difference from district to district.

Radhakrishna Rao in his Article, "Towards controlling the Numbers" in *The Daily Tribune* (31st January, 2000) rightly suggests that a target free approach has now become a part of the population control drive. To what extent this approach will contribute to the success of population control, no one is sure as yet. Sociologists, however, are clear in their perception that when literacy, health, hygiene and economic improvements get high priority, family planning stands a better chance of success.

The document prepared for the International Conference on Population and Development has recognised in its programme of action that "the main message for improving individual well-being comprises two elements: to provide contraceptive methods within the broader reproductive health services and to advance women's equal participation in education, health and economic opportunities."

Notes and References

1. Annual Report, Ministry of Health and Family Welfare, 1998-99, pp. 7-9.
2. State Family Welfare Bureau, DH & FWS, Reproductive and Child Health, Bangalore, July, 1988, p. 1.
3. WHO, May-June, 1994, p. 30.
4. State Family Welfare Bareau, Bangalore, *op. cit.*, pp. 19-20.
5. WHO, SEARO: Managing Essential Reproductive Health Care, New Delhi, p. 5.
6. B.M. Ramesh, S.B. Ganiger and D.G. Satihal, "Family Welfare Programme under Target Free Approach: A Rapid Survey in Belgaum District, Karnataka, 1998, Population Research Centre, J.S.S. Institute of Economic Research, Dharwad.
7. P.N. Mari Bhat, Target Free Approach to Family Planning Programme: A Rapid Survey in Dharwad District in Karnataka, 1997, Population Research Centre, J.S.S. Institute of Economic Research, Dharwad, pp. i-iii.

ANNEXURE 6.1

OF STATEMENT V

Guidelines to Prepare State Implementation Plan Under World Bank Supported Reproductive and Child Health Project

The categorisation of State have already been intimated to all the States. States are also aware that interventions under the proposed RCH project will be provided as per differential approach finalised with all States.

However, during the State Secretaries' meeting held in September, 1996, some States requested that these interventions may be provided as per categorisation of Districts instead of States, as the districts in States can also be classified as Cat. A, B or C. Separately the problem of States under State Health Systems (SHS) project of World Bank also had to be resolved.

Some of the parameters earlier used for classification of States are not available district-wise from 1991 census data. Keeping in view differing needs and availability of reliable data at State and District levels as also available demographic parameters like CBR and female literacy rate district-wise (for major States only), the districts have been classified after computation of weightage and the same may be seen in enclosed *Statement A*. For some States/UTs where District-wise data is not available the State data has been used for classification.

Interventions have, generally, been provided for on District data except when it became necessary to restrict grouping under State Health Systems or under original classification of States. In some cases strengths available due to inputs under Social Safety Net Scheme for 90 demographically weak Districts have been taken into account.

2. Many interventions under the RCH Project will be made available to all States without any differentiation. These are:

- Orientation Workshops on RCH.
- Facilitation for operationalisation of Target Free Approach.
- Institutional Development.
- Preparation of Annual State and District Training (integrated training as per the plan and requirements of the RCH interventions), Logistics and implementation plans.
- Modified Management information system.
- Additional IEC activities under RCH on Team-Building and Community Sensitisation.
- Urban and Tribal Areas RCH as per the needs of the States based on the pilot studies. (Details to be intimated later).
- Local capacity enhancement, as per the projects submitted separately.
- Setting up of RTI/STI Clinics at left out District Hospitals at

places where STD Clinic under AIDS/STD Programme has not yet been provided. The cost of drugs and equipment per unit will be Rs. 75,000.

3. There are some interventions which will be provided to the States on the basis of classification of the Districts and States mentioned at para 1 above. The facilities/interventions which are being considered for the different category of Districts are given below

Facilities to be Provided in Category "A" Districts

- Provision of RTI/STI drugs at FRUs (*) (Not in the SHS Project States).
- Minor civil work/repairs/maintenance provisions of requisite inputs at FRU/PHC/SCs otherwise being covered under RCH Project @ upto Rs. 10.00 lakh per District for the project period.
- MTP equipments to all FRUs/CHCs not provided earlier will be given.
- MTP equipments in phased manner to all PHCs.
- Upto 2 Lab Teach. for FRUs on contract basis per District for operationalising RTI/STI screening and diagnostic interventions.
- Consultant doctor at PHC as per phasing on fixed day visit basis twice per month @ Rs. 500 per visit. (Government doctors can also be used for this purpose and paid an honorariam on the same term). The expected work of the Consultants during visit will be provided safe abortion services. This facility will be provided upto 75% of PHC only in the initial years with declining phasing as it is assumed that trained doctors are available at other facilities. By the end of 5 years, it is expected that with intensive training, the requirement of Consultant doctors will be reduced to 25% from 75%. Work load norms will be atleast 5 surgical interventions or assisted deliveries out of cases referred from periphery. Minimum of atleast 20 referred cases should be attended by the visiting doctor or each visit. Adequate advance IEC on expected date of visit of doctor should be announced.

Facilities to be Provided in Category "B" Districts

- Provision of RTI and EOC drugs at 1 FRU each (*) (Not in the SHS Project States).
- Minor civil work/repairs/maintenance provisions of requisite inputs at FRU/PHC/SCS otherwise being covered under RCH

Project @ upto Rs. 10.00 lakh per District for the project period.

- Two Lab. Tech. at the FRU on contract basis for lab. diagnosis of STI/RTI apart from other work.
- All PHCs to get MTP equipments in phased manner.
- Consultant doctor preferably lady at PHC on fixed day visit basis twice per month @ Rs. 500 per visit. (Government doctors can also be used for this purpose and paid an honorariam on the same term) as per the phasing of MTP equipment and availability of appropriate facility. The expected work of the Consultants during visit is to provide safe abortion services MTP, ANC, PNC and other Family Planning and Family Welfare Services. This facility will be provided upto 75% of PHC only for the initial years with declining phasing as it is assumed that trained doctors are available at other facilities. By the end of 5 years, it is expected that with intensive training, the requirement of consultant doctors will be reduced to 25% from 75%. Work load norms will be atleast 5 surgical interventions or assisted deliveries out of cases referred from periphery. Minimum of atleast 20 referred cases should be attended by the visiting doctor of each visit. Adequate advance IEO on expected date of visit of doctor should be announced.
- SHS Project States viz. A.P., Karnataka, Punjab and West Bengal have already been strengthened upto Sub-District level. The average institutional deliveries in the districts in these states range around 50% as such, for the PHOs with low institutional deliveries (expected around 50%), the facility of the services of PHN/Staff Nurse will be provided in 50% PHOs to improve institutional delivery, ANC/PHC and screening and referral for RTI. This facility will be limited to the 30 identified Category B Districts in these States. They will be staying at the place of posting for round the clock services. Rental for residence @ upto Rs. 5000 per annum will be provided.
- PHC drug kit for management of essential obstetric care will also be provided to the PHOs where PNH/Staff Nurse have been appointed and are providing round the clock services.

Facilities to be Provided in Category "C" Districts

- Provision of EOC drugs at FRUs (*) (Not in the SHS Project States).
- Minor civil work/repairs/maintenance of FRU/PHC/SCs at Rs. 10.00 lakh per District for the project period.
- MTP equipments to all FRUs/CHOs not provided earlier.

- MTP equipments in phased manner to all PHOs.
- Two Lab. Tech. for selected FRUs on contract basis per District.
- Provision of PAN/Staff Nurse on contract basis in all the PHOs (for 30,000 population) in the 90 Social Safety Net Districts for providing institutional delivery, ANC/PHC, Family Planning and Family Welfare. They will be staying at the place of posting for round the clock services and get rental for residence @ upto Rs. 5000 per annum. Under Social Safety Net Scheme provision was made for providing appropriate infrastructure for such PHCs where this was missing. While a perfect machine may not be feasible, it is expected that 35-40% PHCs in these districts would be having facilities which could not be used with provision of PHN/ Staff Nurse for providing essential obstetric care.
- In other Districts, where delivery room and residential quarters have been built under various projects but remain unutilised, a PHN/Staff Nurse on contract basis will be provided at PHC (for 30,000 population). As per available information only about 25% PHCs in Category C Districts can avail this facility.
- Additional ANMs in a phased manner upto 30% of SOs @ Rs. 3600.00 p.m. will be provided to augment the ability to provide focused attention to safe motherhood in the less developed areas/blocks of these districts in 'C' category. This facility is being restricted to remote and for flung sub-centres in C category Districts of the 8 states originally identified as C category States, i.e. Assam, Bihar, Haryana, Madhya Pradesh, Nagaland, Orissa, Rajasthan and Uttar Pradesh.
- Nominal rental to facilitate the stay of these additional ANMs will be provided.
- A Pilot will be launched for assessing long-term feasibility of referral transport for pregnant women from below poverty line category for their obstetric emergencies to be carried out in 2-3 Cat. C Districts in the 8 States (originally identified as C States) with high infant and maternal mortality.
- All PHOs to get MTP equipments in phased manner.
- Consultant doctor (preferably lady) at PHC on fixed day visit basis twice per month @ Rs. 500 per visit. (Government doctors can also be used for this purpose and paid an honorariam on the same term) as per the phasing of MTP equipment and availability of appropriate facility. The expected work of the Consultants during visit will be provided safe abortion services MTP, ANC, PNC and other Family Planning and Family Welfare Services. This facility will be provided upto 75% of PHC only, as it is assumed that

trained doctors are available at other facilities. By the end of 5 years, it is expected that with intensive training, the requirement of consultant doctors will be reduced to 25% from 75%. Work load norms will be atleast surgical interventions or assisted deliveries out of cases referred from periphery. Minimum of atleast 20 referred cases should be attended by the visiting doctor of each visit. Adequate advance IEC on expected date of visit of doctor should be announced.

- PHC drug kit for management of essential obstetric care will also be provided to the PHCs where PHN/Staff Nurse have been appointed and are providing round the clock services.

(*) Identification of two FRUs per District is left to the States. However, it is advisable that these facilities (FRUs) be chosen (a) where availability of manpower is assured; (b) equipment kits were provided under CSSM or where these can be shifted from other facilities; (c) infrastructure is already available and Cesarian Section is being carried out; and (d) have good geographic advantage and have defined catchment area to provide referral services.

4. For proper implementation of some of the interventions, it is proposed to phase the interventions by selecting Districts under the Project, taking only those Districts for the interventions, which are prepared to receive the interventions. In the first year of the project, only those Districts should be selected which are able to start the proposed activity positively in the second half of the year of the project. All the pre-requisite activities like training, gaps in infrastructure, manpower, etc., should have been attended to under State MNP where relevant e.g., infrastructure. The phasing of the Districts for some of the major interventions are given at *Statement 'A-i'* and total number of Districts proposed under phasing is given at *Statement 'C'*.

5. While preparing the interventions for the States, assumptions used by this Ministry described in pre-paragraphs and below may also be kept in mind by States while preparing the State Implementation Plan and phasing of various interventions and districts over the five year project period.

Source: Department of Family Welfare, Government of India, Reproductive and Child Health, Vol. I, New Delhi, March 1997.

CHAPTER 7

INFORMATION, EDUCATION AND COMMUNICATION

"If genuine change is desired it will occur only through the social mechanisms for change which the community has established and to which it is accustomed. People are eager to change behaviour if they perceive the change as beneficial . . . . It is the fallacy of modernity that we believe, we communicate through bonds of mutual confidence. It is the prime task of the health communicator to facilitate a state of communal trust and also avoid Pseudo information."

—World Health

Information, Education and Communication

The creation of awareness is integral to the process of social development. The possibility for the power of communication to liberate the minds and potential of people to critical awareness is real in every field linked to human development, and the generation of public will hinges on effective communication of information and ideas that relate to people's needs, aspirations and capacities for progress in thought and action. In this sense, getting the development process started is largely the task of information, education and communication.

The communication aspect of a national family planning programme is generally termed as IEC-Information, Education Communication. The Year Book (1986-87) of Family Welfare Programme in India has rightly mentioned that the success of the Family Welfare Programme depends primarily upon the voluntary and widespread acceptance of the concept of small family and delayed marriages and well spaced and properly linked births are an effective way of achieving this objective. Mass education and Media activities, accordingly, were given multi-dimensional and integrated thrust through Information-Education-Communication activities in the form of a comprehensive package of social transformation . . . to bring behavioural and attitudinal changes in the people so as to enable them to adopt family planning as a way of life. In brief, we can simplify it, and can call it simply as communication function. Sometimes, the activities under IEG are also referred to as "Mass Communication", "Mass Education", "Mass Education and Media."

Donald J. Bogue has rightly said that IEG is a term widely used to identify the activities of family planning programme to inform the public and stimulate them to adopt contraception.[1] In every technical component of the Family Planning Programme provided by family planning workers, there exists a corresponding educational aspect, which has to be imparted more or less simultaneously, so as to enhance the continuing usefulness of the services provided at the time of need. This would have permanent value.

An added importance of communication in family planning resulted from the experience and studies which indicated that pure clinical approach did not bear fruit. A. Govindachari has mentioned some of the findings of the studies, which have brought to notice the limited impact of clinical approach. These are:

(i) The population reached by the clinics was very limited.
(ii) Education on family planning in the clinics was mostly through individual contacts. There was no organized community education.
(iii) The educational efforts were mostly directed towards women, since the clinics normally have female social workers. Husbands, who are important from the point of view of decision-making in family planning, especially in an Indian cultural context, were not given due attention.
(iv) Couples felt shy to visit clinics for fear of identification by their friends and neighbours.
(v) The working hours of the clinics were found to be inconvenient, especially for the low income groups.
(vi) There was a lack of social support for the programme due to inadequate involvement of the community.
(vii) People generally prefer to obtain contraceptives in an informal way which does not involve formal recording procedures and publicity. This was not possible in a clinic situation.
(viii) There was very little involvement of other supporting staff, like the village level workers, extension officers, etc., in the family planning programme.[2]

Today, Family planning programmes around the world are applying a broad range of service delivery and communication strategies. To make family planning services and supplies more accessible, conventional clinic-based programmes have been supplemented by innovative approaches to services delivery. These include community-based outreach, social marketing through commercial outlets at subsidized prices, and employment-based programmes organized or supported by employees or Unions. Extensive communication campaigns, combining a variety of modern and traditional mass-media are spreading family planning awareness and encouraging more people to seek out family planning services.[3]

INTRODUCTION

The Information, Education, Communication (IEC) component of

National Family Welfare programme is mainly to create an effective communication strategy, to inform the masses about the means and measures of Family Welfare Programme, educate them about the perils of over-population and motivate and persuade them to adopt small family norm, using all possible channels of media.[4]

In a Family Planning organisation, external communication is very important in the implementation of its programme, as information about the utility and means of planned parenthood through appropriate choice and correct use of contraceptives by the eligible married couples is important. Moreover, communication being two-way process brings to the attention of the management the needs, reactions and complaints of the people concerned for necessary initiative or remedial actions. The external communication process needs to be guided by considerations of relevance of information, the choice of communication channels and the existing understanding capacity (education, etc.) of the people concerned outside the organisation. Moreover, it should not by any means be only one sided, i.e., from the organisation to the people. The reverse flow of information from the people to the organisation would make the latter to judge the impact of the programme as well as provide the basis for any changes in the strategies of the Programme. Here again, barriers and disruptions in the two-way communication process have to be dealt with appropriately.

Broadly speaking, communication is the means by which intentions of the programme are classified to ensure fruitful results. It may even be looked upon as the means by which special information inputs are fed into social systems. It is the means by which behaviour of the personnel engaged in the programme is modified; change is effected, information is made productive and goals are achieved.[5] Barnard has aptly viewed it as the means by which people can be linked together in an organisation to achieve the objectives of the programmes.[6] Communication is a universal phenomenon among living beings. Newman and Summer have viewed communication as an exchange of facts, ideas, opinion, or emotions by two or more persons.[7]

Family Planning Communication implies a number of actions starting with identifying the audience, assessing needs and channels for response, identifying specific messages especially in areas of resistance to change in attitude and behaviour, selecting complementary media for optimal combination, producing communication materials and refining messages and techniques after pre-testing, revision and re-testing, dissemination of communication, continuous support through stages of programmes implementation mainly to ensure community involvement and participatory monitoring and evaluation. Since, Family Planning is a challenging and arduous task, communication technology must be well planned. A successful communication effort blends the use of traditional communication media with the modern, brings together the channels of government communication with those of the community and of voluntary organisations and a variety of other groups, Family Planning ideology can be registered in the minds of the people not simply by providing the information on Family Planning, but because people can be told that they exist, shown that they work and encouraged (and empowered) to try them and make them work for themselves. This is the nature of the support which communication lends to a family planning programme.

ESSENTIALS AND ASPECTS OF MASS MOTIVATION CAMPAIGN

Essentials

Dr. John Hubley quoted by Gloria Gorden in his Article, "Let's Communicate" in *World Health* (January-Feb. 1989) has rightly described the essentials of Communication.

- Promote actions which are realistic and feasible within the constraints faced by the community.
- Build on ideas, concepts and practices that people already have.
- Repeat and reinforce information overtime, using different methods.
- Use existing channels of Communication such as songs, drama and story-telling, and be adaptable.
- Entertain and attract the attention of the Community.
- Use clear, simple language with local expressions and emphasize short-term benefits of action.
- Provide opportunities for dialogue and discussion to allow learner participation and feedback on understanding and implementation.
- Use demonstrations to show the benefits of adopting practices.[8]

E.M. Rogers mentions the following essentials:

(i) Family Planning Communication campaigns should be preceded by extensive planning of the strategies to be followed.

(ii) A Consumer Orientation in family planning communication activities will be more effective in achieving the objectives of the National Family Planning Programme.

(iii) A new family planning communication approach should be launched on a small scale pilot project basis.

(iv) Social research can perform an important function in more effective family planning communication, (a) by providing feedback for the design of communication messages through pre-testing; and (b) by yielding evaluative data about the efforts of communication activities.[9]

CHANNELS OF COMMUNICATION

(a) Radio

Radio has been in use since long. It has been effective as a means of communication. Since the start of the programme on a regular basis in May 1967 on All-India Radio, there have been many challenges as it was a new and sensitive issue. All types of methods have been tried on Radio and even today the importance of Radio as a means of popularising F.P. Programme is enormous. To quote G.K. Mathur, "It is through this common sense and realistic approach that All-India Radio is trying to create a massive awareness base which may serve as a take-off platform for ever widening acceptance of actual family planning methods. In all our programmes we have stressed that the family planning campaign is a people's programme for the total well-being of the family. It is from this angle that a distinction has been made between the programmes directed towards scarcely populated areas, like hill areas, desert areas, off-shore islands, etc. and programmes meant for over-crowded cities and densely populated areas. In order to avoid any possible resistance to the broadcast of family planning programmes on a fixed-time basis, they introduced the family planning themes in-between various programmes, thus taking the listener unawares."

All-India Radio produces and broadcasts in different formats such as group discussions, interviews, spot recordings, feature plays, etc. in different languages and areas. The Commercial Broadcasting Services (CBS) have been broadcasting the programme 'Haseen Lamhe' regularly, as well as one minute spots over various channels in Hindi and regional languages.

(b) Television

Television has become very popular. S.K. Sharma in an Article, "Role of Television in Promoting Family Planning" has rightly said that, "In fact, the potential impact of television, as a means of informing the people is greater than that of any other means of mass communication. With television, as with the motion picture film, we can hear what is to be done, can see it done and can see the results. Unlike the motion picture, television conveys the feeling of immediacy. In this sense, it combines radio's intimate quality with the motion pictures' ability to magnify the smallest detail which all can see.

(c) Films

Government of India, Publicity Division has been making documentary and other films on various themes of F.P. activities. Parmod Pati has mentioned that, Films Division has produced so far a number of films on subjects relating to family planning. A good number of films are now under production. A large number of news-reels have already exhibited slogans relating to family planning. Only a few of these are purely informational, for they are factual and principally of interest value without any attempt in conveying a specific educational message. They focus attention on food problem or housing *vis-a-vis* the rise in population. They talk of education facilities or employment and rise in population. But most of the remaining films are designed primarily to motivate, to encourage and inspire the audience to particular action in accepting new ideas and changing attitudes in accepting the norm of a small family or a means to space children or even to accept methods to completely limit further procreation. Some of the films help to put information about a particular means of contraception in the right perspective while the others keep on emphasising the massage "if you have two that would do." Not all these films can be claimed to be outstanding. While an occasional film is made with a festival jury in mind, most of these films meet the needs of the communicator fully so far as family planning education is concerned.

An integrated IEG strategy, mixing inter-personal communication with multi-media contents was developed. Activities were given multi-dimensional and integrated thrust to increase the outreach and impact of Reproductive and Child Health and Family Welfare messages with the objective of bridging the gap between awareness and acceptance.

As part of the new strategy to utilise the services of eminent film-makers, the Ministry has assigned eminent directors, Shri Amol Palekar and Shyam Benegal's two feature films, i.e. 'Kairee' and 'Teri Godi Hari Bhari Rahe' respectively.

(d) Advertising and Visual Publicity

The Directorate of Advertising and Visual Publicity (DAVP) releases press advertisement and arranges exhibitions at various centres throughout the country. Special attention is given to the places of intensive multi-media campaigns.

(e) Song and Drama Division

To educate the masses about family welfare issues, Song and Drama Division organises live entertainment programmes like puppet shows, dance, dramas, folk recitals, mythological recitals, traditional plays, magic shows, etc. Special Programmes to sensitise people regarding the Pulse Polio Immunisation programme are also being organised by the field units, so that greater number of people can bring their children up to the age of 5 years for the extra doses of Polio drops. More than 15,000 variety shows were organised during the year 1998-99 itself.

(f) Press Information

PIB conducts field visits of journalists for the coverage of family welfare activities. It organises special briefing and seminars for journalists. A Scheme to sensitise 'Opinion Leaders' by holding one day session on various aspects of family welfare issues, was instituted in 1993-94. Under this scheme, 10421 opinion leaders of various categories including members of Zilla Panchayats, panchs, private practitioners, teachers, etc. were exposed to family welfare issues. Now, it is proposed to be implemented through State/Regional Health and Family Welfare Training Centres.

(g) Personal Communication

Changes in knowledge, attitudes, behaviour, habits and customs can be brought about by personal as well as impersonal methods of FP education. These methods have certain advantages and disadvantages. While personal methods involve face-to-face interaction the impersonal methods do not require such a close personal contact. Personal methods are indeed more convincing and generally more successful. However, the success of personal methods greatly depends on the establishment of a good rapport between the FP educator and his recipients. The impersonal methods are relatively simpler and even less time-consuming. The radio, the newspapers, the posters, and the pamphlets, etc., can all play an important role in imparting FP education. Experience with personal and impersonal methods of FP education have revealed that if both the methods are used simultaneously one can obtain better results than simply using one or the other method. The most important aspect in the adoption of the programme is the use of inter-personal relationships.

Mr. Manu N. Kulkarni has rightly said that "the information transfer among the poor households takes place through indirect mechanisms like gossip among men in tea and bidi shops and gossip sessions of the women when they gather around a village well, pond, bathing ghats and temples. The health matters affecting poor women like pregnancy, maternity, child spacing, family planning, etc. are not talked out openly. When Public Health advertisement makes such information 'open', a sense of shyness and distrust is shown by these poor women and the "closeness" of information is lost. Unfortunately, glasnost does not work when it comes to information sharing on private health. Private health is not like DDT spraying for malaria eradication. The chances of Private health information sharing are better when it is shared through informal gossip sessions, inter-personal communication, folk media or street theatre. Commercial advertisements cannot penetrate the antenna of the poor and the deprived."[10]

Thus, we see that communication, i.e., dissemination of information is only one important element in FP education. The adoption or acceptance may not take place simply by communicating FP information. A study conducted by United States Public Health Services has revealed that, "unfortunately knowledge alone does not motivate a person to act in accordance with it. He may well know the correct answers to questions without really believing and accepting such information as the basis for his own action."

Dr. Gisela Gastrin, a Finnish physician mentions in his article, "How Education Helps". "People can be motivated to adjust their outlook towards health and disease, but before this can happen their negative attitudes have to be countered with factual information. Education needs to be a part of a comprehensive programme in which responsibilities involving the health authorities and others are clearly delineated and resources allocated."[11]

It was mentioned by Dr. E. Berthat in his article, "A new Role for Teachers" that besides information and motivation, action is indispensable. He said that "Information and motivation are not enough; it remains for governments to ensure that a good health infrastructure is available to all the people. Health education has to convince the men and women who are responsible for taking decisions that health is a basic raw material for their country's eventual social and economic development."[12]

A Family Planning educator as a persuasive communicator can make the best possible use of the personal methods of FP education. But he has to see that the messages which he is delivering get mentally registered with his recipients. Actually, he can present his message and then wait until he gets the requisite response from his recipients. D.F. Skinner has distinguished between two types of approaches to the learning situation, as 'operant behaviour' and 'respondent behaviour'. The two situations have also been described as involving instrumental learning and conditional learning. In 'instrumental learning situation', which involves 'operant behaviour', the FP educator will present his message and then wait for the receiver to make a correct response. When the receiver makes this response, the FP educator will attempt to fix the response by the appropriate award or reinforcement. On the other hand, in 'conditioned learning situation' which involves 'respondent behaviour', the FP education presents his message in such a way that he elicits the response that he wants from his recipients and thus the stimulus that originally served to elicit the response becomes the reinforcing or rewarding element in conditioning. Undoubtedly, conditioning is much more efficient than instrumental learning. It is, however, necessary for the FP educator to be aware of both kinds of situations since the condition for using 'respondent behaviour' may not be present in the persuasive situation. The FP educator has to be aware that the recipients of his messages differ in the ways in which they learn a given response. They may give different responses essentially in the same situation because of certain specific reasons.

Educational methods to promote family planning currently used by Health and Family Planning workers are often dialectic in character, prescribing "dos" and "don'ts" and are not a convenient medium for structured learning. Doubts have been raised about their effectiveness. They do not provide a learning environment within which people can examine whether the recommended procedures fit into their culture, are feasible in terms of cost and of life styles, and are not socially and psychologically counter-productive. In addition, family planning workers often use in appropriate and unrelated visual aids, which have been prepared without keeping in mind the local perceptual patterns of population groups or with insufficient regard to the relevance of these materials to the objectives they are intended to serve.

Everett M. Rogers[13] has maintained that most family programmes have taken too narrow a view of communication in the past They define the province of family planning communication in terms: (1) of only mass-media channels, and (2) of only the communication skills of producing family planning messages. Both functions, of course, are indeed the responsibility of the communication specialist. But, he should do much more, by engaging in activities that include: (1) inter-personnels, channels, and (2) the formation of communication strategies based upon social scientific understanding of behavioural change.

We know that the goals of family planning programmes cannot be reached by using mass-media channels alone. The audiences for such channels are too limited, the attention-getting powers are inadequate, and the motivating and persuading abilities of the mass-media are severely restricted. Research investigations consistently indicate that interpersonal channels are necessary to convince most individuals to adopt family planning methods. So, the province of family planning communication should include word-of-mouth interaction from peers who have previously adopted. By family planning communication, we do not just mean mass-media channels, they are often mediated and interpreted by opinion leaders to a large audience of receivers. So, mass media and interpersonal channels are impossible to separate in their functions and effects, even if we tried to do so.

(h) Local Community Groups

In this strategy, the doubts and misgivings hampering the promotion of family welfare measures are dispelled and popular support for the programme enlisted. Andreas Fuglessang, while admitting the role of information in motivating group action, has warned the need of guarding against Pseudo information. To quote him:

> "If genuine change is desired it will occur only through the social mechanisms for change which the community has established and to which it is accustomed. People are eager to change behaviour if they perceive the change as beneficial . . . . It is the fallacy of modernity that we believe, we communicate through bonds of mutual confidence. It is the prime task of the health communicator to facilitate a state of communal trust and also avoid Pseudo information."[14]

Mothers' Clubs in Korean villages play an important role, (1) in facilitating family planning communication, (2) in the general community development of these villages, and (3) in contributing toward women's equality. Local community groups could be important in reaching national family planning goals in other nations.

Mother's clubs for family planning communication are also being tried out on a pilot project basis in the Philippines and in Bangladesh, and are widely used in Colombia. Other types of local community groups can also be used for family planning communications, such as agricultural cooperatives, local units of political parties, farmers' associations, etc. Or, as in the "Extra Drive" approach used since 1971 in the province of East Java in Indonesia, strong local leadership in the village is used as a motivational force; here a local group with regular meetings is not used, but a temporary, once-only meeting of all target couples performs a similar function. The "group planning of births" in the People's Republic of China also depends for its success on encouraging the adoption of family planning methods and lowering fertility, on a once-a-year public meeting followed by continuous peer pressure to encourage parental implementation of the group birth plan.

All these examples illustrate a general proposition that local community groups can be an essential tool in family planning communication by providing motivation for the adoption of family planning methods and for their continued use to reduce fertility. In most Asian nations, there is presently no government development apparatus that reaches to the local level of social organisation in village. Local groups provide a mean for government to deliver services to the mass population and to change strongly-held beliefs and behaviour.

We must popularise such clubs in India and make trade unions, Mahila Mandals, Youth Organisations and students' associations active in this direction, as has been the experience in many other countries.

Donald J. Bogue rightly says that taking all factors into account, the group meeting in which some entertainment such as a film or film strip is shown, followed by group discussions, or comment by local leaders, combines many desirable features and is probably one of the best ways (if not the best) to bring information in family planning to a village or neighbourhood.

(i) Mahila Swasthya Sangh

Greater emphasis is being laid on inter-personal communication to encourage community participation, particularly for the women-folk through Mahila Swasthya Sangh (MSS) in villages with a population of over 1000 or 200 households in plain areas and for population of 500 or more in hilly terrain, including the North-Eastern States. The Auxiliary Nurse Midwife (ANM) is the member-Secretary of MSS. The MSS comprise five grass-root level functionaries and 10 prominent women from the village community. The field level functionaries of education are also the members of MSS. MSS are being constituted since 1990-91 at village level. A nominal amount of Rs. 1,200 per year is allocated for arranging its monthly meetings.

We can, thus safely say that in order to ensure the success of family planning programmes, the IEC activities must make use of all the communication skills and technology. P.T. Piotrow has rightly said that to enable couples to make informed choices, information about family planning methods must come through many media, leading ultimately to person to person contacts between clients and providers.[15]

CONCLUSIONS AND RECOMMENDATIONS

Without evaluating the impact of FP education programmes on the bulk of the people, one cannot possible identify positive as well as negative aspects of the programme. An objective evaluation of the FP education programme alone can help one improve guidelines for future action. Cost-benefit analysis should be an integral part of this evaluation, so that one may assess how available resources have been utilized. Through objective evaluation, one may also be able to curtail mass production of ritualistic FP education material as produced by various FP education bureaus. The amount thus saved can be effectively utilized for a more purposeful and meaningful health education programme.

FP education is the most difficult task as habits, usages and customs are deeply entrenched. But, FP administration would fail in its purpose, if it could not produce social change, as it is easier to destroy our villages than to change our customs. (Bosnian Proverb quoted in John I. Hanlon, Principles of Public Health Administration, St. Louis, 1960, p. 375). Professional training helps the FP experts to deal with the health changes effectively. Their pharmacopoeia in both fields must be strong in order to translate the findings of biological investigations into social application. So over and above each technical act, there is a corresponding education function which doubles the value of the act, increases its efficiency and endows it with real human and social value.[16]

We now give some concrete suggestions, which can enable effective communication and information

1. Strengthen Media to Cover Populous Areas Through Audience Segmentation

A recent study conducted by Monis Raza has indicated that the couple protection rate varies from 62 to 68 in different areas. Therefore, there is a need to segment the population areas so that more attention can be paid to low acceptability areas. To quote E.M. Rogers, "We conclude that audience segmentation strategies, which delineate sub-categories of the total audience and aim special messages at them, offer important potential for family planning communication effectiveness."

Joung Whang rightly stresses that sound communication strategies at the grass-roots level require segmentation of individual clients of the community into specific categories, according to geographical and social accessibility, kind of media available to identified clients, particular language and symbols familiar to them level of understanding, level of motivation already attained, level of aspiration, etc. There is a need of Audience research to get feedback, ready reference and analysis for programme planners on various aspects pertaining to audience composition, its habits, tastes, preference, exposure, extent of coverage, impact of the programme.

2. Adequate and Reliable Information based on Research in Bio-medical Aspects of Family Planning

The National Perspective Plan For Women (1988-2000 AD) has rightly stressed the need to educate and inform the people about Family Planning on the basis of genuine research and findings so that they can choose right methods. To quote the Perspective Plan:

> "It is unfortunate that the family planning policy is oriented towards fertility concerned with providing a means for women and men to have control on their own bodies. . . . Research studies have shed light on the fact that the knowledge regarding Family Planning/Methods is low despite the huge amounts of money spent on propaganda. The only method known to all is sterilization. The high rates of abortion show the desire and need of the women for family planning and the failure of the family planning information and services to reach them in time. Laproscopic operations are being performed in several family planning camps without proper care and follow-up. Consequent problems tend to create apprehension among people. More intensive propagation of spacing methods together with innovative strategies for delivery of supplies has to be taken up and spread of information about temporary methods should be accorded high priority."

B.L. Raina has rightly mentioned that it is essential: (a) to understand human reproductive processes; (b) to find out means for modification, adaptation and control of these processes; (c) to know the complexity of human behaviours and its consequences; and (d) to mobilize our knowledge so gained for achievement of our social aims. The knowledge of reproductive processes is still limited. Species differences make the problem more difficult.

3. Research to make Mass Communication More Effective

There is a need of continuous research in the areas of FP Programme Communication activities. Reliance on mass media can reach only to those few who constitute the elite group. If the family planning programme was based only on elite participation, the public relations tools could have some utility because the rest of the population did not matter. But when the success of F.P. Programme is based on total participation, the public relations tools have got to be redevised. There has been no organized attempt to find out new tools and techniques of Public Relations based on a scientific study of the nature of the Public to be reached. The problem calls for intensive research programme to delineate channels of communication for reaching the public. To quote Dinesh Chandra Dubey and Kamla Gopal Rao, "With no pretence of giving a comprehensive review of needed research in mass communication for popularizing family planning, the foregoing review only seeks to highlight some of the important areas of research. While most of research findings in mass communication have been extracted from studies in highly urbanized, modern, western cultures, the authors feel strongly that the insights derived from these studies need to be tested out for their validity in the transitional societies and in developing societies."

4. Impart Training Programmes for Family Planning Education

S.S. Bharara has nicely said that 'The population programme essentially has multi-disciplinary and multi-dimensional characteristics. These disciplines fall within four categories, viz., (i) demography and statistics, (ii) biomedicine, (iii) social and behavioural sciences, and (iv) administration and programme planning. Accordingly, the personnel engaged in the family welfare programme are drawn from these disciplines and are demographers, statisticians, doctors, nurses and other paramedical workers; social scientists, social workers and extension educators; and planners, administrators, supervisors, evaluators, etc. Each discipline represented must be integrated into the whole of the programme in the most effective and efficient manner. Personnel from these disciplines have to be available in adequate number at the front line of action, as well as at other levels of administration, supervision and planning. It necessarily implies that the roles and responsibilities of these personnel will vary according to the level at which they function, even though the ultimate goal remains very much the same. All the personnel, therefore, become co-ordinated parts of a machinery, working as a team, in co-operation with each other, by fully synchronizing their activities. This is what a training programme has to cater to, and produce personnel who will be able to function accordingly.

The roles of each group of functionaries at different levels being so varied, training programmes have to develop correct role-perceptions among the workers and, accordingly correct role-expectations among their supervisors and those higher up in the echelons of administration. The higher the degree of role consensus, the lesser the chances of role conflicts, job dissatisfaction and frustrations.

5. Develop Effective Public Relations

One of the important functions of family welfare administrators is the development of cordial, equitable and harmonious relationships with the beneficiaries to ensure their welfare and participation. The public relations is the establishment of a climate of understanding. The purpose of public relations is not only to supply information, but also to encourage an understanding and co-operation between the social scientists, social workers and beneficiaries.

The management of any public agency should not only employ competent media specialists—those who handle press contacts, prepare news releases, write radio scripts, and carry on other information activities—but it should also create a favourable image of help both inside and outside the agency.[17] The family welfare programmes have not received desired publicity through the publicity media. Our inquiries have shown that the poor coverage was not due to apathy of the press or other media of publicity but due to lack of communication and inadequate release of information on the subject. Publicity is very useful or even essential not only to highlight the programmes and achievements of the organization but to enlist the cooperation of a large number of employees and the goodwill of public, in the implementation of family welfare programme. Many well intentioned and technically sound family welfare programmes, aimed at solving family welfare problems, have been frustrated by lack of popular acceptance and community participation. To quote a WHO Report, "It has been observed that such programmes are either not actively associated or passively ignored because they do not belong to the population they are designed to help; they are rather seen by the population as imposed external programme that belong to the government and consequently deserves and require little, if any, of the population's attention, action, or other response."[18]

Some of the measures which are suggested for improvement of public relations are:

- The help of local office of the press information bureau may be utilized to release photo-features from time to time.
- Local stations of All-India Radio be persuaded to include talks and discussions of family planning work specialists in the field of family welfare. Sometimes, discussions have much better effect than straight talks.

It is desirable to celebrate "Family Welfare Day" in the country every year during which, on a selected theme, publicity can be given through all available media of publicity. "Family Welfare Day" should be observed by all agencies in the field of family planning work from the village to union level on committed basis.

It may be worthwhile introducing printed "news letter" by every State, which can be sent to all State Boards, the Central Board and voluntary organizations concerned, highlighting the major events or developments in the field within their states during the month.

Another dimension of Public Relations in the area of Family Welfare is counselling the people and also those implementing Family Welfare Programmes. Primary Objective of all family services is to ensure that every individual becomes a well adjusted and productive member of a society. Effective delivery of these services depends, not merely on the material resources or well conceived programmes, but also on the quality of the personnel implementing them. So, there is a need of developing good rapport with the personnel responsible for implementation through counselling is defined in the "Encylopaedia of Social Work of India" as a professional activity associated with the process of helping individual or groups with their various problems and extending to developmental ends.

Successful Field Counselling depends on the following factors:

1. The counsellor should be a mature person, with broad outlook; wide interest and sensitiveness to the behavioural pattern and needs of the persons he/she deals with. These qualities are essential for development of a positive relationship, which is an indispensable tool, in addition to knowledge and counselling skill.
2. A field counsellor should have faith in voluntary and State action and their capacity to effectively render family welfare services.
3. A field counsellor is a dynamic and constructive leader with keen sensitivity to the community needs, feelings and attitudes and the capacity to stimulate the agency and the community to work towards goals, established through mutual and continued interaction between the two. He should be a catalytic agent of planned change, rather than a victim of the system.
4. Effective field counselling requires that the counsellor has knowledge of relevant family planning welfare activities of minimum standards for their family of other social services of National, State and Local levels and of Field Counselling Technique.[19]

Thus, public relations including counselling can help in promoting Family Welfare activities. Due care should be taken that the public relations should not degenerate into a propaganda machinery. "Public relations activities must be honest, truthful, open, authoritative and responsible, they must be fair and realistic; and they must be conducted in the public interest." Due safeguards are therefore necessary to make public relations effective for two-ways and authentic communication nerves of family welfare agencies. This traffic can be best organised by professional public relation men, but at the lowest levels of administration, the administrative personnel must do their own public relations. According to F.C. Gem, "It is not enough for mass media to be blaring forth statement in Government's policies and programmes. There must be deliberate and organised attempts also to assess the needs of people to listen to their grievances and to redress them. And the people, particularly the uneducated people must be treated with courtesy instead of being shouted at and compelled to shell out bribes."[20] All this requires dedicated, scientific and well-conceived public relations work.

6. Understand the Area of Operation

Before launching any F.P. programme, the family planning personnel must assess the local problems and must possess the knowledge about the beliefs, conceptions and misconceptions which the people have formed about F.P. activities. It needs to be stressed that the cultural context of F.P. education programme is of the greatest importance in the Indian situation. The social scientists can help the family planning workers through their studies and research.

7. Effective Administrative Machinery to Impart Family Planning Education

There is a lot of wastage and corruption in the conduct of Mass Education in F.P. Programme. Some activities like Drama, Folk Songs, Puppet shows remain only on the paper and thus the huge amount meant for the purpose is either wasted or embezzled. Vehicles supplied for this purpose are wrongly used.

After independence, the family welfare administrative machinery of India advanced considerably, both in magnitude and direction. Administrative efficiency is the most urgent demand of the day. Most of the grievances of the citizens are because of the apathy of the administration and lack of dynamic administration. An international group of public administration experts has also stressed upon this, "Dysfunctional and inapplicable administrative structures, systems and practices must be replaced. Nothing less than dynamic organizations, resourceful management and streamlined administrative processes will suffice . . . the torturous the consuming routines, special privileges, corruption, indolence and insolence often encumbering any governmental bureaucracies and civil services have no place in development administration. This calls for continuous action to foster honesty and integrity and to weed out corruption as well as to develop preventive measure."[21]

8. Develop Attractive Mass-Media Material

No doubt, a vast majority of our people is still unable to read and write. But, literacy is definitely spreading. More importantly, the printed word influences the literate opinion leader in the village like the teacher, panchayat chief, etc. who will be amongst the first to adopt family planning and who will be able to influence his untutored brethren.

9. Motivate Extension Personnel

The quality of the F.P. operations run by Government would be dependent to a great extent upon the quality of extension workers engaged in their operation. Personnel move the administrative machinery. To quote Mrs. Indira Gandhi: "If Government has to do more for the people, its employees must play a more dynamic and more creative role, as the instrument for implementing government policies and programmes."[22]

An extension group cannot work with their heart in it unless they are adequately motivated with reasonable remuneration and prospects of advancement. The emoluments paid to F.P. personnel have been less than those paid to professionals in comparable pursuits, while the task of successful extension is one of the most difficult. If the Extension workers are motivated, this would generate loyalty, co-operation and team work, essential for the achievement of the goals of F.P. Programmes.

Whenever there is a failure of the family planning programme, we generally attribute it to the illiteracy, ignorance and irrational attitudes of the people. On the other hand, we should make a fresh assessment of what the obstacles to family planning success actually are. In order to tackle these problems, IEC can help a great deal in promoting positive attitudes. The obstacles should not be considered as insurmountable barriers. Within each State and Union Territory, there is a need to set-up communication research project to provide information needed to replan the IEC activities to tide over the difficulties. Lyle Saunders has suggested the following change in IEC activities in future:[23]

(i) Family Planning communicators in the future are likely to be more focused on communities as audiences are more concerned with trying to change collective beliefs and values than with informing individuals;

(ii) They may find it necessary to spend more time providing information demanded by more strongly committed political leader, justifying and defending the spread of sterilization and abortion and developing public support for ideas and activities that may be initially unpopular;

(iii) They will be concerned with explaining new kinds of contraceptives and a variety of incentive and disincentive measures;

(iv) They will find themselves working more closely with other special interest communicators in efforts to integrate development programmes and trying to maximize the accuracy and reliance of family planning information provided by communicators with other major interests;

(v) They will have a role to play in changing the image of family planning as a health matter and may both contribute to and learn from the promotional activities of those on the commercial sector who are distributing contraceptives;

(vi) They will be helping to formulate and implement new communication strategies; and

(vii) They may have some new interesting tools to work with its current trends on communication technology.

10. Multi-disciplinary Integrated Approach to Promote Effective Communication

12th joint conference of central council of health and family planning suggested that the revised strategy predicates on multi-disciplinary integrated approach. Addressing the areas beyond family welfare and mobilizing all development agencies and sectors of society directly inter-facing with the people to join in the task of family welfare promotion is a *sine-qua-non* for its success. The communication support for this work will now accordingly have to be through a multi-dimensional integrated thrust.

This requires a far broader vision for family welfare than has prevailed so far. On the one hand, family welfare communication will need to be embedded in primary health care messages and on the other, form an organic part of a core package of social development issues, particularly those relating to female literacy, employment status, age of marriage and child survival:

(i) Therefore, it is necessary that the State MEM organizations and State Education Health Bureau make more co-ordinated use of manpower and material to put out programmes and messages of health and family welfare in an integrated fashion, integration where possible and in any case functional co-ordination of these two units must be done immediately. Along side efforts must be initiated to ensure that health and family welfare IEC efforts link up and co-ordinate with the media efforts for women and child development, adult and non-formal education and youth activities. The budget for Health and Family Welfare IEC must be substantially enhanced.

(ii) The gap between widespread awareness and limited practice of family welfare also calls for different communication approaches which concentrate on effecting behavioural changes more rapidly. Therefore, at the present stage of the programme, greater use must be made of all inter-personnel channels and appropriate training and orientation of all developmental workers to bring about their involvement with family planning. Equally, the reorientation of Health and

Family Welfare workers to enable an internalization of the broader perspective is important.

(iii) With the country presently going through a communication revolution, all media channels must be fully utilized to create an enabling ethos for the programme and as a means to vault the barriers of illiteracy and ignorance. Greater family welfare acceptance is noted where there is greater exposure to media. Towards this end, the Council recommends urgent steps to be taken to ensure greater access to television and radio for the most critical target groups, who presently form the media-deprived class. This is to be done through promotion of group listening and community viewing situations. A pooling of resources for all departments to create such an access must be considered. The greater use of television, film, radio and traditional media must be encouraged to create a synergy between mass media and inter-personal channels. In the case of television, which is a government medium, maximum support must be ensured to health and family welfare issues by earmarking minimum time for programmes on health and family welfare; weaving of appropriate messages in the regular serials and other-sponsored propagation of public service messages on health and family welfare at prime time.

(iv) Altogether, information must move to another plane from general to the specific, giving the how and why on what is required to be done so as to empower people to act on their own behalf. The spirit of family planning communication has to communicate information, not publicity and propaganda. The States may, therefore, like to ensure that the budget for media work are more effectively utilized on developing information, education and communication materials.

(v) As a part of the effort to bring about total mobilization of society and wider involvement of everyone in the programme, strenuous efforts must now be made to secure free publicity and promotion of the family planning programme and its objectives through every possible source. Free display at sports stadiums, bus panels and other commercial channels should be actively solicited and engineered.

(vi) All communication materials and messages must be pretested before application in the field. The pretesting should be done through quick and ready methods so that material can be corrected at appropriate stage.

(vii) Some immediate administrative measures are necessary to revitalize the IEC programme. There are large number of vacancies in the State media set-ups, particularly at the field level. These must be filled in the shortest possible time. The media staff working in the States should be utilized for intensifying IEC programmes, instead of deputing them for routine clerical jobs.

An efficient extension F.P. service, capable of winning people's confidence as their friend, philosopher and guide, takes decades to build up. Careful selection and training, morale-building, service conditions, rational organization—these are the bricks and mortars of the extension officers. Close co-ordination with research, input supply, marketing and guidance, and employment of an effective combination of communication techniques are prerequisites for the successful functioning of the F.P. service. Various management tasks involved in building up such extension service need strengthening.

Notes and References

1. Donald J. Bogue, "A Five Year Information—Education Communication Perspective to meet the Population, Health, Food Crises, 1975-80", in *Family Planning Resumed,* p. 117, Vol. 1, 1977, No. 1.
2. A. Govindachari, 'The Role of Extension Education in Family Planning', in *Aspects of Population Policy in India,* New Delhi, 1969, pp. 124-25, Population Reports Series, Number 35, November 1987, p. 2.
4. Annual Report of the Health Ministry of the Health and Family Welfare, 1998-99, p. 73.
5. H. Koontz and C. O'Donnell, "Principles of Management: An Analysis of Managerial Functions", London, McGraw Hill, Kogakusha Ltd., 1972, pp. 538-40.
6. Chester, I. Barnard, "Functions of the Executive", Cambridge; Harward University Press, 1968, pp. 226-27.
7. W.H. Newman and C.E. Summer, "The Process of Management Concepts Behaviour and Practice", Anglewood, Cliffs, N.J., Prentice Hall, 1961, p. 59.
8. *World Health,* Jan.-Feb. 1989.
9. F.M. Rogers in *Joung Whang,* ed., pp. 130-31.
10. *The Economic Times,* March 9, 1989.
11. WHO, *World Health,* Nov. 1975, p. 14.
12. *Ibid.,* May 1979, p. 25.
13. F.M. Rogers, Management of Family Planning IEC Activities, in *Joung Whang,* (ed.), pp. 116-17.
14. Andreas Fuglesang, "Fold Wisdom and Pseudo Information", in *World Health,* Jan.-Feb. 1989, pp. 6-7.
15. Population Reports, Series 1, Number 35, Nov., 1987, p. 16.
16. WHO Technical Report Series, 1954, No. 89, p. 4.
17. Felix, Nigro A., Modern Public Administration, *op. cit.,* p. 205.
18. *WHO Chronicle,* 30 (1976), pp. 177-78.
19. Central Social Welfare Board, Field Counselling Service, A Pilot Project, 1974, New Delhi, p. 13.
20. F.C. Gera, "Need for Public Relations in Administration", in *IJPA,* Vol. XXI, July-Sept. 1975, pp. 545-56.
21. United Nations Public Administration in the Second United Nations Development Decade, *Ibid.*
22. Presidential Address by Mrs. Indira Gandhi delivered on October 22, 1971, at the Annual Meeting of IIPA, New Delhi.
23. Lyle Saunders, Family Planning Resource, Vol. 1, No. 1, pp. 30-31.

PART III

POLICY-MAKING AND PLANNING

CHAPTER 8

POLICY-MAKING FOR HEALTH ADMINISTRATION

The formulation of realistic and scientific health policy will go a long way towards better planning of health services, however meagre may be our resources. This would ensure health facilities for all especially the people inhabiting the rural areas, urban slums and tribal areas.

—Author

Policy-Making for Health Administration

NATURE AND JURISDICTION

Nature and Significance

Policies may be thought of as the main system which provides the framework for the accomplishment of intended objectives. Formulation of policies involves making explicit, the various assumptions which are made with respect to the basic premises and the priorities of needs and allocating the finances accordingly. Besides, policies are intended to spell out the parameters in the context of which organisational decisions are to be made. Policy is very essential in administration, for it gives a concrete shape to the political and social objectives which the government lays down in the form of laws, rules, regulations, etc. Davis states: "A policy is basically a statement either expressed or implied of those principles and rules that are set-up by executive leadership as guides and constraints for the organization's thought and action. Its principle purpose is to enable executive leadership to relate properly the organization's work to its objectives."

Policies may be looked upon as general guides to action. They may be verbal, written or implied. They set the overall boundaries for action by individuals or groups in an organisational setting. They indicate the framework within which executives may make decisions for the performance of organisational action. According to Ishwar Dayal: "Policy prescribes the aims, the objectives, the targets that would be used to achieve the objectives. Operationally, the policy statement, in this sense, must specify the expected results, the measures for achieving them and mechanism or method with which the results are expected to be achieved. . . . Policy formulation refers to that aspect of administration which is concerned with defining the objective and determining the choice of action. Decision-making refers to the process by which this policy is determined."[1]

DEFINITION OF HEALTH POLICY

The aim of health policy is to secure a fundamental change in health status of people to help break the circle of poverty encircling the masses in the developing world and liberate the population to secure the change that they have chosen and in which they participate. It includes the decisions on medical education, health facilities, health coverage, medical research, choice of systems of medicine, etc. It also includes the decisions as regards the relative role of the government, the private and voluntary agencies in the promotion of health care. The health policy must be made with relevance to the time dimension. It can be a long-term policy, e.g., provision of comprehensive health care to all by the year 2000, or a medium-term, e.g., providing elementary care to all by 1990, or immediate, i.e., covering half the population by 1985 and so on. In the developing world, there is no comprehensive health policy encompassing all the components affecting the health status of the people. There are piece-meal policy decisions about a particular aspect of health care administration. Besides, there is no continuity in the formulation of health policy because of the change of political leadership. Ministry of Health and Family Welfare and the State Health Departments must come out with a Health Policy which can provide a decent health care to all especially the people living in rural areas, urban slums and the tribal areas in 21st century.

The objectives of the policy of health care delivery system are described as under:

1. To provide universal coverage and enable the whole population to have access to the type of services best suited to their state of health, richness or disablement.
2. To provide comprehensive, preventive, curative and rehabilitative health services for whoever requires them, without financial or other bars and making the best possible use of the available scientific and technological knowledge.
3. To reduce the cost of treatment, giving priority to primary care and services of a preventive and ambulatory type and reserving hospital treatment for those who need it. The hospital standard should correspond to the average standard of living of the population covered.
4. To decentralize health care through a system of levels of care designed so that each person enters the system through the level best equipped to provide the form of treatment most suited to his individual needs and that all services, from the primary up to the specialized level, are accessible to whoever

needs them through an information and referral system.

5. To organize the "health team", composed of professional, technical and auxiliary staff in various disciplines who assume responsibility for the health of the community, acting individually at different levels but with their activities coordinated through an effective system of communication and supervision.

Relationship between Policy-making and Planning (Refer Chart 8.1)

Planning and policy-making are inter-related. Policy determines the principle for action and planning provides the instrument for the application of policy and review. Policy decisions are needed in the planning process and in defining its goals and limitations (Chart 8.1).

CHART 8.1

Relationship between Policy and Plan

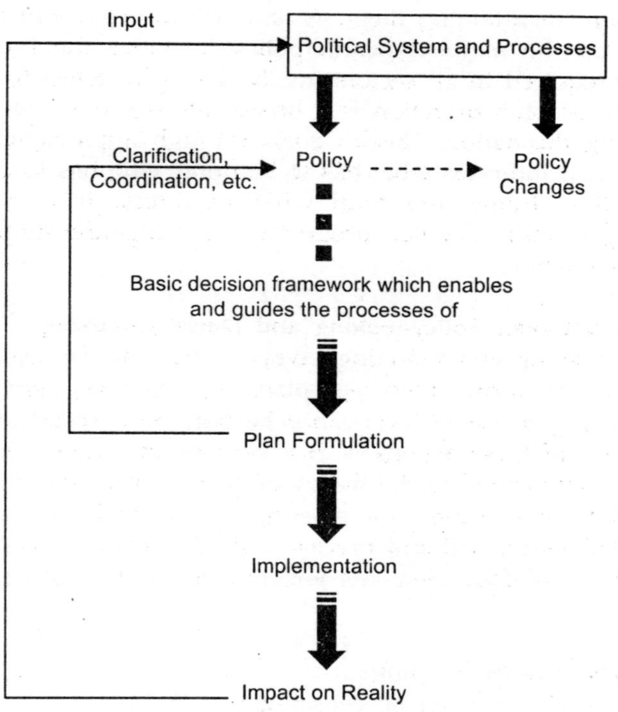

Therefore, planners who ignore policy only jeopardize the good results of their endeavours. On the other hand, a planning process has various possible feedback effects on policy. For example:

(a) it requires explicit policy statements, thus bringing certain subjects to the political arena;

(b) it should reflect the rationale of the policies, show how they can be implemented, and indicate their financial and other implications;

(c) it provides the policy-making with instruments for dialogue, coordination, mobilisation of resources; and continuity of action; and

(d) its impact on the national situation should influence future policy-making.

The Executive Board of WHO has stated (Health for All, Series No. 2, p. 14) that:

> "National policies, strategies and plans of action form a continuum, and there are no sharp dividing lines between them . . . . "A national health policy is an expression of goals for improving the health situation, the priorities among those goals, and the main direction for attaining them. A national strategy, which should be based on the national health policy, includes the broad lines of action required in all sectors involved to give effect to that policy. A national plan of action is a broad inter-sectoral master plan for attaining the national health goals through implementation of this strategy. It indicates what has to be done, who has to do it, during what time frame and with what resources. It is a framework leading to more detailed programming, budgeting, implementation and evaluation."

Relationship between Policy-making and Decision-making

Policy-making and planning involve decisions. Decision-making is the core of policy formulation and planning. Man has been performing the act of taking decisions ever since he became a social animal but a scientific study of these actions is of a very recent origin. During World War II, some studies led to the theory of decisions. Today, the process of decision-making has become the essence of any productive activity. It is an act of intelligence, will and precision. B. Governay suggests that there are a minimum of four elements which when put together result in a decision:

(a) There must be choice.
(b) The choice must be conscious.
(c) The choice must be oriented by various purposes.
(d) The choice must lead to an action.

It is essential to understand the meaning and art of decision-making to formulate scientific and sound health policies. Webster's dictionary defines decision-making as 'the art of determining in one's own mind upon an opinion or courses of actions'. According to W. Brooke Groves, "Decision-making is the selection from two or more reasonable possibilities of a course that will, at the time and under the circumstances, provide the suitable solution of the problem at hand."

It is essential for the policy-makers to keep in mind the five steps mentioned below while taking decisions. (Refer Chapter 8 for decision-making).

Thus we see that decision-making is an important constituent of the processes of policy-making and planning as the decisions weave individual choices into a web of relationship which constitute a policy. According to Herbert A. Simon, decision-making comprises three principal phases: (i) finding occasions for making a decision; (ii) finding possible courses of action; and (iii) choosing among courses of action. The first phase has been described as intelligence activity, the second phase as design activity, and the third phase as choice activity. This analysis of the process of decision-making has special reference for the policy-makers and planners in the Government as they are to ensure that the policies based on such decisions are not only correct and just but must also appear to be correct and just to the people at large.

Existing Health Policy

A Statement on the "National Health Policy" was laid on the Table of both the Houses of Parliament on the second November 1982. The National Health Policy was discussed at length in both Houses and was approved by the Rajya Sabha on fourth August 1983, and the Lok Sabha on 22nd December, 1983. The Policy lays stress on the preventive, promotive, public health and rehabilitative aspects of health care services to reach the population in the remotest areas of the country, the need to view health and human development as a vital component of overall integrated national socio-economic development, decentralized system of health and care delivery with the maximum community and individual self-reliance and participation. The policy also lays stress on ensuring adequate nutrition, safe drinking water supply and improved sanitation for all segments of the population. The policy sets out specific goals to be achieved by 1985, 1990, 1995 and 2000 A.D. in pursuance of the national commitment for the attainment of the goal of Health For All by 2000 A.D.

R.K. Sapru in his Article, "Health Care Policy and Administration in India" in *IJPA*, July-Sept. 1997 is right in his criticism of the present Health Policy to quote him:

> The preceding analysis of the health care policy and administration indicates that although India has adopted the NHP in the contest of the world-wide objective of "Health for All by 2000 AD" now re-oriented towards "Health for Under Privileged", yet the country is nowhere near attainment of this objective. Efforts since 1974

have not yielded results in consonance with the health care objectives. As such, sustained efforts are needed to improve the health status of the people in order to raise it to the acceptable Standards. Considering the efforts so far made in the field of health by the Centre and States, one comes across the major gaps in the current health policy requiring urgent attention.

Ninth Plan has felt the need of formulating New Health Policy to suit the changed conditions in 21st century.

"2000 AD is just two years away. The time is therefore, appropriate for review of achievements against the set goals in the National Health Policy. During the last two decades there have been major changes in disease profile, health care infrastructure and health care seeking behaviour of the population. Several newer technologies for diagnosis and management of health problems have become available. These, in turn, have widened the gap between what is possible and what is feasible and affordable at the level of the individual and the country. Increasing expectations of the population, rising cost of diagnosis and treatment and diminishing resources have brought into fore the issue of how to meet the rising health care costs. The essential inter-linkages between health services delivery and health manpower development are still not fully understood and operationalized. Taking all these into consideration it is essential that the National Health Policy undergoes a re-appraisal and re-formulation so that it provides a reliable and relevant policy framework not only for improving health care, but also measuring and monitoring the health care delivery systems and health status of the population during the next two decades."

Suggestions to Improve Policy-Making (Refer Chart 8.2)

Before this new policy is adopted, it is suggested that the general administrators and health experts should keep in mind the genuine health needs of the people and motivate the political actors to formulate balanced health policy based on scientific methods. The health administrators must keep the following facts in mind to frame effecitve, efficient and relevent health policies.

1. Policies should be made in Consonance with the Objectives

By goal or objective is meant the end towards which action is directed. Since a policy is a guidance for action, it is reasonable to expect that a policy indicates the direction towards which action is guided, either explicitly or implicitly. For this reason, students of policy sciences often define public policies as a programme of goals and objectives.

2. Absence of Contradictions and Inconsistencies

It is necessary for public administators to help in making policies purposeful and goal-oriented, and to assist in defining goals and

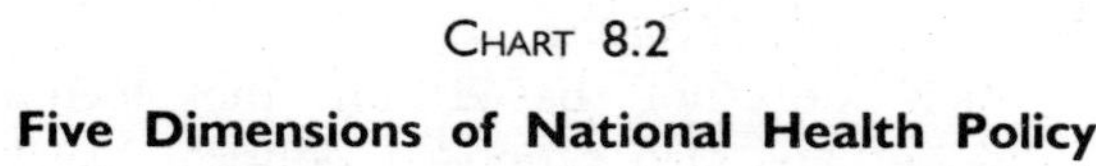

CHART 8.2

Five Dimensions of National Health Policy

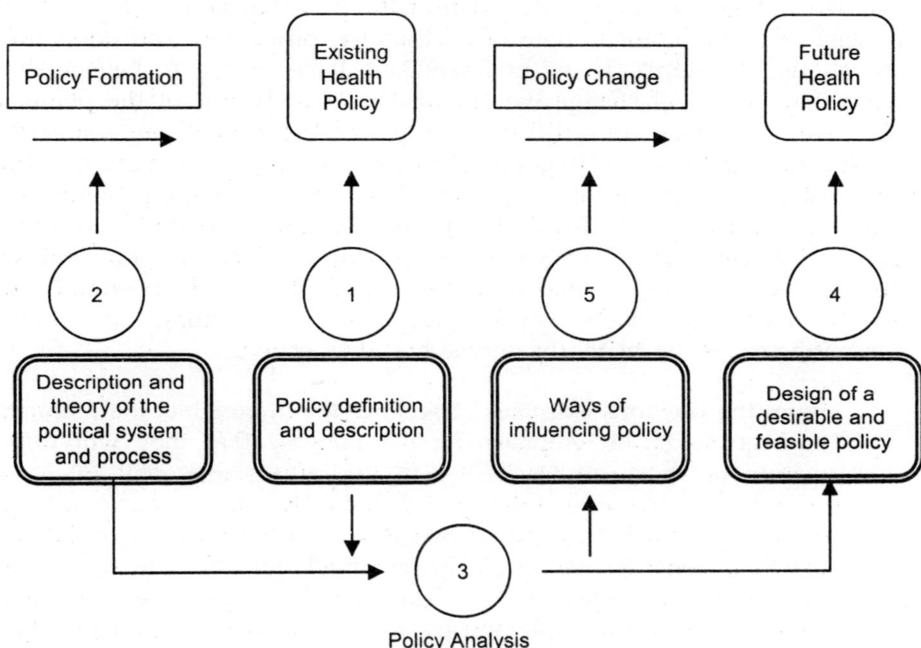

objectives clearly, in making them concrete and also quantifiable if possible and in removing, to the extent possible, any contradictions and inconsistencies.

3. Temporal Dimensions

The modern world is rapidly changing. So, our policies must not remain constant but should change with the change in times. A UN report suggests the following three points:

(a) It is a well-known fact that a public policy, in order to be effective, must not be too little or too late;

(b) Time sequence is an essential part of a successful policy. An effective policy should comprise not only what a government should do but also when to do one thing after another. Timing is often an essential factor for the success or failure of a policy; and

(c) Synchronization is another timing element. Something, for example, what is required is not only that action '2' should follow action '1' but also that action '3' should be taken at the same time as action '4'.

4. Feasibility, Probability and Possibility

Policies which are not based on the technical, economic, administrative and perhaps also proposed political feasibility should be avoided unless it is the specific wish of the policy-makers to adopt such policies. It is important to note that feasibility, probability and possibility are all relative terms. If the policy-makers have reason to believe that what they plan will change the circumstances in favour of the planned objectives, then they are justified in the planning for what may appear to be 'Improbable' or even 'Impossible' to the experts who assume that the circumstances will remain constant. For the developing countries, estimates by experts on feasibility, probability and possibility are often poorly informed guess-work, in part owing to lack of sufficient or decisive evidence and in part owing to a high degree of uncertainty. In a UN document which warns against 'paper planning' and blind commitments to the blatantly impossible, it is stated:

> From the previous extremes of seeking the impossible, the planners may go so far in emphasizing the possible that they will think mainly of short-run feasibility. In this effort, they will often be encouraged by economists who have become accustomed to fighting utopia with myopia, that is with 'hard nosed' calculations of small benefits that might be obtained quickly. The result can easily be that instead of planning for the impossible, they will focus upon most possible and feasible of all, namely, the inevitable. This is the fallacy of epiphenomenal planning. Here the main advantage is that the planners can take credit for any minor progress that might have taken place.

5. Relevant Forecasts and Projections

According to a UN report "Forecasting and projections are important for public policy-making mainly for two reasons. First, as just indicated, policy is a guidance for action that lies necessarily in the future. Therefore, no rational approach to policy-making is possible without some basis for making assumptions about the future. Forecasting and projection can assist policy-makers in this respect. Secondly, public policies should be used, if at all possible, to avoid crisis rather than to meet crisis and may have to devote most of its resources to crisis management. At the same time, a government which is under constant pressure from immediate crisis may not be able to devote its attention and resources to the future in order to prevent the recurrence of crisis. This is a vicious circle which a government should break, and it can succeed in doing so only by assigning suitable priority to forecasting the future."

6. Appropriate Administrative Machinery

Within the central policy cluster there should also be special arrangement for ensuring that appropriate administrative machinery is established for:

(a) policy and plan implementation,
(b) reporting and feedback,
(c) evaluation and control, and
(d) the adjustment and revision of policies, plans and programmes.

This would ensure effective relationships between policy formulation and policy implementation.

7. Understanding the Implication of Policy

Policies must be interpreted and explained, to all members of the organisation. What people do not understand they cannot use correctly and are likely to distrust. Therefore, there is a need to explain it to all persons to whom it applies.

8. Environmental Considerations

Policy is based on actual information or factual data which can be collected from a number of sources by applying different methods. But, before the data can be changed into a policy, many factors have to be taken into consideration e.g., policies must be made in accordance with the provisions of the constitution and the laws enacted by the legislature; these must also be made in accordance with the social, political, cultural, economic and ethical environment prevailing in the country; these must also be linked with the agencies interested in the same policy to have maximum utility and effectiveness; these must also be made in accordance with the opinion of the public otherwise they (the people) would not cooperate with the government in their executive.

Five Dimensions of National Health Policy

Dr. Karan Singh has rightly said that, "if the nation wants a first class health care service with special emphasis on nutrition and child health and the combating of communicable diseases, it will have to readjust its priorities so that adequate inputs are made available during the current and subsequent periods."

Perhaps never before the need to reassess our priorities was as great as it is today. The formulation of realistic and scientific health policy based upon our realistic assessment understanding of our health needs and problems and approaches to deal with them will go a long way towards better planning of health services, however meagre may be our resources.

While reviewing the national health policies the following issues need consideration:

1. Geographical coverage of the population with at least all the essential components of primary health care and the corresponding referral system.
2. A system of financing health care ensuring that all strata of society have an equal opportunity to avail themselves of such care.
3. Coverage of particular population groups, such as mothers and children, working women, school children, workers, and the elderly, and any particular risk group.
4. Preferential allocation of health resources to under-privileged population groups.
5. Facilities available.
6. Rational referred system.
7. Improvement of the human environment by progressive providing safe drinking-water to the whole population, building up waste disposal system, and ensuring clean air.
8. Improvement of communicable and non-communicable diseases.
9. Securing adequate food production and supply and proper nutrition.
10. Community mobilization in planning and development, including promotion of collective responsibility for the health and health care of the community and its constituent families and individuals.
11. Relevant health technologies.
12. Development of human and financial resources for health.

Besides, the existing national health policy has not laid down any programme of action like National Policy on education. There is no mechanism to monitor the implementation of health policy. There are a number of the deficiencies in the existing national health policy.

The government of India should appoint a team to review the existing National health policy and suggest the New policy based on actual and perceived needs of the people. This can be examined at various levels before sending it to Parliament for their comments, discussion and approval. A health policy for 21st century should not be designed by tinkering the current health policy here and there, but should be designed afresh to take into account the past performance and potential problems to be encountered in the 21st century.

Ninth Five Year Plan has made a modest plan to improve upon the targets fixed in National Health Policy upto the year ending 2000. However, there is a need to formulate new health policy to suit the changed circumstances in new millennium.

Note and Reference

1. Ishwar Dayal, "Organisation for Public Policy in government," a paper submitted to the Seventeenth Conference of the Indian Institute of Public Administration, 30 Oct., 1973.

CHAPTER 9

PLANNING FOR HEALTH CARE ADMINISTRATION

> Health Planning is in essence an organised, conscious and continual exercise to select the best available alternatives which can meet the health needs of the people.
>
> —Author

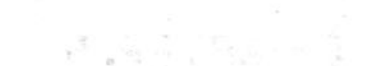

Planning for Health Care Administration

MEANING AND DEFINITIONS

Planning of community health services means the careful analysis, intelligent interpretation and orderly development of these services, in accordance with modern knowledge, techniques, and experience, to meet the health needs of a nation within its resources.[1] A health plan is a predetermined course of action that is firmly based on the nature and extent of health problems, from which are devised priority goals.[2] Health planning is an aid to political and administrative authorities to decide how health services can be modernised and improved to provide effective and decent health care to the community. Health planning is not an independent exercise, it is an integral part of the overall socio-economic development. National Health Planning has been defined as the orderly process of defining community health problems, identifying unmet needs and surveying the resources to meet them, establishing priority goals that are realistic and feasible and projecting administrative action to accomplish the purpose of the proposed programme.[3] Planning is essentially a process of making choice between available alternatives at all levels of decision-making. Planning is the exercise of intelligence to deal with facts and solutions as they are and find a way to solve problems. Planning is, in essence, an organised, conscious and continual attempt to select the best available alternatives to achieve specific goals. As expressed by Ackoff (1970, p. 1):

> "Planning is one of the most complex and difficult intellectual activities in which man can engage. Not to do it well is not a sin, but to settle it for doing it less than well is."

According to Dr. Montoya:

"Health Planning is the phase of the total process which leads from the policy statements to the concrete identification of the populations whose needs and demands will be served; the indication of the types of activities that will be performed for those populations, with their general attributes, and the specification of the type of instruments that will be required to carry out the activities."[4]

DEVELOPMENT OF HEALTH PLANS (Refer Chart 9.1)

Planning is a rational process which involves a number of steps. It is a highly complicated process. We discuss here the important steps which may be kept in mind while planning health services at any level, i.e. Union, State or Local. Whatever be the methodology of planning, these basic steps are essential. The details of these steps may vary from country to country.

1. Pre-Planning

Effective health planning would depend upon the interest of the government as manifested by clear policies framed by the political authorities and the health legislation enacted by the legislature. Besides, there should be an infrastructure to plan for health care. Administrative capability and skill in planning is the most important attribute of the health planning. The twenty-first session of the Regional Committee of South-East Asia held a technical discussion on National Health Planning in 1968. They mainly concentrated their deliberations on the pre-planning stage. The main recommendations of the technical discussion were:

(a) Even though there are health planning units at present in some countries of the Region, it is necessary to strengthen these units as well as the relationship that exists between them and the National Planning Units.
(b) It is necessary to develop urgently realistic health plans as a part of development plans. This apart from other advantages, make it possible for funds for health aspects of development projects to be obtained from the resources of such projects.
(c) In the pre-planning stage, the government should establish health planning units and health administrators should be adequately represented on the national planning bodies.
(d) Heads of planning units should be given a formal course of training.[5]

2. Analysis of Health Situation

The first step at this stage involves:

CHART 9.1

Health Planning

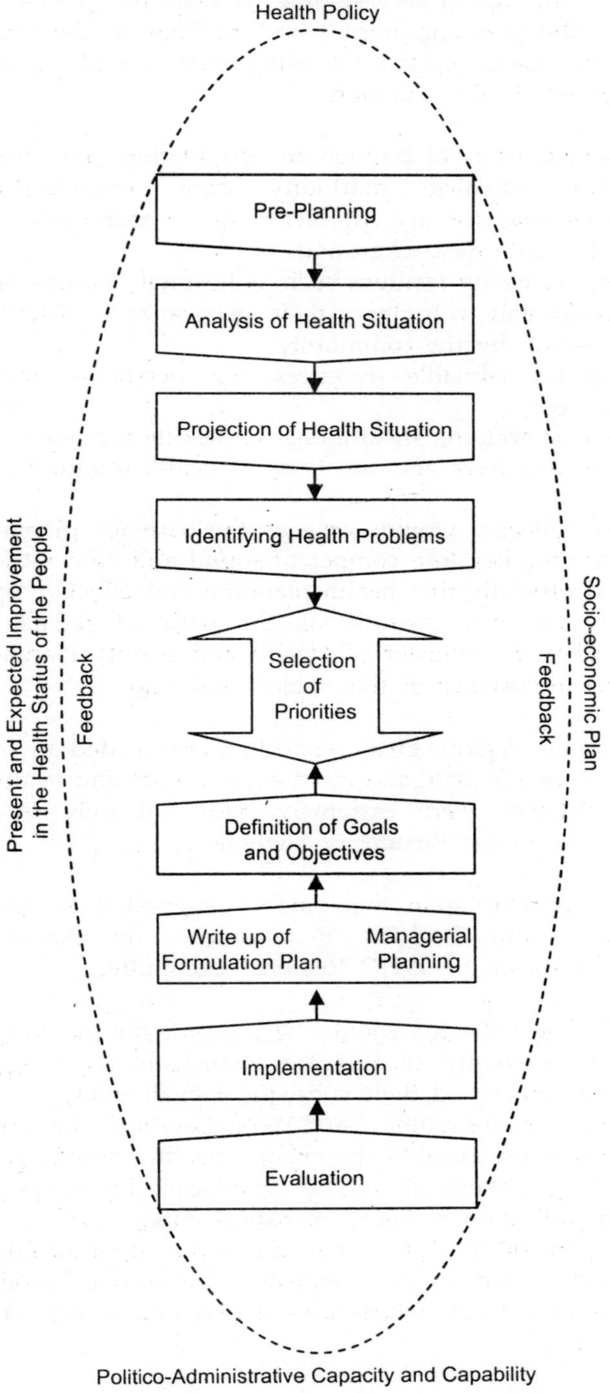

Health Policy

Pre-Planning

Analysis of Health Situation

Projection of Health Situation

Identifying Health Problems

Selection of Priorities

Definition of Goals and Objectives

Write up of Formulation Plan

Managerial Planning

Implementation

Evaluation

Present and Expected Improvement in the Health Status of the People

Feedback

Socio-economic Plan

Feedback

Politico-Administrative Capacity and Capability

Assessment of the Present Health Situation

This relates to a time from which the planning is to be done. It is nothing but setting up of a base line to help the planners to make projections for the planning period and to help in the evaluation of plans. Generally speaking, the following data would be required to analyse the present health situation:

(a) Characteristics of population—population (age, sex) cause of death statistics, morbidity data, environmental data responsible for the problems of environmental threats to health, cultural background.
(b) Data on health facilities such as hospitals, clinics, etc.—public, private and voluntary, their geographical distribution and utilisation by the community.
(c) Data on available resources, e.g. personnel, material, and finance.
(d) Data on training institutions for health personnel.
(e) Data on nature and functions of health organisations.

The data collected would serve as the base for planning. Health statistics provide the key to a competent sound and efficient planning. It has been stated officially that health planning and effective operation of health services are only possible on the basis of reliable statistics.[6] Dr. Chandrasekhar, Ex-minister of Health and Family Planning (India), emphasised the importance of this subject and said:

> "All over the region, greater efforts were needed to have better, further, more adequate and more reliable vital and health statistics. Health statistics were extremely poor not only in India but undoubtedly in the Region as a whole."[7]

We can improve upon this data as suggested by the technical discussion on Health Statistics Requirements for National Health Planning by experts of the WHO Regional Committee:

(1) The data collected should be relevant for planning purposes and sufficiently reliable for a realistic planning of health programmes and their subsequent evaluation.
(2) Closer coordination and collaboration between health statisticians, health planners, health administrators and decision-makers should be established for proper collection and utilisation of health statistical data.
(3) In view of the inadequate development of health statistical services and scarce statistical resources, production of superfluous data which are not required or utilised should be avoided.

(4) Training of health statistical personnel—at the professional, intermediate and lower levels—should be continued and strengthened.
(5) Data-processing facilities should be developed and strengthened.
(6) The most desirable form of organisation of health statistical services at the national level would be an adequately staffed single unit, preferably one of the same rank as other technical divisions of the Ministry of Health or of the Directorate of Health Services. Such a unit should coordinate all the health statistical activities in the country.
(7) An endeavour should be made to extend the coverage of cause-of-death statistics, but, where it is not possible to have the cause of death certified by a physician, it was felt that the reporting by auxiliary and lay personnel could be accepted.[8]

The second step under analysis is projection of the health situation over the plan period. This can be done on the basis of assumptions which can predict as to what is likely to happen at the end of plan period.

3. Identifying Health Problems

On the basis of the projected data, we can enumerate the health problems which need to be tackled by the plans.

Current problems faced by the Health Care System, as analysed by Ninth Plan include:

1. Persistent gaps in manpower and infrastructure especially at the primary health care level.
2. Sub-optimal functioning of the infrastructure; poor referral services.
3. Plethora of hospitals not having appropriate manpower, diagnostic and therapeutic services and drugs in Government, voluntary and private sector.
4. Massive interstate/interdistrict differences in performance as assessed by health and demographic indices; availability and utilisation of services are poorest in the most needy states/ districts.
5. Sub-optimal intersectoral coordination.
6. Increasing dual disease burden of communicable and non-communicable diseases because of ongoing demographic, lifestyle and environmental transitions.
7. Technological advances which widen the spectrum of possible interventions.
8. Increasing awareness and expectations of the population regarding health care services.

9. Escalating costs of health care, ever widening gaps between what is possible and what the individual or the country can afford.[9]

4. Selection of Priorities

Resources in the developing countries are limited. Mydral has forthrighly said, "The now widely used term 'Developing countries' is one of these diplomatic euphemisms. . . . the really important aspect of their situation and the meaning that seeks expression is not that they are developing, but they are under-developed, that they need to develop, and that they ought to develop, and in some cases are planning to develop."[10]

J. Brijant has also pointed out that, "The rates of economic growth for many of the less-developed countries provide a sombre picture for their future. They indicate that now and in the foreseeable future resources will be desperately limited. Indeed these limitations are relentless determinants of design of health services."[11]

Thus, available resources are insufficient to meet the needs of the people. Therefore, there is a need to select the pressing and urgent problems. There are a number of factors (economical, technical, financial, social, political, administrative, ethical, etc.) which must be taken into consideration while laying down the priorities. This can be decided with the help of techniques like cost-benefit analysis, cost-effectiveness. Priorities have to be determined at different levels. The first level is determination of priorities among various sectors of the economy. This would depend, to a large extent, upon the political philosophy of the government.

5. Definition of Goals and Objectives

Goal is the direction in which the plan is to proceed and the term is used more in the case of long-term planning. Goals formulated are generally broad. A goal is usually described in terms of:

(a) what is to be attained;
(b) the extent to which it is to be attained;
(c) the population involved;
(d) the geographic areas in which the proposed programme will operate; and
(e) the length of time required for achieving these goals.[12]

The objective is a precise statement of the ends intended to be achieved. We must build the hierarchy of objectives, i.e. ultimate, intermediate and immediate. Immediate objectives are further divided into effort objectives and performance objectives (targets).

6. Write-up of Formulated Plan

After deciding the priorities, goals and objectives, the next major step is to prepare a write-up of the plan. This may contain a schedule (time sequence for the plan to be implemented) and procedures (a set of rules for implementing the plan) and other details so that evaluation becomes easy and meaningful.

Before we embark upon the planning of health services, we must keep in mind the finances allocated for health. The finances allocated from 1st to 8th Plan vary from 3.3 to 1.75 percent for health and .01 to 1.50 percent for family planning which is quite inadequate. Ninth Plan should allocate more resources.

7. Strategy

Strategy should be defined. Ninth Plan has laid down the following approach to be followed in Ninth Plan:

(i) An absolute and total commitment to improve access to, and enhance the quality of primary health care in urban and rural areas by providing an optimally functioning primary health care system as a part of the Basic Minimum Services;

(ii) To improve the efficiency of existing health care infrastructure at primary, secondary and tertiary care settings through appropriate institutional strengthening, improvement of referral linkages and operationalisation of Health Management Information System (HMIS);

(iii) To promote the development of human resources for health, adequate in quantity and appropriate in quality so that access to essential health care services is available to all so that there is improvement in the health status of community, periodically organise programmes for continuing education in health sciences, update knowledge and upgrade skills of all workers and promote cohesive team work.

(iv) To improve the effectiveness of existing programmes for control of communicable diseases to achieve horizontal integration of ongoing vertical programmes at the district and below district level; to strengthen the disease surveillance with the focus on rapid recognition, reporting and response at district level; to promote production and distribution of appropriate vaccines of assured quality at affordable cost; to improve water quality and environmental sanitation; to improve hospital infection control and waste management;

(v) To develop and implement integrated non-communicable disease prevention and control programme within the existing health care infrastructure;

(vi) To undertake screening for common nutritional deficiencies especially in vulnerable groups and initiate appropriate remedial measures; to evolve and effectively implement programmes for improving nutritional status, including micro-nutrient status of the population;

(vii) To strengthen programmes for prevention, detection and management of health consequences of the continuing deterioration of the ecosystems; to improve linkage between data from ongoing environmental monitoring and that on health status of the population residing in the area including health impact assessment as a part of environmental assessment in developmental projects;

(viii) To improve the safety of the work environment and workers' health in organised and unorganised industrial and agricultural sectors especially among vulnerable groups of the population.

(ix) To develop capabilities at all levels for emergency and disaster prevention and management; to implement appropriate management systems for emergency, disaster, accident and trauma care at all levels of health care;

(x) To ensure effective implementation of the provisions for food and drug safety; strengthen the food and drug administration both at the Centre and in the States;

(xi) To increase the involvement of ISM&H practitioners in meeting the health care needs of the population;

(xii) To enhance research capability with a view to strengthening basic, clinical and health systems research aimed at improving the quality and outreach of services at various levels of health care;

(xiii) To increase the involvement of voluntary, private organisations and self-help groups in the provision of health care and ensure inter-sectoral coordination in implementation of health programmes and health-related activities; and

(xiv) To enable the Panchayati Raj Institutions (PRI) in planning and monitoring of health programmes at the local level so that there is greater responsiveness to health needs of the people and greater accountability; to promote inter-sectoral coordination and utilise local and community resources for health care.[13]

8. Implementation

Plan implementation is an integral part of the planning process. It requires responsibility for translating the objectives of health plan into action. However, looking from the broader point of view, plan implementation requires cooperation, coordination and commitment at all levels of the implementing machinery starting with the Ministries of Health at the Union and State levels through to the various non-secretariat organisations in the field at the district, block or village level.

It is at the implementation level that the difficulties creep in resulting in lower output. Implementation must be watched properly and timely action should be taken to improve administrative, technical, financial or personnel inadequacies.

9. Monitoring or Managerial Planning

In developing countries, there is a large gap between planning and implementation. Monitoring can help in improving the situation through advance fixing of targets to be achieved in a short period of time. We can compare the achievement targets with the targets planned. If there is a gap between the two, we can locate the reasons and take remedial action. Monitoring helps to verify whether the performance is according to the time schedule.

10. Evaluation

Evaluation is a built-in device to measure the effectiveness of health planning. "Evaluation measures the degree to which objectives and targets are fulfilled and the quality of the result obtained. It measures the productivity of available resources in achieving clearly defined objectives. It measures how much output or cost effectiveness is achieved. It makes possible the re-allocation of priorities and of resources on the basis of changing health needs."[14] Dr. J.E. Asvall, Deputy Director, Bureau of Hospitals, Director General of Health Services, Oslo, Norway in his article, "Evaluation of Public Programme" mentions the problems of evaluation of health programmes. He says that inadequate evaluation is a serious weakness in health services. A key factor to the improvement of the whole health care system, evaluation has not so far been developed in the country to such a level that it fulfils the requirements of planning and management.[15] The ultimate test of evaluation should be perceptible change in the health status of the people and improvement of the quality of life. In a Foreword to the Fifth Five Year Plan, 1974-79, Prime Minister, Mrs. Indira Gandhi writes:

> "A plan is ultimately neither a mere catalogue of schemes nor a sophisticated exercise in numbers. It is a charter of the progress of a people who refuse to be overwhelmed by the magnitude and vast variety of their problems and difficulties but are courageously struggling to map out a programme of action which will step by step and year by year help to overcome them."[16]

Constraints on Health Planning

There are a large number of factors which stand in the way of effective health planning. We should try to overcome or minimise these constraints. These are as follows:

(a) Lack of adequate health information system for planning and monitoring and ultimately for evaluation.

(b) Natural resistance to change.

(c) The relatively low priority often accorded to health by political decision-makers and the public.

(d) The frequency of governmental, political, and administrative changes, with concurrent changes in commitments to support the plan.

(e) The imperfect state of the art of planning, i.e. absence of trained health administrators and planners, and particularly the lack of precise tools to measure need, demand, cost and benefit.

(f) The 'long time' lag between planning and implementation, particularly as regards the supply of additional health manpower and the enactment of necessary legislation.

(g) The traditional division of health professionals into compartments and the resultant lack of adequate inter-professional communication.

(h) The inflexibility of educational system.

(i) Inefficient administrative practices that limit the flexibility of the budgets, promote fragmented programmes, and result in inappropriate personnel system.

(j) Inadequate coordination of planning between the various ministries and departments concerned with socio-economic development.

FORMULATION OF HEALTH PLAN IN INDIA

Planning Machinery at Various Levels

Let us now discuss in brief the planning machinery responsible for the formulation of health plan in India.

India has perhaps the largest tradition of planning in any non-socialist country. The nearest parallel to it in Western Europe is the French System of planning. The main difference, however, is that India has a federal structure of Government and achievement of socialist pattern of society is her avowed objective. The Planning Commission was established in March 1950, the Commission was required:

(a) to make an assessment of material, capital and human resources as well as formulate development plans for the most effective utilisation of these resources for improvement of social human and economic conditions in the country;

(b) to indicate the obstacles in the way of planned economic and social development in the country and suggest ways and means to the government to deal with them;

(c) to suggest any change or addition to the administrative system for effective implementation of development plans proposed by it and approved by the government; and

(d) to carry out appraisals, from time to time, of the progress achieved in implementation of the development plans by the administrative agencies or departments concerned and to suggest ways and means for improving the scale and quality of this implementation.

The Commission comprises a number of members at its head as well as a body of experts, administrators and house-keeping personnel which constitute its secretariat. So far as the members are concerned, some of them are whole-time while a few are part-time. For the preparation of Ninth Plan, for instance, there were 7 members, out of which 5 were whole-time experts including Vice-Chairman while 4 were *ex-officio* i.e., Prime Minister, the Finance Minister, the External Affairs Minister and the Planning Minister. There is, however, no fixed strength and thus the exact number of members may vary from time to time, depending upon several factors.

The Secretariat of the Commission includes three wings:

(i) General Divisions, (ii) Subject Divisions, and (iii) House-keeping Divisions.

There are at present 12 general divisions which concern themselves with the studies relating to the Plan as a whole. The branches are: (a) Perspective Planning, (b) Statistics and Surveys, (c) Economic Research, (d) Socio-Economic Research, (e) Plan Coordination, (f) Programme Administration, (g) Multi-level Planning, (h) Project and Information, (i) Scientific Research, and (j) Plan Information and Publicity.

There is also a Programme Evaluation Organisation which scientifically evaluates the results achieved in terms of the objectives and targets of various Sector plans, State plans, programme and projects which together comprise the National Development Plan.

Then there are 14 Subject Divisions: (a) Agriculture, (b) Land Reforms, (c) irrigation, (d) power, (e) Transport, (f) Communication, (g) Education, (h) Employment and Manpower, (i) Health and Family Welfare, (j) Housing and Urban Development, (k) Industry and Minerals, (l) Village and Small Scale Industries, (m) Social Planning, and (n) Social Welfare.

These divisions maintain intimate relationship with their counterparts in the Central Ministries and State government departments. They collect, process and analyse relevant information and data as well as sponsor research for use by the Commission in the formulation of sector plans and programmes.

The House-keeping Divisions deal with records, Accounting and Routine Administration.

The Subject Divisions carry out most of the Planning excercises. Each Division utilises working or expert groups on which the concerned

Ministry is represented. At the Central level, a Health Planning Section was created in the Employment and Social Services Division of the Planning Commission in October 1951. In April 1956, it was made a separate and independent division. As a 'Subject Division' it helps the Planning Commission in the formulation of the health programmes and projects to be incorporated in the five-year and annual plans. It assists in evaluating performance. It carries out studies of special interest to health planning, e.g. manpower requirements of health programmes. The division works in close cooperation with the Ministry of Health and Family Welfare so that there may be an intimate relation between planners and those who carry out policies. Each division utilises working or expert group for preparation of the plan in their respective fields. The directions given to working groups are of a general nature in the beginning but becomes much more specific as the preparation of a five-year plan proceeds towards completion. The planning unit in the Ministry of Health and Family Welfare has the following functions:

(a) compilation of national five-year health plan and supporting material;
(b) development of strategy for getting plans accepted and financed;
(c) preparation of the central, annual health plan and discussions with the Planning Commission and the Ministry of Finance;
(d) discussion and coordination with States on matters relating to planning developments and the financing and implementation of plans; and
(e) submission of progress reports on planning schemes to the Planning Commission.

Thus, the health plans prepared by the Division in collaboration with the Ministry of Health and Family Welfare is reviewed by the members of the Planning Commission and is integrated with the total plan.

Most of the health work is carried out at the State level. Health services are primarily the responsibility of the State. State Planning Boards have been set-up in many parts of India. These boards are to prepare the draft State plans by bringing about consultations between the experts, ministers, and other decision-makers as well as by seeking the views and demands of the district administration and other organisations. Except in a few States, the State planning boards have, however, yet to establish their role in a meaningful manner. They lack adequate expertise and creativity. Their position as the 'thinking tank' of the Government on social and economic problems has yet to demonstrated and proved. *The Tribune* Editorial has rightly stated that:

"In most States, the Planning Boards, like several 'autonomous' Corporations, have been made sanctuaries for disgruntled, defeated or troublesome politicians who tend to treat Plan funds as discretionary grants. Sinecures were deemed necessary to ensure the political support of such politicians in the struggle for ministerial survival amidst recurring toppling drives.

Inevitably, such political accommodation has led to the minimum involvement of economic experts who alone should comprise State Planning Boards. It is time the pollution of planning through politics was ended."[17]

The programme advisers are responsible for coordination and cooperation between the Union Ministry of Health and Family Welfare, the Planning Boards at the State level, the Planning Bureau of the State Departments of Health, especially as regards the allocation of resources and the determination of priorities during the five-year plan. The various groups concerned have strong preferences and influences. The programme advisors have to reconcile these conflicting interests without much friction. The Planning Commission submits the plan to the National Development Council. The Council comprises the Prime Minister as the Chairman and the Chief Ministers of States as Members while the Members of Planning Commission are its *ex-officio* members. Several Ministers of the Central Government may also be invited by the Chairman to attend the meetings as non-members, in order to put forward their viewpoints on matters within their respective ministerial jurisdiction. The Council may set-up a Committee for various subjects of fields of planning. The main functions of the Council may be summarised as:

(a) To formulate and prescribe guidelines for the preparation of the National Plan as well as to suggest ways and means for mobilisation of resources for the Plan.
(b) To discuss and scrutinies the draft National Plan as prepared by the Planning Commission.
(c) To examine policy question arising in regard to the Plan.
(d) To review relevant questions relating to the implementation of the Plan.

The decision of the National Development Council along with the draft National Plan are sent to the Cabinets and legislatures of all the Governments in the country for discussion. These high powered organs of the Government have thus the final voice in regard to the nature and scope of plan as well as for the strategy and resources for its implementation.

How can we plan for attaining an acceptable level of health for all in 21st Century? The Government must make an unequivocal political commitment including required legislations and introduce the health reforms (as suggested by the expert agencies) that are essential if the delivery of health care to all by the legendary of new century is to become a reality.

The health administrators lack the art of health planning. This results in giving low priority to the programmes directly or indirectly affecting health services. In the past, the health administrator has rarely made a contribution in the planning process to the totality of the plan. He has been advocating only for expenditure on health services without realising that the programmes of education, agriculture, community development, etc., also contribute indirectly to the health of the people. To quote Myrdal:

> "From the Planning point of view the effect of any particular policy measure in the health field depends on all the policy measures and is, by itself, indeterminate. This means that it is impossible to impute to any single measure or set of measures a definite return in terms of improved health conditions. A generalised model, in aggregate financial terms, visualizing a sum of inputs of preventive and curative measures giving rise to an output of improved health conditions, cannot be of any help in planning."[18]

Thus, there is a need of training health administrators in the art of planning. The WHO has been encouraging the training of health administrators in institutes of health administration. Strangely enough, it was found that most of the health experts trained in the art of planning were not engaged on the activity resulting in the wastage of the resources of the sponsoring organisation and the training institutions. It is suggested that the young people from the health departments may be selected, trained and made responsible for planning. In the developing world the senior positions are occupied by elder people who do not want to be trained. Thus, there is a need to create a special cadre for health planners beside imparting general training for health planning to all. The training institutions should not be satisfied with their passive role of training health experts in the art of health planning but should see that the knowledge provided during training is being made use of effectively and the situation is improving.

The health administrators lack the techniques of management and personal qualities which are essential for successful health planning. Planning is a complicated and complex process and health administrators have to convince all concerned for developing meaningful health planning. There are still a number of problems requiring solutions with regard to coordination, communication and inter-relationships between the many individuals and organisations involved. The head of the health planning team and the health project officers will have to develop considerable skill in the political, administrative and technical areas. The health administrators will have to work hard in preparing health plans acceptable to policy-makers.

Health planning methods need modifications to suit the social, political and economic environment prevailing in the country. We have already discussed in brief the different methods being used in different countries. The understanding of health planning process and methodology in different countries throughout the world will equip the health administrators with a broader horizon of health planning. There is still plenty of room for innovation to develop new patterns and variety of approaches. The health administrators should not adopt blindly any approach which has been successful in some countries. They must find out the methods most suitable to the macro-environment prevailing in their own countries.

The health planning should be based on the needs of the population. A population base, in contrast to an institutional disease, or diagnostic base, is absolutely necessary for objective planning and evaluation.

The health planning should encourage people's participation. People should form an integral part of planning process. V. Subramaniam writes:

> "A people's plan cannot be a people's plan unless it has an inbuilt flexibility so that adjustment and mid-term corrections are possible in the light of several factors and circumstances which come to the fore during the implementation of the programme.[19]

CONCLUSION

During the Ninth Plan efforts will be further intensified to improve the health status of the population by optimising coverage and quality of care by identifying and rectifying the critical gaps in infrastructure, manpower, equipment, essential diagnostic reagents and drugs. Efforts will be directed to improve functional efficiency of the health care system through:

(a) Creation of a functional reliable health management information system and training and deployment of health manpower with requisite professional competence.
(b) Multi-professional education to promote team work.
(c) Skill upgradation of all categories of health personnel, as a part of structured continuing education.
(d) Improving operational efficiency through health services research.
(e) Increasing awareness of the community through health education.
(f) Increasing accountability and responsiveness to health needs of the people by increasing utilisation of the Panchayati Raj institutions in local planning and monitoring.

(g) Making use of available local and community resources so that operational efficiency and quality of services improve and the services are made more responsive to users' needs.[20]

Notes and References

1. WHO, *Technical Report Series*, 215, 4, (1961).
2. WHO, *Public Health Paper*, 46, p. 9.
3. WHO, *Public Health Paper*, 44, p. 15.
4. Dr. Montoya, "Programme Technology in the Context of Health Planning", Unpublished.
5. Gunaratne, *op. cit.*, p. 10.
6. WHO, *WHO Chronicle*, 1966, No. 20, pp. 301-9.
7. WHO, SEARO, 20th Session of the WHO Regional Committee for South-East Asia, New Delhi, October, 1970, p. 101.
8. WHO, SEARO: SEA, RC 24/16 Rev. I, 1 October, 1971, p. 38, Annex. 4.
9. Ninth Five Year Plan, 27, *op. cit*, p. 139.
10. G. Myrdal (1968), Asian Drama, an Inquiry into the Poverty of Nations, New York, Pantheon, Vol. 3, p. 1841.
11. J. Brijant, 1969, Health and the Development World, Ithaca and London, Cornell University Press, p. 26.
12. WHO, *Public Health Paper*, 41, p. 31.
13. Ninth Five Year Plan, *op. cit.*, pp. 140-41.
14. WHO (1967), *Technical Reports Series*, No. 350.
15. WHO, *WHO Chronicle*, Vol. 27, No. 1, pp. 3-5.
16. Government of India, Planning Commission, Fifth Five Year Plan, 1974-79, New Delhi, p. vii.
17. *The Tribune*, Chandigarh, 1 August, 1979.
18. G. Myrdal (1968), Asian Drama, an Inquiry into the Poverty of Nations, New York, Pantheon, Vol. 3, p. 1618.
19. Subramaniam, V., "The Citizens and Planning" in the *Indian Journal of Public Administration* (New Delhi), Vol. XXI, No. 3, July-Sept., 1975, p. 57.
20. Ninth Five Year Plan, *op. cit.*, p. 139.

CHAPTER 10

PLANNING NURSING EDUCATION AND ADMINISTRATION

> The nurse is a person who has completed a programme of basic nursing education and is qualified and authorised in her country to supply the most responsible service of a nursing nature for the promotion of health, the prevention of illness and the care of the sick.
>
> —International Council of Nurses

Planning Nursing Education and Administration

A. NATURE AND CLASSIFICATION OF NURSING PERSONNEL

Significance

The institution of nurses is the backbone of the organisation that provides health services to the community at large. Nursing is a vocation, implying dedication to the service of suffering mankind and a missionary service to be rendered at any hour of the day and night as the need arises. It is a demanding and exacting profession. The ideal relations of a doctor, patient, nurse and the medicine are the four pillars upon which a cure must rest.

Definition of Nursing

A study carried out by the International Council of Nurses defined nursing as:

> The nurse is a person who has completed a programme of basic nursing education and is qualified and authorised in her country to supply the most responsible service of a nursing nature for the promotion of health, the prevention of illness and the care of the sick.[1]

Nursing in its brodest sense, may be defined as the provision of nursing care to individuals, families or communities in connection with the restoration or preservation of health, and comprising the nursing component of the organised health care and preventive services. Such care may be provided by personnel ranging from the nursing aide to the professional nurse and nurse-midwife. The National League for Nursing has adopted the following principles of nursing care:

> Nursing care encompasses health promotion, the care and prevention of disability, and rehabilitation, and involves teaching, counselling and emotional support, as well as the care of illness. Nursing care is an integral part of total health care and is planned and administered in combination with related medical education and welfare services. Nursing personnel respect the individuality, dignity and rights of every person regardless of race, colour, creed, national origin, social or economic status.[2]

The following is a statement taken from the Code of Ethics as Applied to Nursing published by the International Council of Nurses:

> Nurses minister to the sick, assume responsibility for creating a physical, social and spiritual environment which will be conducive to recovery and stress the prevention of illness and promotion of health by teaching and example. They render health service to the individual, the family and the community and coordinate their services with members of other health professions.

The words and expectations appear to vary a great deal, and, as with many other professional groups, the nurses' role is a shifting one. A unique function of the nurse has been identified as ". . . to assist the individual, sick or well, in the performance of those activities contributing to health or its recovery (or to peaceful death that he would perform unaided if he had the necessary strength, will or knowledge. And to do this in such a way as to help him gain independence as rapidly as possible."[3]

From these definitions, we infer that nursing is—to nurse the patients or to serve the patients. It is the duty of the nurse to ensure the healing touch of sympathy for the patients. In view of these, Florence Nightingale felt a nurse should be chaste, sober, honest, truthful, trustworthy, punctual, quiet, cheerful and kind.

Categories of Nurses and their Education

There are a large number of categories of nursing personnel depending upon the duration and purpose of training and the level of general education. Let us discuss these categories briefly:

1. Auxiliary Nurse-Midwives

This category of nurses are trained to function as multi-purpose workers in rural areas. Their functions are: care of the sick, home visits, treatment of minor ailments, maternal and child health care, family planning follow-up, nutritional education, etc. The entrance qualification for training to such category is Middle Standard and the age between 18-

30 years. The duration of the training is two years and includes shorter and simpler courses in nursing and midwifery. Students are provided stipends and free accommodation.

2. Lady Health Visitors' Course

This is of 1/2 year's duration. This is a modified Auxiliary Nurse-Midwives Course with more emphasis on maternal and child health. The minimum entrance qualification is matriculation.

3. General Nursing and Midwifery

Minimum education is matriculation with 45 per cent aggregate marks, having science subjects. Duration is 31 years. They are trained to function efficiently both in hospitals and in the community. It is also called Grade Nursing Course.

4. B.Sc. Nursing Degree Course

This is a University Programme, in General Nursing and Midwifery of 4 years' duration. Educational requirements are higher secondary or intermediate with science subjects. Degree programmes are conducted in colleges of nursing in our country at Delhi, Bombay, Bangalore and Chandigarh.

5. Post-Certificate B.Sc. Degree Course

This course is conducted for diploma-holders in seven colleges of nursing in India. Duration of this course is two years.

6. Masters in Nursing

This is of 2 years' duration and is conducted at Delhi, Vellore, Chandigarh and Bombay.

7. Specialised Courses

A large number of specialised courses are conducted for diploma-holders. They are:

(a) Ward Sister's Course for efficient management in the wards.
(b) Public Health Nursing is for better community health services.
(c) Tutor's Course.
(d) Administration in Nursing.
(e) Operation Theatre Training.
(f) Paediatric Nursing.
(g) Psychiatric Nursing.
(h) Orthopaedic Nursing.

These are essential for efficient functioning of specialised departments.

8. Nurse Technician

This category includes Senior Dressers, Assistant Nurses and Community Nurses. More than one but fewer than three years of nursing education and training is required with a minimum of nine years of general education.

9. Nursing Aides

This category at present includes servants, messengers or other personnel actually performing certain nursing functions. Although aids must be literate, formal training is not generally required, since they are trained on the job to assist in patient care.

On examining critically, we find that it is illogical to classify all the personnel engaged in the assistance of health care as 'Nursing Personnel'. We must restrict the classification of nursing personnel to the nurses formally trained to do the job. We may give different names to the personnel helping the nurses. This would enhance the status of nursing personnel and would focus our attention on a definite category of personnel. The numerous categories of nurses diffuse functions and responsibilities. Dr. Gunaratne, the present Regional Director of the South-East Asia Regional Office of WHO observed that Sri Lanka had experienced some difficulties because of the numerous categories of nursing personnel, including staff nurses (who underwent three years' training), emergency nurses (with only three to six months' training), assistant nurses, nursing aides and ward attendants. The Government intended to have only two categories of personnel-staff nurse (a fully qualified nurse) and ward labourer (who would have nothing to do with patient care). The same is the problem in many countries. There is a need of rational classification of nursing personnel so that their duties may be clearly demarcated.[4]

In order to provide incentive and motivation to nursing personnel, five per cent of the seats in the proposed short-duration course of medical education may be reserved for the nursing personnel who fulfil the minimum qualifications and have set good standards of service. This would also attract good candidates to this profession.

Changing Concept to Meet Present Needs

There has been a change today in the concept of nursing care. In the words of the WHO Expert Committee on nursing, "Minor modifications of existing nursing systems will be inadequate to meet new situations and demands in a rapidly changing society. . . nursing must break with some of its traditions as well as alter existing stereo-types."[5]

The current trend is to involve the nurse in the planning. implementation and evaluation of health programmes rather than simply expecting from her a subservient role in patient care. This requires a great change in the contents and methodology of nursing education. The present nursing education does not encourage research. The nursing journals contain articles of descriptive nature. There is a need to encourage research among the post-graduate nursing students and the faculty members to prepare them for senior in the health care delivery system. In a report of an international seminar on Research in Nursing. Brotherston has summarised the position thus:

> Whereas the ability and opportunity to carry out research must be limited to a minority in any profession, an urgent and understanding sense of the need for research should be part of the mental equipment of every member of any profession worthy of the name.

He further adds that there is a need for the profession to cultivate research-mindedness which he defines as, "readiness to look analytically at the events or working methods, a willingness to encourage scientific study or experimentation and an ability to accept the proven conclusions and act accordingly."[6]

Research is a fundamental function of a profession which is necessary to ensure its growth and progress. The professional competence of nursing personnel also greatly depends on the availability of research reports based on basic as well as applied researches. A recent book on *Essentials of Nursing Research* by Notter says that "Research is serious business. It should not be entered into lightly, but neither should it be feared." Nursing research in India still remains neglected.

In order to keep the nursing service up-to-date it is necessary to organise programmes of in-service education and training for all nursing personnel as a means of improving the quality of patient care. The contents of these programmes may be carefully scrutinised. At present, wherever such programmes are being carried out, they are few and lack in seriousness and purpose.

The literature available for the study and research in nursing services and administration is in the context of the developed world and is written by the writers and their professional associations from the developed world. This situation needs to be improved by rejuvenating the nursing professional associations to inculcate professional standards among their members and produce stimulating literature in the context of the needs of their countries. Dr. Chitt (Thailand) while speaking in the Regional Committee meeting of the WHO suggested that steps should be taken to stimulate the establishment and development of professional nursing associations. The essential part to be played by them in the overall growth of the profession has not been fully appreciated even by the nurses themselves.[7] Besides, the nursing associations can help in building professional standards for the professional growth of their members. According to Gardner:

> Standards are contagious. They spread throughout an organisation, a group, or a society. If an organisation or group cherishes high

standards, the behaviour of the individual who enters it is inevitably influenced.[8]

The future of the nursing profession is in the hands of its members who must strive for creativity, academic excellence and the pursuit of a lofty standard in their professional activities.

Critical Appraisal of Nursing Education

The quality of nursing education needs immediate change so that qualitative nursing care can be assured. The following facts and suggestions can be taken into consideration to improve the situation.

1. There should be two categories of nursing personnel—Graduate Nurse and an Auxiliary Nurse/Midwife. The nursing aides may not be included while classifying or defining nursing services.

2. The entrance qualifications should be higher secondary with science. At present, there is no admission policy, i.e., a fixed criteria for admission to nursing schools. It was learnt from direct interviews of some nurses that "merit is no criteria to get admission in a nursing school. Those who have political and other pressures get admitted leaving the best available candidates." It is suggested that nursing schools and colleges should declare their admission policy to ensure fairness, impartiality and proper selection. This would go a long way in improving the nursing profession.

3. All nursing education should be continuous and not terminal. Besides, the in-service training programmes may be arranged to keep them abreast of the latest development. The nursing leaders do not appreciate the need for higher education among nurses as they think that nurses are to carry out only routine and mechanical duties which, as already mentioned in the earlier part of this chapter, is quite short-sighted and wrong. A nursing superintendent of a big hospital informed the present author that the nurses did not need higher education as they were responsible only for elementary activities like bed-making, sponge-bath, noting the temperature, pulse-rate, respiration, etc. The same view is held by the doctors in a hospital about the status of nurses. Mrs Narinder Nagpal, Secretary, Trained Nurses Association of India, in her article, 'Noble Profession in Neglect' in *The Tribune* (Nov. 15, 1979) rightly mentioned,"The nursing profession is treated as an auxiliary to the medical profession. We have been telling the medical men that they should leave the nursing profession to the nurses. But, so far we have not met with success." This is the reason why most of the nursing superintendents and hospital authorities are not in favour of deputing their nursing personnel for higher education. Some nurses even seem to feel that they are not allowed to improve their qualifications so that they may not become more qualified than the existing nursing leaders thereby posing a professional threat. It is strange to find that most of the nurses have improved their general qualifications through correspondence

courses or by appearing in examinations in a private capacity. Many of them have completed the university degree courses while some of them have passed M.A. examinations from first rate universities. It is suggested that correspondence courses in B.Sc. Nursing may be instituted by some universities to ensure professional growth of nurses otherwise they would be misutilising their energy for improving general qualifications.

4. Nursing schools and colleges should be independent institutions. There may be arrangement for formal and informal coordination between the hospital and the nursing institutions. This would save the exploitation of nursing students—perhaps relieve them from excessive clinical work and thus neglects of their studies. Miss Simmone Liegeois, Secretary, International Committee of Catholic Nurses, New Delhi, has rightly mentioned that the shortage of nurses led to the use of student nurses for services much to the detriment of theoretical instructions. This problem needed to be studied in order to raise the quality of basic training.[9] Besides, nursing schools should adopt some hospitals to enlighten and develop the existing nursing personnel with the latest developments in the field of nursing education and administration. The nursing personnel in the hospital should be encouraged to study in the library so that they keep themselves aware of the latest developments.

5. The nursing teachers of right quality and calibre should be prepared. Some research degree may be instituted. This would encourage research among the nursing educators. Their conditions of service must be the same as of lecturers in a college. Besides, the time devoted by them in the nursing institutions is about 9 hours which is too much. This leaves no time for research and library reading. They must be encouraged to do independent work by reducing their duty hours.

6. Most of the nurse educators interviewed by the writer were unaware of the system of health care prevailing in the country. They were only equipped in the paper they were teaching. It is suggested that an independent paper on "Health Care Administration" may be started to inform them of all the developments in this sector from the international to the local levels.

7. Whenever a new post-graduate course in a particular medical specialty is started for doctors—a course for nurses and other workers should also be started simultaneously to prepare a team and provide effective services to the patients.

8. The school and college subjects may include 'Nursing' as one of the papers which can create interest among the students to pursue this profession.

The dearth of nurses especially really well qualified and the unsatisfactory standards of education are because of the poor status of nursing as a career. Besides, the teachers of nursing institutions are not at par with their counterparts in schools and colleges. Professor P.K. Devi has suggested that: "In order to improve the image of nursing, the profession has to consider three aspects. First, the independent way in which nursing benefits humanity, by taking crucial decisions at critical times where timely action by nurse-in-charge has led to saving of life, e.g., early diagnosis of fatal complications like pulmonary oedema, embolism, collapse, hyper-pyrexia, etc. Secondly, administrators must recognise the place of nursing in the medical team and nurses must prepare themselves to take their due place and accept this challenge. Thirdly, economic rewards must be commensurate with the nature of their responsibilities. Employment conditions must not be laid down unilaterally, nursing personnel must have a voice in determining how best and efficiently their services can be utilised."[10]

9. There is a need of introducing principles of management and administration of health care in the curriculum of B.Sc. and M.Sc. Nursing. At present, the principles of administration are taught without making them understand their application in the provision of health care. It is suggested that an independent paper on 'Health Care Administration' may be started at B.Sc. and M.Sc. levels.

10. There is a need to open more colleges/schools for imparting nursing education. The delegates at the Third All India Nursing Education Conference held at Chandigarh from 14 to 16 November 1979, strongly demanded a sizable increase in the number of seats in nursing colleges to tackle the growing need for nursing personnel in the country. The conference also urged that the nursing education curricula may be improved so that nurses are able to manage minor ailments on their own.

Indian Nursing Council: We may mention here briefly the role of the Nursing Council. It is a statutory body constituted under the Indian Nursing Council Act, 1947. The Council is responsible for regulation and maintenance of a uniform standard of training for nurses, midwives, auxiliary-nurse-midwives and health visitors. The Council prescribes syllabus and regulations for various nursing courses. In every meeting, the council discusses the issues pertaining to education and training of nursing personnel. Recently, the Council organised a workshop of the Registrars of the State Nursing Councils and Secretaries of the Examining Board from 8th August to 13th August 1983, at New Delhi, to review and study the functioning of various councils. At the 36th Meeting of the Council held on 16th April 1983, many issues were discussed. Some of them are:

(a) recognition of the B.Sc. (Nursing) degree granted by P.G.I., Chandigarh, College of Nursing, Ludhiana, and College of Nursing, Trivandrum;
(b) to approve the recruitment rules for various posts of nursing personnel prepared by the Nursing Education Committee at its meeting held on 8th and 9th February 1983; and
(c) to incorporate section 23 of the Indian Medical Council Act, 1947, regarding registration in the Indian Nurses Register.

B. PLANNING NURSING SERVICES

Meaning of Nursing Service Administration

According to Shanks and Kennedy, "Nursing Service Administration is that organisation through which nurses in a hospital or another type of health agency are able to provide the best possible nursing care for patients in the hospital or under the jurisdiction of another type of health agency.[11]

According to Finer:

> Nursing Service Administration is a coordinated system of activities which provides all of the facilities necessary for the rendering of nursing care to patients. Nursing Service Administration is the system of activities directed towards the nursing care of patients and includes the establishment of overall goals and policies . . . Administration is the selection, provision and employment of resources for a purpose—the fulfilment of which is desirable or compulsory.

Objectives of Planning

The objectives of planning of the Nursing Service should be:

(a) to ensure total patient care;
(b) to see that the nursing component at the operational level is properly organised;
(c) to ensure optimum utilisation of nursing services by avoiding non-nursing duties of nurses;
(d) to provide a congenial environment for the professional development of the nursing personnel;
(e) to encourage staff education and training so that they can take up positions of higher responsibilities in the future;
(f) to ensure effective participation of all nurses through team work in the planning and implementation of nursing services and the total hospital plan;
(g) to promote effective public relations through effective communication; and
(h) to evaluate the quality of the nursing service.

In order to achieve these objectives, we need nursing administrators who possess administrative capability, capacity and ability; good professional knowledge and skill; good communication skills, problem-solving ability and a scientific attitude enabling them to be involved objectively.[12]

Indices of Nursing Care

Some of the indices that have been used as measures of nursing care are discussed here. At least two indices will be needed for each kind of service studied, one for the total staff per care unit, and one for the staff pattern, or the proportion of each category of personnel, per care unit or per service.

1. Indices of Total Nursing Supply

(a) The ratio of number of nurses to total population is a crude index that is useful in comparing the supply of nurses in one country with that in another. Within a country, it is useful only if hospitals and health services are uniformly distributed throughout the country.

(b) The ratio of number of nurses to number of physicians is helpful in ensuring the realistic allocation of medical and non-medical tasks.

2. Indices of the Nursing Staff Pattern

(a) The ratio of the numbers in any category of nursing personnel to those in any other category is a useful index in analysing the quality of nursing service.

(b) The percentage of total staff in each category is a useful way to express levels of nursing because it makes comparison possible between more than two levels.

3. Indices of Hospital Nursing

(a) The nursing time provided per patient per day is the most useful and realistic index since it takes account of occupancy rates, working hours, and days absent from work. It is also easier to interpret since it provides a picture of the amount of care each patient receives, but requires more information and is more difficult to compute. The following steps are involved in the computation:

Step 1. Find the average number of days worked per year by a nurse by subtracting from 365 the total number of days taken, on the average, as annual leave, sick leave, holidays, and regular days off.

Step 2. Find the average number of hours worked per year by a nurse by multiplying the average number of days worked by the number of hours per working day.

Step 3. Multiply the hours worked per year by a nurse by the total number of nurses to obtain the total number of nursing hours per year.

Step 4. Divide the total number of nursing hours per year by

365 to obtain the number of nursing hours per day.

Step 5. Divide the total number of nursing hours per day by the average daily patient census to obtain the number of nursing hours per patient.

(b) The number of nursing hours per hospital bed per day is calculated as above except that in step the total number of nursing hours per day is divided by the total number of hospital beds.

(c) The number of hospital beds per nurse is easily computed and is a useful rough index. It is not an accurate measure of the amount of service given, because it does not reflect differences in hours worked, absence from work, number of shifts in a 24-hour period, hospital occupancy, or the condition of the patient.

(d) The average daily number of patients per nurse is an index having the same advantages and disadvantages as (c) above except that it reflects differences in hospital occupancy and is therefore a little more accurate.

(e) The number of nurses per 20 (or 50 or 100) hospital beds or patients provides a rough indication of the staff needed for planned new facilities. It may be preferable to use the number of beds or patients in an average nursing care unit rather than an arbitrary figure of 20, 50, etc.

4. Indices of Public Health Nursing

(a) The number of persons per public health nurse is a useful index where health services are well developed and distributed fairly uniformly over the country.

(b) The number of live births in the population per nurse or midwife may be a useful index when the major emphasis of a particular programme is on maternal and child health, as with the number of persons per public health nurse. It is unsuitable for use in planning when coverage of the population is limited and distribution of services uneven.

(c) The number of public health nurses per health centre of a given size is a practical index that allows plans for nursing to keep pace with the programme of a developing health centre. It is not as useful for purposes of comparison between countries or different kinds of services.

(d) The number of hours or minutes of nursing service per activity (e.g., home visit, clinic, consultation, immunization, etc.) is a useful index if the plan of action for the health plan is drawn up in terms of activities. An accurate calculation must be based on a time study.

5. Indices of Nurse-Teacher Supply

(a) The number of students per nurse-teacher is a good rough index for use in planning recruitment and training programmes for nurse-teachers.
(b) The number of nurse-teachers per education and training programme of a given type is also workable index. For a realistic school staffing plan, both this and the preceding index must be used.

Planning Nursing Services

Nursing in 1948 lacked the status of a profession in most of the countries in South-East Asia. This can be seen from the figures by the Regional office:

> For Afghanistan's 12 million population, there were 44 mid-wives and 303 nurses (1954); Ceylon (now Sri Lanka) with a population of 8.25 million had 1785 midwives and 2056 nurses (1953); for India's 375 million population, the figures were 17,000 and 22,100 (1954); Indonesia had 1035 midwives and 5548 nurses for 79.5 million (1954), and Thailand, 915 and 3874 for its estimated 19.5 million people (1954).[13]

The third session of the Regional Committee passed a resolution and requested the Regional Director, "to take active steps in collaboration with governments, to promote the expansion of training facilities, particularly through the provision of specialised international staff and essential teaching equipment."[14]

Since then the governments with the help of the WHO have been striving to prepare an adequate number of nurses with good training arrangements. The conditions are the worst in Nepal where there is yet one professional nurse per 52,755 people and one auxiliary per 22,570 people. However, the conditions are better in Sri Lanka and Thailand. The conditions in India and Burma are satisfactory. Still, the doctor/population ratio is better as compared to nurse population ratio in the developing world while in the developed countries, the nurse/population ratio is six times the doctor population ratio.

Thus, the staffing of the services in the developing countries at a reasonable level of adequacy and efficiency obviously calls for vast expansion of nursing education and training. Besides, these countries must take energetic steps to build-up a nucleus of highly trained nursing personnel for manning positions of administrative and teaching responsibilities. This requires effective planning and should include all the steps required to develop health manpower plans. As stated in a WHO Health Paper, "Systematic planning for nursing is the orderly development of a system of nursing that will enable the most effective service possible to be provided with the resources available. Such a system will be based on an analytic study both of the nursing service currently provided and that needed in proposed health services."[15]

C. PLANNING A NURSING UNIT OF A HOSPITAL AND PUBLIC HEALTH NURSING

Need and Functions

The nursing unit is an integral part of the hospital complex. The hospital is divided into blocks and each block is divided into wards. A ward is that area of the hospital where all the amenities—physical, social and especially medical care—are made available to make the patients feel at home till they are discharged. In other words, a ward is a temporary home for the patients admitted there. Evidently, there is a need to ensure a healthy environment to help early recovery of the patients and to win their confidence. In each ward, there is a nursing unit to take care of the patients for all the 24 hours. The efficient planning of this unit would ensure maximum care of the patient. The broad categories of functions that should be discharged by the nursing unit are:

(a) Meeting personal needs of the patients.
(b) Efficient ward management.
(c) Proper maintenance of records of the patients.
(d) Provision of basic institutional services.
(e) Availability of diagnostic and treatment equipment.
(f) Arranging formal and informal health education of the patients and their relatives.

Planning a Nursing Unit

Planning is preparation for action. The proper advance planning would ensure best patient care. Dimock defines planning as "the use of rational design as contrasted with chance, the reaching of a decision before a line of action is taken instead of improving after action has started."[16]

The aspects of planning a ward include—Space Planning, location of Nursing Unit, Materials Planning, Personnel Planning, etc. The planning here must be practical and operational and not theoretical. In the words of Millet, "Planning is the process of determining the objectives of administrative effort and of devising the means calculated to achieve them."[17]

Hudson succinctly defines it as "the process of devising a basis for a course of future action."[18]

In each nursing unit, planning may be done to provide the following basic facilities:

(a) Patient rooms with attached or separate toilet and bathing facilities.

(b) Nurse's duty room.

(c) Treatment area.

(d) Waiting room for the relatives.

(e) Storage of linen and other supplies and equipment.

Besides, there is a need of manpower planning i.e., identification of actions which personnel have to take in order to perform activities, and identification of positions by which personnel requirements may be grouped to determine types, number and qualifications.

Administration of a Nursing Unit

The American Hospital Association and National League of Nursing Education (1950), Hospital Nursing Service Manual, New York, indicates the following steps to administer the ward:

(1) Assisting the patient with those physical services necessary for his well-being and comfort which he cannot do for himself or cannot do unaided, and planning such services to meet his individual needs as they are affected by his physical condition and his emotional reaction.

(2) Observing, recording, and reporting to the physician for the 24-hour period the physical, emotional, and mental symptoms which may have significance in diagnosis and in the direction of therapy.

(3) Preparing the necessary equipment for and assisting the physician with diagnostic tests and therapeutic measures.

(4) Giving medication and carrying out treatment prescribed by the physician.

(5) Observing the patient for reactions which may follow treatment, and taking the necessary measures to combat them, should they occur.

(6) Assisting in providing a clean, orderly, well-ventilated environment for the patient, and protecting him from infections, accidents, and fire hazards.

(7) Helping the patient to feel secure in his new environment and to adjust himself to his condition and to any limitations he may have as a result of his illness.

(8) Teaching the patient how to maintain and improve his health and to carry out his treatment when he goes home.

(9) Establishing good rapport with the patient's family and his friends.

(10) Meeting emergency situations and unforeseen situations with promptness and good judgement.

(11) Making contacts for the patients with others concerned with his care, such as the medical social worker, the dietician, the

occupational therapist, or the clergy, or nursing agencies when he leaves the hospital.[19]

Planning Public Health Nursing

Public Health nursing is a recent development. The real foundation of health can be laid if the public health nursing is properly developed. This is meant to provide preventive and promotive health education. The objective of planning public health nursing may include:

(1) health counselling to individuals, families and community groups;
(2) provision of nursing care when necessary, and teaching and supervision of others providing nursing care;
(3) assistance during physical examination and medical, diagnostic, and preventive procedures;
(4) promotion of environmental sanitation in homes, schools and industry;
(5) case-finding related to the agency's programmes, and participation in epidemiological investigation;
(6) cooperation in community studies and other special research of the agency; and
(7) participation in educational programmes for nurses, other professionals, and members of the community.[20]

Nurses and Primary Health Care

Besides we must plan the use of nurses in the promotion of primary health care.

The International Council of Nurses (ICN) representing nurses throughout the world, supports the present WHO/UNICEF concept of Primary Health Care (PHC). In so doing, ICN affirms the commitment of nurses to effect changes in nursing education, practice and management which are conducive to the implementation of PHC.

ICN recognises that to effect the necessary changes in the nursing contribution, nurses must continue to influence governments in their own countries to take the following action (ICN/78/142/E):

- review the role of nursing personnel in the context of the primary health care approach within the national health services, and the overall development of the country;
- develop a health manpower system which is relevant to the country and its need;
- review legal instruments which protect the public and health personnel;
- involve nurses in the policy-making, planning and management at national and local level;
- utilise nurses as teachers and supervisors in PHC activities;

and

- utilise suitably prepared nurses in PHC research and as project planners/participants when planning, implementing and evaluating PHC programmes.

ICN declares its intent to cooperate, at international level, with government and non-governmental organisations, and at national level with its member associations, in making PHC an effective reality.

A Case Study of the Ward Administration of a Teaching-cum-Research Hospital— P.G.I., Chandigarh

The whole hospital has been divided into blocks. Each block is further divided into wards. The overall responsibility of planning, implementation and supervision of nursing personnel vests in the Nursing Superintendent who is assisted by one Joint Nursing Superintendent and one Assistant Nursing Superintendent (see attached Fig.). Below them are 62 nursing sisters and 366 staff nurses.

The main responsibility of administering a ward or nursing unit 15 of the ward sister. She looks after some particular ward as assigned to her. Let us take the case study of *Male Surgical Ward* to understand the dynamics of Ward Administration.

It is located on the 5th Floor, B-Block of the Nehru Hospital, PGI, Chandigarh. It consists of ten cubicles for the patients, class-room, intensive-care unit, a store, a room for doctors and nurses, and nurses' and doctors' duty room (see Fig. 10.1). Let us mention some of the facts about the ward:

Bed strength	74
Number of units	4
Number of patients in each unit	18-19
Number of consultants	3 consultants in each unit
Number of junior doctors in each unit	10-12 in each unit
Total number of medical personnel	60
Nursing Staff:	
Ward Sister	1
Staff Nurses	12
Ward Aide	1
Class IV Employees:	
Ward Servants	4
Sweepers	5

Sanitary Annexes for the ward consisting of
6 Latrines; and
3 Bathrooms.

The working of the ward has been examined on the basis of personal observation, interview and discussion with the staff in the ward

Fig. 10.1

Nursing Organisation of Post-Graduate Institute of Medical Education and Research, Chandigarh

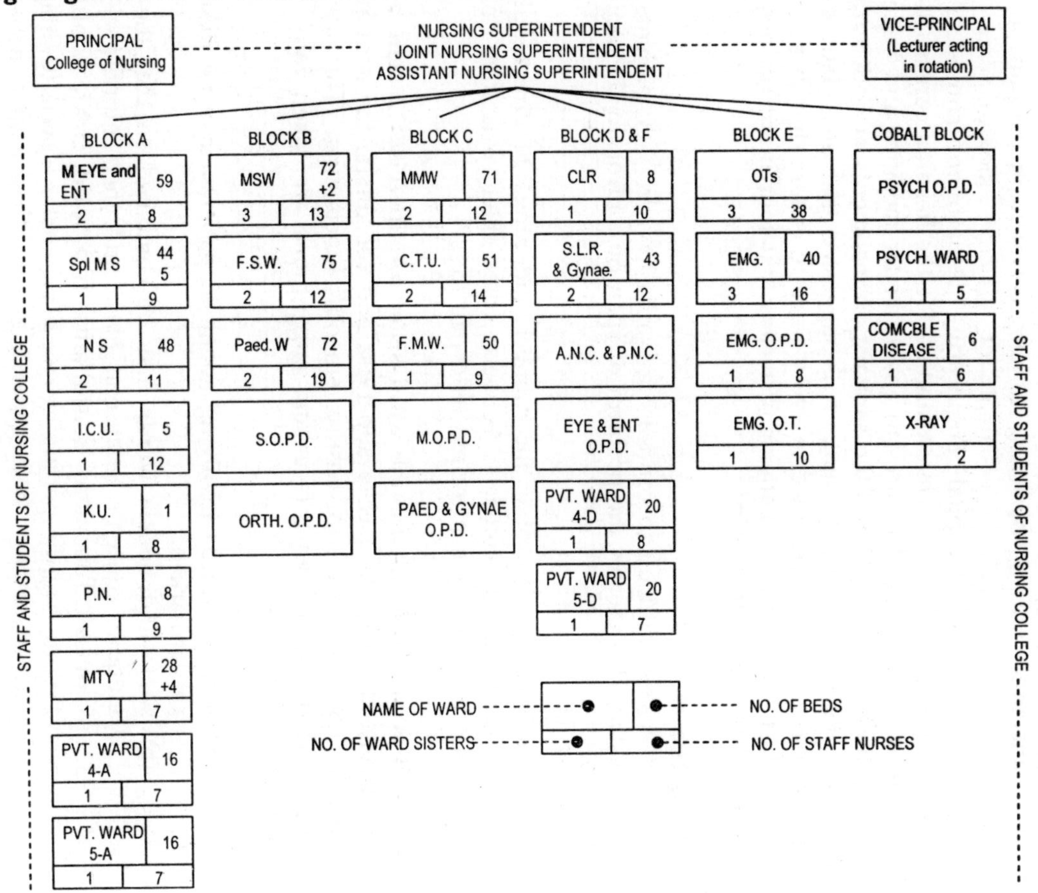

PRINCIPAL College of Nursing

NURSING SUPERINTENDENT
JOINT NURSING SUPERINTENDENT
ASSISTANT NURSING SUPERINTENDENT

VICE-PRINCIPAL (Lecturer acting in rotation)

STAFF AND STUDENTS OF NURSING COLLEGE

BLOCK A
M EYE and ENT 59
2 8
Spl M S 44 5
1 9
N S 48
2 11
I.C.U. 5
1 12
K.U. 1
1 8
P.N. 8
1 9
MTY 28 +4
1 7
PVT. WARD 4-A 16
1 7
PVT. WARD 5-A 16
1 7

BLOCK B
MSW 72 +2
3 13
F.S.W. 75
2 12
Paed. W 72
2 19
S.O.P.D.
ORTH. O.P.D.

BLOCK C
MMW 71
2 12
C.T.U. 51
2 14
F.M.W. 50
1 9
M.O.P.D.
PAED & GYNAE O.P.D.

BLOCK D & F
CLR 8
1 10
S.L.R. & Gynae. 43
2 12
A.N.C. & P.N.C.
EYE & ENT O.P.D.
PVT. WARD 4-D 20
1 8
PVT. WARD 5-D 20
1 7

BLOCK E
OTs
3 38
EMG. 40
3 16
EMG. O.P.D.
1 8
EMG. O.T.
1 10

COBALT BLOCK
PSYCH O.P.D.
PSYCH. WARD
1 5
COMCBLE DISEASE 6
1 6
X-RAY
2

NAME OF WARD — NO. OF BEDS
NO. OF WARD SISTERS — NO. OF STAFF NURSES

STAFF AND STUDENTS OF NURSING COLLEGE

and the patients and their relatives. Let us mention some of the problems which need the attention of hospital authorities for better performance and decent patient care.

1. Defective Construction of the Ward

The ward is made up of cubicles with a brick wall in each cubicle. This type of construction is not good as it is not possible for the ward sister and other nursing personnel to keep a watch on the patients from the duty room which is essential for effective medical care. It is suggested that the Hospital Engineering Department should always involve nursing personnel while planning for the hospital construction or alterations of existing structures to ensure better facilities and better use of the buildings. At present, the sanitary arrangements are not sufficient to meet the needs of the patients. It is suggested that more latrines and bathrooms should be provided in every ward to ensure that there should be at least 1 latrine for 8 patients. It means that four more latrines need to be provided in this ward.

2. Big Size of Ward

It is very difficult to control big wards having 70-80 patients by a ward sister. This creates the problem of span of control. In the words of Dimock:

> The span of control is the number and range of direct, habitual communication contacts between the chief executive of an enterprise and his principle fellow officers.[21]

It is very difficult for the ward sister to supervise 12 staff nurses effectively. Besides, she has to supervise and coordinate the activities of doctors and sweepers to ensure smooth functioning. This can be improved if the following facts and suggestions are taken into consideration:

(a) Smaller wards involving about 40 patients may be designed or earmarked.

(b) Male and female wards may be combined so that the consultants concentrate at one place and their number can be reduced. Too many consultants in a ward create confusion. Private wards pertaining to a particular specialty may be located nearer their general wards. This would make the inter-ward coordination easy and more manageable. This experiment has been a great success in some of the hospitals like General Hospital, Sector 16, Chandigarh. Even in this very hospital, this arrangement exists in cardio-thoracic ward.

3. Lack of Effective Inter-personnel Relationships

As we already know a ward has a large number of personnel-doctors, nurses, sweepers, etc. The efficiency of the ward depends upon the team spirit among all these persons without any distinction of status. Most of the staff members interviewed were of the view that there is absence of harmonious relationship among the personnel working in a ward as all individuals think in terms of their own interest rather than that of the group. It is suggested that the hospital authorities should see that the ward is conceived of as a team or group of people so related that the efforts of each duly contribute to the best patient care and most satisfying to all. The trend should be to encourage the growth of informal relations which would create better understanding and appreciation of each other's role. Such an atmosphere would germinate administrative vitality and ensure access to group opinion by extending and broadening the avenues of institutional planning and thought. Henry Fayol (1841-1925) recommended the principle of *esprit de corps*, i.e., in union there is strength. The organisation ought to function as a team and every team member should do his best to accomplish organisational goals.

4. Defective Materials Management

The efficiency of the ward depends to a great extent upon the proper and timely supply of equipment and goods by the Central Supply and Laundry Departments. There is lack of coordination between the wards and the supportive services. On holidays, wards either do not get the supply or get partial supply resulting in poor performance. It is suggested that the personnel of Central Supply and Laundry Departments may adjust their duties on holidays and compensation may be provided to them in lieu thereof.

5. Pilferage of Goods and Poor Maintenance of Equipment

It was told to the writer that the doctors do not use the equipment carefully resulting in great losses. Nursing personnel are considered by them as servants. It is suggested that the doctors may be taught health economics and the proper use of equipment as we cannot afford wastage. The main reason of the mounting cost of hospital expenditure is the improper utilisation of hospital resources.

Besides, the Class IV employees do not care much for the orders of the ward sisters and nurses. These employees are under the direct control of the Medical Superintendent. This vitiates the principle of 'Parity of responsibility and authority.' The ward sister has no effective control over the sweepers, etc. Herbert A. Simon has rightly said that, "Those who have the authority to issue orders should be willing to accept responsibility for the consequences."[22]

How can we expect responsibility from the ward sisters without granting them sufficient authority? There is a need to inculcate discipline among the employees which would generate obedience, application, motivation, energy and respect.

6. Low Morale among Nursing Personnel

If we examine the hospital structure, we find that the hospital authorities have not given due status to the nursing personnel—the backbone of the hospital system. Staff nurses get the chance of being promoted to nursing sisters but the avenues of promotions are blocked after that. A sound policy of promotion fosters a feeling of belonging and dedication among the personnel and leads to building up of healthy traditions and conventions. It is suggested that more posts of Assistant Nursing Superintendents, Deputy Nursing Superintendents may be created, to provide suitable avenues of promotion. Besides, the ratio of ward sister to staff nurse may be decreased to 1:6 from 1:12 at present. This would provide better avenues of promotion to staff nurses. Moreover, the hospital authorities should encourage higher education among nurses and provide facilities for their growth. Henry Fayol has rightly said that: "a sign of good administration is the steady methodical training of all employees required at all levels."

Most of the nurses were very sore and mentioned that they are not encouraged to undergo higher education. It is suggested that the nursing personnel should be encouraged to undertake higher education and their promotion avenues may be increased by increasing their status in the hospital system. Most of the nurses feel that there is hardly any job satisfaction. It was mentioned by (Mrs) Nagpal in her interview to *The Tribune* (Nov. 15, 1979), that when the patient is cured, it is the doctor who gets the credit. "The nurse who must have spent hours together by the patient's bedside is more often than not ignored."

7. Unsatisfactory Nurse/Patient Ratio

The present ratio of 1 nurse to 12 patients is against the recommended norm 1:3. Secondly, the number of staff nurses on night duty further decreases as compared to day time. It is a strange paradox as the patients feel more necessity of medical care during night hours. This need to be by appointing more nurses. It should be practised at least in Central Institutes which are to set standards for other hospitals.

8. Non-nursing Duties by Nursing Personnel

There are many duties which are clerical and can be performed by non-technical personnel. Most of the nursing personnel in the ward were having 40 per cent of their work which was non-nursing. This would result in the wastage of resources. It is suggested that the hospital should appoint a committee to demarcate the nursing duties so that they can devote more time to patient care and non-nursing duties may be transferred to other personnel.

D. PLANNING NURSING ORGANISATION AND ADMINISTRATION

After the formulation of the plan, the organisation is designed to implement the plan. According to Mooney, "Organisation is the form of every human association for the attainment of a common purpose."[23]

> And this is what Dimock and Dimock have to say of organisation. "Organisation is the systematic bringing together of inter-dependent parts to form a unified whole through which authority, coordination and control may be exercised to achieve a given purpose. . . . Organisation is both structure and human relations."[24]
>
> Herbert A. Simon has concluded:
>
> . . . . Organisation affects the people who work for it in five different ways:
>
> (i) The organisation divides work among its members; by giving each employee a particular task, it limits and concentrates his attention on that task. . . .
> (ii) The organisation establishes standard practices: by working out detailed procedures, it relieves employees of the need to determine such procedure, each time they use crossways;
> (iii) The organisation transmits authoritative decisions by despatching such decisions downward, upward and crossways;
> (iv) The organisation provides a communication system; and
> (v) The organisation trains and indoctrinates its members by providing for the internalization of influence relating to knowledge, skills and loyalties; training enables employees to make decisions as the organisation would like them to be made.[25]

It would, therefore, be of utmost significance to stress that organisation is not merely a structure; in fact, it embraces a structure as well as the human beings who man and run it in order to realise the pre-conceived objective.

Organisation can be formal and informal. According to Simon, formal organisation means, "a planned system of cooperative effort in which each participant has a recognised role to play and duties and tasks to perform. The key to the whole process is effective cooperation among the persons engaged in the operation."[26]

But the actual working of any organisation is not according to the formal plan. The informal relationship of the persons working in the organisation may be different from the formal expected relationship. It is better to encourage informal relationships among nursing organisations to promote decent patient care.

Keith Davis has enumerated the following five practical benefits which can be derived from informal organisations which may be kept in mind by the Nursing Superintendent and other hospital administrators.

1. It blends with the formal organisation to make a workable system for getting the work done.
2. It lightens the workload of the formal manager and fills in some of the gaps in his abilities.
3. It gives suggestion and stability to work groups.
4. It is a very useful channel of communication in the organisation.
5. Its presence encourages the manager to plan and act more carefully than he would otherwise.[27]

Likert has called this general principle, the principle of 'supporting relationships', in which decision-making, leadership, motivation, communication and control move together. He states, "the leadership and other processes of the organisation must be such as to assume a maximum probability that in all interactions and all relationships with the organisation each member will, in the light of his background, values, and expectations, view the experience as supportive and one which builds and maintains his sense of personal worth and importance.[28]

Thus, the Nursing Superintendent and other top nursing personnel should strive as far as possible to create the atmosphere of an informal organisation which would develop the genuine feeling of goodwill and mutual trust among the nursing personnel. It should not be understood that the Nursing Superintendent should not follow the formal plan. The idea is to supplement the good elements of formal organisation with informal organisation to get the best out of the employees.

There are many aspects or problems which must be taken care of while planning an organisation. Let us discuss some of them which are important—

(i) Authority and responsibility—Development of team nursing.
(ii) Delegation and decentralisation.
(iii) Public relations.
(iv) Communication.
(v) Coordination within the nursing unit and coordination with the entire hospital system.
(vi) Supervision and control.
(vii) Personnel management.

Authority and Responsibility

Authority is the right or power of a person to command other people to do things and to get work done from them. This authority in a hospital organisation relating to nursing services is exercised by the Nursing Superintendent subject to the overall control of the Medical Superintendent/Director. It requires complete understanding of the decisions by the Nursing Superintendent and communicating them to the subordinates for implementation. Responsibility means a charge for which one is responsible or accountable. Since it would not do just to hold a person responsible for performing a task without first giving him/her the authority necessary to get the job done, responsibility should always be coupled with commensurate authority. If a Nursing Superintendent and her team is to perform efficiently, she should know what her job is and with how much authority she has to perform it. This parity is not mathematical but rather co-extensive, because both relate to the same assignments. According to Ernest Dale:

> Authority should be equal to responsibility. That is, if a man is responsible for the results of a given operation, he should be given enough authority to take the action necessary to ensure success.[29]

The trend today is to make use of authority in collaboration with colleagues—developing team work. Team nursing is a plan of nursing care which makes possible utilisation of all levels of personnel to provide optimum patient care. The nurse should be a team member. This means that the nurse is to be totally integrated into the function of the team. It means involvement of all nursing personnel in the planning and implementation of patient care. It implies "expert planning and assigning of the duties to be performed by all those concerned with the care of the patient, so that nursing will be improved and the entire staff will function smoothly, efficiently and happily."[30]

The team leader must ensure effective communication to ensure effective participation. We can represent the merits of team work with the help of the diagram.

Thus, the fuller staff participation is important both as a means of tapping the practical and intellectual resources of all the nursing personnel for the benefit of the organisation and as a way of making work in the organisation more meaningful for each nurse.

Such participation though theoretically available in one form or the other is practically non-existent. Most of the nurses interviewed revealed that the nursing leaders allow superficial participation which serves as an eyewash indicating the presence of distrust in the mind of the nursing leaders. The consequences of this can be represented with the help of the Schematic Chart.

The following advantages would result from the participative management:

- participation yields personal commitment and involvement of

Fig. 10.2

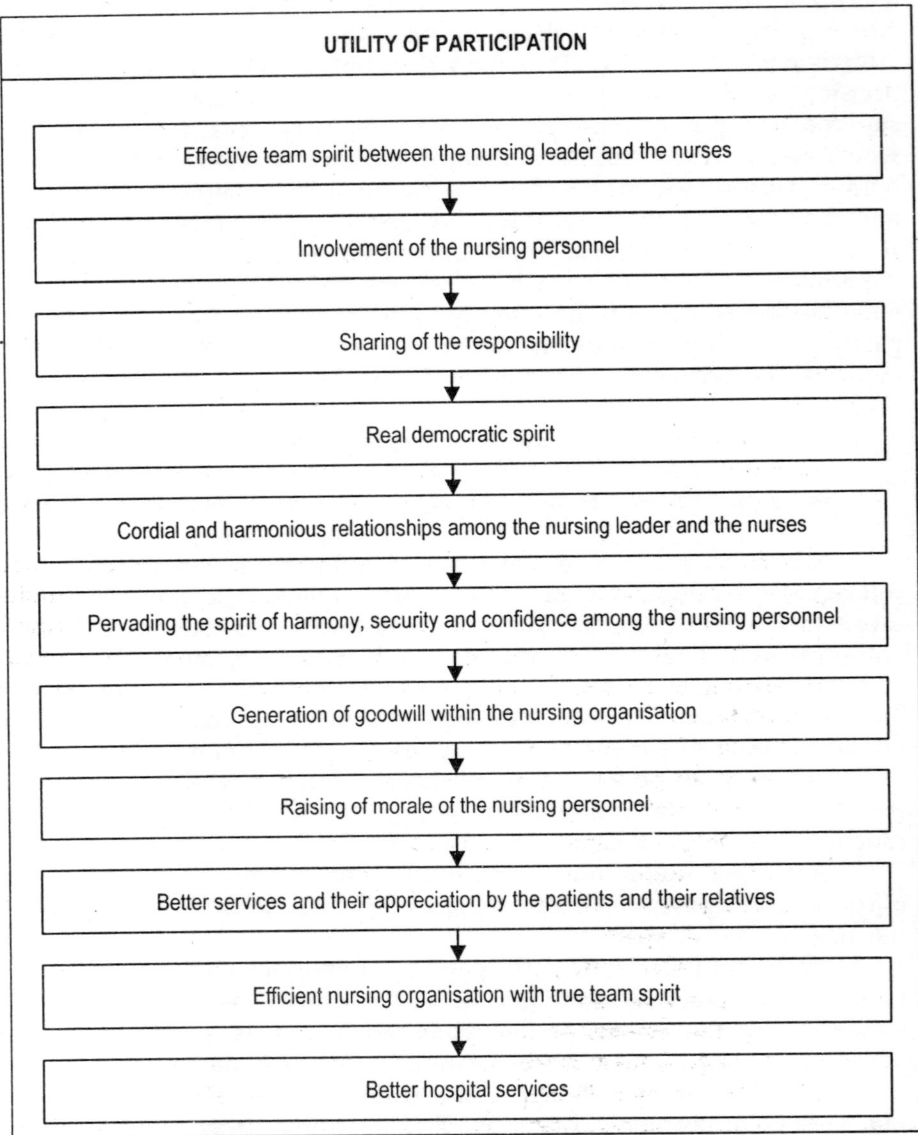

nurses toward organisational goals;

- participation produces the free flow of communications for an informal work force and atmosphere;
- control systems are primarily for self-monitoring and guidance and not needed for external control;
- it produces a high degree of mutual respect and trust among organisational members;

- through participation a nursing superintendent is likely to obtain stronger motivation towards an objective. Even those who disagree will feel compelled to loyalty by the sheer weight of the group opinion; and
- a high degree of confidence is shown in subordinates which facilitates interpersonal processes.

Therefore, we should encourage nurses' participation in the promotion of patient care. An employee's participation would build his morale and ultimately his efficiency. An ILO document mentions that the individual worker "is not just a cog in the very big wheel, but that his personal effort is essential for the achievement of the overall production plan."[31]

The research theory in social organisational psychology has also suggested that participation in group decision-making enhances satisfaction among members and removes tensions. Micheal R. Cooper and Micheal T. Wood have shown that satisfaction is affected by the participation. Satisfaction was greater where participation was complete than where it was partial.[32]

There is a need to practise 'Management by objectives' to ensure fruitful participation. Management by objectives shifts the focus to goals, to the purpose of the activity rather than the activity itself. It is a process whereby the superior and subordinate personnel of an organisation jointly identify its common goals and ensure performance. The Nursing Superintendent must encourage such concepts to develop among nurses. The Nursing Superintendent/Nursing leaders should check the nursing organisation in the context of the essentials of a good organisation to ensure parity between authority and responsibility.

(a) Clear definition of objectives.
(b) Systematic grouping of related activities.
(c) Maximum delegation of authority.
(d) Minimum layering.
(e) Clear demarcation of line and staff functions.
(f) Unity of command.
(g) Correct span of control.
(h) Proper conditions of work.
(i) Provision for easier communication.

For a Nursing Superintendent it is one thing to have the legal right to command, and quite another to have effective direction over the nursing personnel. The former is a matter of formal power. The latter is largely a matter of appeal and influence. It requires, first of all, evidence of interest, intelligence, and energy. Unless there is single-mindedness that will enable the Nursing Superintendent to generate and sustain a general concern for the fufilment of the goals of his/her programme he/

Fig. 10.3

Implications of Lack of Participation

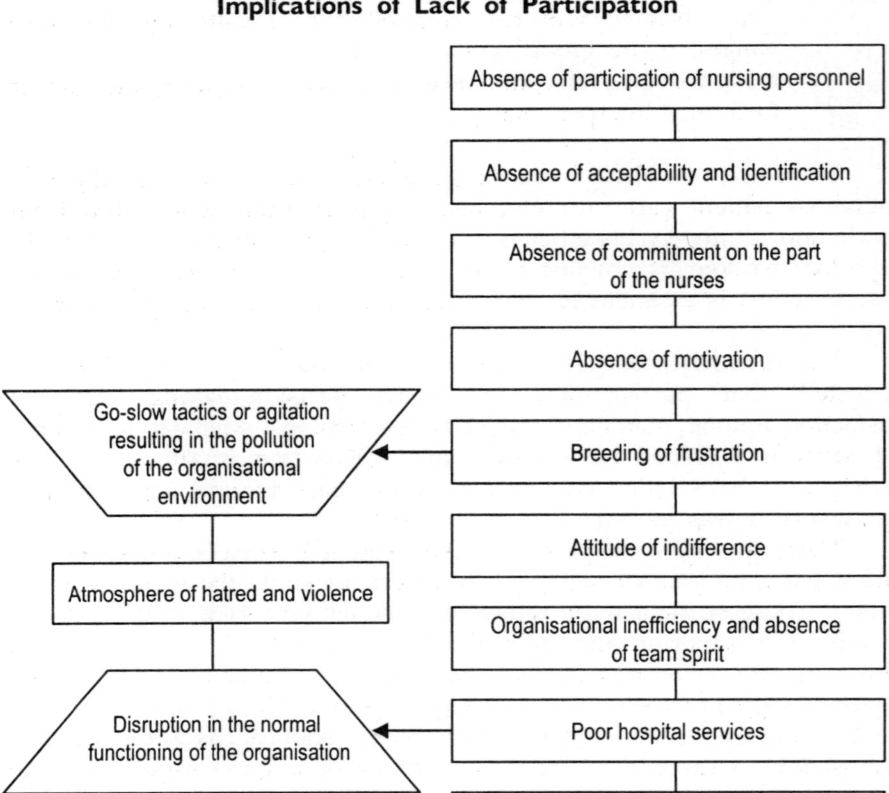

she cannot hope to assert the authority that signifies the true leadership.

These qualities—interest, intelligence, and energy—are fundamental to strength of personality. But they must also be in balance. Unless the individual's traits are so combined that they enable one to win and hold the devotion of other colleagues, one will have little chance of meeting the demands made on him or her. The nursing personnel must be able to feel that they know the Nursing Superintendent and can trust her because she is the leader of their team. More specially, an executive must have that quality about his or her personality which enables him or her, without sacrificing integrity of purpose, to lubricate human relationships.

Let us understand the psychological reasons for participative management with the help of extracts from the scholars of organisational psychology. This would help the Nursing Superintendent and hospital authorities to manage their personnel efficiently.

McGregor categorised the traditional motivational assumptions as theory X, a string of self-consistent notions about human nature. Firstly, the theory X assumes that the ordinary man is selfish, lazy and stimulated by only economic rewards. Secondly, the average man is not interested in work unless goaded by the superior. Thirdly, the individual and organisational goals are contradictory and tend to clash against each other. Fourthly, the average man is devoid of self-discipline and self-control. Finally, he tends to submit himself to the control and direction of others and avoids responsibility.

McGregor, however, points out that man's motivation is far too complex and varied to be explained away wholly by the aforementioned assumptions. In line with other thinkers of social psychology school, McGregor describes his alternative model of motivation as theory Y. The assumptions of theory Y may be stated as:

1. The average man is not really against doing work.
2. The ordinary man can show self-control and self-direction, depending upon the involvement in the work he is doing.
3. The average man craves self-actualisation and it is the responsibility of the management to provide genuine conditions for satisfying his creative abilities and yearnings.
4. The ordinary man, under suitable conditions, would willingly shoulder responsibility.
5. The average man is capable of making significant contributions to the solution of many administrative problems but his potentialities are not fully utilised.

McGregor's assumptions in theory Y roughly correspond to what Maslow and Argyris have stated about human motivation. The running theme of all these thinkers has been to show that adequate attention has not been paid, so far, to the actual potentialities, creativity and responsible behaviour with which the ordinary man is endowed. That way, McGregor has successfully discarded the assumptions of classical school of thoughts. Douglas McGregor has rightly given his preference for theory Y which helps in true organisational building and development. He states:

> Theory X leads naturally to an emphasis on the tactics of control—to procedures and techniques for telling people what to do, for determining whether they are doing it, and for administering rewards and punishments. Since an underlying assumption is that people must be made to do what is necessary for the success of the enterprise, attention is naturally directed to the techniques of direction and control. Theory Y, on the other hand, leads to a preoccupation with the nature of relationships, with creating an environment which will encourage commitment to organisational objectives and which will provide opportunities for the maximum exercise of initiative, ingenuity, and self-direction in achieving them.[33]

Elton Mayo and his colleagues who pioneered the Human Relations' school also recognised and emphasised the use of techniques as given in theory Y. They outlined the following principles, which may be followed by the Nursing Superintendent and other top personnel of the hospital to develop and maintain sound organisational health:

(i) The need for recognition of the 'human' element and the well-being and motivation of the working teams.
(ii) Good supervision is exercised with proper understanding of the subordinates.
(iii) It is important to have proper communication and consultation between the managers and the workers. This creates a sense of participation and involvement among the employees. There should be means of keeping the management informed of what the employees are thinking, fearing, hoping and equally of keeping the employees informed of what the management is thinking or proposing to do.
(iv) The Hawthorne experiments showed that economic incentive is far less powerful than the personal or social incentives.
(v) The flow of work and arrangements of operations should give full play to the informal organisation of the workers.

In Argyris' view an organisation following these principles would be able tó achieve efficiency as well as keep its employees satisfied. He says:

> Every individual has 'psychological energy' to expand. Exerting that energy in a way that helps him fulfil his own social and egoistic needs is what motivates an individual. Therefore, provided a company is structured in such a way that an individual is able to meet these self-fulfilment needs, the psychological energy will be used in the company's interests. If the reverse is the case the psychological energy can easily be used to thwart the company's aims.[34]

This would promote dynamism. To quote Howard P. Smith:

> Dynamism in an organization cannot be declared by fiat, nor can it be generated by the artificial insemination of imposed systems, procedures, and job demands. The enthusiasm people express about their jobs, about each other, and about their organization is a priceless corollary of effective management. Without it, the whole management effort can easily become a kind of drudgery, never moving beyond a mechanical process with little sense of personal involvement. A spirit of dynamism in the organization, a sense of

personal involvement in the organization's affairs, is particularly necessary as the setting for meaningful appraisal and development because of the high personal relevance of this activity. Good leadership is the real determinant of such a spirit.

Thus, we can say that the Nursing Superintendent must encourage participative management among nursing personnel to raise their morale. Such a situation will be conducive to the growth and development of nursing personnel and they, in turn, would do their best to provide decent patient care. In such a situation, the energy and initiative among the nursing personnel would be self-generating. Besides, all their latent potential energy would be changed into kinetic energy which can be utilised for the promotion of health among the persons visiting the hospitals.

Delegation and Decentralisation

The decentralisation and delegation can lighten the burden of the Nursing Superintendent and enable her to devote attention to important aspects of planning, policy-making and coordination. She should clearly make use of delegation and decentralisation through Sisters and Staff Nurses to achieve the objective of best patient care. According to Fayol, "Everything that goes to increase the importance of subordinate's role is decentralisation. Everything which goes to reduce it is centralisation."

Let us first understand the meaning of delegation and decentralisation and their utility.

Delegation is a process whereby a superior divides his total work assignment between himself and subordinates or operative personnel in order to achieve both operative and management specialisation. It is the entrustment of responsibility and authority to others and the creation of accountability for performance. It is to be clearly understood that delegation is not a process of abdication. The person who delegates does not divorce himself from the responsibility and authority which he entrusts.

There are three aspects of delegation: "the entrustment of work of responsibility to another for performance, the entrustment of powers and rights, or authority to be exercised and the creation of an obligation, or accountability, on the part of the person accepting the delegation to perform in terms of the standards established."[35]

Speedy and realistic decision-making is one of the essentials of efficient administration. In a big and complex organisation like the hospital, the number of decisions to be taken from time to time is so large and the points at which decisions are to be implemented are so many that it becomes necessary to distribute decision-making powers among a number of organs, rather than concentrate in one organ. This is expected to prevent the emergence of bottlenecks which bedevil highly centralised power structures. Thus, one of the important problems of organisation is to reconcile the administrator's desire for centralised control for the sake of uniformity and certainty of decisions and actions, with the people's view that administration should be so organised as to deal with the needs of the different segments of the society in an effective manner.[36]

Effective decision-making can be facilitated by decentralisation and delegation of powers. The word decentralisation is derived from Latin.[37] In modern times, it has been so widely and differently used that, as Norman D. Palmer says, it has become less precise.[38]

Decentralisation is a twin process of deconcentration and devolution. In deconcentration, a superior officer, in order to make his department function effectively and efficiently, delegates to his subordinate field officials the power to act in his name without transferring to them the authority he enjoys.[39] Devolution, which also implies dispersal of authority, is a process wherein power is transferred from one organ of government to another by means of a piece of legislation or constitution. A certain sphere of jurisdiction, either functional or territorial, is set apart for a legally-constituted body which while administering its authority, enjoys "some power of self-determination."[40]

Besides, proper delegation of authority promotes effective control over operations, due to a clear definition of responsibility and action at each level. When decisions are no longer to be referred up the line, the delay in execution is minimised.[41]

Such delegation can prove to be of considerable value. It can lighten the burden of the Nursing Superintendent and enable her to devote her attention to more important things. The Sisters/Staff Nurses under her may feel more responsible and act more effectively if they are entrusted with responsibility and authority.

The importance of delegation was also stressed by Goddard:

> "Delegation of responsibility and authority is an important aspect of successful administration, to place the responsibility for decision at the lowest possible organisational level in order to attain decision as speedily as possible. No administrator can do in detail all the work he is administering, for by definition an administrator manages the work of others. Therefore, the principle of delegation of responsibility should be followed to the utmost extent consistent with efficiency and coordination of policy. The responsibility and authority of individuals should be clearly defined in writing, and the authority placed in each position must correspond to the responsibility which the position carries."[42]

Public Relations

Public relations is the establishment of a climate of understanding. It means interpreting the programme of an organisation to the public and *vice-versa*. According to J.L. McCany:

> Public relations in government is the composite of all the primary and secondary contacts between the bureaucracy and the citizens and all the interaction of influences and attitudes established in these contacts.

According to Harwood:

> Public relations may be defined as those aspects of our personal and corporate behaviour which have a social rather than private and personal significance.[43]

The purpose of public relations is not only to supply information, but also to encourage an understanding and cooperation between the citizens and the public servants. This is very important in a hospital situation as the patients and their relatives are demoralised and psychologically insecure. It is the duty of every member of the nursing personnel to maintain public relations in the hospital at various stages of contact with the patients and the visitors.

At present, we find a great deal of alienation between the patients and nursing personnel. A large number of patients who were contacted in various hospitals were of the view that the attitudes and behaviour of the nursing personnel were negative and they lacked sympathy and courtesy. Some even went on to say that their tone was biting and insulting. This has undermined the legitimacy. effectiveness and credibility of the hospital system in our country. We need to promote harmony and mutual trust among the patients and hospital authorities. The objectives of public relations should be to increase prestige and goodwill and to protect the life of the organisation by safeguarding it against unwarranted attacks as well as to remove the genuine complaints and grievances of the people. This would be possible only if all the employees of the hospital, especially the nursing personnel, make it a point to remove the prevailing in the minds of the people about the nature and scope of hospital services.

To improve understanding between the citizens and the hospital personnel, public relations need to be developed in an effective manner to create favourable community opinion towards the hospital services. This would create confidence in the minds of the people towards the competence, fairness, honesty, impartiality and sincerity of the hospital personnel.

Communication

Communication is central to the exercise of authority in an organisation. In the words of Ordway Tead,

> Communication is the touching of mind by mind, of person with person whether it be one man, to a thousand. . . . It can include conversation, interview, dialogue, visual technique carefully used.[44]

This is of great significance as any wrong communication or misunderstanding can be responsible for the death of the patient. There is a need to issue orders, instructions and prescriptions to be implemented clearly, simply and understandably. The Nursing Superintendents should not think that their job ends after conveying the commands to the subordinates. He or she should encourage effective participation from the nursing personnel to ensure proper understanding.

Most of the nurses complain that the Nursing Superintendent issues orders as these are received from hospital authorities above her. She does not take pains to understand the implications resulting in confusion. It is her duty to clarify the details of the orders before passing these on for implementation. Nursing Superintendent and Sisters may keep the following facts in mind to achieve effective communication:

(a) Clarity of Thoughts

The first *sine qua non* of good communication is that the idea to be transmitted must be absolutely clear in the mind of the communicator. It must spring from a 'clear' head. It should be understood by the nursing personnel so that it may be fully appreciated and acted upon.

(b) Attach Importance to Action Rather than Words

In all communication, actions are more significant than words. Example is better than precept. A Nursing Superintendent or Sister who is not punctual cannot succeed in enforcing the time-rules on the subordinates.

(c) Participation

In this connection the essential is that both the parties (communicator and the recipient) should participate in the communication. It is the only way to make the communication effective.

(d) Transmission

In this connection the communicator must plan carefully what to communicate, to whom to communicate and how to communicate. How can the Nursing Superintendent/Sister communicate with the workers when they themselves do not know or cannot understand all the facts about the new plans? Further, delegation of authority without responsibility breaks down the spirit of communication.

(e) Keep the System always Alive

The system of communication should be kept open and alive all the year round. It is only by honest attempts that good communicative relations can be developed.

(f) Cordial Employer-Employee Relations

Effective communication requires good employer-employee

relations which enables mutual appreciation of different viewpoints.

According to Terry, eight factors are essential to making communication effective:

(a) Inform yourself fully.
(b) Establish a mutual trust in others.
(c) Find a common ground of experience.
(d) Use mutually known words.
(e) Have regard for context.
(f) Secure and hold the receiver's attention.
(g) Employ examples and visual aids.
(h) Practice delaying relations.

According to Millet, seven factors make communication effective viz., it should be clear, consistent with the expectation of the recipient, adequate, timely, uniform, flexible and acceptable.

To quote Goddard:

> Efficient communications are essential to all aspects of effective administration. Staff must be adequately and currently informed about plans, methods, schedules, problems, events and progress. It is necessary that instructions, knowledge, and information be passed on for practical application to all concerned, and that they be so clearly presented as to make misinterpretation or misunderstanding impossible. Proper and adequate communication is not just in one direction; it requires a two-way passage. Administrators must be certain that they know and understand the problems of workers for whom they are responsible. Communications must flow from the bottom upwards, as well as from the top down."[45]

Because of the lack of proper communication and resultant misunderstandings, we observe a lot of conflict among the nursing personnel and between the nursing personnel and other staff working in the hospital. This causes a lot of inter-personal rivalries and jealousies. Such conflict may not be treated as an evil. According to Mary Parker Follett, it is possible "to conceive conflict as not necessarily a wasteful outbreak of incompatibilities, but a normal process by which socially valuable differences register themselves for the enrichment of all concerned."[46]

According to her, there are three ways of dealing with conflict. She says, "By domination only one side gets what it wants; by compromise neither side gets what it wants; by integration we find a way by which both sides may get what they want."[47]

She favours integration through uncovering the conflict and bringing the whole thing into the open. The Nursing Superintendent and hospital authorities should encourage methods to remove conflicts in a positive manner.

Coordination

In the nursing organisation, different nurses perform different duties because of the adoption of specialisation and division of work to achieve maximum results. This is possible only if all the nurses work to achieve the common purpose—welfare of the patient. This can be achieved by devising a proper system of coordination. According to J.C. Charlesworth:

> "Coordination is the integration of the several parts into an orderly whole to achieve the purpose of the undertaking."[48]

It is the centripetal force in administration. It is the duty of the Nursing Superintendent to ensure this coordination among the different wards in the hospital and among the nursing personnel in the same ward through effective communication and sharing responsibility. Besides, the Nursing Superintendent has also to coordinate with the hospital authorities. This is very important as she has to plan her activities only in consonance with the total needs of the hospital. She has to liaison with the different departments, e.g., Stores, Central Steriles, Pharmacy, Dispensary, Registration, Laboratories, etc. to ensure smooth functioning.

Where the central purpose of the organisation is known, understood and considered to be worthy by the workers, it binds them together as a coherent group and unifies their separate efforts into a common endeavour to realise the goal. A stimulating leadership of Nursing Superintendent/Nursing Sisters can create enthusiasm among the nurses for the common cause and spur them to overcome difficulties.

Ideally, coordination should be achieved through voluntary co-operation of the members of an enterprise. Each member should be ready and willing to adopt his work to secure unified action. Coordination can be secured by:

(a) instilling dominant objectives among the members of the group;
(b) developing generally accepted professional standards and norms making it easy for nurses to work with one another enthusiastically;
(c) promoting informal contacts to supplement formal communication;
(d) encouraging Nursing Sisters to maintain close contact with nurses working under them; and
(e) using group methods for informal exchange of ideas and views.

Supervision and Control

Planning, communication and supervision are the three main steps in the process of directions. Like every other aspect of organisation, supervision is also becoming very complicated and complex. The responsibilities of a supervisor has increased and of a good supervisor it is expected that he should have the qualities of head and heart. There is an old saying, "that which is not inspected is not done." Hence, inspection, overseeing and supervision, arise in response to needs inherent in the functioning of an organisation.

Supervision is a compound word and its two parts are 'super' and 'vision' which means overseeing. In a hierarchical organisation no one can claim to work without proper supervision. Generally, each officer is given certain powers and responsibilities and is supposed to be responsible to the officer above him for proper execution of the decisions and use of delegated powers. Moreover, for proper functioning of an organisation it is very essential that there should be proper coördination and link among different parts and organs of an organisation. It is also to be ensured that departments of an organisation do exactly the same work which is expected of them. In common parlance, by supervision we mean direction accompanied by authority. In a broad sense we mean superintendence and overseeing. Margaret Williamson has defined supervision as a process by which workers are helped by a designated staff member to learn according to their needs, to make the best use of their knowledge and skills and to improve their abilities so that they do their jobs more effectively and with increasing satisfaction to themselves and the agency."

The purpose of supervision and control is to ensure that the purpose of the organisation is being fulfilled. In nursing organisations, the supervision and control is still on the old philosophy i.e., to find faults and award punishments. The purpose of supervision is not only to inspect and inquire but to encourage and inspire, and thus achieve team work. To quote Pfiffner:

> The supervisor on the lower levels secures cooperation and production by de-emphasizing his own ego, stimulating group participation, and encouraging the maximum satisfaction of individual egos that is consistent with coordination.[49]

The supervisor should have training in human relations, public relations and human dynamics. Supervision and control should ensure higher efficiency through clarification and encouragement by the supervisors. John D. Millett rightly observes:

Supervision is more than a process, it is a spirit which animates the relationship between levels of organisation and which induces maximum administrative accomplishment, or when unsuccessful, generates administrative paralysis. Effective management is concerned to realise the first and to avoid the second.[50]

According to Newman and Summer, "The aim of control is to

assure that the results of operations conform as closely as possible to established goals."[51] Henry Fayol says that "Control consists in verifying whether everything occurs in conformity with the plans adopted, the instructions issued and principles established. It has for its object to point out weaknesses and errors in order to rectify them and prevent recurrence."[52]

Nigro has identified the following aspects of the supervisor's job:

(i) To satisfy the employees' desire for recognition.
(ii) To keep them informed.
(iii) To allow subordinates to make as many independent decisions as possible.
(iv) To avoid invading the specialist's bailiwick.
(v) To keep the door open for conference and consultations with subordinates.
(vi) To accept the probability of being unpopular with at least a few subordinates.
(vii) To avoid over-optimism.
(viii) To assure the proper interpretation and execution of orders.
(ix) To abolish useless regulations.
(x) To recognise that assistants will sometimes be more intelligent than oneself.
(xi) To make no promises that cannot be fulfilled.
(xii) To expect loyalty and give it too.
(xiii) To avoid discrimination even in favour of a friend.
(xiv) To resist undue pressure and fight for the interests of subordinates.

According to Chester Bernard, subordinates obey authoritarian command only when: (1) they understand what the order is and what purpose to achieve through their collective effort; (2) they feel in their cognition that the command is consistent with the organisational purpose and obeying that they are trying to be moral beings respecting a commitment; (3) they realise and understand that the command is the authority as issued and is compatible with their personal interests. If they see some gain or their personal interests are served in obeying the command, they generally accept it; (4) they know that they are qualified, competent and capable of complying with the orders. In other words, the nature of the command is such that they are mentally and physically fit to execute it.

The Nursing Superintendent and other nursing leaders must understand the implication of the true meaning of supervision and control, if properly understood, supervision and control would ensure good healthy cooperation among the nursing personnel. Such a situation would be beneficial and rewarding both to the supervisors and employees working under them. The Nursing Superintendent should see that the supervision and control should promote better understanding and cooperation rather than conflict, jealousies, heart-burning, enmity, which are detrimental to the smooth functioning of an organisation, through her role as a friend, guide and philosopher.

Personnel Management

Management of nursing personnel—recruitment, training, promotion, conditions of service, etc.—is an area which holds the key to the success of health care administration especially the hospital services. Bacon, philosopher and administrator, has rightly said:

> It is vain for princes to take counsel concerning matters if they take no counsel likewise concerning persons; for all matters are as dead images; and the life of the execution of the affairs lies in the good choice of person.

Therefore, the first and foremost task is to pay attention to the administration of personnel in nursing organisations if we expect the effective performance of such organisations.

Several steps, however, need to be taken if the health systems are to succeed in their avowed attempt to attract, retain and utilise the best talents available in the country. This includes healthy internal environment, competitive wage structure, potentialities of rapid growth and advancement and opportunities to create change/challenge and work for the promotion of decent health care.

In spite of the inherent merits of attending to personnel management, nursing manpower planning has not received due attention in the hospital management in spite of the expansion and diversification of hospital services. The image of the hospital services depends to a great extent upon the requisite skills, aptitudes, integrity and organising capacity of the personnel working in the hospitals. In order to optimise the performance of the nursing personnel as a component of health care administration, we have to harness, coordinate and channelise their capacities and energies in meaningful and fruitful ways.

It is very difficult to deal with all aspects of nursing personnel management as it is a subject by itself. We may mention here briefly one of the serious challenges facing the performance of nursing organisations i.e., unsatisfactory terms of employment. The importance of pay or compensation is very great for every employee. The standard of living and the social prestige of an employee depends to a great extent on the pay he draws. A man chooses his career on the basis of pay which he expects to receive. Rightly does Mason Haire remark, 'Pay in one form or another is certainly one of the mainsprings of motivation in our society."[53]

The tempo of challenging and arduous tasks to be undertaken by the nursing personnel can only be accelerated in case they have the right number of employees, with the right level of talent and skills, in the right job, at the right time, performing the right activities and to achieve the right objectives. But the health care systems cannot attract such talented and motivated nursing personnel unless they are able to provide good conditions of service and good status.

Because of the poor conditions of service, it is very difficult to attract better qualified people to take up the nursing profession. Besides, their avenues of promotion are very limited. A staff nurse can be promoted to a Ward Sister and it is very difficult to be promoted beyond that as the positions are very limited. The status of Nursing Superintendent in a hospital is very low which affects the morale of the nursing personnel. In many hospitals, it is the Superintendents who are all in all. The Nursing Superintendents are mere decorative pieces. They have no authority. Even the Nurses' duty rosters are made by the Medical Superintendents. This leads to a deterioration in the quality of Nursing care. It is suggested that the status of Nursing Superintendent should be raised to the level of Medical Superintendent and more avenues of promotion may be made available to Nursing Sisters. It has been the feeling of most of the nursing personnel interviewed by the writer that, "inadequate salary structure, poor service conditions, want of scope for career development, long duty hours, are the general features of employment causing frustration and low morale."

Thus, an adequate and sound salary structure together with healthy working conditions is the *sine qua non* for the organisational efficiency and effectiveness. Otherwise, as the Administrative Reforms Commission aptly observes, the lack of those conditions has been:

> "one of the major factors for strikes, agitations, inter-service tensions and rivalries, indifferent attitude to work, poor performance, frustration and low morale of the employees."[54]

In other words, the aim of health care systems should be to create and maintain such conditions whereby an employee feels like giving his best, gets satisfaction out of his job and is suitably rewarded. Besides, the conditions of service, the personnel management may look after the following aspects of nursing personnel:

(a) to treat the nursing personnel as partners along with the other members of health and medical team;
(b) to help the nursing personnel reach self-actualisation and thereby help release their creative energy for the promotion of health;
(c) to create facilities for continuous growth, development and training of nursing personnel to make them fit for higher jobs;
(d) to ensure adequate working arrangements and maximum participation in management and decision-making of the

health system by nursing personnel;

(e) to provide institutional safeguards for redress of grievance by nursing personnel;

(f) setting good professional standards by senior nursing personnel; and

(g) development of unity, energy, initiative and loyalty among nursing personnel.

Notes and References

1. International Council of Nurses (1965), Special and Committee reports presented to the IGN Board of Directors and Grand Council meetings in Frankfurt, June 1965, p. 6.
2. National League for Nursing, What People can Expect of Modern Nursing Service?, New York, 1959.
3. Henderson, Virginia (1969), Basic Principles of Nursing Care, Geneva, International Council of Nurses, p. 4.
4. WHO, SEA/RC/19/2, p. 96.
5. WHO, *Technical Report Series*, 1966, No. 347, p. 7.
6. Brotherston, J.H., Research Mindedness and the Health Profession, quoted in *International Council of Nurses*, Learning to Investigate Nursing Problems, London, 1960, p. 24.
7. WHO, SEA/RC/21/2, p. 111.
8. Gardner, John W., *Excellence*, New York, 1961, Harper and Brothers, p. 74.
9. WHO, SEA/RC/21/2, p. 111.
10. The First All-India Nursing Education Conference, Chandigarh, April 19-24, 1971, *Proceedings of the Conference*, p. 26 (Address of Prof. P.K. Devi, P.G.I., Chandigarh).
11. Mary, Shanks D., and Dorothy, Kennedy A., The Theory and Practice of Nursing Administration, London, McGraw-Hill, 1965, p. 3.
12. Herman Finer, Administration and the Nursing Service, New York, 1952, The Macmillan & Co., p. 19.
13. SEARO, Summary of Vital and Epidemiological Statistics, 1956, New Delhi, p. 28.
14. WHO, SEA/RC/3/R8, September 1950.
15. WHO, *Public Health Papers*, 44, p. 18.
16. Dimock and Dimock, Public Administration, Rinehart, New York, 1956, p. 83.
17. Millet, Government and Public Administration, the Quest for Responsible Performance, New York, McGraw-Hill, 1959.
18. Seckler Hudson, Organization and Management: Theory and Practice, The American University Press, Washington DC, 1957, p. 102.
19. American Hospital Association and National League of Nursing Education (1950), *Hospital Nursing Service Manual*, New York.
20. Goddard, H.A., Principles of Administration applied to Nursing Service, World Health Organisation, Geneva, 1958, pp. 35-36.
21. Dimock and Dimock, *op. cit.*, p. 110.
22. Herbert, Simen A., Administrative Behaviour, 2nd Ed., New York, the Macmillan Co., 1958.
23. Mooney, J.D., Principles of Organisation, p. 1.
24. Dimock and Dimock, Public Administration, p. 104.
25. Simon, H.S., Administrative Behaviour: Study of the decision-making process in administrative organization (2nd Ed.), New York, Macmillan, 1960.
26. Simon H., Public Administration, p. 5.

27. Keith Davis, Human Behaviour at Work, 4th Edition, New York, McGraw-Hill, 1972, pp. 257-59.
28. Rensis Likert, The Human Organisation, New York, McGraw-Hill Book Co., 1967, p. 103.
29. Ernest Dale, Management—Theory and Practice, 1973, Tokyo, McGraw-Hill, p. 149.
30. Elizabeth Jones and Joan Grube Ellsworth, "An Experiment in team assignment", *The American Journal of Nursing*, 49, 146 (March), p. 34.
31. ILO, International Labour Conference, 33rd Session, Provisional Records, p. 34.
32. Micheal, Cooper R., and Micheal, Wood T., "Member participation and commitment in group decision-making on influence satisfaction and decision riskness", *Journal of Applied Psychology*, Vol. 59, No. 2, April 1974.
33. Douglas McGregor, *op. cit.*, p. 132.
34. Fayol, Henri, General and International Management, London, Pitman, 1956, p. 26.
35. Lyndall Urwick, The Element of Administration, New York, 1953, pp. 41-42.
36. James, Charlesworth C., Government Administration, New York, 1951, p. 207.
37. Arthur, Machmohan W., Delegation and Autonomy, New Delhi, 1961, p. 15.
38. Norman, Palmer D., "Experiments in Democratic Decentralisation in South Asia", *The Indian Political Science Review*, Delhi University, Vol. 1, Oct. 1966-March 1967, Nos. 1 and 2, p. 49.
39. White, L.D. (Ed.), Encyclopaedia of the Social Science, The Macmillan Company, 1951, Vol. 5, p. 43.
40. *Ibid.*, p. 18.
41. *Ibid.*, p. 16.
42. Goddard, H.A., Principles of Administration Applied to Nursing Service, World Health Organisation, Geneva, 1958, p. 85.
43. Harwood, Childs L., An Introduction to Public Opinions, *op. cit.*, p. 2.
44. Ordway Tead, The Art of Administration, New York, McGraw-Hill, 1951, p. 45.
45. Goddard, H.A., Principles of Administration Applied to Nursing Service, World Health Organisation, Geneva, 1958, p. 85.
46. Mary Parker Follet, Creative Experience, New York, Longman's, 1924, pp. 101-2.
47. *Ibid.*, p. 300.
48. J.C. Charlesworth, Government Administration, N.Y., Harper and Brothers, 1951.
49. Pfiffner John M., The Supervision of Personnel, Human Relations in the Management of Men, N.Y., Prentice-Hall, 1951, p. 215.
50. Millett John D., *op. cit.*, p. 122.
51. Newman and Summer, The Process of Management, p. 561.
52. Henri Fayol, General and Industrial Management, p. 107.
53. Mason Haire, *et. al.*, "Psychological Research in Pay: An overview" in *Personnel Administration*, Paul Pigos and Charles A. Myers, New York, 1969, p. 491.
54. ARC, Report of the Study Team on Promotion Policies, Conduct Rules, Discipline and Morale, Vols. I and II, Delhi, 1967, p. 72.

PART IV

ORGANISATIONAL FRAMEWORK FOR IMPLEMENTATION OF HEALTH POLICY

CHAPTER 11

ADMINISTRATION OF PRIMARY HEALTH CARE

"Essential health care made universally accessible to individuals and families in the community by means acceptable to attain through their full participation and at a cost that the community and country can afford. It forms an integral part both of the country's health system of which it is the nucleus and of the overall social and economic development of the community."

—World Health Organisation

Administration of Primary Health Care

Primary Health Care is essential both for developed and developing countries especially developing. Alastair Andusen visualises this need. He rightly says,[1] people who live in most of the world's industrialized countries tend to take their health services as much for granted as the water that comes from the tap, the electricity that gives them light at the press of a switch, or the public transport that gets them to work or school.

For the less privileged countries, a health service is far from being one of the accepted facts of life. It tends to concentrate on urban areas and caters in particular for the wealthy sections of the big cities. Frequently in these countries the rural masses are deprived of adequate health care.

He further gives a detailed definition of Primary Health Care in *World Health,* July 1976 says[2]: Primary Health care integrates at the community level, all the elements necessary to make an impact on the health status of the people. It calls for measures that are simple and effective in terms of costs, technique and organization, that are easily accessible, and that improve living conditions. It should use available local resources including manpower, material and funds generated within the community itself as well as strictly essential resources allocated by the government. It should be fully integrated with the national health system and with the other sectors involved in community development—agriculture, education, public works, housing, communications.

Primary health care activities should be carried out by trained health auxiliaries and should reflect real problems and community concerns, and should be based on practicable, modern, scientific knowledge and health technology, as well as accepted and proven traditional healing practices. The treatment of everyday minor injuries, advice and instruction to pregnant and nursing mothers, childhood immunization against common infectious diseases, provision of safe water supplies, building of latrines and waste disposal systems—all these come within the purview of primary health care. At the same time, a higher echelon of medical care should be available to which serious or dubious cases can be referred.

A. NEED, MEANING AND SCOPE OF PRIMARY HEALTH CARE

Need

According to Dr. Manuel Carballo, "Rural communities the world over have tended to share a common predicament, namely that relative to urban areas they have been undeserved and, in many respects, have experienced a quality of life and health inferior to that found in large towns and cities. In terms of overall national investment directed towards them or of the self-development they have been encouraged to generate, rural areas have historically been at a disadvantage and have enjoyed less well developed communication infrastructures, educational facilities and health-related services."[3]

It appears that the benefits of modern medicine would accrue to only a small population. The Regional Director of South-East Asia Region affirmed that most of the governments in the Region recognise that despite every effort to extend the provision of basic health services to the population, during the last three decades, the achievements have not been impressive. In view of this situation, systematic health planning and country health programming have, in some countries, resulted in the formulation of primary health care projects as integral part of the basic health services.[4]

Thus, the health care administration in developing countries has failed to meet the minimum health care needs of its people. Dr. N.R.E. Fendall has nicely explained the short-falls of health care system: "If I were asked to compose an epitaph on medicine throughout the twentieth century, it would read: brilliant in its discoveries, superb in its technological breakthrough but woefully inept in its application to those most in need. Medicine will be judged, not in its vast and rapid accumulation of knowledge *per se*, but on its trusteeship of that knowledge. We are now experienced and all that remains is the problem of translating what is common knowledge and routine medicine and hence practice, to the world. The implementation gap must be closed."[5]

The basic question which needs to be answered is: What model of administration on health care can meet the health care needs of all the people in the developing world? What are the constituents of such a model? Past experience has amply made clear that by adoption and uncritical transfer of the model health systems from the developed to the developing world, the basic health needs of the people in the developing world cannot be fulfilled. Henry R. Labouisse, Executive Dirctor of UNICEF, vehemently held while submitting to the First International

Conference on Primary Health Care, "The developing countries have come to realise that the conventional approach inherited from industrialised countries was hopelessly inappropriate when it came to meet, within a reasonable period of time, the health care needs of these vast populations. And the industrialised countries themselves after making spectacular advances in the field of medicine and building up services with expensive facilities, sophisticated technology and highly specialised personnel, are now finding themselves burdened with ruinous medical care systems with which they are unable to provide proper health protection to their own very numerous people. So, there has to be change everywhere."

It has been recognised and accepted that the health care services which exist in most parts of the world have not been meeting the basic needs of very large groups of the population especially in the developing countries.

Meaning and Strategy

The most effective and acceptable form of health system for the people in the developing world has to the community itself. Development is indigenous to each society and builds primarily on a country's resources mainly land and people. Each country must develop its own model to social fulfilment. This will enlarge the capacity of individuals and communities to create and innovate. The mobilisation of the energies and resources of the people especially the rural poor themselves emerges as the key factor in increasing their productivity and self-reliance. Such mobilisation assumes the formation, adaptation and strengthening of community structures. Since each country differs from others in its recources and needs, the concept of Country Health Programme (CHP) must be practised by every country. It is a pragmatic approach which tailors the services precisely to the national situation. In his Preface to the Annual Report for 1975 Dr. Mahler said that, "Such programming is a long-term process, not a one-time intensive planning effort. In order to attain the systematic development of health programmes and services, countries that have not already done so well need to set-up permanent mechanism for formulating health policies and translating these policies into operational programmes. This implies a continuing process of planning, implementing, monitoring, controlling, evaluating and replanning—a truly new approach for most countries and the need for appropriate mechanism to launch the venture and maintain its dynamism which will continue for the foreseeable future." Community Health Programming would give high priority to the needs of the undeserved. Thus, the developing countries must design their own health care delivery models to provide primary health care to all its people. Let us now define the meaning and essential features of such care, commonly known as Primary Health Care.

Nature af Primary Health Care

The WHO defined Primary Health Care as "essential health care made universally accessible to individuals and families in the community by means acceptable to attain through their full participation and at a cost that the community and country can afford. It forms an integral part both of the country's health system of which it is the nucleus and of the overall social and economic development of the community."[6]

The first International Conference on Primary Health Care defined it as "essential health care based on scientifically sound and socially acceptable methods and technology made universally acceptable to individuals and families in the community through their full participation and at a cost that the community and country can afford to maintain at every stage of their development in a spirit of self-reliance and self-determination." There are many different ways of defining primary health care. The 28th World Health Assembly accepted the working definition of primary health care. According to this definition primary health care is taken to mean, "A health approach which integrates at the community level all the elements necessary to make an impact upon the state of health of the people. Such an approach should be an integral part of the national health care system. It is an expression or response to the fundamental human needs of how a person can know of and be assisted in the actions required to live a healthy life and where a person can go if he or she needs relief from pain or suffering. A response to such needs must be a series of simple and effective measures in terms of cost, technique and organisation which are easily accessible to the people in need and which assist in improving the living conditions of individuals, families and communities. These include preventive; promotive, curative and rehabilitative health measures and community development activities."[7]

In short, we can say that primary health care is an approach which integrates at the community level all the elements necessary to make an impact upon the health status of the people.

Primary Health Care should not be understood as primitive care. lt uses simple administrative structures, procedures and operates within the community but "it is an essential first level in a scale of services and is in no way inferior." It is providing the benefits of modern medicine to the community through better methods based upon the socio-economic conditions prevalent in each country. It was mentioned by a delegate from Switzerland. "To wish to promote primary health services does not signify the establishment of two parallel or juxtaposed systems of which one is for the poor and the other, the classic system, more complex, more sophisticated, is reserved for the rich. The goal is to set-up a system where primary health care forms the base of a structure accessible to all, upon which other levels of care can be grafted and can develop."

Gururaj Mutalik in his articles, "The Challenge of PHC" rightly says that Primary Health Care—the vital key for attainment of our goal—

has two essential dimensions. First and foremost, it is an upward movement of the community towards a better quality of life for its members, primarily through its own efforts but of course with assistance from the government's developmental activities in various sectors. Secondly, primary health care is also the ultimate extension of the health care services to the health and home of every member of the community. The whole, in this regard, is truly larger than the sum of these two parts. It is only when these two fundamental facets are woven into an inextricably interlinked process that this magic key can unlock the doors towards better health. The spread of primary health care that is seen in the countries of the South-East Asia Region today is indeed very encouraging.

Jagdambi Prasad Yadav in his presidential address delivered at the Twentieth Convocation of IIPA (Bombay, 15 July 1978) defined the philosophy of the Primary Health Care as: "The philosophy of the community health workers' scheme is to place people's health in people's hand. It is well-known that in most parts of rural India even rudimentary public health facilities are lacking from times immemorial. The CHW's scheme is designed to take health care to door-steps of people. It is hoped that the community health workers will bridge the gap between rural community and health care—preventive, promotional and curative."

Speaking on the new health policy, Shri Morarji Desai, former Prime Minister of India, said, "Whatever development we want to do in the country depends upon the capacity of the people to do their work efficiently and to go on increasing their productive capacity in any field of work, that they can take up. And if this is to be done, health becomes a very primary condition. Unless a person enjoys fairly good health, it will not be possible for him to do work efficiently. It is, therefore, necessary for us to see that the people of the country are enabled to maintain their health in a fairly good manner, so that they are able to follow their work and profession efficiently and live also a healthy life."

Essentials

1. Primary Health should be shaped around the life styles of the people to be served.
2. The local people should be actively involved in planning health care so that it suits their needs and priorities.
3. The health care offered should make maximum use of community resources.
4. Primary Health Care should not only deal with the prevention and cure of disease but also promote health, in the community; in the family and in the individual.
5. All health interventions should take place in or as near as possible to the patient's home and be carried out by the worker most simply (but adequately) trained to give the

treatment in question.

6. Other services, in particular supplies, supervision and referral and technical support should be designed to support the needs at the local level.

Principles (Refer Chart 11.1)

Primary Health Care is part of human development in social, educational and economic spheres. It rests on the following 8 principles:

CHART 11.1

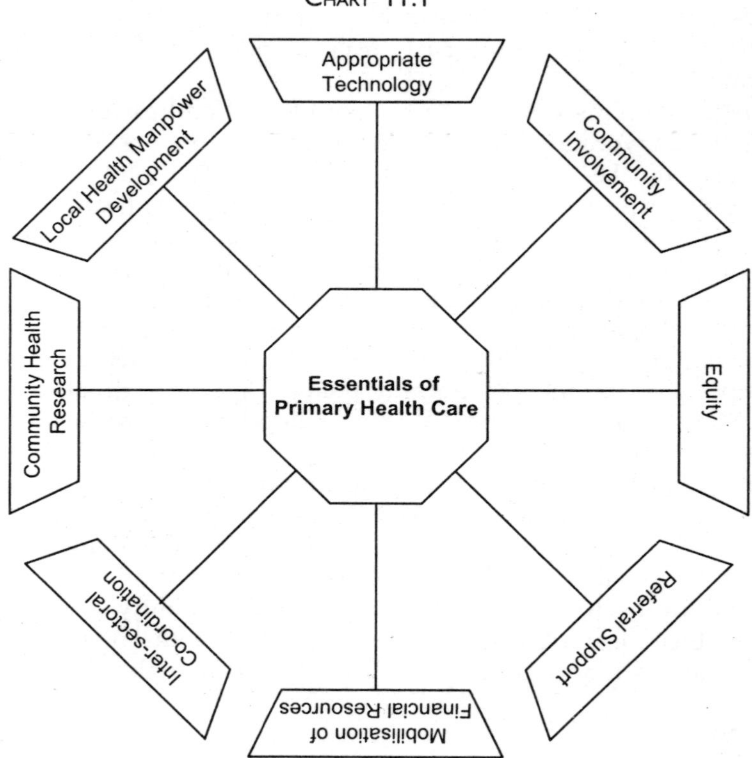

1. Equitable Distribution

Health services should be available to all sections of the society with special attention to the needy and vulnerable groups. Primary Health Care aims at correcting urban-rural imbalance and bringing health services as near to people's homes as possible. It should be supported by higher level of health care to which the needy can be referred.

2. Community Involvement

The involvement of individuals, families and communities in promotion of their own health and welfare, including self-care, is an essential ingredient of Primary Health Care. The community should participate in the planning, implementation and maintenance of health services.

3. Multi-Sectoral Approach

One of the basic tenets of Primary Health Care is that full health cannot be provided by the health sector alone. It requires the joint efforts of the health sector and other health-related sectors. Primary Health Care should be set in context of integrated development to include health, housing, transport, water and sanitation, nutrition, agriculture, education, community development including women's development.

4. Appropriate Technology

This does not mean cheap, primitive technology for the poor. It calls for scientifically sound materials and methods that are socially acceptable, directed against relevant health problems. The examples are domiciliary treatment as against sanatorium treatment for Tuberculosis patients, sputum examination for mass Tuberculosis screening, immunisation by the health workers through outreach sessions, ORS, simple weighing scales, growth monitoring cares, collection of blood smear for malaria control programme.

5. Prevention of Disease and Promotion of Health

This is the basic strategy of Primary Health Care. All activities use this strategy as it is cost-effective to prevent diseases than to treat the same.

6. Development of Effective Referral Support

This is a need to develop proper referral support of secondary and tertiary levels.

7. Medical and Health Services Research including Innovative Approaches

8. Health Manpower Development

Primary health care requires development and mobilisation of resources, especially trained medical staff.

Elements

In 1978, WHO identified eight elements of Primary Health Care:

1. Promotion of food supplies and proper nutrition.
2. Education about health problems and their control.
3. Safe water supply.
4. Basic sanitation.
5. Mother and child health including family planning.
6. Immunisation against infectious diseases and injuries.
7. Prevention and control of locally endemic diseases.
8. Treatment of common diseases and injuries.

The Primary Health Care in India is being carried out through sub-centres, Primary Health Centres, Community Health Centres, Village Health Guide Scheme, Trained Birth Attendants, etc. By the end of March 1996, in India there were 1,32,727 sub-centres, 21,853 Primary Health Centres, 2424 Community Health Centres (these are upgraded Primary Health Centres to cover a population of 80,000 to 1.20 lakh having 30 beds). Sub-Centres are manned by one Male Multi-purpose Health Worker (M.P.W.) and one Female Health Worker (A.N.M.). Village Health Guides numbering 3.21 lakhs work in the village (1 Village Health Guide for 1000 population).

Every ministry appoints from time to time committees including expert committees to advise that Government on a particular issue or a number of issues. The views of these committees have an important influence on the formulation of policies. When the advice of these bodies is accepted by the Government, it may take the form of a policy either through the legislative enactment or executive orders. Let us now discuss the role of some of the important committees appointed by the Government of India to look into the issues of health care administration.

Bhore Committee, 1946

The Government of India appointed this committee in 1943 to survey the then existing health conditions and health organisations in the country and to make recommendations for the future development.

The health of the nation (British India), as it stood in 1946, was revived by the Health Survey and Development Committee (Bore Committee). The Committee reviewed the nation's health under:

1. Public Health
2. Medical Relief
3. Professional Education
4. Medical Research
5. International Health

The report of the Bhore Committee was published in 1946 on the eve of India's Independence, and the proposals for the health programmes were made to provide, among others, the following:

(a) No individual shall fail to secure adequate medical care because of inability to pay for it.
(b) In view of the complexity of modern medical practice, the health services should provide, when fully developed, all the consultant, laboratory and institutional facilities necessary for proper diagnosis and treatment.
(c) The health problem must from the beginning lay special emphasis on preventive work.
(d) The need is urgent for providing medical relief and

preventive heath care to the vast rural population of the country.

(e) The health service should be placed as close to the people as possible in order to ensure the maximum benefit to the community to be served.

(f) It is essential to secure the active cooperation of the people in the development of the health programme.

(g) The report in this long-term programme recommended a primary health unit for a population of 20,000, a secondary unit for a population of 6,00,000 and a district headquarters organisation for a population of three million. The committee in its short-term programme recommended a primary unit for a population of 40,000, a secondary unit for a population of one and half million, and a district headquarters organisation for a population of three milllion.

(h) Recommended a three-month training in preventive and social medicine to prepare social physicians who would guide the people to a healthier and happier life.

This report continues still to be an important document in the field of health care administration.

Mudaliar Committee, 1962

In 1959, the Government of India instituted a "Health Survey and Planning Committee" called the Mudaliar Committee to survey the programme made in the field of health since submission of the Bhore Committee's Report and to make recommendations for future development and expansion of health services.

The Mudaliar Committee found the quality of services provided by the primary health centres inadequate and stressed the need to strengthen the existing primary health centres before new centres are created. It also stressed the need to strengthen sub-divisional and district hospitals so that these could effectively function as referral centres. The main recommendations of the Mudaliar Committee were:

(a) Consolidation of advances, efforts and achievements made in the first two five-year plans in the field of health.

(b) Equipping district hospitals with specialist services.

(c) Need of regionalisation of health services i.e., setting up of regional structures between the State and District headquarters.

(d) Each primary health centre should serve not more than 40,000 people.

(e) The quality of care provided by the primary health centre needs improvement.

(f) Integration of medical and health services should be achieved as already suggested by the Bhore Committee.

(g) Constitution of an All-India Health Service on the pattern of Indian Administrative Service.

Chadah Committee, 1963

This committee was set-up by the Government of India in 1963 under the Chairmanship of Dr. M.S. Chadah, the Director General of Health Services, to study the arrangements for the maintenance phase of the National Malaria Eradication Programme. The Committee recommended that:

(a) The vigilance operations of the National Malaria Eradication Programme should be the responsibility of the general health services i.e., primary health centres at the block level.
(b) Vigilance operations through monthly home visits should be implemented through basic health workers. The norm of one basic health worker per 10,000 population was recommended.
(c) The basic health workers should look after additional duties of collection of vital statistics and family planning, in addition to malaria vigilance. Three to four such workers may be supervised by a Family Planning Health Assistant.
(d) The general health services at the district level should undertake the responsibility for the maintenance phase.

Mukerji Committee, 1965

The Committee was appointed by the Government of India to review the strategy for the family planning programme. The major recommendations of the committee were:

(a) There should be separate staff family planning programme and the family planning assistants should look after family planning work exclusively.
(b) The basic health workers should not be utilised for the family planning programme.
(c) The Malaria Eradication activities should be separated from the family planning, so that the latter can concentrate on family planning programme.

Mukerji Committee, 1966

The States were experiencing difficulties to shoulder the whole burden of maintenance phase of malaria and other mass programmes like family planning, smallpox, leprosy, trachoma, ete., due to paucity of funds. A committee was constituted under the Chairmanship of Shri B. Mukerji, the then Union Secretary, Health, to work out the details 'Basic Health Service' which should be provided at the block level and some consequential strengthening required at higher levels of administration.

The Committee recommended the following additional staff for the various agencies administering health services in the country:

I. Primary Health Centre

1. Basic Health worker	1	for 10,000 population
2. Health Inspector	1	for every four basic health workers
3. Clerk	1	
4. Laboratory Technician	1	

II. District Health Organisation

1. Upgradation of the post of Administrative Officer sanctioned under the Family Planning Programme.

2. Health Supervisor	1	for every 10 primary health centres subject to a maximum of one per district.
3. Public Health Engineer	1	for 2 or 3 districts.
4. Sanitary Supervisor	1	

III. District Hospital

1. Administrative Officer	1	

IV. Urban Areas

1. Basic Health Workers	1	for 15,000 population
2. Health Inspector	1	for 5 basic health workers.

Jungalwalla Committee, 1967

The Committee on 'Integration of Health Services' was appointed in 1964 under the Chairmanship of Dr. N. Jungalwalla, the then Director of National Institute of Health, Administration and Education, New Delhi, to examine the various problems including those of service conditions. The major recommendations made by the Committee were:

Integration of organisation and personnel in the field of health from the highest to the lowest level in the service through:

(1) Unified cadre,
(2) Common seniority,
(3) Recognition of extra qualifications,
(4) Equal pay for equal work,
(5) Special pay for specialised work, and
(6) No private practice but good service conditions.

The Committee did not spell out steps and programme for the integration recommended by it and left the matter to the States to work out the set-up. It, however, defined the integrated health service as:

(a) Service with a unified approach for all problems instead of segmented approach for different problems.
(b) Medical care of sick and conventional public health programmes functioning under a single administrator and operating in a unified manner at all levels of hierarchy with due priority for each programme obtaining at a point of time.

Kartar Singh Committee, 1973

The Committee on 'Multi-purpose workers under Health and Family Planning' was constituted by the Government of India in 1973 under the Chairmanship of Shri Kartar Singh, the then Additional Secretary, Health, Government of India. The Committee's terms of reference were to study and make recommendations on:

(1) The structure for integrated service at the periphery and supervisory level;
(2) The feasibility of having multi-purpose, bi-purpose workers in the field;
(3) The training requirements for such workers; and
(4) The utilisation of mobile service units set-up under family planning programme for integrated medical, public health and family planning services operating in the field.

The main recommendations of the Committee were:

(a) The present Auxiliary Nurse Midwives be replaced by newly designated 'Female Health Workers' and the present day Basic Health Workers, Malaria Eradication Assistants and Family Planning Health Assistants to be replaced by 'Male Health Workers.'
(b) The programme for having multi-purpose workers should be first introduced in areas where malaria is in maintenance phase and smallpox has been controlled and later to other areas as malaria passes into maintenance phase or smallpox controlled.
(c) For proper coverage there should be one primary health centre for a population of 50,000.
(d) Each primary health centre should be divided into 16 sub-centres, each having a population of about 3,000-3,500 depending upon the topography and means of communication.
(e) Each sub-centre should be staffed by a team of one male and one female health worker.
(f) There should be a male health supervisor to supervise the

work of 3-4 male health workers and a female health supevisor to supervise the work of 4 female health workers.

(g) The present day lady health visitors to be designated as female health supervisors.

(h) The doctor incharge of a primary health centre should have the overall charge of all the supervisors and health workers in his area.

Shrivastava Group Report, 1975

The Shrivastava Group also known as "Group on Medical Education and Support Manpower" was appointed by the Government of India in 1974 under the Chairmanship of Dr. J.B. Shrivastava, the then Director General of Health Services, Government of India. The terms of reference of the group were:

(a) To devise a suitable curriculum for training a cadre of the Health Assistants conversant with basic medical aid preventive and nutritional services, family welfare, maternity and child welfare activities so that they can serve as a link between the qualified medical practitioners and multi-purpose workers, thus forming an effective team to deliver health care, family welfare and nutritional services to the people.

(b) Keeping in view the recommedations made by earlier Committees on Medical Education, specially the Medical Education Committee (1968) and Medical Education Conference (1970) to suggest suitable ways and means for implementation of these recommendations and to suggest steps for improving the existing medical educational processes so as to provide due emphasis on the problems particularly relevant to national requirements.

(c) To make any other suggestions to realise the above objectives and matters incident thereto.

After carefully examining various reports and papers relevant to the subject including the recommendations of as many as 12 Conferences and Committees held earlier, the major recommendations of the group were:

(a) A nationwide network of efficient and effective services suitable for our conditions, limitations, and potentialities should be evolved.

(b) Steps should be taken to create bands of para-professional or semi-professional health workers from the community itself to provide simple protective, preventive and curative services which are needed by the community.

(c) Between the community and the primary health centre, there should be two cadres—health workers and health assistants. (1) Health workers should be trained and equipped to give simple specified remedies for day-to-day illness. (2) Health assistants would work as intermediaries between the health workers and the Primary Health Centre. The health assistants should be located at the sub-centres. Like the health workers, they should also be trained and equipped to give specific remedies for simple day-to-day health problems. While they will have a supervisory role over the health workers, they would also function as health workers in their own areas and carry out the same duties and responsibilities, but at a higher level of technical competence.

(d) The Primary Health Centre should be provided with an additional doctor and a nurse to look after the maternal and child health services.

(e) The possibility of utilising the service of senior doctors at the medical college, regional, district or taluka hospitals for brief periods at primary health centre should be explored.

(f) The Primary Health Centre as well as taluka, tehsil, district, regional and medical college hospitals should each develop living and direct links with the community around them, as well as with one another within a total referral services complex.

(g) The Government of India should constitute under an Act of Parliament a Medical and Health Education Commission for coordination and maintaining standards in medical and health education on the pattern of University Grants Commission.

Alma Ata Declaration (1978)

In the International Conference on Primary Health Care, jointly organised by the WHO and UNICF in Alma Ata, USSR in September 1978, fundamental principles of health development were enunciated and a declaration was made which was by the 30th World Health Assembly (1977). This is popularly known as Health for All (HFA) and it is to be achieved through primary health care approach in a spirit of social justice and as a part of overall development. (see Appendices I and III for Alma Ata Declaration and Alma Ata Recommenations).

National Health Policy

A statement on the "National Health Policy" was laid on the Table of both the Houses of Parliament on the second November 1982.[8] The National Health Policy was discussed at length in both Houses and was approved by the Rajya Sabha on fourth August 1983, and the Lok Sabha on 22nd December, 1983. (Refer Appendix I for the Statement on National Health Policy). The Policy lays stress on the preventive, promotive, public health and rehabilitative aspects of health care and points to the need of establishing comprehensive, primary health care services to reach the population in the remotest areas of the country, the need to view health and human development as a vital component of overall integrated national socio-economic development, decentralised system of health care delivery with the maximum community and individual self-reliance and participation. The policy also lays stress on ensuring adequate nutrition, safe drinking water supply and improved sanitation for all segments of the population. The policy sets out specific goals to be achieved by 1985, 1990 and 2000 A.D. in pursuance of the national commitment for the attainment of the goal of Health For All by 2000 A.D. The Government has been to come out with a New Health Policy to meet the health needs of the people in 21st century. Sixth conference of Central Council of Health and Family Welfare held from April 8 to 10, 1999 at New Delhi came out with a draft National Health Policy to remedy the weakensses in the existing National Health Policy (see Appendix IV for Draft Health Policy). In addition, Govenment of India has enacted National Population Policy, 2000, which is an attempt to improve the quality of life of the people through population control.

Basic Concepts: Parameters for Assessment of Primary Health Care

I. Availability of Health Services

The availability of health services is a major factor of the accessibility of services, and is taken to mean the physical presence of a health service provider who constitutes a primary entry point to the health service system, either providing the service directly, or providing referral to another health care provider at an appropriate facility level.

II. Accessibility of Health Services

"Accessibility" is taken to mean the composite of the characteristics of health services which facilitate or obstruct their utilization by potential consumers. Accessibility also incorporates such factors as the availability of needed drugs and supplies; affordable costs to consumers who seek and receive services, including service cost, transportation cost, and cost in time, and social factors relating to the consumer provider interaction, such as the service provider's attitude towards and rapport with consumers.

III. Acceptability and Acceptance of Health Services

The proof of accessibility and acceptability of health services is "acceptance" of health services that is the actual utilization of health services or the expressed demand for services by consumers.

W.A. Hassouna in his article, "A Strategy against Poverty" says that in most developing and some developed countries, governments have been the major providers of preventive and curative health care. These services used to be accessible to the poor since they were provided without charge. But the unprecedented escalation of the cost of health services in the last ten years and the adoption of economic reforms which usually resulted in sizeable reductions of allocations for health services have greatly reduced the access of the poor to government health services. Such reforms have affected curative more than preventive care since than preventive care since many governments provide the latter free or at minimal cost.

Several ways have been adopted in various countries to increase access to health services, all of which are aimed at reducing the patient's economic burden. Unfortunately, most of the approaches such as health insurance and cost-sharing are geared to helping middle-income groups rather than the poor who cannot afford to pay insurance premiums or even reduced fees, and in many cases will not have the cash to pay for health services when they are seriously sick.

It seems clear that what is needed is a system that ensures for the poor a reasonable access to health services with a minimal economic burden. This could be done by including specific health benefits within a compulsory social insurance system or making available interest-free loans from group savings to be used in case of sickness.

Certainly, increasing access to health services as a strategy for poverty alleviation should be dealt with in a comprehensive manner that takes into account physical, social, cultural and economic factors. The ultimate aim should be to put "reasonable quality of care" at an affordable cost within the reach of the poor, rather than offering low quality of care at cheaper prices. The aim should be to put "reasonable quality of care" at an affordable cost within the reach of the poor, rather than offering low quality of care at cheaper prices.

We must, however, be clear that health for all does not mean that in the year 2000 nobody will be sick or disabled nor does it mean that in the year 2000 doctors and nurses will provide medical repairs for every body in the world. It does mean that health begins at home, in schools, and in working places. It does mean that the people will use better approaches than they do now for preventing diseases and reducing unavoidable illness and disability and better ways of growing up, growing old, and dying, gracefully.

B. GENERAL PRINCIPLES OF PRIMARY HEALTH CARE WHILE DEVELOPMENT OF PRIMARY HEALTH CARE IS LIKELY TO BE

(1) Increasing involvement of the community in all aspects of programming.
(2) Adaptation of local health service personnel to Primary Health Care.
(3) The closer links of health with general development.
(4) Need of national resources and political will to support Primary Health Care.

1. Participation: It Means Self-motion

Such participation can be mobilised if the community is properly educated. This education would help them pinpoint the obstacles to development. In the field of health, this would enable them to diagnose their health problems and to deal with their problems in the most effective way. When the community is enlightened, every man and woman would become a secret teacher. Man's energy is tbe most powerful tool of health and socio-economic development.[9] "It does not tally with reality to view the political and administrative environment solely in terms of a Central Government acting upon an inert periphery."[10] According to Professor Ramalingaswami, Director General ICMR:

> "An indigenous health system based on community health derived personnel is needed in which the services are economical, acceptable, continuous and belong to the people."[11]

Community participation must not become an amorphous and abstract slogan like all other socio-political entities; a community comprises different and often conflicting interests. Community participation will only have real meaning when a democratic and genuinely participatory system prevails political power must be in the hands of the people and not in those of interested groups, such as local chiefs and property holders. The poor individually cannot stand up or speak up for their rights and privileges and remain meek spectators in the development process. So, participation by the majority is possible only if they are mobilised. Mobilisation should be done tactfully. To gain the confidence of the poor, we must guard against the strong opposition by the power group in the village.[12]

2. Adaptation of Local Health Service Personnel to Primary Health Care and their Utilisation

The Primary Health Care envisages the provision of health care through trained personnel indigenous to the community. This worker is chosen from the village and by the village and trained to deliver elementary integrated health service. Such workers properly trained through well-designed short-term courses can provide effective, acceptable and inexpensive health care to the community. According to WHO: "Primary Health Care is likely to be most effective if it employs means that are understood and accepted by the community and applied by community health workers at a cost the community and the country can afford. These community health workers, including traditional practitioners where applicable, will function best if they are properly trained socially and technically to respond to the community's expressed health needs. The skills that community health workers require and their consequent training will vary widely throughout the world. But whatever their level of skill, it is important that they understand the real health needs of the communities they serve and they gain the active confidence and hacking of the people."[13] Professor V. Ramalingaswami while receiving the Leon Bernard Foundation Award stressed that this system of community-based health services employing auxiliaries must not be understood by the people as "providing inferior medicine to the rural poor." He went on, "An Auxiliary is a health educator, a rudimentary physician, a social worker and a preventive person, all in one. . . . The education and training of auxiliaries is the most challenging task that medicine faces today. Auxiliaries served to bridge the catastrophic separation between hospital-based, fragmented, episodic medicine and mass public health. The principles of educational science and technology must diffuse into their training programmes. It is on our willingness and ability to experiment with auxiliary training programmes that the chances of success will depend. The moment modern medicine penetrates the social veil in developing countries, that it is the moment of triumph of modern medicine. Here is medicine in the raw, medicine rooted in the reality of rural life."[14]

3. The Closer Links with General Development

Community health actions cannot be effective in isolation. These must be linked with the effort of total community development. These should be supported by a community-based organisation. As WHO has stated, "since Primary Health Care is an integral part both of the community's health system and of overall economic and social development without which it is bound to fail, it has to be coordinated on a national basis with the other sectors that contribute to a country's total development strategy."[15]

4. Need of National Resources and Political Will to Support Primary Health Care

National resources are needed to support primary health care. We have to find resources partly from the community and partly from the national exchequer. We have to change priorities of investment in the interest of the poor. The responsibility of the state must be there to provide continuous support in terms of technical knowledge, guidance and supervision, training, supplies and maintenance, the solving of specific problems, and the care of patients referred to other levels of the health system. The presence of a supportive health service infrastructure is essential for primary health care. Political leadership must also understand and appreciate the needs and aspirations of the rural poor. We are sure to provide an acceptable level of health to all the people by the year 2000 if each government has the political initiative, courage boldness, innovation to reorient for the population, its health priorities according to their socio-economic conditions.

5. Health Information System in Relation to Primary Health Care and Community Development (See Chart 11.2)

Information is the planner's raw material, forming the basis for the diagnosis structuring his objectives and permitting him to evaluate the programme's efficiency and effectiveness which have been planned. The degree to which a planner can be successful in terms of the provision of primary health care services will depend upon the degree to which he is able to obtain information about them which is valid and reliable. The term system has been defined as a coherent, integrated whole, being a combination of a number of entities or elements. Similarly, in the information area there are a number of elements which have to be considered in an integrated manner, as components of one system so that they are viewed in totality as means of providing the health administrator with required formation in the appropriate form and at the appropriate time. These elements are:

Input (data).
Analysis and Processing Storage and retrieval Output Flow.

In order to improve the information for Primary Health Care, the following essential steps should be taken into account:

(i) Analysis of System's Requirements

It analyses in depth the system's requirements. Such an analysis will require answers to questions like:

- What are the objectives of Primary Health Care? What are the activities to be carried out?
- What type of evaluation is required to assess the impact of primary health care?
- Who will collect the data?
- How will the data be collected?
- Where, how and by whom will the data be processed?
- How accurate and reliable should such data be?
- What will be the frequency and timeliness of the report? Who will use the information generated and how will it be used?

(ii) Design of Information System

The next step is the actual design of an information system covering all its five elements already mentioned, in such a manner that it fulfils with minimum cost and delay and in the required form, the information requirements of the health care administrator. The following points may be kept in mind:

(a) The data generated at the primary health care level should

CHART 11.2

Primary Health Care System (A Conceptual Model of the Health Information System with Special Emphasis on the Local Community Level)

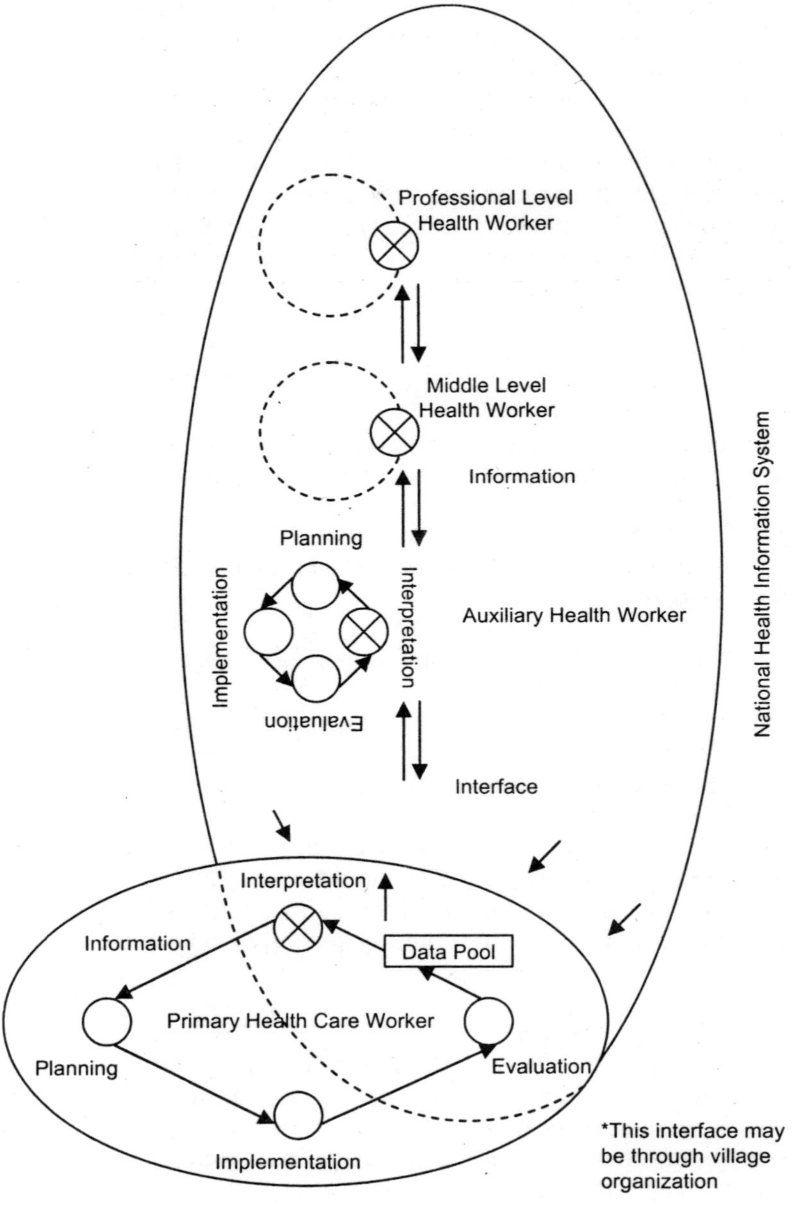

Source: SEA/RC/30/1, p. 47.

correspond to that actually needed for management of primary health care services.

(b) The necessary links between the various sub-systems of the national health information system and the information systems of the other health-related sectors on the one hand and with the primary health care sub-systems on the other, should be provided.

(c) An appropriate method for the processing and analysis of basic data by the supervisors of primary health workers should be designed. The primary health workers may be trained to understand the meaning and the value of the data so that they can play an active role rather than passive transmitters of data.

(iii) Procurement of Necessary Material

The third step is the production of necessary material and the provision of required facilities so that the system could be put into operation, e.g., for a manually operated system the formats have to be produced.

(iv) Installation

The information system should be set-up keeping in mind, to retain as far as possible, the existing procedures and system. It may replace the other components which require change slowly.

(v) Operation and Follow-up

The output of the system is examined against the objectives for which the system was designed. It should be the endeavour to continuously improve upon the system taking into account the changed situation.

This information in primary health care may be supplemented with the case studies carried out by the community. This system of community case study implies a form of popular participation and thus would enhance the utility and scope of primary health care.[16]

C. EXPERIMENTS OF PHC IN DIFFERENT PARTS OF THE WORLD

In this section we would review (on the basis of case studies conducted by the health experts in different parts of the world) the progress of the implementation of primary health care in different parts of the world. After this we shall discuss the progress of primary health care in India.

Experiment of the Soviet (Kazakhstan)[17]

Before the Russian Revolution of 1917, Soviet Kazakhstan was one of the most backward and neglected provinces of Tsarist Russia. Not more than two per cent of the total population could read and write. In the field of health, there was not a single medical institution and the number of medical personnel was negligible.

Today, this region enjoys all the health facilities. Five medical schools and 26 junior medical colleges have helped to train some 40,000 doctors and more than 130,000 intermediate level medical workers. The bed-population ratio is 12:4.

After the revolution, primary health care formed the basis of the health system. It provided service through out-patient and posts staffed by midwives and fieldscher (medical auxiliaries). Each post is staffed by a nurse as well as a fieldscher and a midwife and covers about five hundred people. Those posts enlist the support of the population to carry out health activities. These also train assistants voluntary health workers from the Red Cross Society. The posts are also helped in their work by members of the rural workers' councils, by school teachers, by students, by rural youth groups, and by the managements of collective and state farms. The function of each post is to organise and carry out primary preventive health measures, i.e., immunization, home visiting of patients and new born babies, sanitary inspection of land and installations, primary epidemic, central measures, health education, etc. In addition, the post carries out primary curative measures including treating patients, carrying out instruction of the rural or district physician, or referring patients to the physician for medical advice treatment. There is a medical store attached to every post.

Primary Health Care in Kazakhstan as in all the Republics of the Soviet Union is closely integrated with socio-economic plans of the rural districts and also with the overall medical care system.

Soviet Kazakhstan had 60 years' experience in the organisation and successful development of a national public health system and of primary health care. The conditions under which the people of the Republic were able, virtually from scratch, to build-up a public health service closely resemble conditions in developing countries that are still experiencing the aftermath of colonial oppression. The study of Kazakhstan public health experience should therefore prove useful for all public health administrators particularly for representatives of the developing countries.

Experiments of Columbia[18]

The problems of health in Columbia is typical of the situation in most developing countries. In fact, mortality rate is very high, 45 per cent of the rural population have no access to safe drinking water. The former health system has not been meeting existing demands of the population. Thirty-six per cent of the population in rural and urban slums never or rarely use doctors or hospitals. They are organising a new mode, called M.A.C. system (Modulo de Amplication de Cobertura). Dr. Norberto Martinez explained the thinking behind it. We were aiming at people who had been inaccessible, culturally, economically and geographically to formal health provision. There were rural people and rural migrate living in belts of misery around the cities, not participating in modern economic and social life. These people were not using the health services, so we needed to build a bridge between them and the services by using auxiliaries drawn from their own communities. High technology was not appropriate because it cost much and our resources were limited. Moreover, most people were dying of a basic diseases that could be cured or prevented by using a fairly simple technology without the need for highly qualified personnel. The key to the new system is Columbias own brand of the barefoot doctor selected from the area to be served. These workers are trained for four months and receive an allowance of US $ 850 a month. They serve 3,000 people in the fringe urban areas or 1,000 in the more scattered rural areas. Each group of 6 workers is backed by a MAC health centre to which they can refer difficult cases.

> "It is perhaps too soon to judge just how effective the MAC system will be. But even in its two years, it seems to have reached out to a section of the population previously untouched by the health services. It has made a start on the crucial vaccinations and environmental health campaigns that will prevent so much disease. Above all, it has begun to get people out of their traditional fatalistic attitudes which lead them to suffer patiently, believing that basically nothing could or should be done about it unless they were at deaths door. The marginal millions of Columbians are becoming actively interested in doing something individually and collectively to improve their own health."

Experiments in Thailand[19]

More than half of Thailand's approximately 7500 graduate physicians live and practice in Bangkok. The doctor population ratio was 1:22,070 for the provinces and 1:84,000 for the countryside. The people in the countryside do not have any access to medical care. WHO (UNICEF assisted) provincial health care project was formulated whereby it is planned to train 22,400 village health volunteers, about 200,000 village health communicators, 2800 tambon doctors and 8400 granny midwives during the next five years.

Although Thailand still has a long way to go before health care reaches all its citizens, the adoption of Primary Health Care programmes will do much to alleviate the feeling of hopelessness that many villagers had thought was their inevitable fate.

Experiments of Costa Rica and Mexico[20]

There were no organised health services available in these two countries. The shortage of health workers hampered the development of health services. In 1972 WHO and other agencies began collaborating in a local development effort (PRODESCH) to identify and stimulate the type of activities that could be meaningfully undertaken by the community itself. The progress is going on. They are both examples of how communities with outside support can resolve their own problems and thus can generate enough confidence in themselves to go ahead with other socio-economic efforts.

Most of the countries in Asia, Africa and Latin America have either introduced or are planning to introduce Primary Health Care system to provide health care to the unprivileged section of their countries. This is a challenging task which requires constant, continuous and persistent efforts of their governments and especially the health departments. All these countries may learn from each other's experiences and improve the mechanism of primary health care programmes. If such programmes are successful, it is sure that the health care would be available to all the people in the world by 2000 A.D. without exception.

Primary Health Care in India

The provision of adequate health care to 1 billion people is a challenging task. The Government has been trying to provide health care through primary health centres, dispensaries and mobile units.

The quality and quantity of medical care available is extremely variable—ranging from organised, sophisticated and advanced in urban areas to the most primitive in rural areas. The Fifth Five Year Plan emphasized that the correction of the regional disparities and heavy concentration of health infrastructure and manpower in the urban areas is the imperative of the social justice in the health sector. With this objective a re-orientation of the health programmes and policies was planned as envisaged in the Master Plan considered by the Health and Family Planning Conference held in Delhi in December, 1970. The consensus was that a minimum infrastructure for the entire country particularly in the rural areas should be set-up with the resources available. Many expert committees were appointed from time to time to look into these glaring contradictions during the last three decades. These committees have made some concrete and some general suggestions but because of the implementation crisis in the developing countries, nothing much substantial has been achieved. We are much concerned about these 70 per cent of the people living in rural areas. It is a stupendous task.

Village Health Guide Scheme

The Village Health Guide Scheme was initially started as Community Health Workers' Scheme on 2nd October, 1977 in all the States except Arunachal Pradesh, J&K, Kerala and Tamil Nadu. The Scheme was renamed as Village Health Guide Scheme in 1981, when it was made 100% centrally sponsored scheme under Family Welfare Programme. According to the scheme, the village community selects a volunteer as Village Health Guide, who after training acts as a link between the community and the governmental health system. He/she mainly provides health education and creates awareness on MCH and Family Welfare Services. He/she has to keep track of communicable diseases, treat minor ailments and provide first aid to the patients.

At present, about 3.23 lakh VHGs are reported to be working. Each VHG is paid an honorarium of Rs. 50 per month. The Scheme has recently been reviewed by a committee of experts, which has looked into various aspects of the scheme such as the usefulness of the scheme, the work done by VHGs, capability of VHGs in the context of institutional arrangements available in the country, enhancement of honorarium and other facilities available to VHGs, etc. The committee obtained feedback from the states and visited some of the states to get first hand information and it has submitted its final report/recommendations and the same is being examined in the Ministry.

D. CRITICAL APPRAISAL OF THE HEALTH GUIDE SCHEME IN INDIA

Health Guide Scheme in India has not made much impact so far. It was initiated to provide health care for the people and by the people. A seed can flourish and develop into a full-fledged plant only in a congenial soil and environment. Similarly, Health Guide Scheme can be successful if a sound organisation set-up is provided for its growth. Let us analyse the reasons which are responsible for its failure in the areas where the scheme was introduced. If we want to put the scheme on a sound footing, we may keep the following facts and suggestions in mind.

Health Experts Lack Commitment

There persists widespread negative and unhelpful attitude among health personnel towards the health care of the poorest strata in the rural and urban population. They are not aware of the social responsibility to the society. If the doctors at the primary level are not mentally convinced of the scheme, changes at the grass-roots are unimaginable and impracticable. Most of the doctors and health experts contacted by the writer pointed out that, "Such schemes are unworkable as the community health workers cannot learn much during such a brief training. Instead of being an asset to the health care system, they may reverse the trends and they may create more problems than solutions." Others remarked that, "They are already overworked. They do not find any time to have intimate contacts with the community." A few remarked that, "the present health care system cannot meet the needs of the society. The new system may be given a trial but the care may be taken to plan the scheme effectively before the introduction." The Medical Association has been vocal enough and described this scheme as a "cruel joke." The major hurdle is the opposition to change. Established health associations, institutions and organisations find it difficult to come out from their ivory towers and adjust to change and accept new challenges and responsibilities. Their resistance may be an attempt to defend their false prestige or traditions. Thus, there is a need to convince and train the health experts and their organisations before launching such schemes. We may cultivate a change in their attitudes in the interest of the programme.

At the Golden Jubilee Celebrations of the Indian Medical Association, its President, Dr. J.V.R. Sarma, said that the IMA had not been consulted by Planning Commission in the matter of evolving an effective pattern of rural health care and a national policy on health. He complained that various Governments had instead devised schemes arbitrarily to "suit the fancies and philosophies of changing personalities." If the entire medical manpower could be involved through their professional organisations he was confident that it would be possible to achieve the objective of the scheme. There is an element of truth in this criticism. The Government should not only consult experts before formulating any scheme but should also be able to energize, enthuse and develop a rapport with the professional organisations and, through them, their individual members to take an active part in the community health programmes.[21]

Opposition from Local Practitioners

The scheme is being opposed by the established personnel of traditional system of medicine and local allopathic practitioners. They view this scheme as an encroachment on their authority and prestige. Most of the community health workers interviewed by the writer remarked, "practitioners of all the systems of medicine are making a lot of money by exploiting the illiterate poor in the villages. They think that if the scheme becomes successful, their future existence is uncertain. Besides, they have a strong hold on their clients and through them they spread propaganda against the utility of this scheme." One of the workers went on to the extent, "These practitioners would warn community that those people who would consult the community health workers would be in trouble as they knew nothing." Thus, there is a need to educate these practitioners properly and associate them in the planning and implementation of the scheme.

Insufficient Training to Community Health Workers

The training imparted to the community health workers is quite inadequate. He has a very weak educational base. Dr. C. Parkash, Senior Medical Superintendent, Medical College, Rohtak, remarked about this scheme to *The Tribune*, "The scheme is conceptually sound . . . . Since the success of the scheme will largely depend on the quality of personnel chosen for the job . . . A bare three months' training to a person who had schooling up to sixth standard is not likely to adequately equip him for the job."[22] The same opinion was expressed by Prof. S.P. Gupta,

Professor of Medicine in Medical College, Rohtak."[23] The Indian Medical Association suggested that the qualification for a CHW should be matriculation and that he must undergo at least 15 months' training to acquire the fundamental knowledge needed for his work. He is to be trained in medicine, art of communication, leadership, etc. The people pointed out that the community health workers do not have much education and training to discharge the responsibilities entrusted to them. The success of the scheme would depend upon the confidence of the community in these workers. There is need for screening these workers so that we retain only those workers who can really be effective. Besides, it has also become apparent that the process of retraining is essential in order to fill the gaps in the initial training or to refresh the health and medical knowledge imparted on a poor educational base.

Medical Education is Urban Oriented

There is national commitment to reorient medical education profession and health services, so as to serve the needs of rural people. All the expert bodies have agreed to modify the syllabus of under-graduate medical education so as to produce a basic doctor who would have the ability to cater to the needs of the rural area. It is necessary to make the medical colleges act not as ivory temples in majestic isolation but take on the responsibility for providing total health care for specified segment of the rural population.[24] The aim of medical education should be to promote happiness through better health of most of the deprived hundreds of millions of human beings. With the contemplated changes in the contents of the under-graduate course, the students would be in a position to appreciate the problems of rural people and would develop proper motivation to help them.

Village Community not Educated

Rural people lack functional literacy which is *sine qua non* for any endeavour towards community development. This requires a great effort on the part of the State governments; voluntary institutions and the health administrators should properly educate and enlighten the people. Properly planned programmes of health education would go a long way in propagating the ideals of a primary health care. It was observed by the writer that no regular efforts are being made to educate the public either by the health department or by the CHW. CHW devotes most of his time in providing curative care rather than laying much emphasis on educational approach. We must provide elementary and simple health education to the community. It should be based on indigenous technology. According to Dr. Mahler, the required new type of health education should be, "neither over-sophisticated nor condescending but rather gains the confidence of the individuals and communities by explaining health technology in a language they can understand so that they can participate genuinely in taking decisions concerning their health.

In short, a replacement of passive health education by active health learning." Besides, the beneficiaries should be asked to contribute to the cost of Primary Health Care. Everyone should realise his responsibility towards the health coverage of the community. When the rural people would be contributing, they would like to participate and take interest in its functioning. Some nominal contributions may be taken from the people themselves depending upon their income.

No Mechanism for Community Participation

Community participation is the way to development but how to go about it? In the field of primary health care, it was pointed out by the workers that, "It is impossible to educate all the people by them. They have to carry out their own work, and this is only their part time duty. At present, there is no system to involve the community." It is suggested that we may involve teachers, Panchayat members and their influential men and women to diffuse the health education in the community. The constitution of Youth Clubs, Mother Clubs, etc., as has been done in DRK, may be set-up to promote functional literacy and health education among the community.

Exploitation by Community Health Workers

Community health worker is the pivot of the whole scheme. The success or failure of the scheme would depend to a great extent upon the attitudes, perception and ethos of the workers. It has been mentioned that "These workers are not being selected properly. The selection of Community Health Worker has become a political patronage." Such a scheme would have no chance to grow and ultimately survive if we do not find workers who are committed to bring about a social change in the villages. They must have missionary zeal. Their enthusiasm should not be dampened by unfavourable local conditions. They must have zeal and preservance to reorient the attitudes of the people, otherwise the whole scheme would be a failure. Some people went to remark, "These community health workers have become the agents of the political parties. They are making a lot of money. They want to pose as doctors. They are not easily accessible. They are exploiting the poor people." A section of medical practitioners apprehends that, "half-baked and semi-literate persons masquerading as barefoot doctors will play havoc with the health of the masses." What is the difference then between the private practitioners and CHW workers. It is high time that we select, train and develop our community health workers properly. We must get a system by which we must be able to assess the work of these workers. *The Tribune* editorial, dated 17 July 1975 had rightly commented that, "If pickine cood man is the most important of them all, dumping the bad one is the next most important." We know that even poorly devised machinery may be made to work if manned with well trained, intelligent, imaginative and devoted staff. On the other hand, the best planned organisation may produce unsatisfactory results if it is operated by mediocre or disgruntled people. So, we must find out workers who are committed, willing to accept hardships and prepared to work in a spirit of dedication.

Absence of Political Support to Solve Problems of Rural Areas

The political elite in the country are not sensitive and responsive to their duties. They are busy with manipulation of politics and find hardly any time to look into the problems of the people. Because of instability in politics, there is no continuous, concerted and consistent effort to weed out the obstacles in the path of development. What is required is a strong political will and determination to make these schemes successful. Political elite at all levels must support the cause of the rural poor and help them to enjoy the good standards of life which were promised to them at the inception of independence. Political powers and wisdoms are constantly required in a democratic set-up to resolve any problem arising out of the policies and implementation of the scheme. The political elite may have to take bold and unpleasant steps to reallocate the resources between urban and rural sectors.

No Sound Administrative set-up to Implement the Policies of Community Health

A revolutionary scheme of this type can be successful only if there is proper administrative set-up to implement it. Most of the health experts are of the view that the scheme has been rushed through without examining its requirements. It is suggested that some experts in Public Administration may examine the organisation and procedures which are being used to implement the scheme. They may also examine the problems of coordination, control, supervision and headquarters-field relationships. In the light of the suggestions, the existing scheme may be modified to suit the requirements and the scheme in new areas may be set-up according to new recommendations. One of the very important problem is the poor quality of supervision of the scheme. Multi-purpose health workers who are supposed to be their immediate supervisors lack proper orientation and training themselves. It is suggested that the multi-purpose workers may be given refresher courses to discharge their duties efficiently.

Absence of Proper Evaluation

Evaluation is one of the most important components of any scheme. The good evaluation is to measure the impact of this scheme on health, the process of operations and scheme replicability. When the writer contacted the health experts, they pointed out many difficulties. Most of them observed, "No evaluation machinery has been designed. No methodology has been designed to measure the output. There is no simple information system by which the assessment of the scheme implemented so far can be made." This situation leads to failure in taking timely decisions and lack of feedback. Without an appropriate feedback, the health workers of the PHC level feel frustrated and their function as agents for information becomes meaningless to them. This lack of feedback is probably one of the most important problems in the development of primary health care which need solution. It is suggested that a simple information system may be designed to suit the conditions prevailing in a particular area.

Insufficient Supply of Drugs

The drugs are very costly. Most of the workers mentioned that "The amount of Rs. 600 per year for drugs is too small to meet the demands of the people." It is suggested that:

(a) The Government must strengthen the drug industries in the public sector and manufacture essential drugs at cheaper prices.
(b) The indigenous medicine may be standardised and used to provide cheaper services.
(c) Beneficiaries may be asked to contribute two to five rupees per head per year to make the scheme viable and effective. This would also encourage more participation.
(d) Researches to exploit local flora and fauna as medicine may be encouraged.
(e) More treatment may be suggested through the control of diet and naturopathy which would lead to better health.
(f) The supply of drugs may be made in time to keep the morale of the workers high and win confidence of the people.

CONCLUSION

The experiment of Community Health Workers' Scheme in India has not gone on long enough to reveal all the problems inherent in it. Besides, it has not acquired the sophistication and expertise that one associates with already existing health programmes. There has been great opposition from many quarters. They consider this system as inferior and primitive. But their opposition is based on superficial thinking. There is no substitute for a poor country like India where the people cannot afford the costly medical care system. It may be noted here that even highly industrialised societies are depending upon such schemes to provide effective health care to the community. There is no denying the fact that this is theoretically sound and can help the unprivileged people and deprived communities to take care of their health problems which otherwise would remain unattended to because of financial and professional constraints. The scheme is a vital link in the country's health schemes. The weakness of the scheme is because of the poor design of the implementation machinery which may be streamlined to provide the health facilities for all.

Notes and References

1. Alastair Anderson, "Strengthening of Health Services: Adapt-Don't Adopt", in *World Health,* July 1976, p. 4.
2. *Ibid.*
3. WHO, *World Health,* May, 1978, p. 26.
4. WHO, SEARO: Annual Report of the Regional Director (1966-77), p. 5. (SEA/RC3/30/2).
5. WHO, "The Role of Frontier Workers", *WHO Chronicle,* Vol. 29, No. 1, (January 1975).
6. WHO: *World Health,* "Primary Health Care", May 1979, p. 6.
7. WHO: SEARO: SEA/RC, 30/Sept. 1977, p. 38.
8. Giovanni, Sartori, "Concept Misformation in Comparative Politics", *The American Political Science Review,* Vol. LXIV, No. 4, December 1970, pp. 1050-52 (Pluralism, integrating, participation, mobilisation).
9. M. Soyasal, "Public Relations in Administration: The influence of the Public on the Operation of Public Administration, Excluding Electoral Rights", General Report to the XIIIth International Congress of Administrative Services, Paris, 1965 (Brussels II AS, 1966, p. 47.
10. P. Yadav Ram: "People's Participation: Focus on Mobilisation of the Rural Poor", UN Asian and Pacific Institute, *op. cit.,* p. 6.
11. H. Mahier, "Further Thoughts of WHO Mission", *WHO Chronicle,* 29, 253-56, 1975.
12. Lucan Pye, Aspects of Political Development, p. 64.
13. Ramalingaswami, *op. cit.,* p. 12.
14. WHO, *World Health,* July, 1976, p. 12.
15. For details refer to Chapter VIII.
16. See Chart 11.1 to understand the intricacies of Health Information System in relation to Primary Health Care System.
17. Based on the article, "A Land Transformed", written by Prof. T.S. Sharmonov, Minister, Health of the Kazakh Soviet Socialist Republic, and corresponding member of the Soviet Academy of Medical Science, in *World Health,* May 1978, pp. 4-6.
18. Based on the article, "Building a Bridge" by Paul Harrison, British Journalist and photographer in *World Health,* May, 1978, pp. 7-11.
19. Based on the article, "Medicine Man" by Johan Loftus, a Journalist, *World Health,* Oct. 1976, pp. 17-19.
20. Based on the article, "Generating Self-Confidence" by Manual Carballo, a member of the unit of maternal and child health division of Family Health, WHO Headquarters in Geneva, *World Health,* May 1978, pp. 26-29.
21. *Sunday Standard,* Oct. 1, 1978.
22. *The Tribune,* Oct. 25, 1978, Chandigarh.
23. *Ibid.*
24. India: National Plan for Health Care Services in the Rural Area.

CHAPTER 12

HEALTH CARE ADMINISTRATION AT THE UNION LEVEL: ORGANISATION AND WORKING OF MINISTRY OF HEALTH AND FAMILY WELFARE

"The Central Health Ministry is the pivot round which all the major schemes for improving the standards of health of the nation revolve. All major schemes have necessarily to be sponsored and encouraged by the Central Ministry."

—Pt. Jawaharlal Nehru

Health Care Administration at the Union Level: Organisation and Working of Ministry of Health and Family Welfare

Health and Human Development form integral components of overall socio-economic development of a nation. Amartya Sen in his keynote address to the Fifty-second World Health Assembly, Geneva (18th May, 1999) made strong plea for promoting health to ensure development. To quote him, "How does health relate to development? The first point to note is that the enhancement of health is a constitutive part of the development. Those who ask the question whether better health is a good "instrument" for development may be overlooking the most basic diagnostic point that good health is an integral part of good development; the case of the health care does not have to be established instrumentally by trying to show that good health may also help to contribute to the increase in economic growth.

Second, given other things, good health and economic prosperity tend to support each other. Healthy people can more easily earn an income, and people with higher income can more easily seek medical care, have better nutrition, and have the freedom to lead healthier lives.

Third, "other things" are not given, and the enhancement of good health can be helped by a variety of actions, including public policies (such as the provision of epidemiological services and medical care).

While there seems to be a good general connection between economic progress and health achievement, the connection is weakened by several policy factors. Much depends on how the extra income generated by economic growth is used, in particular whether it is used to expand public services adequately and to reduce the burden of poverty. Growth-mediated enhancement of health achievement goes well beyond mere expansion of the rate of economic growth.

Fourth, even when an economy is poor, major health improvements can be achieved through using the available resources in a socially productive way. It is extremely important, in this context, to pay attention to the economic considerations involving the relative costs of medical treatment and the delivery of health care. Since health care is a very labour-intensive process, low-wage economies have a relative advantage in putting more—not less—focus on health care.

Finally, the issue of social allocation of economic resources cannot be separated from the role of participatory politics and the reach of informed public discussion. Financial conservatism should be the nightmare of the militarist, not of the doctor, or the school teacher, or the hospital nurse. If it is the doctor or the school teacher or the nurse who feels more threatened by resource considerations than the military leaders, then the blame must lie partly on us, the public, for letting the militarist get away with these odd priorities.

Ultimately, there is nothing as important as informed public discussion and the participation of the people in pressing for change that can protect our lives and liberties. The public has to see itself not merely as a patient, but also as an agent of change. The penalty of inaction and apathy can be illness and death.[1]

Chart 12.1 depicts the synoptic view of Health Care Administration in the country from top to bottom.

ROLE OF THE UNION GOVERNMENT

According to the Constitution, the Central Government is concerned only with international health matters, assisting and coordinating State activities, establishing standards and promoting research and professional education. Most other health matters are thus reserved for the States and their health departments, though a few, such as mental health, food adulteration, drugs and vital statistics are on the Concurrent list. The 42nd Amendment to the Constitution has made "Population Control and Family Planning" a Concurrent subject and this provision has been made effective from January 1977. The two Health Survey Committees (Bhore and Mudaliar) reporting in 1946 and 1961, did not recommend an amendment to the Constitution although it was stressed that the Central Government should have greater powers to coordinate the activities of the State authorities dealing with health. Many persons from time to time have stressed that the Ministry of Health should be given more powers to deal with health matters.

> "The Central Health Ministry is the pivot round which all the major schemes for improving the standards of health of the nation revolve. All major schemes have necessarily to be sponsored and encouraged by the Central Ministry."
>
> —Pt. Jawaharlal Nehru

CHART 12.1

Synoptic View of Health System in India

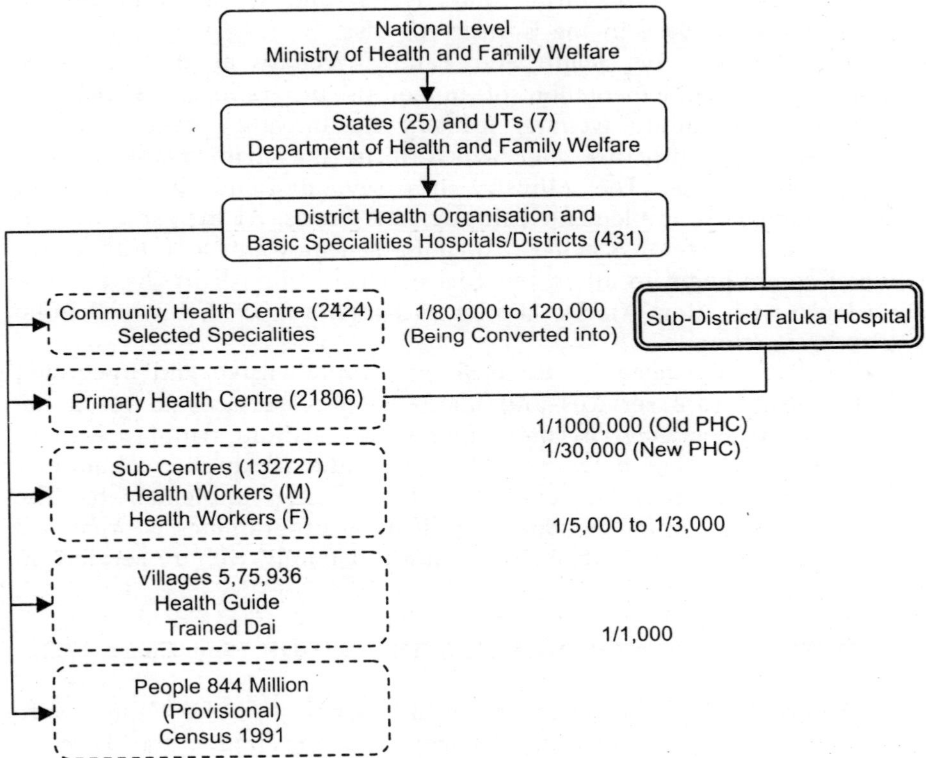

Speaking about the role of the Central Health Ministry, Raj Kumari Amrit Kaur, Minister of Health (1947-57) observed:

> "Health in India is a state subject and the Union Government has mainly as advisory and coordinating function to discharge. The Central Ministry of Health in pursuit of its objective, health for all, has had to initiate countrywide programmes and to coordinate the activities of the various participating States and to see that no State lags behind for lack of Central aid whether in the matter of material or human resources or of technical know-how. In doing this the centre has not arrogated to itself any power of overall control but has maintained the coordinating and advisory function through the Central Council of Health."[2]

The Ministry of Health and Family Welfare plays a vital role in the national efforts to enable the citizens to lead a healthy and happy life. Under the Indian Constitution, the items public health, sanitation, hospitals and dispensaries fall in the State List. Items like population control and family planning, medical education, adulteration of foodstuffs and other goods, drugs and poisons, medical professions, vital statistics including registration of births and deaths and lunacy and mental deficiency find a place in the Concurrent List.

The Ministry of Health and Family Welfare at the Centre is responsible for implementation of numerous programmes of national importance like family welfare, primary health care, prevention and control of major diseases, etc. which form the main plank of our development efforts. The Ministry has several Centrally Sponsored Schemes which are implemented through the States. At the same time, it has also Central Sector Schemes. All these schemes aim at fulfilling our national commitment to attain the goal of Health for All by 2000 AD in accordance with Alma-Ata Declaration of September 1978 to which India is also a signatory.

Realising the need for establishing comprehensive and integrated primary health care services and family welfare services to reach the people's doorsteps even in the remote and far-flung rural areas, an integrated health care delivery system with the maximum community participation has been developed and is being implemented. The administration and implementation of all these programmes is organised through an integrated structure of health and family welfare services in the country.

STRUCTURAL GROWTH AND EXISTING SET-UP (See Chart 12.2)

Before 1947, the medical and health services at the Centre were administered by two separate departments, one under the Director General of IMS and the other under the Commissioner of Public Health. After independence these two offices were amalgamated under the Director General of Health Services and the Post of Commissioner of Public Health was abolished. The Union Ministry of Health was vested with several additional responsibilities, namely, Family Planning, Works and Housing and Urban Development. The functions of Works and Housing and Urban Development were transferred from this ministry. Family Planning was raised to the status of a full-fledged department in 1966, and the Ministry was designated as the Ministry of Health and Family Planning. It is known at present as "Ministry of Health and Family Welfare."

The Union Ministry of Health and Family Welfare is headed by a Cabinet Minister, a Minister of State and a Deputy Health Minister.

The Union Ministry of Health & Family Welfare comprise of the following departments, each of which is headed by a Secretary to the Government of India: (i) Department of Health, (ii) Department of Family

CHART 12.2

Ministry of Health and Family Welfare
Cabinet Minister
Minister of State
Deputy Ministers
Department of Health
Secretary Health
Additional Secretary
Joint Secretaries-(9)
Director General of Health Services
Additional Director Generals (4)
Department of Family Welfare
Secretary
Chief Director (1)
Joint Secretary (3)
Department of Indian System of Medicine and Homoeopathy
Secretary
Chief Ayurvedic and Sidhi
JS (ISM)

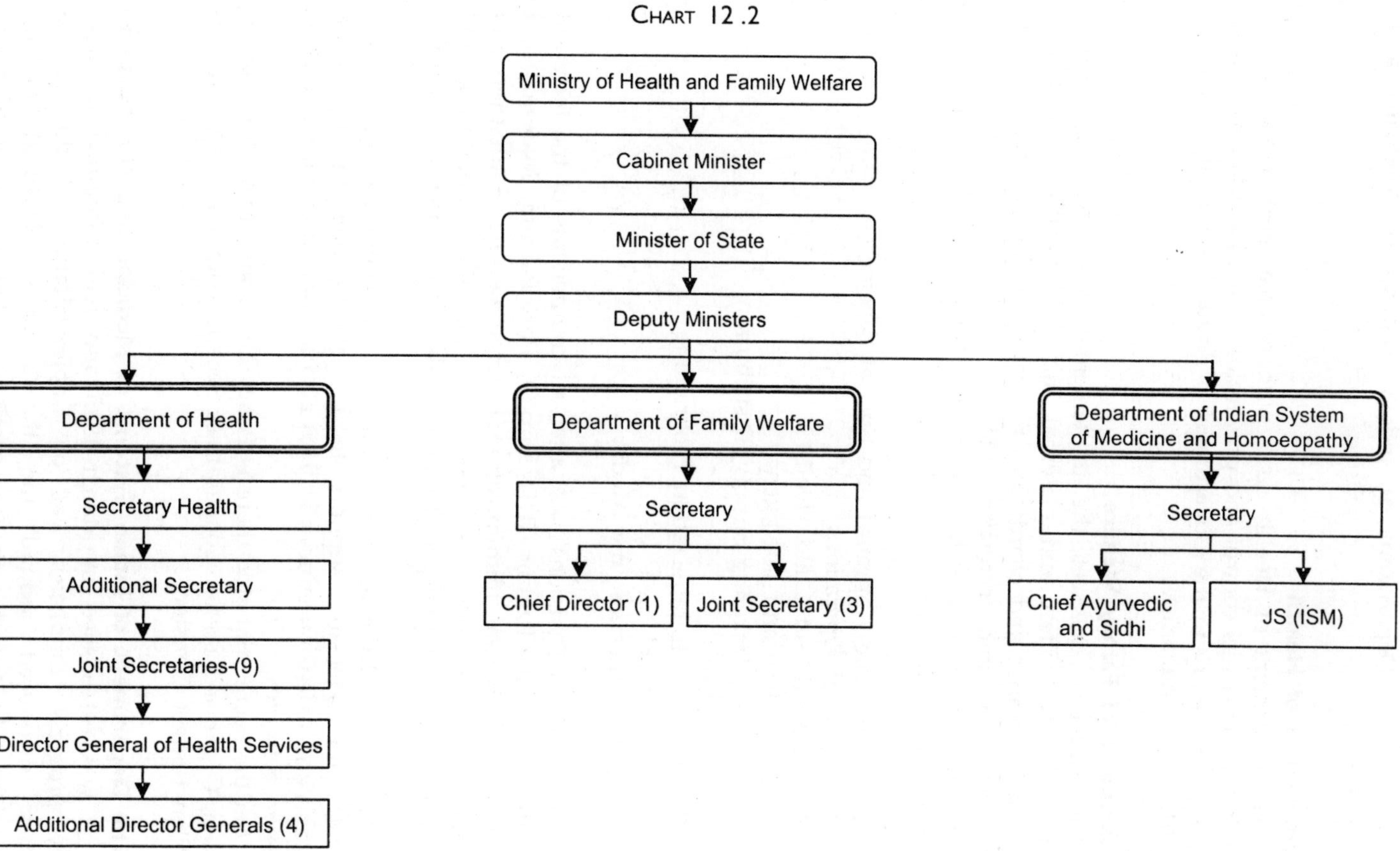

Welfare, and (iii) Department of Indian Systems of Medicine and Homoeopathy.

1. Deapartment of Health

The Department of Health deals with medical and public health matters including drugs control and prevention of food adulteration. It is headed by a Secretary to the Government of India, who is supported by two Additional Secretaries.

2. Department of Family Welfare

The Secretary oversees the implementation of the programmes concerning family welfare and maternal and child health in the States and Union Territories and coordinates the activities and functions of the Technical Divisions and Secretariat side.

On the Technical side, the following Divisions are functioning in the Department of Family Welfare:

1. Programme Appraisal and Special Scheme
2. Technical Operations
3. Maternal and Child Health
4. Evaluation and Intelligence
5. Nirodh Marketing Supply/Distribution
6. Transport
7. Universal Immunization Programme
8. Area Project
9. Mass Education and Media

The Technical Divisions look after all components of the technical programmes viz. Sterilization/IUD/Nirodh, Post Partum, Maternal and Child Health, Universal Immunization Programme, etc. Evaluation and Intelligence Division helps in perspective planning, monitoring and evaluating the programme performance. It also coordinates demographic research.

The Media Division is responsible for providing educational publicity and extension support to the programme through mass education and extension education. It is also looking after the population education activities.

On the Secretariat side there is Policy Division, Aided Programmes Division, Organised Sector, Cooperatives Sector, Voluntary Organisations and Plan Budget Division.

3. The Department of Indian Systems of Medicine and Homoeopathy

It was established in March 1995 and had continued to make steady progress. Emphasis was on implementation of the various schemes introduced around the thrust areas identified by the Department. The thrust areas are education, standardisation of drugs, enhancement of avilability of raw materials, research and development, information, education and communication and involvement of ISM & H in national health care.

FUNCTIONS

Most of the functions of this ministry are implemented through an autonomous organisation called Director-General of Health Services (See Chart 12.3).

The functions of the Union Ministry of Health in terms of specific responsibilities are:

(a) Maintenance of international health relations, administration of port health and quarantine laws.
(b) Administration of Central health institutions, training colleges, laboratories and hospitals.
(c) Promotion and maintenance of appropriate standards of education in medicine, nursing, dental, pharmaceutical and of ancillary health personnel through statutory bodies and coordination and collaboration with various national associations in health programmes.
(d) Promotion of medical and public health researches through the Indian Council of Medical Research and other research institutions and bodies.
(e) Regulation and development of medical, dental nursing and pharmaceutical professions in consultation with the State governments.
(f) Establishment and maintenance of drug standards (including antibiotics) and of control over the manufacture and sale of drugs and biological products.
(g) Collection of information regarding development in the medical and health services in India and abroad to be made available to all State Governments through the Central Bureau of Health Intelligence.
(h) Maintenance of a Central Medical Library.
(i) Promotion and coordination of health activities through the Central Council of Health.
(j) Establishment of close contact with other Ministries in respect of health measures, e.g., Employees' State insurance Scheme, Factories Act, etc.
(k) Coordination of various activities through consultative committees of the Parliament, statutory bodies, committees and associations.
(l) Negotiations with International bilateral agencies.
(m) Planning and organisation of health activities throughout the country in collaboration with the State governments and the

Planning Commission.

(n) Evaluation of health schemes organised in the country.

(o) Assessment of health conditions in the country through health and morbidity surveys and by regular collection of vital and health statistics and spreading of the information throughout the country.

(p) Promulgations of Central enactments on health matters as may be provided by the Constitution of India.

(q) Organisation of health measures as are required for: (i) the control of inter-State spread of communicable diseases, (ii) the sanitary control of inter-State traffic, and (iii) control of food, drugs in the inter-State commerce.

(r) Organisation and maintenance of a Central Health Service.

(s) Establishment of total medical care programme for the Central Government Employees (Central Government Health Scheme).

(t) Carrying out of the functions of health services in the centrally administered areas.

(u) Power to lay down and enforce minimum standards of health administration for these services which are within the immediate control of other departments e.g., Railways, Prisons, Labour, etc.

The functions of the Family Welfare Department are:

(a) To organize family welfare programme through family welfare centres throughout the country.

(b) To create an atmosphere of social acceptance of the programme and to support all voluntary organisations interested in the programme.

(c) To educate every individual to develop a conviction that a small family size is valuable for him or her, and to popularise every known, appropriate and acceptable method of family planning and to leave the choice of method to the individual couple.

(d) To disseminate the knowledge on the practice of family planning as widely as possible through all available publicity and educational measures, and to provide service agencies nearest to the community.

(e) To organise basic research of human fertility, genetics and population dynamics and on the evolution of easy and more reliable method of contraception.

(f) To study the social factors that affect fertility and to take such steps as will reduce the number of children in a family, e.g., raising the age of marriage, education and employment of women, etc.

(g) To coordinate the family planning programme with the child

CHART 12.3

Organisational Structure of Director General of Health Services (GOI)

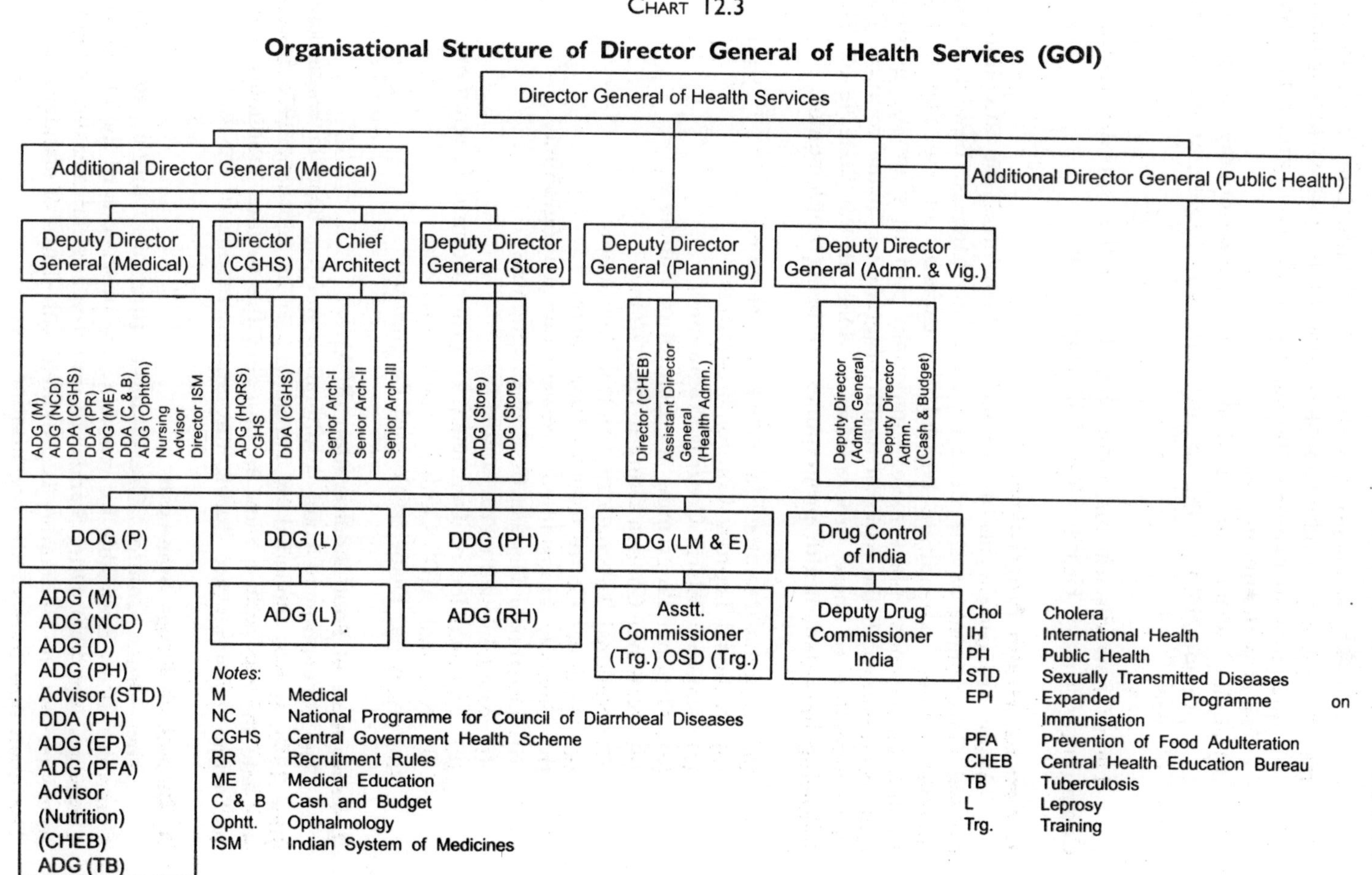

Source: Annual Report of the Ministry of Health and Family Welfare, 1996-97.

welfare and maternal health services throughout the country.

(h) To organise production of contraceptive devices in adequate quantities to maintain the supply at all levels preferably free or at a minimum cost.

(i) India system of medicine and Homoeopathy helps to promote/ISM in the country through training, research and use.

Let us now discuss important activities of the Ministry affecting Community/Primary Health Care at the local level.

1. National Health Programmes

There are certain health problems which need the attention of Central Government as the diseases know no barriers. Besides, these involve a huge expenditure beyond the capacity of the States. The Central Government plays a very important part in planning, guiding and coordinating all the national health programmes in the country. The implementation of these programmes is done at the State level. The following important health programmes are being implemented:

(a) National Malaria Eradication Programme,
(b) National Leprosy Control Programme,
(c) National Filaria Control Programme,
(d) National Programme for Control of Blindness,
(e) National Cholera Control Programme,
(f) National Tuberculosis Control Programme,
(g) National Goitre Control Programme,
(h) Sexually Transmitted Disease Control Programme,
(i) Diarrhoeal Disease Control Programme
(j) Mental Health Programme,
(k) National Iodine Deficiency Disorder Control Programme,
(l) National AIDS Control Programme, and
(m) National Diabetes Control Prograrmme.

2. Prevention of Food Adulteration (PFA)

The Prevention of Food Adulteration Act has been in vogue since June 1955. It was amended by Parliament in its February 1976 Session and late in 1986 with a view to plugging the various loopholes which had come to the surface during the implementation of the Act.

3. Control of Drugs Standards

The Drug Control Organisation functions under the Drug Controller. It is responsible for enforcing the provisions of the Drugs and Cosmetics Act, 1940. Drug Standard Control is a social measure intended to ensure that the community is provided with drugs of standard quality. The main objectives of the organisation are:

(a) Controlling the quality of imported drugs and drugs moving in inter-State commerce;
(b) Coordinating the activities of the State and advising them on matters relating to uniform administration;
(c) Laying down regulatory measures and standards of drugs; and
(d) Granting approval of 'new drugs' proposed to be imported into or manufactured in the country.

It has been conducting training programmes for the training of Drug Inspectors and Drug Analysts concerned with drug standard control.

There is a statutory Drug Consultative Committee constituted under the Drugs and Cosmetics Act, 1940 to advise the Central and State Governments and the Drug Technical Advisory Board on matters tending to secure uniformity in the administration of the Drugs and Cosmetics Act. It consists of representatives of the State and Central Governments.

4. Medical Education

The Centre has set-up regulatory bodies for monitoring the standards of medical education, promoting training and research activities. This is being done with a view to sustain the production of medical and para-medical manpower to meet requirements of the health care delivery system at the primary, secondary and tertiary levels in the country. To achieve the objective, Medical Council of India has been set-up.

The Medical Council of India was established as a Statutory body under the provisions of the Indian Medical Council Act, 1933 which was later repealed by the Indian Medical Council Act, 1956 with minor amendments in 1958 (36 of 1958) and 1964 (24 of 1964). A major amendment in the Indian Medical Council Act, 1956 was made in 1993 to stop the mushroom growth of medical colleges, increase of seats and starting of new courses without prior approval of the Central Government in the Ministry of Health and Family Welfare. The main functions of the council are:

(i) Maintenance of uniform standards of medical education at undergraduate and post-graduate level;
(ii) Maintenance of Indian Medical Register;
(iii) Reciprocity with foreign countries in the matter of mutual recognition of medical qualifications; and
(iv) Provisional/permanent registration of doctors with recognized medical qualifications, registration of additional qualifications and issue of Good Standing Certificate for doctors going abroad to commonwealth countries.

5. Medical Research

Medical Research is co-ordinated through Indian Council of Medical Research (ICMR). It has a network of 21 permanent research institutes and six regional medical research centres distributed throughout the country. During 1997-98 the Council continued research on a wide spectrum of subjects through intramural and extramural project including various multi-centric collaborative projects.

The Council is administered by a Governing Body chaired by the Minister for Health & Family Welfare. The Council receives grant-in-aid from the ministry under Plan and Non-plan for meeting its normal expenditure as well as for plan activities.

6. Health Intelligence

The Central Bureau of Health Intelligence established in 1961 is the agency at the national level, for collection, compilation, analysis, evaluation and dissemination of health statistics. It also disseminates epidemic intelligence to State/Union Territories informing against spread of epidemic diseases and provide necessary intelligence on quarantinable disease to the World Health Organisation according to the International Sanitary Regulations. The Bureau maintains liaison with research institutions in India and abroad and promotes research in health statistics. The Bureau has been giving technical assistance in respect of health statistics to different states.

The Bureau is activity engaged in the monitoring and evaluation of a strategy of 'Health for All' by 2000 A.D. in India. In compliance with the resolution of the World Health Assembly, the Ministry of Health and Family Welfare (MOHFW) has been periodically conducting exercises for monitoring and evaluating the goal of 'Health For All' (HFA). The earlier rounds of monitoring work were carried out in 1982, 1988 and 1994 while the evaluations were undertaken in 1985, 1991 and 1997.

The Bureau has the following objectives:

(a) To centralise collection, compilation, analysis, evaluation, synthesis and dissemination of all information on health statistics for the nation as a whole.
(b) To work out uniform and standard returns so as to get uniform information for efficient interpretation.
(c) To disseminate epidemic intelligence to States and international bodies.
(d) To organise training programmes for personnel in Medical Health statistics in order to meet the expanding needs in the field.
(e) To promote research in health statistics through cooperation with national and international bodies.
(f) To prepare annual report for DGHS and Ministry of Health and Family Welfare.

(g) To publish special issue on different medical and public health problems in the country.

7. National Medical Library

The National Medical Library (NML) under the aegis of Directorate General of Health Services continued to provide wide and efficient access to information to all Health Science Professionals in the country.

8. Facilities for Scheduled Castes and Scheduled Tribes

India is a signatory to the Alma-Ata declaration, 1978 and is committed to achieve the goal "Health for All by the year 2000 A.D." The National Health Policy (1983) accordingly envisages high prioritity to provide health services to those residing in the tribal, hilly and backward areas as well as to endemic diseases affected population and vulnerable sections of the society.

Accordingly, the strategy adopted for meeting the Health care needs of Scheduled Tribes and Scheduled Castes envisages the provision of preventive, promotive and curative services through a network of Primary Health Centres. Rural Dispensaries and at village level through Health Guides and Trained Dais supported by implementation of programme for control of communicable diseases, undertaking of research in diseases to which Scheduled Tribes/Scheduled Castes are generally prone. The mobile dispensaries and camps catering to their needs, at their door-steps are being organised, wherever feasible.

9. Central Government Health Scheme

The Central Government Health Scheme was started in Delhi in 1954 to provide comprehensive care to the Central Government employees stationed at Delhi. The scope of the scheme has been gradually extended over the years to cover cities outside Delhi, Bombay, Allahabad, Meerut, Kanpur, Patna, Calcutta, Nagpur, Madras, Hyderabad, Bangalore, Jabalpur, Jaipur, Pune, Lucknow, Ahmedabad, as well as other sectors of population, such as the employees of the autonomous organisations, retired Central Government pensioners, existing and ex-MPs, ex-Governors, and retired Judges of Supreme Court and High Courts. The services provided are now comprehensive and include:

(1) Laboratory investigations,
(2) Outdoor treatment,
(3) In-patient treatment,
(4) Specialist care,
(5) Emergency services,
(6) Domiciliary services,
(7) Supply of medicines,
(8) Ambulance services,

(9) Ante-natal confinement and Post-natal care,
(10) Optical and dental care, and
(11) Family Welfare Services.

10. International Cooperation for Health and Family Welfare

Various international organisations and the United Nations Agencies continued to provide significant technical and material assistance for many Health and Family Welfare programmes in the country.

World Health *Organisation*

The World Health Organisation (WHO) is collaborating with this country in providing and developing health care facilities. India makes regular annual contribution to WHO.

The WHO provides assistance to Member States on a biennium basis for supplies and equipment, training/fellowship/study tours, short-term consultants, subsidy for Group Educational Activities (Seminars/Workshops/Meetings/Conferences/Studies, etc.) and for participation of Indian experts in various symposia, workshops and seminars organised by the WHO and other international organisations in India and abroad.

World Bank

State Health System Development Projects are being implemented in the following States with World Bank Assistance:

(i) Andhra Pradesh (from 1995 for 6 years) 608 crore;
(ii) Karnataka (1996 for 5 years) 546 crore;
(iii) West Bengal (1996 for 6 years) 698 crore;
(iv) Punjab (1996 for 5 years) 425 crore;
(v) Orissa (1998 for 5 years) 415.58 crore.

The state of Maharashstra has also been cleared by the Bank Board on 8th December, 1998. Besides, small help is rendered by many countries.[3]

CRITICAL APPRAISAL

Ministry of Health and Family Welfare has been striving to improve the status of health of the people in the country. Planned development of over four and a half decades has resulted in improved health facilities. (See Appendix 12.1 for latest statistics).

It has been playing an effective role in co-ordinating the efforts of the State governments and has been supplementing their efforts through national programmes and centrally sponsored schemes. Besides, this Ministry has been providing guidance to the State Health Institutions and Administration. It has also set-up autonomous institutions to guide the

Union and States in the formulation of health policies in their respective fields. Over the years it has become so unwieldy that it is difficult to manage its operations efficiently. These national institutes have become a burden on the exchequer. For example, the Estimates Committee was critical of the performance of AIIMS. It remarked that 19 years after the setting up of the institute—a depressing picture is revealed in the field of medical education in India. Why is it so? it is because of the fact that the persons working in these institutions have been living in ivory towers forgetting about the needs of a common man. Is the common man paying taxes to perpetuate this class of people. The Ministry must find answer to these questions and make its structure relevant to the needs of the society. Dr. Mahler, Director General of the WHO while addressing the senior doctors at the PGI, Chandigarh said that it was a pity that a country like India with its rich intellectual background had still to grapple with basic health problems even 30 years after independence.[4]

According to Tarlok Singh:

> "Whatever the shortcomings of the past two decades and more, and the unbolt rigidities and injustices of our social institutions and modes of thought and behaviour, India possesses resources of unusual richness. We see this on all sides—in the endowments of nature, in economic and technological capacities, in potentials for growth, in the quality and wealth of manpower, in the institutions for research and training, in the available pool of talent and experience. Presently, these resources and energies are being somewhat frittered away for lack of a sense of fundamental directives and failure to build-up a shared national effort. The appraisal of the record of constructive endeavour since independence undertaken in this country supports the belief that it is within India's grasp to eliminate swiftly the worst forms of poverty and, over a period of years, to create a cohesive social order and classless society based on the values of equality, welfare, and mutual cooperation."[5]

There is a need of bold attempt and innovations to set the whole structure in order to subserve the needs of the society. Let us now discuss some facts and suggestions which can help in the improvement of the functioning of this Ministry.

1. Inadequate Facilities

Health facilities in India face many operational difficulties. These include inadequate funding for drugs, supplies and other consumables, shortages of diagnostic facilities and laboratory equipment, and a general deterioration of physical infrastructure. These major constraints lead to a low quality of care and inefficient functioning of the system at first referral units in the district health system. Some innovations have been initiated, based on the concept of community participation (cost-sharing) and through a system of matching grants.[6]

2. Poor Accessibility for Disadvantaged Groups

Modern medicine, today is not within the reach of common man which is a great cause of concern. Policy-makers in the government and especially in the Ministry of Health and Family Welfare need to redefine health policy to ensure on priority of the health care to disadvantaged sections of the society. Dr. Hiroshi Nakajima, Director General of World Health Organisation while inaugurating the meeting on "Policy-Oriented Monitoring of Equity in Health and Health Care, convened from 29 September to 3 October 1997 at WHO headquarters in Geneva stated that the overall gains in health that have occurred around the world are being overshadowed by increasing disparities between rich and poor. Such inequalities are both unnecessary and unjust. To quote him: "equity is a value that governments subscribe to, but do not always make explicit in their policies. The importance of emphasizing this value is that it is often overlooked in today's attempts to tackle the financial problems of health care. Health systems are in turmoil, partly because of severe economic difficulties in some parts of the world. Ministries in rich and poor countries alike have responded to the current pressure by introducing health sector reforms that are market-friendly and encourage competition. Such mechanisms may generate revenue for health, but may increase inequities. The overall gains in health that have occurred around the world are being overshadowed by increasing disparities between rich and poor. The number of people living in absolute poverty now comprises one-fifth of the global population or 1.3 billion people. In health and health care the gap is widening between rural and urban areas, with resources concentrated in the cities. Within the same country, life expectancy and infant mortality rates may vary enormously between regions, and often over 80% of public health expenditures benefit less than 40% of the population.[7]

The government of India must ensure health care to all otherwise, the well-off population may also be affected in the long-run as President Roosevelt rightly stated that "poverty anywhere is a danger to prosperity everywhere." In the new-millennium our policy measures should go in favour of the poor to ensure equality which involves equity in provision and use of health facilities irrespective of income levels.

3. Fragmentation of Sectoral Responsibilities at National Level

Health affects and is affected by other socio-economic factors. There is little coordination between the Ministry of Health and Family Welfare and other ministries to ensure sustained development. Besides, there is no attempt to educate, empower people to ensure equity. To quote World Health Organisation:

> "There are numerous obstacles to the creation of health-supporting environments, not least of which is the fragmentation of sectoral responsibilities at national level. In many countries, health remains the concern of a single ministry rather than a goal to which each sector or ministry contributes in a conscious and coordinated manner. Similarly, traditional boundaries between government and non-governmental organizations, and between the public and the private sectors, hinder the development of strategies and policies informed by an awareness of health and health needs."

This fragmentation can reduce the impact of health-promoting activities, particularly those undertaken at the local level. It is only very limited benefit.[8]

Participation and empowerment are also the key to reducing the gaps between the "haves" and the "havenots." This inequality not only results in disparities in health status but also prevents groups such as women, elderly people, children and indigenous peoples from playing a full role in creating health-supporting environments.

Ensuring that our surroundings are conducive to good health thus means directing effort at all levels, within and between all sectors of society. In so doing we can make the healthier choice the easier choice and lay the foundation for true social and economic development. In the new millennium, we have to empower the people in the real sense, i.e. controlling the system and not merely participating theoretically.

4. Researches Bear no Relevance to Practical Problems

There has been a lack of cooperation and coordination among the institutions engaged in teaching and research. This resulted in disjointed, isolated and rank duplication of scientific research in several national laboratories resulting in waste of scarce resources. The Public Accounts Committee in its 40th Report of the 5th Lok Sabha (1971-72) emphasized the importance of collaboration and coordination among various agencies engaged in medical research with ICMR taking lead and suggested that energetic steps may be taken to enlarge the scope of collaboration to avoid repetitive research.

Besides, over the years, for a variety of reasons the medical research programmes in the country could not follow the path of problem-oriented medical research in priority areas such as nutritional disorders, control of communicable diseases, operational research for providing health care to all, research in medical education, health manpower planning, utilisation of health personnel, research in indigenous system of medicine, etc. The Sixth Draft Plan (1978-83) was also critical of the research policy pursued so far. It was stated that:

> "Medical research in the past had, by and large, failed to lay emphasis on problems of immediate practical importance. Efforts

were mostly towards collection of disjointed and isolated research work by individuals/agencies in the country."

The Estimate Committee in its 102nd Report pointed out that "the purpose of medical research is to bring about results of practical utility in the fight against disease with the maximum expedition possible and that little purpose will be served unless the results of research can find immediate application in the field . . . . It is unfortunate that resources and time and talent of the medical community of the country have not been meaningfully utilized over the years according to well thought out priorities."[9] Thus, there is a need of costing of research projects in terms of time and money likely to be required for their completion. The aim of the research should be to solve health problems of the social significance to the country.

The foreign sponsorship of research projects has not been examined properly before accepting the proposals. The Public Accounts Committee in their 167th and 200th Reports have been very critical of the research projects conducted in collaboration with foreign organizations, e.g. Genetic Control of Mosquitoes Unit Projects, the Bird Migration and Arbovirus studies, the ultra low volume spray experiments, the Pantnagar Microbial Pesticides project and some of the research projects undertaken in West Bengal and Narangwal in collaboration with the John Hopkins University. The Committees are not unwilling to concede the importance of research efforts, the projects examined revealed a rather casual attitude and indifference on the part of the authorities concerned towards foreign supported research in India. The Committee reiterated the imperative need for the utmost care, caution and critical scrutiny before approving foreign sponsorship of research projects undertaken in India, particularly when such projects have military or quasi-military implications of an almost incalculable character. Such researches must be got conducted by the Indian scientists. If the foreign collaboration is indispensable, research ventures should ensure the following:

(a) that such ventures are not only of potential value for the country but are of immediate productive utility;
(b) that the objectives of the projects are clearly spelt out and the research plans are notified in advance so as to avoid any ambiguity;
(c) that the collaborating Indian agency or institution has personnel with the requisite qualification and equipment to concurrently evaluate and monitor the progress of the research;
(d) that the technical and administrative control of the projects and determination of policies vest only with the Indian agencies and personnel concerned;
(e) that all data and materials collected are shared with the

Indian collaborators;
(f) that any kind of secrecy in the conduct of research is eschewed and that the results of the research are made public; and
(g) that all research is conducted in accordance not only with the country's own environmental standards but the international environmental standards as well.[10]

In the new millennium, researches must also be encouraged in the area of equity, quality, telemedicine, etc. to benefit the poor people.

5. Unsuitable System of Medical Education

The objective of a good medical education should be to produce general practitioners, specialists, teachers and research workers. The factors governing this are the curriculum, medium of instruction, duration of course, admission qualifications, the examination system, teacher-students relationship, prospects of teachers and students, etc. Besides, it may be mentioned that the medical education should fit in with the needs of the country and the conditions prevailing there. For instance, 80 per cent of the population of India live in rural areas. The training given to the doctor should enable and motivate him to carry on his work among the vast masses in the villages. We have been designing our under-graduate and post-graduate medical education which can fulfil this basic aim. There has been a big gap between aims and fulfilment. J. Gallagher, Regional Officer for education and training, WHO Regional Office for Europe has expressed concern about, "inadequate communication between educational system for health personnel and the health administrations that use the products of these systems. There is very little understanding of how the manpower training and development needs of health administration can be met in a systematic way."[11]

The Government of India launched Re-orientation of Medical Education Scheme in 1977 with the objective of involving the various medical colleges in the country in the direct delivery of health care services to the rural and semi-rural population. Under the scheme, each medical college in the country is to accept in the first instance, the total responsibility for promotive, preventive, curative health services in three Community Development Blocks in the district in which the institution is situated. The objectives of the scheme are:

(i) To expose the Medical faculty, residents, interns and the students to the Rural Community;
(ii) To train the students, interns and Residents in Community Organisation and Community Participation; and
(iii) To render comprehensive health care to the villages in collaboration with the local Primary Health Centres.

It has been expressed in the Fifth Plan document that teaching in medical colleges still requires a radical change for its orientation towards the need for community care. Medical education over the years has been urban biased. It is hoped that it would be possible to produce medical graduates who are aware of the health problems of the community, who have a sense of compassion and motivation to serve the public and who have ability to effectively meet the urgent needs of the health care problems of the rural masses and the urban-poor.

According to the Estimates Committee:

> "The National Policy should indicate in unmistakable terms the goals to be achieved and the method of accomplishment . . . . Such a policy especially in the context of health being a State subject will help in maintenance of the requisite standards of medical education throughout the country in keeping with the needs of the people"[12]

The Government of India has announced the National Medical Education Policy.

In the new millennium, there is a need to set-up a Health Care Medical Service Commission responsible for planning of medical manpower, medical education, research, training of all para-medical personnel. This Commission when appointed should use Health and Medical Educational Planning as a means of rationalising the education of health manpower. Besides, the Commission may encourage the health administrations to provide the policy and planning backgrounds required for this purpose.

6. Lifestyle Causing many Health Problems

Lifestyles in many countries are also changing radically. Today, more and more people are employed in sedentary occupations in offices and factories, a considerable change from the outdoor labour of earlier times. This has contributed to an increase in morbidity and mortality from heart disease and stroke, the two conditions which are responsible for the majority of premature deaths occurring in the Region. Changes in dietary habits from traditional diets rich in fibre and low in fat, to convenience foods rich in salt, fat and calories and low in fibre, have contributed to the proliferation of these disease. Such dietary habits are also associated with cancers of the breast, rectum and prostrate.

7. Implications of Privatisation and Globalisation for Better Health Services

It is important to note, however, that the implications of globalization for public health are not all negative. The diffusion of modern technologies and ideas between countries presents promising opportunities for improving global health in the future. Recent advances in telecomunications techology, for example, have resulted in global communications links which are unprecedented in world history. Communications technology can be exploited for health purposes, which include: telemedicine, interactive health networks, disease surveillance systems, communication links between health workers, human resource development and continuing education, and distance learning.

In summary, a strong case can be made that the globalization of public health represents an important trend for the 21st century. Although some transnational health problems have historical precedents, many new issues are emerging which are unique to our time. The 1997 Kyoto conference on climate change underscored the fragility of the world's ecosystem, and showed how interdependent the health of all of humanity has become. Shared global problems transcending state borders call into question conventional paradigms which divide countries into North and South, or developed and developing.[13]

We had gone a long way in promoting better health in 20th century. With the new developments, we should ensure decent health care to all in the new millineum so that people can enjoy good quality of life and not simply adding of years.

Notes and References

1. Amartya Sen, Health in Development, in *Bulletin of the WHO*, Vol. 77, No. 8, 1999, p. 623.
2. Borkar, G., Health in Independent India (Revised Edition) 1961, Ministry of Health, New Delhi, p. ix.
3. *Ibid.*, p. xvii.
4. *The Tribune*, Chandigarh, February 24, 1979.
5. Tarlok Singh, India's Development Experience, Macmillan India, 1974, Delhi; pp. 453-54.
6. WHO, Health Situation in the South-East Asia Region, 1994-97, p. 186.
7. WHO: Final Report of meeting on Policy Oriented Monitoring of Equity in Health and Health Care, Geneva, 29th Sept.-30th, 1997, p. 2.
8. WHO: *World Health*, 51st Year, No. 2, March-April 1998, pp. 22-23.
9. Lok Sabha Secretariat: Estimates Committee, 102nd Report, (5th Lok Sabha), New Delhi, 1975, pp. 92-94.
10. Lok Sabha Secretariat, Public Accounts Committee, Fifth Lok Sabha, 200th Report, 1976, New Delhi.
11. J. Gallagher: "Educational Planning and Health", in *WHO Chronicle*, 30: 70-71 (1976).
12. Lok Sabha Secretariat: 102nd Report, Estimates Committee, (Fifth Lok Sabha), p. 4.
13. WHO: Globalisation and Public Health: A New Challenge for WHO, *World Health*, March-April, 1998, p. 25.

CHAPTER 13

HEALTH CARE ADMINISTRATION AT THE STATE LEVEL

Health, according to the Constitution of India, is a State subject. The main responsibility for providing health services to all people lies with the State Health Department with the assistance of local health organisations wherever these exist, e.g., Corporations, Municipalities, Panchayati Raj, *ad-hoc* statutory bodies like the Mines Board of Health, Employees State Insurance Corporation and so on.

—Author

Health Care Administration at the State Level

We have already the tools to prevent most of today's biggest killers. Yet, while knowledge and technology continue to advance, fairness is lost when their benefits are distributed. There is a widening gap between urban and rural areas and among population groups within the state.

Health, according to the Constitution of India, is a State subject. The main responsibility for providing health services to all people lies with the State Health Department with the assistance of local health organisations wherever these exist, e.g., Corporations, Municipalities, Panchayati Raj, *ad-hoc* statutory bodies like the Mines Board of Health, Employees State Insurance Corporation and so on.

The executive machinery of the government at the State level is headed by the Governor. Article 163 of the Constitution provides for a Council of Ministers with the Chief Minister as its head to aid and advise the Governor. The business of the government of the State (viz., law and order administration, the developmental functions like general administration, local government, public works, irrigation, health, education, cooperation, etc.) is allocated by the Governor amongst the Ministers in accordance with the provisions contained in Article 166(3) of the Constitution.

We shall now discuss the organisation of State Health Department in one State of the Indian Union, i.e., Punjab.

ORGANISATION OF STATE HEALTH DEPARTMENT (See Chart 13.1)

(a) Political Head

In the State of Punjab, a Minister of a Cabinet rank is the political head of the Health Department. He has to bear a heavy responsibility for formulating policies and monitoring the implementation of these policies and programmes.

CHART 13.1

Organisational Structure of Health and Family Welfare Services at State Level

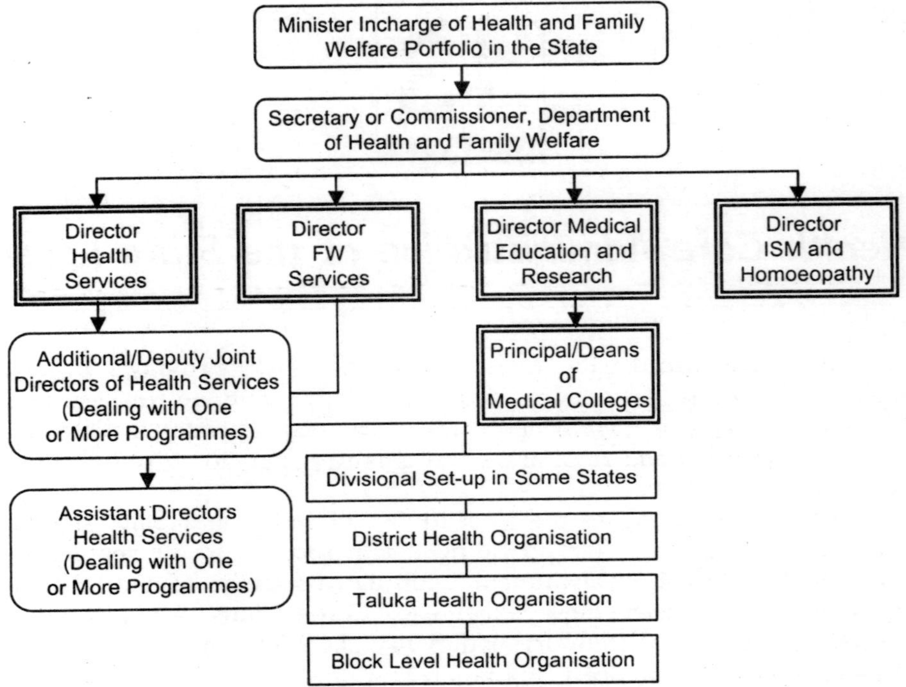

The Health Minister has to perform both types of activities, viz., political as well as administrative. These can be broadly discussed as follows:

(i) As a member of the State Legislature, it is his duty to support and safeguard the total policies of the Government because of the collective responsibility of the cabinet.

(ii) As a member of the Ministry, he brings all the bills pertaining to his Department for the approval of the legislature.

(iii) As political head of the Health Department, he acts as an executive and administrator. He has to see that the policies approved by the legislature are faithfully implemented.

(iv) He is the custodian of the interests of the people in general and of his constituency in particular.

(v) As a member of the Government, he performs ceremonial duties.

As far as the administrative functions of the Minister are

concerned, we find that for a number of reasons these activities do not receive the time and attention they deserve. Being busy with political activities, the Minister does not find enough time for administrative works. Lack of professional knowledge and lack of aptitude are the other contributory factors.

It was also pointed out by the Administrative Reforms Commission that there was a growing feeling among the public that most of the ministers lacked interest in efficient discharge of their administrative duties and did not possess the aptitude required for the purpose. The Administrative Reforms Commission in its report on State Administration recommended that, "the head of Council of Ministers (the Chief Minister) should, in selecting his colleagues, give special attention to considerations of political stature, personal integrity, intellectual ability and capacity for taking decisions and sustained application to work. Further, in assigning a portfolio, due regard should be paid to the aptitude and capacities of an incumbent."[1] The suggestion of A.R.C. must be accepted by the Chief Ministers to bring about innovations in political leadership.

(b) Administrative Head

In order to keep a record of the policies framed by the political heads and to watch over their implementation and execution, the State administration has to take the help of an office which is known as the state secretariat. The word 'Secretariat' refers to the complex of departments which vary from State to State.

The Secretariat organisation of the State Health Department, Punjab, is presently headed by an IAS officer of the rank of Commissioner who functions as Secretary to the Government in the Department of Health and Family Welfare. He is assisted by 3 Joint Secretaries and one Under-Secretary along with other administrative staff.

The main duties and responsibilities of the health department are as under:

(i) Assisting the Minister in policy-making, in modifying policies from time to time and in the discharge of his legislative responsibilities;
(ii) Framing draft legislation and rules and regulations;
(iii) Coordination of policies and programmes, supervision and control over their execution and review of results;
(iv) Budgeting and control of expenditure;
(v) Maintaining contact with the Government of India and other State Governments; and
(vi) Overseeing the smooth and efficient running of administrative machinery and initiating measures designed to develop greater personnel and organisational competence.[2]

(c) Technical Head

Below the State Secretariat, there are Executive Departments. These departments are headed mostly by the specialists and are concerned with the supervision, coordination and control of the policy framed by the State Government. Based on our personal observation and discussion, it was revealed that notwithstanding the apparently clear demarcation of functions as between the secretariat and the Executive Department a lot of duplication and overlapping still persists between the Secretariat (Health Department) and the Executive Department. This results in too much interference in the day-to-day functioning of the Executive Department. As a matter of policy the Secretariat should restrict its activities only to policy-making.

The Executive Organisation of the Health Department in Punjab is headed by the Director, Health Services, who has under him four Joint Directors—Joint Director (Family Welfare), Joint Director (Food and Drug), Joint Director (Employees' Social Insurance) and Joint Director (Administration), three Deputy Directors, responsible for inspection and supervision of all the National Health Programmes and Medical Institutions in their respective zones of four districts each and five Programme Specialists, of the rank of Assistant Directors to deal with specific programmes like leprosy, eradication of Malaria, planning, etc. Besides, the Director has the assistance of an Accounts Officer, who is on deputation from the State Finance Department. Similarly, he has the transport officer to control the operations of the large number of transport vehicles. The Joint Directors except the Joint Director (Administration) also have Assistant Directors under them to help them in the discharge of their duties. The Director and all other officers of the Department except the Joint Director (Administration) belong to the Provincial Health Service. The Joint Director (Administration) belongs to the Punjab Civil Service cadre and is on deputation to the Health Department. Apart from allopathy, the Indian System of medicines, namely, Ayurveda, Homoeopathy and Unani systems are also now beginning to receive proper attention. Their functioning is being regulated by the Director Ayurveda, Punjab. This Directorate constitutes a separate organisation and deals with all the three indigenous systems of medicines. Recently there has been separate Directorates of Medical Education and Family Welfare. The area of medical education which was integrated with the Directorate of Health Services at the state, has once again shown a tendency of maintaining a separate identity as Directorate of Medical Education, who is answerable directly to the Health Secretary/Commissioner of the state. Directorates of Medical Education and Research are found in the States of Jammu & Kashmir, Punjab, Haryana, Maharashtra, Karnataka and others. These four Health Directorates provide technical knowledge to the Secretary and the Minister. They also coordinate, supervise and control the implementation of health programmes and projects. The success or failure of the health department depends upon the leadership of the Directors of various systems of medicine.

DISTRICT LEVEL

The district is the most/crucial level in the administration and implementation of medical/health services. At the district level there is a District Medical and Health Officer (DMHO) or Chief Medical Officer who is overall responsible for the administration of Medical and Health Services in the entire district and for the implementation of all the national health and family welfare programmes. He is assisted by the Additional District Medical and Health Officers or Deputy District Medical and Health Officers along with other district officers for various national health programmes in the district. Their number varies from state to state.

Each district has been divided into two or more sub-revenue divisions. In each sub-division, there is a Senior Medical Officer who is overall in charge and is responsible for supervising the activities of all health and family welfare programmes in dispensaries and Taluka Hospitals of the sub-division. He is assisted by Health Supervisors and Health Education Officer.

FUNCTIONS

The following health services are provided at the state level:

1. Rural Health Service through Minimum Needs Programme;
2. Medical Development Programme;
3. M.C.H., Family Welfare and Immunisation Programme;
4. National Malaria Eradication Programme and National Filaria Control Programme;
5. National Leprosy Eradication Programme;
6. National Tuberculosis Control Programme;
7. National Programme for Control of Blindness;
8. Prevention and Control of Communicable Diseases like Diarrhoeal Disease, Kyasanur Forest Disease, Japanese Encephalitis, etc.;
9. School Health Programme;
10. Nutrition Programme—Education and Demonstration;
11. National Goitre Control Programme (Iodine Deficiency Disorder);
12. Laboratory Services and Vaccine Production Units;
13. Education on Environmental Sanitation;
14. Health Education and Training Programme;
15. Curative Services through Major Hospitals; and
16. National Aids Control Programme.

Let us explain some of the health facilities with an example of Punjab

(a) Medical Institutions

As on 31.3.98 there had been 2229 Medical Institutions in the State which included:

1.	Hospitals	208
2.	Hospitals-*cum*-community Health Centres	12
3.	Primary Health Centres-*cum*-Community Health Centres	39
4.	Community Health Centres	56
5.	Primary Health Centres	445
6.	Subsidiary Health Centres/Dispensaries/Clinics/Centres	1469

Out of these institutions, one hospital and eight dispensaries were functioning outside Punjab State but they were under the administrative control of Punjab Government.

On an average a medical institution was available within a radius of 2.697 kms. Similarly, the population served per medical institution as on 31.3.98 was 10,426.

(b) Number of Beds

During the year 1998-99, 25,094 beds were provided for indoor treatment to the patients in all the 2229 medical institutions. The bed strength in rural as well as in urban areas is given as per Table 13.1 below:

TABLE 13.1

Area	*Number of beds*	*%age of beds*	*%age of beds to medical institutions*
Rural	10697	42.63	79.64
Urban	14397	57.37	20.36
Total	25094	100.00	100.00

(c) Medical Care

During the year 1997, 10,462,384 out-patients received medical treatment at the out-door departments in various medical institutions of the State as compared to 10,253,381 out-door patients during the preceeding year.

(d) National Family Welfare Programme

The area of Punjab amounts to merely 1.57% of the country. Almost 5.50 lakh children are born every year and annual deaths count approximately 1.50 lakh, making a net annual increase of 4 lakh persons. In other words, double of Patiala city is added every year to the population of Punjab. 1503 children are born daily, 469 persons die everyday, leaving daily demographic gap of 1034 persons. As a result, during the past 4 decades of socio-economic development, the State had diverted more than half of the GNP growth to the needs of 12 million people added to the population count.[3]

CRITICAL APPRAISAL OF WORKING OF THE HEALTH ADMINISTRATION AT THE STATE LEVEL

We have already examined the organisation and functions of the Punjab State Health Department. From the quantitative analysis, it becomes quite clear that the department is doing well. On qualitative examination, it appears that the progress is superficial, unplanned and not directed to the needs of the clients. We give here some facts and suggestions which can help in the improvement of the organisation and functions of the health administration at the State level.

I. Serious Imbalance between the Rural and Urban Areas

There has been an imbalance in the availability of medical facilities and health manpower in rural area. Rural people have become conscious of their rights. They demand and deserve good quality health services. Even the Government itself is critical of this situation. It was stated officially that "It is an unfortunate fact that thirty years of health services development resulted in concentration of 80 per cent of medical manpower and facilities in urban areas where just 24 per cent of the total population resides. Paradoxically enough, Punjab's rural areas where 76 per cent of the State's total population lives, were getting just 20 percent institutional health services. Even 80 per cent of the total health budget was being spent on urban hospitals, etc. So the challenge of providing primary health care services to the ruralites was quite sizable in magnitude."[4]

What is being done to ensure health care to the rural people? The State governments are diverting more funds to develop infrastructure for providing health care to the rural people especially during the last five years. The basic question is how to ensure whether the rural people are being benefited or not. It is a common ill of Indian Administration that the people are not getting benefits because of the apathy of the personnel associated with the programmes. It is high time that we must ensure the fruitful working of our health schemes benefiting the villagers. Otherwise there is a likelihood of this imbalance increasing further. Health programmes could no more look mere political lollipops. These ought to be structured and designed in a fashion that meets the needs of the people. In the next century, we have to improve the health centre for the rural people otherwise there can be violence.

2. Status and Role of the Director of Health Services

In the execution of health policy, programmes and activities, persons who have an exceedingly important role to play are the Directors of Health Services. Thus, a great deal depends on their competence, method of approach and managerial ability. If they have the right kind of leadership qualities, there is no reason why they should not succeed in the implementation of programmes under his control. If one has to identify factors affecting the role or performance of a Director of Health Services at the State level, one cannot possibly miss the most important factor related to his relative inferior position as compared to the prestigious position of the Secretary of Health Services. The Secretary/ Deputy Secretary/Under-Secretary of Health Services as a rule is a senior member of the Indian Administrative Service. The Director is generally the senior most member belonging to the State Medical Service cadre. The issues which involve them in conflicts range from decision-making regarding health programmes to their actual implementation in the field. The director often feels that by virtue of his professional knowledge and competence his judgement is better than the judgement of his administrative counterpart. The domination of technocrats by the administrators in their day-to-day work has been debated in many national forums. The scientists feel that if they are given the freedom to decide, they can take much more interest and take rational decisions. The Administrative Reforms Commission (1666-70) pointed out: "An effort is needed to match jobs with the men possessing the needed qualifications, which means that the preference for the generalist, pure and simple should give place to a preference for those who have acquired competence in the concerned field."[5]

The Fulton Committee which was set-up in Great Britain in 1966 and which submitted its report in 1968 similarly said, "Many scientists, engineers and members of other specialist classes get neither the full responsibilities and corresponding authority, nor the opportunities they ought to have. Too often they are organised in a separate hierarchy while the policy and financial aspects of the work are reserved for a parallel group of generalist administrators, and their access to higher management and policy-making is restricted. In the New Civil Service a wider and more important role must be opened up for specialists trained and equipped for it."[6]

Mr. P. Lal in his article, "Saving bye-bye to bureacracy" in the Sunday *Tribune* rightly sensed the role of specialists in 21st century. To quote him: The bureaucratic system worked well when organisations were static, challenges small, expectations low, knowledge limited and information confined to local areas. Turnover of her individual's relations with people, institutions and ideas was also quite manageable. However, with the advent of the age of information technology some three decades back when computers came of age, knowledge burst upon the planet globally. What happens in one corner of the world now becomes known instantly in another. Internet has provided access to the common man, to information earlier available to specialists and professionals. High speed decisions are required to be taken by men and organisations.

As the governance and management functions require more and more of inputs from specialists—systems analysts, computer programmers, engineering specialists operation researchers—the importance of the latter increases and their advice and opinion cannot be brushed aside by the top management. Thus, they acquire a new decision-making function.

Says Professor William H. Read of the Graduate School of Business at McGill University, USA, "More and more of specialists do not fit neatly together into a chain-of-command system and can not wait for their expert advice to be approved at a higher level." They assume the role of decision-maker, they may well consult the ground level worker but would merely inform the top-executive who nods and accepts as the system benefits the organisation.

Thus, the specialists should be given parity with the Indian Administrative Service in the matter of conditions of service. Besides, they must be given top positions at the policy-making levels in Government. This would raise the morale of the technocrats and would improve the efficacy of the Government.

3. Absence of Comprehensive Health Legislation

In the States, legal provisions in regard to health lies scattered over a number of acts. At present, there is only one State—Tamil Nadu—which has a comprehensive public health Act satisfying reasonably the requirements of the modern health administration. The present corpus of health legislation is inadequate resulting in piecemeal decisions. Regulations are lacking in many vital subjects. In several respects the legislation is ineffective and outdated. There is need for comprehensive legislation embracing all aspects of health in a State. This would result into good health polices and plans.

4. Medical Education not Oriented to Rural Needs

A group on medical education and support manpower set-up in 1974 noted with concern that "Medical Education in India over the years has been essentially urban-oriented, relying heavily on curative method and sophisticated diagnostic aids, with little emphasis on preventive and promotional aspects of community health. Programmes of training in the field of nutrition, family welfare planning, maternal and child health have tended to develop in isolation from medical education and thus do not subserve the total needs of the community. Although the number of doctors has speedily increased over the successive plan periods, the alienation of doctors from the rural environment has deprived the rural communities of total medical care." The same feeling was voiced in the Fifth Five-Year Plan. The Sixth Plan also went on to point out that, "the basic problem is to produce a doctor who will be able to provide good health care and medical service to the community and will be able to work effectively in rural areas." Thus, it is high time for the State governments to take policy decisions to reorient medical education with a view to progressively make the training of the medical students more community-based. It is suggested that the internship of medical college students may be arranged in villages. The students may be asked to execute a bond to serve in the villages atleast for a period of five years. The curriculum may be curtailed and may be oriented to the community needs.

5. Lack of Community Health and Health Administrative Researches

Huge sums of money are poured out annually on clinical hospital-based research in most States of India. One would not under-estimate the importance of this type of research because it adds to knowledge. However, one has to think in terms of defining the priorities of research. A country, where the bulk of people are living in the rural areas, should normally involve the greater number of doctors doing researches in community health. India is one country which cannot boast of even a single good epidemiological study of such communicable diseases as tuberculosis, from which a sizable number of people suffer every year. In fact, the area of community health research does not encourage clinicians to work in the rural areas. The problems of community health, no doubt, are vast and intriguing. Yet, the country cannot afford to ignore them. India lives primarily in the villages and it is the villagers who are the recipients of probably the poorest quality of medical care. The future of India also depends on the progress made in the villages, particularly in the area of health. One has to watch and see how different States plan and administer their health programmes so that their rural beneficiaries are not outnumbered by their urban beneficiaries. Thus, the present trend of our spending on curative medicine research has to change in favour of community health research particularly in the rural areas. This is a challenge which no State of India can afford to ignore.

Further, the health administration at the State level is poorly equipped. Most of the health administrators have got no training in the modern knowledge of management. There is no effort on the part of the personnel working in health departments to use modern methods to improve health care delivery. Moreover, the health departments, training institutions, medical colleges, nursing colleges do not seriously concern themselves with finding methods for optimum utilisation of resources. Health services research should be multi-disciplinary, involving not only medical professionals and experts but also system analysts, operational researchers, social scientists, health economists, public administrators, anthropologists, etc. The State health department may encourage research in consonance with priority problems of its health care delivery system. The health department may encourage researches which affect programme delivery. Some areas are mentioned below:

(a) Health manpower, their training, development, utilisation, availability, needs and demands, etc., including experimentation with the development of various categories of health manpower.
(b) Equipment, materials, etc., their availability, utilisation, needs and demands.
(c) Organisational and management process in health and family welfare services, their linkages, etc., including referral systems.
(d) Performance and impact of health and family welfare services.
(e) Needs and demands of population for health and family welfare services.
(f) Perception, attitude, utilisation factors (promoters and barriers) effecting utilisation, etc., of population towards health and family welfare services.
(g) Problems and bottlenecks in the existing organisational systems and redesigning of existing systems to eliminate the same.
(h) Information systems for health and family welfare.
(i) Cost-benefit and cost-effectiveness analysis of health and family welfare services, programmes and projects.
(j) Cost-analysis of health and family welfare services, programmes and projects.
(k) Development and testing of technology suited to the Indian health scene and needs.
(l) Studies focused on the interphase between community and health services organisations.
(m) Studies on health status and social and economic development.
(n) Materials Management in a hospital.
(o) Working of Intensive-care units.
(p) Cost of running hospital services.
(q) Staffing of emergency services.
(r) Utilization of operation theaters.
(s) Enlisting of community participation.
(t) Development of planning and management techniques.
(u) Identification of goals and priorities of the health services.

6. Absence of Well-Designed Management Information System

Many State governments have performed the ritual of setting up statistical bureaus dealing with health. Huge health statistics have also been collected but these have been put to a bare minimum use in terms of utilising this information for developing a realistic health care delivery system. Thus, the ever-widening gap between accumulation of health statistics and their utilisation for improving health services has of late acquired new significance. While in the developed countries management information system is increasingly being given the importance it deserved, in the developing countries it has not yet become an integral part of the state health system. It would indeed be very profitable for all the States to organise data banks and critically examine the quality of their health services. Because of the many uses of health statistics in scientific analysis, planning, administration and evaluation, the health statistician must begin to think in terms of a fully coordinated health information system, in which all relevant data are collected, compiled, stored, retrieved, analysed and published.[7]

However, the Health Information System has to be planned properly. A Health Information System was defined by Conference on Health Information Systems held by WHO in Copenhagen from 18-22 June 1973, as:

> "A mechanism for the collection, processing, analysis and transmission of information required for organising and operating health services and also for research and training."[8]

We must ensure the accuracy of data, otherwise the whole of our planning would go wrong. Goddard has rightly said, "One of the greatest possible contributors to wastage of our precious resources, whether at the local, national or international levels, is the failure of those at any level of administration, and at all stages in the management of the activity, to base all decisions on verifiable facts. There should be no tolerating errors in administrative action which occur because someone failed to get all of those facts. In the evolution, execution and control of work plans, obtaining the factual evidence should always be the first step."[9] Mahdi Elmandjra in his article, "Informatics and Telematics: The Future" in *World Health,* Aug./Sept. 1989 warns the use of borrowed systems. To quote him, "he says that knowledge—which has become the most strategic raw material in all the domains of human activity—is simply information produced by sound research and managed by people well-trained in the pursuit of clear objectives and goals. Informatics is of course not a panacea especially if it is used as a purchased gadget and implanted as a foreign body in an environment which does not meet its minimum conditions. Yet it represents today the most efficient instrument which man has so far invented to help him to analyse and solve problems."

7. Inadequate Financial Resources

It is one thing to define health needs of a given population and another thing to adequately plan health services in accordance with their needs. No aspect of planning health services appears to be more important than the consideration of finance. The paucity of financial resources because of poor allocations has often proved to be a major obstacle in the execution of health programmes. With the meagre resources, one cannot expect much. At present the health department of Punjab is being allocated only 3-4 per cent of the total resources for the promotion of health. The task of providing health care to improve the quality of life of the people is challenging. The State governments must allocate at least 10 percent of their total budget for health. Besides, there is a need to make the best use of the resources already allocated.

However, financial resources mobilized through alternative mechanisms, such as cost recovery and user fees, are minimal at this stage, being less than 10% of the total recurrent health expenditure. It has therefore become increasingly difficult to meet the unprecedented rising costs of health care.[10]

8. Non-availability of Dedicated Doctors/Workers to Serve in the Villages

The doctors prefer to serve in the cities than in the villages. When they are forced to work in the villages, their mind is always in the cities. This results in lower efficiency of the Primary Health Centres. It is suggested that the Government while selecting the students for medical education must ensure that a large number of students should come from villages, i.e., rural areas. The missionary zeal may be cultivated among the doctors during their education so that they take up the rural assignments with dedication.

(i) Need for Human Resource Development to Inject Creativity and Dynamism among Health Personnel

The provision of Health Care at lower levels is not a mechanical process, it is a human enterprise and its success will depend ultimately on the skill, the quality and motivation of the persons associated with it, e.g. Medical Officers. Workers of Health at the lower echelons of Health Administration are vital link between people and the health care system.

The quality of personnel appointed to take care of health care activities, levels of efficiency, motivation and enthusiasm have not been maintained at a high level and there is lack of devotion to duty on the part of the medical and paramedical personnel. Complaints by the citizens regarding inefficiency and lack of devotion to duty on the part of medical and para medical personnel have become quite articulate, and many people are even losing confidence in the existing primary health care system thereby widening the credibility gap.

HRD is concerned with organising, in systematic fashion, the goals, objectives, priorities and activities of manpower development in order to ensure that the right number of staff with the appropriate skills are provided at the right time to meet the requirement of the work to be done.

There should be only one yards stick to judge the effectiveness of Manpower Development, namely, continuous improvement of the status and the quality of health of the population with the least friction to those who supply the services and the most satisfying to those who receive it. We have to achieve all this with the minimum cost and maximum efficiency.

(ii) Need of Developing Missionary Spirit Among the Health Personnel

The problems of public health are challenging as it can be gauged from the statistics already enumerated. It is very difficult to solve these problems with bureaucratic and inhuman attitude. It requires hard work, sympathy, and tolerance on the part of the health personnel engaged in this arduous and challenging task. Most respondents felt that the personnel working are fulfilling only their legal duties, and that too reluctantly. We do not need highly specialised people in these areas. We, however, require dedicated people with missionary zeal to serve the people suffering from illness. Prof. J.S. Neki has rightly said in the context of health personnel which is true for all categories of personnel:

> "To help, to heal, to reconstruct, to comfort—and all along the line to act with compassion—all these bear testimony to the moral consciousness of the doctor. Whatever the new strains imposed upon medical ethics, this structure will survive and continue to guide doctors in their professional conduct . . . . Legal and judicial obligations they have, of necessity, to fulfil. But these are not genuine ethics. Genuine ethics has to be ingrained into character and does not have to depend upon external controls.[11]

R.S. Pathak, Former Chief Justice of India rightly mentions:

> "The vitality of an ethical dimension in the discharge of public responsibilities is essential to a developing nation. In a developing nation, the release of nascent national energy is a great moment. It provides the power necessary for building of a nation.[12]

9. Under-utilisation of Indigenous System of Medicine

Indian health problems are of such magnitude that if left only to the allopathic system of medicine, one cannot possibly hope to achieve much success. In the past, a policy of drift has been followed with regard to Ayurveda and other Indian systems of medicine. The supporters of Ayurveda and Homoeopathy feel that this system could not get a chance to demonstrate its utility. It has been claimed by the practitioners of the indigenous system of medicine that the facilities provided to them have been too patchy and the services were inadequately supplied to prove the true worth of the system. The Punjab government has shown its keenness to promote the system but the tempo is very slow. The government should take a bold decision to encourage these systems which can provide health care to a large number of people with little cost.

10. Unsatisfactory Management of Employees' State Insurance Scheme

Employees' State Insurance Scheme has not been functioning well. The shortage of doctors and medicines is the common ill of these institutions. There had been complaints from the beneficiaries about the malfunctioning of these hospitals. It was mentioned in *The Tribune* by C.M. Kumbhkarni with reference to E.S.I. Hospital, Jullundur:

> "The indoor patients take their meals like beggars on paper and towel. The hospital is provided with stainless steel utensils but these are kept under lock and key."

Besides, it is widely felt that there is a lot of corruption among the doctors working in these hospitals. The State government must tighten the control over these hospitals and monitor the reactions and feelings of the patients to streamline the functioning of the ESI scheme.

11. Poor Nutritional Status of the People

Punjab is an economically well-off State but the majority of the people suffer from diseases arising from nutritional deficiencies and malnutrition.

The following recommendations were made by the South-East Regional Committee to solve the problems of nutritional deficiencies which need the immediate attention of the State health department:

(1) Nutrition activities should be recognised as crucial components of health programmes, particularly of those directed at the mother and child.
(2) The nutrition activities of health programmes should be very clearly defined and their implementation at all levels and especially at the local level, should receive sufficient attention and allocation of resources.
(3) In the package of services, nutrition should receive the same priority as other components, so that it is not relegated to a position of secondary importance as has been many times the case.
(4) The delivery system for nutrition activities catering to the needs of the under-served population should be rationalised applying the principles of primary health care and using

primary health workers within the context of national health administration.

(5) Nutrition education relevant to the local situation as a part of health education of the community and its inclusion in formal and non-formal education need to be improved.

(6) Service-oriented nutrition research to solve public health nutrition problems must receive priority.

(7) To fulfil the inter-sectoral and intra-sectoral responsibilities of health in nutrition, the role of the nutrition unit at the central level of the health services needs to be considerably strengthened with its increased participation in health planning and programming.

Finally, there are a large number of other problems in the areas concerning Health Planning, Health Manpower Planning, Health Project Management, Hospital Management, Administration of Health Education and Environmental Sanitation Programmes which would be discussed in the relevant chapters.

12. Lack of Community Participation in Health

Community participation is perceived as a dynamic partnership process that is reinforced by information feedback. Health personnel are responsible for explaining and advising, and for providing clear information on health options. Community participation enables people to become agents of their own development, instead of being passive beneficiaries of development aid. The channelling of a community's human resources generated by the health volunteer movement is advantageous to both the health care providers and the recipients. Volunteers in community health activities not only bring health services to the community, but also act as agents for health development.

Social preparation of and capacity building in the community are prerequisites for mobilizing communities for health activities. This could be supported through information, education and communication (IEC) materials in both electronic and printed media, the formation of support groups, shared efforts of health volunteers through village exchange visits, and the development of joint plans of action and intersect oral activities at village level.[13]

Community health development through education is a critical issue that requires an investment of time and resources by the health care system.

In the new millennium, State Health Department must change its emphasis from merely examining files sitting in the offices but should ensure implementation of the programmes through personal visits, monitoring, regular guidance. We have to discard the old method of paper approach to action approach in new millennium. In the 21st century, Health Departments must be guided by the motto, "words written or spoken are of no use unless but to action."

The big task in new millennium is not only to enable change but to communicate it as widely as possible. Can the field functionaries dream what the headquarters policy-makers dream. Such congruence is sure to fillip progress

In the new millennium, the State Government has to play a more dynamic role through Panchayati Raj System, Municipal Government in ushering new era of health development by exploiting local resources. This can be achieved through transparency, accountability and good governance. People's empowerment is the only answer to solve many national and bureaucratic ills from which the system suffered.

Notes and References

1. GOI: Report of Administration of the State Level Administrative Reforms Commission, New Delhi 1969, p. 10.
2. *Ibid.*, p. 19.
3. Government of Punjab, Deptt. of Planning, Annual Plan, 1979-80, p. 112.
4. Government of Punjab, Bold Planning and Solid Action: Health Services in Punjab, 1979.
5. Administrative Reforms Commission, Report on Personnel Administrative, New Delhi, Manager of Publication, 1969, p. 10.
6. Report of the Committee of Civil Services (The Fulton Committee), Cmnd: 3638, London, H.M.S.C., 1968, p. 12.
7. Forrest E. Linder, Director, International Programme of Laboratories for Population Statistics, School of Public Health, University of North California at Chapel Hill, N.C., USA, "Recent Trends in Health Statistics" in *WHO Chronicle*, 30: 58-63 (1976).
8. M.R. Aderson, Honorary Director, Medical Information Unit, Wessex Regional Hospital Board, Winchester, U.K.: "Health Information System" in *WHO Chronicle*, 1974, 28, 52-54.
9. H.A. Aderson, Principles of Administration Applied to Nursing Service, World Health Organisation, Geneva, 1958, p. 84.
10. SEA/RC20/pp. 39-40.
11. J.S. Neki, "Medical Ethics: A view point from the Developing World", *World Health*, July 1979, p. 15.
12. R.S. Pathak, Ethics in Public Life: Some Observations in *IJPA*, July to Sept. 1995, p. 265.
13. WHO: SEARO: Health Situation in the South-East Asia Region, New Delhi, 1994-97, p. 193.

CHAPTER 14

DISTRICT HEALTH CARE ADMINISTRATION

The District is the most peripheral fully organized unit of local government and administration. It is geographically compact and every part of it can normally be reached within a day. The District is often the natural meeting point for "bottom-up" Planning and Organization and "top-down" planning support. It is a place where community needs and national priorities can be reconciled. We can develop here good planning for a small area and ensure implementation.

—Author

District Health Care Administration

The District is the most peripheral fully organized unit of local government and administration. It is geographically compact and every part of it can normally be reached within a day. The District is often the natural meeting point for "bottom-up" Planning and Organization and "top-down" planning support. It is a place where community needs and national priorities can be reconciled. We can develop here good planning for a small area and ensure implementation.

District level health structure is a middle level Management Organisation and has been set-up to provide an organic link between state level health infrastructure as well as regional level infrastructure on the one side and district level and lower level health institutions on the other side. District health administration is the nerve centre of health infrastructure as upon its efficiency depends the efficiency of primary health care to a substantial extent.

Eighth General Programme of work covering the period (1990-95) Geneva, WHO (Health For All, Series No. 10) defines District Health System as:

> A district health system based on primary health care is a more or less self-contained segment of the national health system. It comprises first and foremost "a well-defined population living within a clearly delineated administrative and geographical area. It includes all the relevant health care activities in the area, whether governmental or otherwise. It therefore consists of a large variety of interrelated elements that contribute to health in homes, schools, workplaces, communities, the health sector, and related social and economic sectors. It includes self-care and all health care personnel and facilities, whether governmental or non-governmental, up to and including the hospital at the first referral level, and the

appropriate support services, such as laboratory, diagnostic, and logistic support. It will be most effective if coordinated by an appropriately trained health officer working to ensure as comprehensive a range as possible of promotive, preventive, curative, and rehabilitative health activities.[1]

The term district is used in a generic sense to denote a clearly defined administrative area which commonly has a population of between 50,000, where some form of local government or administration handles many of the responsibilities for central government sectors or departments, and where a general hospital for referral support exists. The actual organization of district health systems depends on the specific situation in each country and each district, including the administrative structure and personalities involved. Nevertheless, the general principles for developing such systems are based on the Declaration of Alma-Ata and the global strategies for health for all. They incorporate the elements of equity, accessibility, emphasis on promotion and prevention, intersectoral action, community involvement, decentralization, integration of health programmes, and coordination of separate health activities.[2]

The head of the District Organisation is designed differently in different states of India, e.g. Chief Medical Officer or District Health Officer, or District Health and Family Planning Officer. He has under him a lot of staff to supervise, co-ordinate and control the field activities as well as report to the headquarters. In some of the states of the Indian Union, District Health System has been entrusted to the control of Panchayati Raj System, while in others, it is still under the total control of the state Government.

There has been a tendency in developing countries including India to allocate more and more powers to union and state Governments resulting in centralisation and lack of initiative at local levels. In recent times, there has been a trend to decentralise health system to ensure fruitful results. Through decentralisation, lower level units can meet local variations in ecological, geographical, economic, social and cultural conditions (e.g. 73rd and 74th Amendments of the Indian Constitution).

A. DECENTRALISATION IN HEALTH CARE SYSTEM

Speedy and realistic decision-making is one of the essentials of efficient administration. In a big and complex organisation, the number of decisions to be taken from time to time is so large and the points at which the decisions are to be implemented are so many that it becomes necessary to distribute decision-making powers among a number of organs, rather than let it concentrate in one organ. This is expected to prevent the emergence of bottlenecks which bedevil highly centralized power structures. Thus, one of the important problems of organisation is to reconcile the administrator's desire for centralized control for the sake of uniformity and certainty of decisions and action with the people's view that administration should be so organised as to deal with the needs of the different segments of the society in an effective manner.[3] Decentralisation has many other advantages.

(a) Decentralisation Lightens the Works of the Upper Echelons in Administration

Most of the personnel at top level remain too busy and thus cannot devote time to everything they do. The result is mere signing.

(b) Decentralisation Promotes Quick Disposal of Work

Decentralisation can promote quick disposal of work as the decision-making authorities are in the field itself.

(c) Decentralisation Generates Interest among Employees

Decentralisation generates participation which increase the motivation of employees as they get the opportunity to express themselves and not simply act as ordered. In the words of J.C. Charlesworth, "Decentralisation has a more important justification than mere administrative efficiency. It bears directly upon the development of a sense of personal adequacy in the individual citizen, it has spiritual connotations."[4]

(d) Decentralisation Develops Leadership

Through decentralisation, opportunity is provided to people to put their ideas into practice. This gives a boost to experimentation and creativity which are the essential qualities of leadership. According to Dimock and Dimock, "Decentralisation permits to less standardisation and hence allows more variation and experimentation, more freedom to innovate and choose, encourages more experience and a wider scope for initiative, both of which stimulate leadership."

(e) Decentralisation Promotes Effective Supervision and Control

Control and supervision become easier at lower levels since operations are being done at lower levels.

In a WHO document, "Strengthening Ministries of Health for Primary Health Care", a question is raised about the extent of decentralisation to provide primary health care. The answer goes in favour of decentralisation to districts.[5]

How far down the line should decentralization go? Should it stop at large geographical areas, such as regions or states, or should matters be taken further down, to the provincial, district or municipal level? Answers are necessarily tentative. In part they depend on the system's initial degree of centralization. If it is built downwards from a "top-heavy top", then decentralisation to a small number of regions could be indicated. Human resource constraints may add force to such a strategy.

There may, for example, be few health planners, appropriately trained district medical officers, PHC nursing supervisors, pharmacists, or administrators with a broader understanding of management. It is easier to assemble a few teams of capable officials than to find the expertise to staff large numbers of them. Some countries which have decentralised to lower levels have been seriously hampered by a lack of appropriate skills, especially in administration and management (Sudan). Yet there are also factors to be considered which point the other way.

Larger (and fewer) decentralized units will find it harder to ensure the required adaptability, flexibility, and efficiency and to promote devolution of power and accountability towards the grass-roots, where the services operate. There is growing evidence that an important cause of the limited efficiency of the health care system is often found at the "district" level i.e., the level from which the basic PHC services are organised and managed, and where the primary back-up services are situated. The weakness of district level organization often leads to the breakdown of support and supervision, to shortage in essential supplies, and to lack of facilities for training (and retraining) grass-roots health workers.

Conversely, strong and well-organised district health teams with access to relevant information sources appear to be an esential ingredient of the PHC approach. It may even be argued that district PHC teams are the key units of the entire organizational structure, and that their leaders are placed in the most critical positions of the health sector. Such teams can be responsible for all basic health care activities for the promotion and sustaining of community involvement, and for the operational link-up between PHC and hospital activities. The district, therefore, needs resources and authority under its own control to be able to fulfil its tasks properly. Decentralization should go down all the way to the district, wherever possible.

Even a review of primary health care system by World Health Organization, resulted in a resolution (WHO 39.7) in May 1986 in which it urged countries to strengthen further the health system infrastructure based on primary health care, laying particular emphasis on district health systems based on primary health care, and defining targets for the integrated delivery of essential elements of primary health care until all districts and all elements were covered. It also called on WHO to intensify support for countries in this regard.

In order to facilitate a common understanding, the WHO Global Programme Committee in 1986 defined the district health system based on primary health care as "a self-contained segment of the national health system comprised of a well-defined population living within a clearly delineated administrative and geographical area, whether urban or rural. It includes all institutions and individuals providing health care in the district, whether governmental, social security, non-governmental, private, or traditional. A district health system therefore consists of a large variety of interrelated elements that contribute to health in homes, schools, work places and communities, through the health and other related sectors. It includes self-care and all health care workers and facilities, up to and including the hospital at the first referral level and the appropriate laboratory, other diagnostic, and logistic support services. Its component elements need to be well coordinated by an officer assigned to this function in order to draw together all these elements and institutions into a fully comprehensive range of promotive, preventive, curative and rehabilitative health activities."[6]

With regard to development, the objectives of the WHO Programme on Strengthening District Systems are to improve the quality of life and reduce mortality and morbidity by strengthening the effective implementation of primary health care in participating countries, with due consideration to equity, effectiveness, efficiency, and flexibility within the context of national, regional, and global strategies for reaching the goal of Health for All.[7]

(f) Government Responsibility for District Health System

1. Government should strengthen support and encouarge the decentralization process to give necessary autonomy and responsibility to district health systems and to ensure the development of an appropriatte network of facilities, including at least one first referral hospital in each health district, together with the first contact services without which the hospital cannot function coherently and efficiently.
2. Governments should ensurre that first referral hospital have a high degree of technical and administrative competence and equipment to deal with clinical problems that cannot be handled at the health facility at first contact level. These hospitals should be equipped with reliable laboratory, imaging services, a pharmacy, and a blood bank. In this way further referrals up the chain can be reduced and rationalised.
3. Governments should ensure effective supervision, communication and control.
4. District Health System should provide leadership to motivate Personnel at the perephery level.
5. Governments should develop networks of urban primary health facilities so that the services of urban hospitals at first referral level may be used more rationally and efficiently.
6. Governments should review the allocation and use of hospital resources, and encourage the mobilization of additional sources of revenue for individual district health systems. Local financial resources should as much as possible, be retained and administered locally.
7. District Health System should ensure that the equipment

remain functional.

8. Governments should ensure that no capital investment is made unless the attendant recurrent expenditure can be assured.
9. District Health System should supply drugs of good quality and in time to field centres.
10. In order to reduce and rationalise referrals to hospital, governments should ensure that adequate diagnostic facilities are extended to health centres and other community-based units, together with appropriately trained personnel.
11. Governments should design training curricula for health workers involved in district health care to suit changing environment.
12. District health system should be transparent and responsive.

B. ORGANISATIONAL STRUCTURE OF DISTRICT HEALTH SYSTEM

District Health System is under the control of State Health Department. The head of the district health system, generally called, chief medical officer, is directly responsible to the state health department and is not accountable to elected Panchayati Raj Institutions. This system has many disadvantages as it is bureaucratic in style and functioning, secondly, it has no mechanism to involve the people, thirdly, health system is not in tune with the needs of the people. Let us explain with an example of District Health System in Punjab.

The district is the most/crucial level in the administration and implementation of medical/health services. At the district level there is a District Medical and Health Officer (DMHO); Chief Medical Officer who is overall responsible for the administration of medical and health services in the entire district and for the implementation of all the national health and family welfare programmes. He is assisted by the Additional District Medical and Health Officers or Deputy District Medical and Health Officers along with other district officers for various national health programmes in the district. Their number varies from state to state.

Effective development strategies require a process of planning and implementation which enables local people and officials to equally express their needs and to share in deciding what is to be done. Neither party has control. Their motivation is based on the desire to satisfy both personal (individual, family, community) needs as well as compatible joint project objectives. To the extent that communities and outside agents view the rewards they receive from performance as supportive of their personal objectives, they will be productive within the limits of their individual and group capacities and within the restraints placed upon them by their situation. One of the rural development manager's tasks is that of analyzing the situation to determine the most appropriate conditions and resources which can lead to improving the situation and the equitable merger and attainment of personal and project needs.

This process of analysis, likewise, should be done not just by the manager but also on an equal basis with the people, incorporating popular knowledge as much as possible. This consultative process must go much deeper than the usual diplomatic and technical channels, for it must first and foremost involve people below the level of government officials; it must involve people in non-government organizations and in the communities. Thus, we come to the need for partnership, that is, for a means of enabling people to work together in a spirit of mutual trust and respect which encourages people to volunteer information and resources because that they believe they are being taken seriously. Partnership is thus a means for improving the process of development by creating linkages which will bring more people into the process, which will provide better information and participation, and which will more widely disperse responsibility for decisions.[8]

Let us now explain the District Health System with an example from Karnataka. Establishment of three-tier panchayat raj system is the first step towards decentralisation of power. It provides for a Gram Panchayat, Taluka Panchayat and Zilla Panchayat. The Zilla Panchayat or District Panchayat has authority over the entire district except the urban areas under municipal or city or town councils (See Chart 14.1).

There is provision for transfer of power and functions and devolution of funds to Panchayats. Practically all the development programmes are transferred to the District Panchayat and an officer of the rank of the collector is the Chief Executive Officer of the Zilla Panchayat.

It has an elected president and vice-president from among its elected members. Elected members alone have a right to vote. There are associate members too who are nominated and can only discuss and express their views in the meetings of Panchayat. The Chief Executive Officer of the rank of collector is posted to Panchayat who acts as an *ex-officio* Secretary of the Panchayat and has a pivotal role. This district panchayat functions through various committee structures and the Health Committee is one of the important committee to work for health development (See Chart 14.2).

Thus, Zilla Parishad with Taluka and Gram Panchayats are ushering in democratic decentralisation of administration. They are the active instruments at people's level. The panchayat system is taking strong roots and providing a solid base for building up and strengthening the decentralisation of the planning process. The District Planning Board (DPB) provides a forum for all sectors and organisations engaged in development work including panchayats to pool their efforts and assist in evolving a well coordinated and participatory approach to planning.

The Karnataka Panchayat Raj Act, 1993, which is now in force in

CHART 14.1

Organisational Structure of Panchayat Raj Institutions

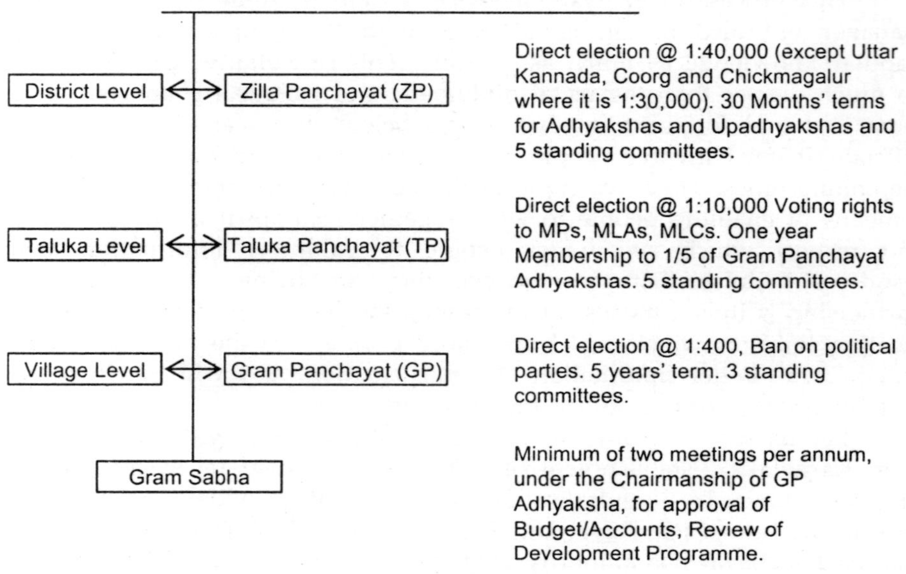

CHART 14.2

Committee System in Panchayat Raj Institutions

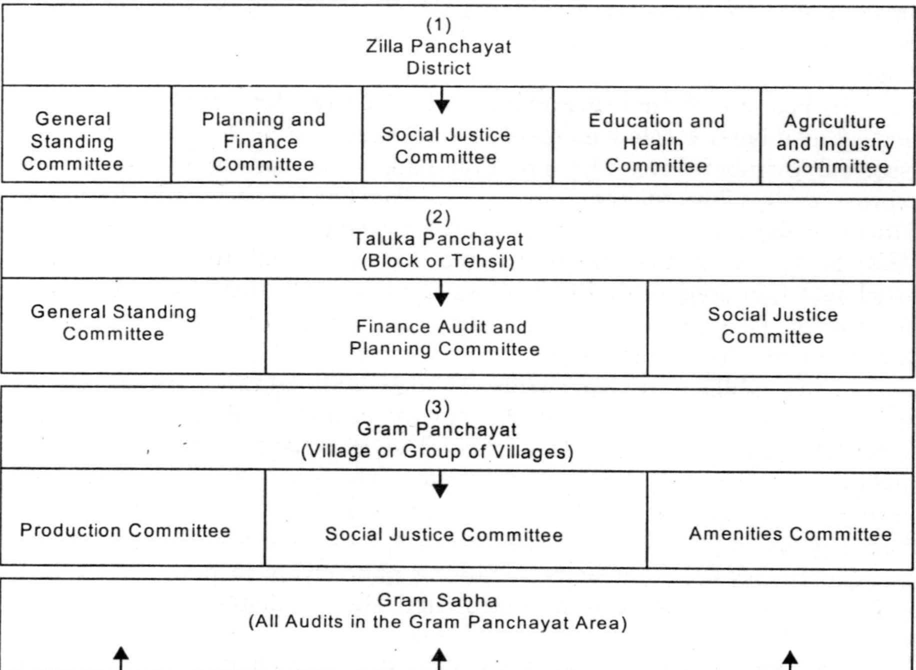

the State, specifies the following functions to be performed by the Zilla Panchayat, in respect of Health and Family Welfare, at the district level—

(1) Management of hospital and dispensaries excluding the District hospital and other hospitals under the direct management of Government (above 50 beds);
(2) Implementation of maternity and child health programmes;
(3) Implementation of family welfare programmes; and
(4) Implementation of immunization and vaccination programmes.

The Taluka Panchayats deal with:

(1) Promotion of Health and Family Welfare programmes;
(2) Promotion of immunization and vaccination programmes at the Taluka level; and
(3) Health and sanitation at fairs and festivals.

At the village level, the Gram Panchayats deal with implementation of family welfare programmes, preventive measures against epidemics, regulation of sale of food articles, participation in immunization programmes, licensing of eating establishments and regulation of offensive and dangerous trades. Apart from operating the District Sector budget, the Zilla Panchayats also implement such State Sector schemes as are entrusted to them by Government.

The State plan and centrally sponsored or assisted schemes and the normal schemes of the district are budgeted accordingly. Only innovative district specific schemes have to be funded under decentralised district planning for which either DPB provides 100 percent discretionary funds or funds flow under incentive outlay where local community has to contribute on 50:50 or 25:75 basis of its proportion of the funds or from special outlays for backward areas. Otherwise, the district budget is proportional to the number of institutions functioning in the district and the norms set for Central and State programmes being operated in the district under various approved budgetary heads of expenditure. Each programme officer at district level is drawing and disbursing officer and there is no integrated budget for the district. The delay in release of budget is generally normal constraint affecting the utilisation.

Administrative Machinery

Below this political set-up, there is administrative health machinery to implement the Plans made by ZP. This machinery also helps PRI system in the formulation of Health Plans as well. The district administrative machinery under ZP consists of the Chief Executive Officer (CEO), an IAS officer, as head of the administrative organisation.

Besides CEO, the ZP secretariat comprises of 2 Deputy Secretaries in-charge of administration and development respectively, a Council Secretary for organising ZP meetings, a Chief Planning Officer to assist in planning exercise and a Chief Accounts Officer to supervise the money transactions in the ZP (See Chart 14.3). There are field officers, i.e. Executive Officer, Block and Development Officer and G.P. Secretary. Besides, there are departments headed by specialists. Let us explains with the examples of one of the Districts, i.e. Dakshina Kannada, where there are 17 departments (See Chart 14.3).

CHART 14.3

The Administrative Structure of Panchayat Raj Institutions

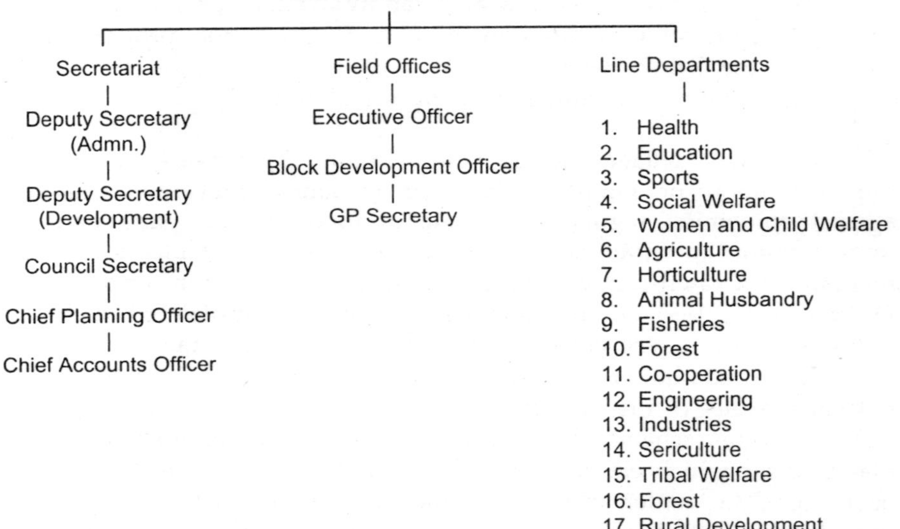

Role of Chief Executive Officer of ZP

Chief Executive Officer (CEO) has to play a great role in ushering the benefits of democratic decentralization. However, CEO's tenure is not fixed and in practice is very short and hence, it is very difficult to maintain continuity and interest in programmes. We can explain with the help of a case study of CEO in the district of Dakshina Kannada.

Since inception in 1987 to 01.04.98, there have been 9 incumbents to the post of CEO, with an average tenure of one and a half year. The CEO is expected to provide requisite linkage between the elected representatives and administration personnel within the ZP, between the District Administration and the State Government. The Chief Executive Officer attends every meeting of the ZP and has right to attend the meeting of any committee thereof and to take part in the discussion, but does not have the right to move any resolution or to vote.

It is also very difficult to control and co-ordinate so many departments. Specialists who head the District Departments find it very difficult to meet the CEO as the post is burdened with many departments.

District Health Department

It may be interesting to note that the Health Department in the district is the second biggest department. For example, in Dakshin Kannada, out of total employees of 14,184, 3130 belong to health, more than 20 percent of the total. In Group A, out of 216 employees, 137 belong to Health Department, more than 50 percent. Thus, CEO has to devote a lot of time to the Health Department in the District.

Functions of District Health and Family Welfare Officer

The district officer with the overall responsibility for health is designated as the District Health and Family Welfare Officer (DHO).

In a district the overall responsibility of implementation of health care delivery system, lies with the DHO who is assisted by a number of other district officers (Family Planning, Health, Malaria, T.B., U.I.P., etc). (See Chart 14.4). These district officers are declared as "Head of Office." The Head of office is declared by the head of department under certain rules framed by the State Government/Central Government. The head of office has overall responsibility of carrying out all office functions. In this task he is assisted by Administrative Officer/Office Superintendent/ Office Assistant. The office work is allocated amongst the employees of the office by dividing them into different sections, i.e. Establishment, Accounts, Stores, Statistics, Transport, General, etc. The number of employees in a section depends upon the workload in that section and the number as well as the nature of section may vary from office to office depending upon the type of work and the quantum of work.

In line with the government of India guidelines in the implementation of minimum needs programme the State has revised its Health Policy and decided to establish a 3-Tier Health Infrastructure, viz. Sub-Centres, Primary Health Centres and Community Health Centres to provide health for all under the overall supervision and control of District Health System. (See Chart 14.5)

Role of DHO

DHO is given authority and is therefore responsible for other people, money and resources allocated to health. Authority in the managerial context of a DHO is usually identified with the legitimate base of power. It may be defined as the legal right to command action by others and to enforce compliance. A DHO, however, might gain compliance in a number of ways through persuasion, sanctions, requests, coercion, co-operation or force. The responsibilities of a DHO are made clear by the State Health Administration through the statement of

CHART 14.4

Organisational Structure of Health Department

- **District Health and Family Welfare Officer**
  - Dy. CMO/ Medical Officer (FW & MCH)
  - Assistant District Health and Family Welfare Officer (HQ)
  - Assistant District Health and Family Welfare Officer (Sub-Division Level/Dy. CMOS)
  - District Malaria Officer
  - Senior Malaria Officer
  - Senior Medical Superintendent
    - Medical Officers of Dt. General Hospital and other Govt. Hospitals
  - District Leprosy Officer
  - District Health Education Officer/DMEIO
  - Medical Officer (District Lab.)
  - Medical Officers of Primary Health Centres (Co-ordinators at PHC Level)
  - District Tuberculosis Officer (TB Centre)
  - District Nursing Supervisor
  - Gazetted Assistant
  - Assistant Statistical Officer
  - Lady Medical Officers/II MO of Primary Health Centres
  - Service Engineer (Mobile Workshop)

"Function, Duties, and Responsibilities of DHO." In the absence of such role description, it may lead to role ambiguity and ultimately to role conflict where role boundaries have an overlap. The working relationship with other district health offices, district hospital and other programme officers has to be clarified and clearly understood. In fulfilling his responsibilities, the DHO often delegates authority and responsibility to other district health officials. By delegation, we meant conferring authority from DHO to another in order to accomplish particular activity/programme. Of course, such delegation has, in most districts, been very limited. When a DHO delegates authority and responsibility, it can never be abdicated. That means, the DHO cannot throw the blame on others to whom he has delegated. Ultimately, it is the DHO who is accountable for everything in the district health services delivery.

For every recognized position in any organization, there is an

CHART 14.5

Primary Health Care Infrastructure at District Level

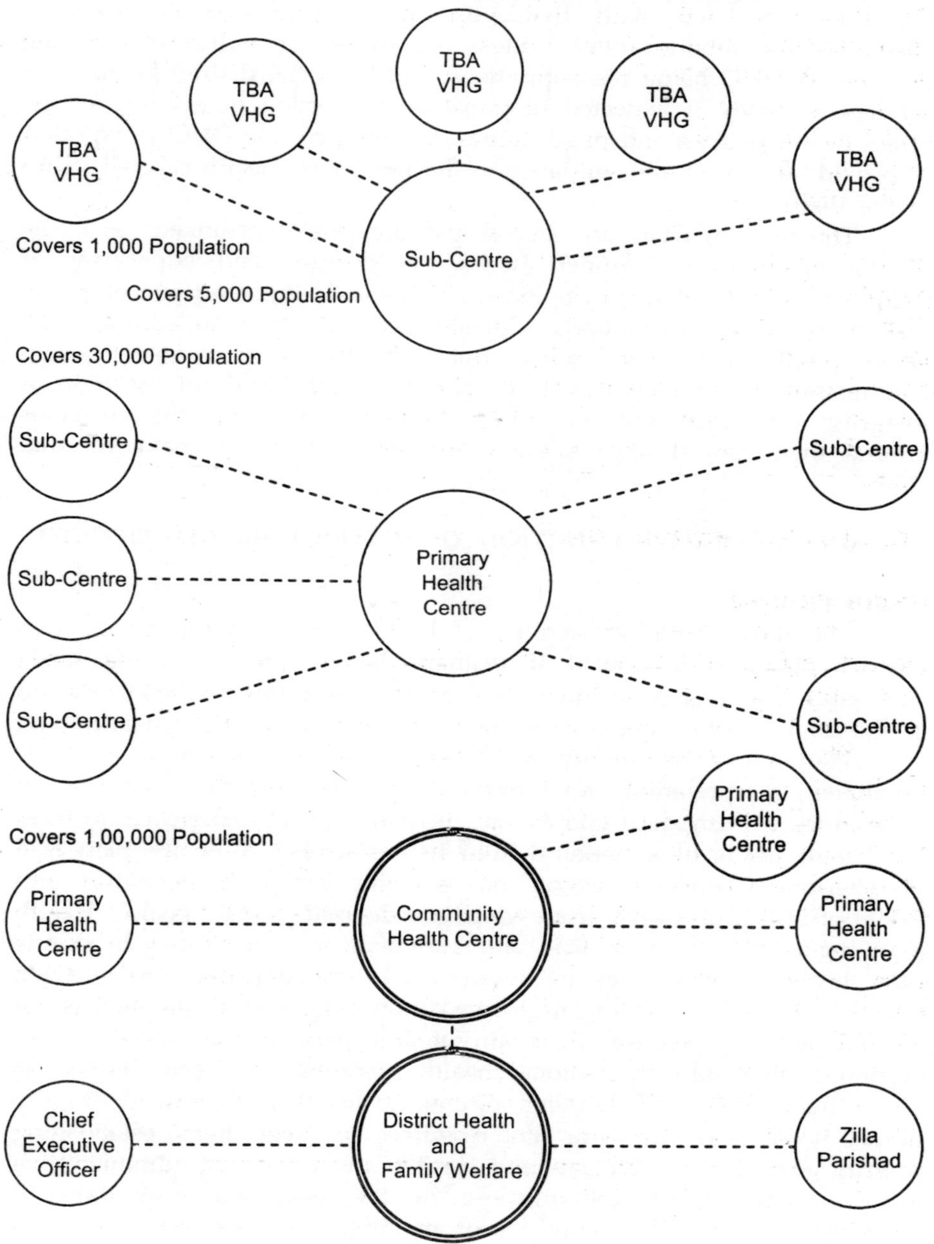

expectation widely shared by members of organization as to what would be the behaviour of persons who occupy that position. What a typical occupant of a given position such as DHO is expected to do, constitutes the role associated with that position. A role can be seen as encompassing, among other things, the duties or obligations of the position. A DHO being the supreme authority of the district health care services structure is expected to translate into action in his district the broad health policies and programmes. In doing so, the DHO is expected to provide direction and guidance to the peripheral health care structure in the district.

The roles of DHO are several and they are inter-linked; he is the district health-action planner: he is the director and supervisor of peripheral health structure in his district. He is the manager of entire district including lower levels of health care structure. In addition, the DHO might also have other roles in the district development administration and activities. DHO should create "prideful tradition of integrity, excellence and fellowship. Human beings breathe an ethos around them almost unconsciously and these traditions make for that ethos."

C. ADMINISTRATIVE FUNCTION OF DISTRICT HEALTH OFFICER

Health Planning

The most important activity of DHO is to plan for the district. District planning is crucial if primary health care is to be made successful. Planning is an intellectual exercise to adopt the health system to the district environment to achieve the goals of primary health care.

Planning of community health services means the careful analysis, intelligent interpretation and orderly development of these services, in accordance with modern knowledge, techniques, and experience, to meet the health needs of a nation within its resources.[9] A health plan is a predetermined course of action that is firmly based on the nature and extent of health problems, from which are devised priority goals.[10] Health planning is an aid to political and administrative authorities to decide how health services can be modernised and improved to provide effective and decent health care to the community. Health planning is not an independent exercise. It is an integral part of the overall socio-economic development. National health planning has been defined as "the orderly process of defining community health problems, identifying unmet needs and surveying the resources to meet them, establishing priority goals that are realistic and feasible and projecting administrative action to accomplish the purpose of the proposed programme."[11] Planning is essentially a process of making choice between available alternatives at all levels of decision-making. Planning is the exercise of intelligence to deal with facts and solutions as they are and find a way to solve problems. Planning is, in essence, an organised, conscious and continual attempt to select the best available alternatives to achieve specific goals. As expressed by Ackoff (1970, p. 1):

> Planning is one of the most complex and difficult intellectual activities in which man can engage. Not to do it well is not a sin, but to settle it for doing it less than well is.

According to Dr. Montoya:

> Health Planning is the phase of the total process which leads from the policy statements to the concrete identification of the populations whose needs and demands will be served; the indication of the types of activities that will be performed for those populations, with their general attributes, and the specification of the type of instruments that will be required to carry out the activities.[12]

1. Implementation

Plan implementation is an integral part of the planning process. It requires responsibility for translating the objectives of health plan into action. However, looking from the broader point of view, plan implementation requires cooperation, coordination and commitment at all levels of the implementing machinery in the field at the district, block or village level. It is at the implementation level that the difficulties creep in resulting in lower output. Implementation must be watched properly and timely action should be taken to improve administrative, technical, financial or personnel inadequacies.

2. Intersectoral Action

District Health Officer should promote intersectoral action to attain full impact of health services.

3. Leadership

The District Health Officer should provide leadership to the personnel working with him and at lower levels. Leadership is an indispensable phenomenon associated with the effective functioning of the district health services.

The attributes that are required in district health leadership may be briefly summarised as: technical competence, missionary zeal, the capacity to motivate others, the capacity to communicate with others, the ability to get along with people, cultural adaptability, the capacity to organise and manage, the capacity to inspire confidence in others, patience and dignity. Besides a leader must believe in the ideals of the organisation, be willing to accept hardships and prepared to work in a spirit of service. His ambition and enthusiasm should not be dampened by local conditions which may not provide him with the necessary facilities.

4. Supervision

Planning, communication and supervision are the three main steps in the process of direction. Like every other aspect of organisation supervision by district health team is also becoming very complicated and complex. The responsibilities of a supervisor have increased and a good supervisor is expected to have the qualities of head and heart. There is an old saying that "which is not inspected is not done." Hence inspection, overseeing and supervision arise in response to needs inherent in the functioning of an organisation.

The purpose of supervision and control is to ensure that the purpose of the organisation, i.e. provision of primary health care are being fulfilled. In most organisations, the supervision and control is still based on the old philosophy, i.e. to find faults and award punishments. The purpose of supervision is not only to inspect and inquire but to encourage and inspire, and thus achieve team work.

5. Communication

District Health Officer should ensure effective communication among all the members of the staff at district and lower levels. This is essential to create sound understanding.

Effective communications are essential to all aspects of effective administration. Staff must be adequately and currently informed about plans, methods, schedules, problems, events and progress. It is necessary that instructions, knowledge, and information be passed on for practical application to all concerned, and that they be so clearly presented as to make misinterpretation or misunderstanding impossible. Proper and adequate communication is not just in one direction. It requires two-way passage. Administrators must be certain that they know and understand the problems of workers for whom they are responsible. Communications must flow from the bottom upwards, as well as from the top down.

6. Co-ordination

The District Health Officer must ensure co-ordination among all aspects of health care, at all levels and among all sections.

Coordination implies the prevention of both duplication and overlapping so as to avoid administrative wastes of efforts, manpower and resources and to pool resources and experiences in dealing with problems and in achieving common objectives. Coordination which is a means to an end and not an end in itself must be considered in relation to its practical purposes which is to facilitate better performance and greater administrative efficiency in the system. To ensure efficient and economical functioning of an organisation, coordination is not only desirable but even essential. For the same reason inter-organisation coordination is advisable, especially when the activities of the various organisations concerned are of a complementary nature.

7. *Control*

The most important activity of District Health Officer is to control the activities of the district health office.

The objectives of control are as under:

(a) to ensure that the work has been accomplished according to stated objectives within budgetary and time limits,
(b) to enable the administration to identify the causes of work deficiencies, and
(c) to enable the management to suggest remedial action, i.e. to improve upon the system.

For control to be effective, it must be—

(a) Timely—Control needs to be exercised timely, otherwise there can be additions in problems.
(b) Simple—Control mechanism should be simple so that it can be easily adopted to make amends.
(c) Flexible—It should be flexible as too rigid control may be self-defeating.
(d) Minimal—Control must be exercised rarely but must be thorough. Whenever, it is done, all aspects need to be diagnosed.

8. *Finances*

The distribution of finances within the district needs to be ascertained and alternative ways found of using available finances equitably.

9. *Delegation*

Delegation has been defined as "inventing subordinates with authority to perform the manager's job on the manager's behalf."

The starting-point in the delegation process is to examine the district health officer's own job description. Some of the jobs that have to be done can be assigned to a subordinate. Delegation can be encouraged by including a specific mention of the function in the job description of the district health officer, e.g. assignment of work to others.

10. *Monitoring*

Monitoring is the process of measuring, coordinating, collecting, processing and communicating information of assistance to management and decision-making. The sources of information used in monitoring health activities include monthly, quarterly, and annual reports from health centres and hospitals, data on notifiable diseases and special surveys. Good information systems are required for effective monitoring. There is a practice to collect unnecessary information resulting in wastage of human and material resources. It must be emphasized that the problem is not a shortage of data—there is often too much—but the fact that little useful information can be gleaned from them.

D. FUNCTIONING OF DISTRICT HEALTH SYSTEM

(a) Headquarter-Field Relationship

The important function of District Health System is to Control, Supervise and Co-ordinate the activities of various field agencies, viz. CHCs, PHCs, and Sub-Centres to ensure their smooth functioning and providing: (a) Preventive, (b) Promotive, (c) Curative, and (d) Rehabilitative health services. This is achieved by DHO and his staff through: (a) Field reports, (b) Inspections, and (c) Meetings. District Health System has to submit reports upward to Divisional and State headquarters.

(b) Field Reports (See Chart 14.6)

These are prepared according to set guidelines to facilitate the comparability of reports on related matters and reduce as far as possible, the element of subjectivity. The reports are occasionally sugar-coated. Information that will evoke a favourable reaction is played up and the lapses are glossed over without some standard guide forms, it is all too tempting for reporters to inject extraneous bits of information. [13]

A large number of reports and returns are procured from the field by District Health Office. Let us mention here some of them:

1. Household and Family Register.
2. Village Register.
3. Target Couple Register.
4. Sterilisation and IUD Register.
5. Oral Pill and Nirodh Distribution Register.
6. Sterilisation and IUD Follow-up Register.
7. MCH Register.
8. Malaria Blood Slide Proforma.
9. Malaria Positive Case Register.
10. Stock and Distribution Register.
11. Birth and Death Register.
12. Sub-centre Clinic Register.
13. Health Worker Male Diary.
14. Health Worker Female Diary.
15. Health Worker Monthly Report Proforma.
16. Supervisor Compiled Report Proforma.
17. Monthly Report on Health and Family Welfare Programme.

All the reports after compilation at the District level are sent to the Division level and from there to the State level.

CHART 14.6

Headquarter-Field Relationships through Health Management Information System

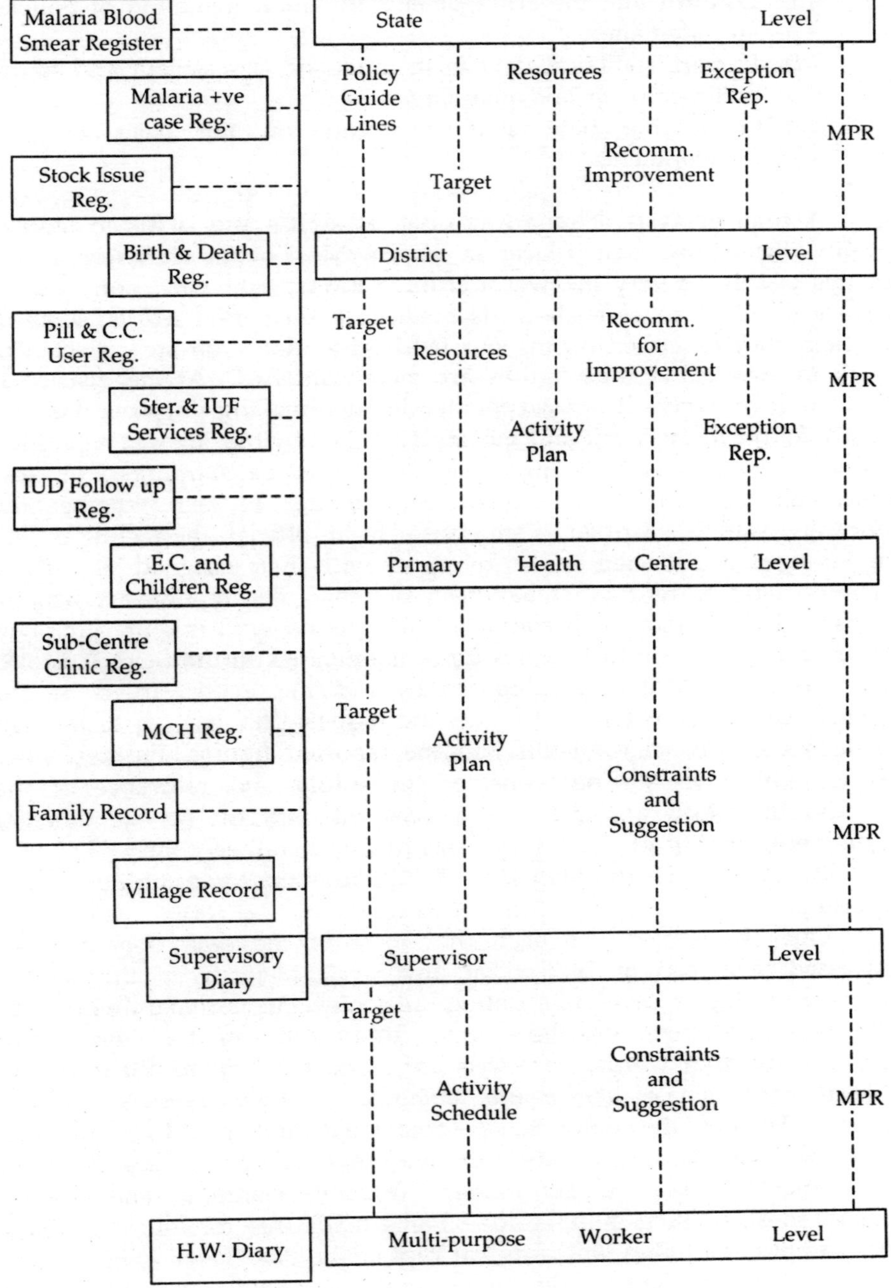

The purpose of report is to:[14]

(a) Measure the progress in the field.
(b) Locate problems in the field.
(c) Confirm that the arrangements for implementation of policies are adequate.
(d) Prepare statistical data for comparison, assessment and future policy-making and planning.
(e) Guide the field staff in future on the basis of past developments.

A brief analysis of reporting done by CHCs and PHCs to District Health office shows that it lacks in quality. Most of the staff responsible for this task has a very lukewarm attitude towards the collection of data, leave aside their concern about its quality. In their own words, some of the field staff remarked during our field visits that 'data are collected to check the work and thus figures are mostly inflated.' At the district or the State level where it is used for the decision-making purpose, data are mostly found inconsistent and incomplete. The obvious answer submitted by the concerned staff is 'proforma needed to be simplified' or 'less information should be collected'. As a matter of fact, whether the concerned staff is a worker, a supervisor or an official, the feeling is that the information collected has no relevance with their assigned jobs. Thus, attention paid to its quality has been minimal. The reports are usually prepared by a person with statistical background who is quite junior in status and has a very little exposure of happenings in the field. It is also observed that whatever is prepared by him/her is forwarded by the responsible officer to the next higher authorities. This has led to the gap between the real achievements and the reported figures. Further, since district authorities do not consider the utility and relevance of the records maintained and the reports received with the service delivery component, quality of the information has been rather poor.

Besides, the Health Staff feels that there is not much utility of such reporting.

Our observation has been that most of the data does not get processed, analysed or utilised at any level. Majority of the reports submitted to higher level after noting the achievements remain within the files and thus there has been very little utility of the information collected. In other words, no efforts are made to compare the resources utilised with that of the results obtained (cost-effectiveness or cost-benefit). Further the data is so fragmented and objectives of data collection are so vague and limited that excepting matching of achievements with the set targets (Family Planning and Health Programmes), nothing more is done. Same holds true for follow-up data. For example, the follow-up cards are kept at the PHC level whereas field workers are supposed to do follow-up in the field. As a result, the follow-up cards are either not prepared or are incomplete or not updated.

One of the reasons for the indifferent attitude of the workers towards information system is that very little administrative monitoring at the field level is done by the district authorities. The only monitoring which has been made as a regular feature of the family welfare programme is whether targets have been met and respective feedback is given. Again, feedback is mostly to warn the staff, if achievements do not commensurate with the targets or to congratulate those who have completed the targets. This is not adequate. To make the system effective and increase its use, adequate processing and appropriate analysis is needed.

Reporting and its analysis cost time and money. Therefore, only standardised, authenticated and useful reporting may be used to have genuine field control and field development. For this purpose, there is a need of designing and installing Management Information System to suit the needs of the organisation. This would hasten the exchange of information between headquarters and field. Besides, it would help in improving efficiency in operational functions, controlling organisational performance, and supporting intelligent planning by providing such information to the decision-makers which is most relevant, accurate, complete, concise, timely, economical, reliable and efficient. In addition, the use of electronic gadgets can speed up the flow of information. In this context, district information centres set-up by the Government of India can serve as an effective link between headquarters and the field agencies.

(c) Supervision and Inspection of Field Organisations

The effectiveness of workers depends largely on the supervision they receive from district staff. In other words, quality of work is directly related to the degree of supervision. High degree of supervision improves the quality of work; poor supervision leads to poor work. So good supervision is very important for health workers, health guides and Dais. Even well trained highly motivated health workers eventually become discouraged and ineffective when supervision is lacking. Objectives of Supervision are:

To help subordinates to do their job skillfully/efficiently, develop subordinates capacity to the fullest extent, to guide/assist in meeting pre-determined work objectives (targets), to promote effectiveness of subordinates, to motivate subordinates and maintain high morale and promote teamwork.

In addition to formal reporting, observation and inspection are indispensable if field operations are to be kept under effective control and the mistakes made in one field are not to be repeated in another. The inspection should not be conducted for isolated activities as is the practice in most of the organisations, but should combine together all the issues needing attention at the field level. This combination of aims is necessary partly because travel costs have to be kept within the limited budgetary allocations and also to economize the use of staff time.[15]

However, in practice, inspections are not planned and no use is made of reports prepared, i.e. no action is taken upon them. The inspection is a formality and done hurriedly.

In spite of all these handicaps, the cumulative insight gained by the headquarters over field offices through observation and inspection helps in developing good relationships between headquarters and field agencies, as well as in effective evaluation.[16]

(d) Meetings between the District and Field Staff

One of the most common and useful techniques of improving workers' performance is staff meeting. It is held by supervisors at various levels of an organisation, who are responsible for getting the work done through a group of individuals placed under them. Staff meetings are productive if staff members participate freely, feel responsible, and contribute to the achievement of the organization's goals. Staff conference may be held for different purposes. A staff conference may be called for: (a) for giving staff members certain information or to explain certain decisions taken at higher levels and to clarify certain points or doubts; (b) for solving problems arising out of day-to-day work situations for which the supervisor may have to draw upon the skills and talents of staff; and (c) for giving instructions about a new skill which may need detailed explanation and demonstration. Thus, as staff conference is not always a single-purpose meeting, and the supervisor who calls and conducts it must be aware of the variety of objectives, each of which may require different patterns of leadership and participation. If staff meetings are planned and held regularly they contribute to the development of teamwork.

The purposes of meeting are to discuss and solve a problem, communicate information, plan and organize, evaluate staff performance, evaluate the health services, coordinate the work of a health team, give training, motivate health workers and seek intersectoral meetings.

Every staff members should prepare for participation in a meeting. They should study the agenda and note carefully the topics to be covered. They should think about the items in terms of their own information and experience, and plan to share their ideas with others. They should feel free to make suggestions regarding the topics discussed during the meeting. Staff members should remain open-minded to listen to others' reactions and accommodate the ideas of others. They should follow the discussions carefully and make notes of important decisions.

E. FACTS AND SUGGESTIONS

While district health systems have been developed and

strengthened in varying degrees, a number of critical issues and problems remain: (i) thus the main emphasis has been on coverage, and quality of performance has been neglected; (ii) Policy guidelines are inadequate to support planning and implementation at district level; (iii) decentralization is rare; (iv) the roles, responsibilities, and procedures of district health staff are poorly defined and their leadership and management expertise is usually weak; (v) the integration of vertical programmes is still facing difficulties, and unipurpose workers, who have been trained as multi-purpose workers, continue to give preference to their earlier programmes; (vi) there are deficiencies in collaboration within the health sector, and between the vertical programmes and the general health services; (vii) much of the information generated at district level is neither for the district health managers, nor required for decision-making, monitoring, and evaluation at district level, but only for transmission to the upper echelons, from which feedback is rarely provided; (viii) community involvement in health is weak and attempts to foster leadership capability in the community are inadequate; (ix) in district development committees, insufficient attention is paid to identifying health problems that require intersectoral action, and individual sectoral priorities and different administrative structures often prevent the pooling and sharing of resources between sectors; and (x) finally, there are not enough financial or skilled human resources, at the district level, and those that are available are usually neither equitably distributed nor efficiently used.[17]

Based on the discussions in the preceding paras, we seek to highlight various issues affecting district health system and also propose suitable suggestions to make this system effective.

I. Democratic Decentralisation not Effective in Practice

An experience of democratic decentralisation has not been fruitful as expected. Our elected representatives are not the persons who want to serve their area without selfish motives. They, in connivance with district bureaucracy want to exploit the system. In the new millennium, we have to ensure total transfer of power to people so that they can watch their interest and weed out bogus elected leaders and corrupt officials.

(a) Lack of able and mature leadership among office-bearers at all levels of PRIs; need to strengthen their competence and capability through education and training.
(b) Mismatch of functions and resources; need for augmenting resources through local mobilisation and participation.
(c) Inconsistencies in the PR Act, 1993; need for amendments to clarify issues to ensure a stable institutional framework of PRIs.
(d) Absence of continuous contact between the elected representatives and the people; need for people's association and organisations.

(e) Misconceptions about PRI's obligations for rural development; need for promoting self-reliance in the community.
(f) Lack of genuine will and faith in decentralization; need for transfer of full powers and authority to PRIs.
(g) Lack of cordial official-non-official relationship; need for creating harmonious conditions conducive to rural development.
(h) Undue interference by vested interests and pressure groups on PRI system; need for empowering the disadvantaged sections through education and awareness.

2. Poor Quality of Health Care

In the new millennium, quality is becoming an essential part of the health system in both developed and developing countries. Quality Assurance in Health Care is not a programme. Quality Assurance is a process, which is continuous one. Quality of Medical Care is an index of Civilization. Health Care Quality is being demanded and expected and providers are judged by it. Quality is tangible and measurable. It is cost effective. Quality is as simple as doing one's job better continuously. There is a great pressure from patients and general public for quality health care which is based on certain standards, accreditation, certification and bench marking. The quality of health care needs continuous improvements in services. Quality of health care should be effective, efficient, technically sound, safe and accessible. A WHO report of a meeting held in Indonesia recommended the following to improve quality health care:[18]

(1) Ensure that quality of health care is an integral part of health services delivery at all levels of health care covering public and private sectors;
(2) Organize advocacy/awareness workshops on quality assurance for policy-makers, administrators and the leadership of health care to get their commitment for quality assurance;
(3) Establish a coordinating mechanism for quality assurance activities at national constitute a multi-disciplinary task force of national experts to provide advice on technical aspects of quality assurance;
(4) Initiate quality assurance of health care in selected hospitals and in primary health care through the district health system approach, document the experiences and expand gradually to more health care facilities;
(5) Organize national strategic planning workshops with technical assistance from WHO;
(6) Formulate guidelines to set standards and select national key indicators on quality assurance to monitor compliance and measure performance;

(7) Invest on building local capacity in health care quality through the creation of a critical mass of expertise within the country;
(8) Mobilize potential resources from within the country including support from international agencies; and
(9) Ensure that orientation on quality assurance be integrated in both basic and in-service training programmes of all health care professionals.

3. Lack of Equity in Health Care

In the new millennium, we have to change our priorities to benefit the most deprived from the health services. We must plan and implement our health system to ensure quality health care to the poorest section of the society. Mahatma Gandhi has rightly suggested the providers of health care that "if modern medicine is to be humane, then compassion and wisdom on the part of clinicians are attributes that are needed perhaps as never before." First of all, an attitudinal change among health service staff has to be brought in so that they can make the patients feel important, wanted, cared and well looked after. This change in affective domain must start early as part of the teaching objectives for all medical and paramedical students. They should be made to realize that the hospitals of medical colleges need the patients for clinical teaching; thus the academia is dependent on patients and not *vice versa*.

Empowerment of patients will lead to medical uprising of the society by creating an educated and health awareness, informed and health conscious, striving to improve their quality of life with justified use of their rights. They can curb exploitation in the name of medicine and ensure a decline in quackery.

The empowered can be easily motivated and channelised to enlist support for health programmes and achievement of health goals. Thus, health programmes will be a truly peoples' programme since indifference will cease to exist in health matters. Voluntary participation in health activities will increase.

We have to empower the poor people so that they can take their due from health care system. As long as the services do not reach the needy people, there cannot be any perceptible change in the health status of the people. Services are not to be merely accessible but must reach those most in need.

Today, there is great alienation between the goals of District Health System and the personnel working in them resulting in inefficiency, tensions, conflicts, and low morale. Personnel system needs overhauling and reform to suit the health needs of the poeple in the next century. We may not get the result from the existing health personnel in the district without bringing about changes in them to usher an era of hardwork, ethics, responsivness and transparency.

4. Resistance of Bureaucracy to Change to Suit the Needs of Democratic Decentralisation

However, the greatest contribution of PRIs is breaking the hegemony of a few and empowering the masses. The concepts of transparency in administration and accountability to the people have a potential for being translated into reality through PRIs. The public mandate for a partyless development-oriented institution forces us to unlearn our present practices and beliefs.[19]

It is for the government to take certain tough decisions in overhauling the work culture and infusing ethics in administration. It is argued that appropriate action be initiated by policy-makers, administrators, political and social scientists to overcome the obstacles undermining the potential of these local institutions.

We know that, it is easy to move the mountains than to change the minds of the people, without such changes, impact of Primary Health Care would be temporary and ineffective. Shri R. Srinivasan, Secretary (Health), Government of India in his message to Regional Review meeting Primary Health Care System Development for Southern Zone held at Bangalore on 22-23 February, 1990 said that "These tasks cannot be achieved by mere investment of further resources for buildings, residence, training centres, etc. but call for both professional and local accountability to the community. Unless the health care work force in a district remains accountable to the community and takes a large hand in health education and public information. Primary Health Care System can never do justice to its challenges. Within Government, even though the departmental organisation assigns specific responsibility at different levels, all policy level functionaries must keep the above considerations fully in mind."

For democracy to be successful at the national level, the grass-roots organisations have to be strong. PRI system has to respond to the felt needs of the people. The citizens have to have faith in the efficacy of the administrative system so that the distance between people and the government is reduced.[20]

5. Primary Health Care Delivery Programme not Effective in District

(i) Implementation of national health programmes is weak. In particular, the routine operations should be managed well, campaigns should be properly organised and integrated well with other health activities.

(ii) Promotive health programmes such as health education, school health, nutritions, food adulteration and environmental sanitation are usually neglected. District officials should be able to plan, implement and monitor them well.

(iii) Epidemic control activities need to be streamlined.

(iv) District has to perform several functions to support

functioning of PHCs which at present suffer because of resources and lack of support. These include:

- guidance/supervision to PHCs,
- exercise financial and administrative powers,
- maintenance of equipment,
- supplies,
- allocation of staff,
- appraise performance of PHCs systematically, scientifically and objectively,
- assess training needs of MOs, and
- create favourable community environment for health workers and PHCs to function.

6. Inadequate and Non-functional Infrastructure

Committed and reputed NGO's may be involved in the development of primary health care system by handing over certain proportion of infrastructure facilities, namely, sub-centre or primary health centre along with building, funds and staff with relatively more management freedom to VOs/NGOs depending upon their capability of funds, staff, etc. after ascertaining their credibility.

Mechai Viraavaidya in his article, "Utapped potential" in *World Health* rightly states, "The NGO sector has the potential to be a much greater force than it is at present . . . . A working partnership between government agencies and NGOs can make tremendous progress in the next fifteen years."[21]

NGO-supported and organized health care services must be an integral part of the total health system of a country, including the referral system.[22]

7. Lack of Enlightened Community Participation and Involvement

Although academics, voluntary organisations, government and funding agencies and UN agencies have promoted and supported the participation concept of development and much has been written and spoken about participation, authentic participation of the poor has hardly taken place in real life situation. People's participation in development process has been elusive.[23] Same is true about participation of the people in health services.

To quote WHO: Community participation is a political process insofar as community members acquire a say in decision-making about health and health care issues that affect them, and a measure of control over the persons that are supposed to serve their needs. Community participation in this sense raises the most serious organizational problems, and even dilemmas, for ministries of welfare.[24] Community participation also has political implications when community members are involved in monitoring the services from which they are supposed to benefit.

They can demand that the necessary attention be paid to the needs of the people at the grass-roots, and of those expected to serve them. The mechanisms of community involvement are also important to give the responsible authorities at the district level adequate information about the grass-roots functioning of the health care system: without direct inputs from the communities, those authorities may only receive information from the very system they are supposed to control.[25]

Ministry of Personnel has also realised the neglect of elected bodies from being given the real power to monitor. To quote: "The agenda for real empowerment of elected local bodies, has largely not gone beyond conforming legislation in most states-centralised system for planning and service delivery often through functional agencies still persist, and the local self-government bodies and the elected functionaries are not able to function with adequate control over local functions and resources.[26]

8. Intersectoral and Intrasectoral Co-ordination Lacking

The concept of primary health care encompasses the overall socio-economic development of communities concurrent to the improvement of the health status. Therefore, the health sector cannot function in isolation when implementing primary health care programmes. More important and relevant to the technical discussions is the acceptance by other sectors involved in the socio-economic development—agriculture, housing, public works and communications, education, mass media—that they cannot work in isolation, to the exclusion of the health sector. The establishment of intersectoral coordination is therefore an important primary health care approach.

Aleyco El Bindari Hammad in his Article, "Intersectoral Co-operation in Primary Health Care" in *World Health* rightly mentions that "the broader aim of increasing well-being and resistance to disease as a whole while promoting and maintaining good health will require the combined efforts of many sectors not immediately related to health."[27]

9. Universities are Engaged in Traditional Activities

Universities, must act as bridges between the community and the Government. In Karnataka we have half a dozen universities and large number of medical colleges who can help in the promotion of Primary Health Care. In May, 1984, World Health assembly chose the theme, "The Role of Universities in the Strategies for Health for all." To quote:

> Universities are seeking new relationships with health policy-makers, extending the concept of health care beyond that of the individual to that of whole communities, and adapting their under-graduate curriculum to ensure that education equips students to undertake those supervisory and managerial roles which have not hitherto been seen as appropriate for health professionals.[28]

Now at last, the universities seem prepared to lend whole-hearted backing to three of the main imperatives of Health for all: political commitment to social equity, community participation and the use of appropriate and affordable technology.[29]

10. Stereotyped Health Management System

The challenge of Health for All calls for a permanent and systematic managerial process, ranging from planning and policy-making, in collaboration with other sectors, to implementation, monitoring and evaluation, for the development of an effective health system. The managerial process entails the formulation of a health policy with defined priorities, and the preparation of programmes and budgets to put the policy into effect. It also calls for the assessment of manpower requirements and the formulation of plans to train the requisite manpower, together with the integration of well-formulated programmes into the general health system. A dynamic civil society and a professionally trained and dedicated civil service (Insulated from political interference) are the twin pillars of a constructive relationship between State and Society.[30]

Mr. M.G. Devashayam, ex-IAS officer, in his Article, 'Good Administration' in the *Daily Tribune* mentions the components of responsible administration. These are:

(i) Openness in the sense of having wide contact with the people administered;
(ii) A sense of justice, fair play and impartiality in dealing with men and matters;
(iii) Sensitivity and responsiveness to the urges, feelings and aspirations of the common people;
(iv) Securing the honour and dignity of the human being, however humble he or she might be;
(v) Humility and simplicity in the persons manning the administrative machinery and their easy accessibility;
(vi) Creating and sustaining an atmosphere conducive to development, growth and social change; and
(vii) Honest and integrity in thought and action.[31]

11. Lack of Reliable and Scientific Referral System

At present, the referral system does not function effectively. This is due to the following reasons: (i) Overloading of hospitals with self-referrals; (ii) lack of confidence in lower-level facilities because of perceived low quality of care; (iii) lack of organisational and management links between hospitals at various levels. An effective referral system has to be designed by focusing on three important areas: the structure of the referral system, management co-ordination and quality improvement.

The District Health System has the potential capacity and means to deliver decent health services to the people. However, the administrative system and the ethos and perceptions of the personnel working there do not possess confidence in achievement.

A visit to various health offices at District, revealed the poor functioning of these offices. People mentioned the following problems faced by them in dealing with the officials:

(i) Unhelpful attitude,
(ii) Inordinate delay in transacting business,
(iii) Corruption amongst the officials,
(iv) Shortage of medicine,
(v) Faulty procedure,
(vi) Intentional delays,
(vii) No arrangements for persons on leave, and
(viii) Improper behaviour.

In the new millennium, we have to change the District Health System as envisaged in World Health Assembly Resolution WHA 39, in terms of its structure, approach, methodology to meet the health needs of the people. We have to appoint persons who have vision, vitality, deduction, clarity and who can get the results and not simply move the papers.

In the new millennium, District Health System has to introduce new technology of Telematics, and ensure equity and quality in health care.

A Report of a WHO Inter-country Workshop on Telemedicine for Health Development in the 21st century, Bangkok, Thailand, (30 March-3 April, 1998) defines the meaning, use and give recommendations to promote telemedicine. To quote (WHO: SEARO, Report of WHO Inter-country Workshop on Telemedicine For Health Development in the 21st Century, Bangkok, Thailand, 30 March-3 April, 1998, pp. 1-21).

Health Telematics is defined as a composite term for health-related activities, services and systems carried out over a distance by means of information and communication technologies for the purpose of global health promotion, disease control and health care, as well as education, management, and research for health.

The process of planning which includes the formulation of policy and strategies is followed by the choice of technology, which is implemented in three phases. The first phase of implementation includes the development and adoption of standards and laying down of specifications to meet the health telematics strategies. Standardization is required at different levels varying from Data Standards; Technical Standards; Work Standards, and Equipment Standards to Training Standards and Professional Standards. The second phase deals with the selection of computing hardware, peripherals, telecommunication infrastructure, operating and utility software, while the third phase concentrates on procurement, implementation, training and support.

Health Telematics raises certain ethical issues, such as the acceptability of transmitting personal information across cultural boundaries; young doctors getting professionally affected, and the confidentiality of the relationship between the patient and the treating doctor. Full cooperation of the medical and paramedical staff involved, as well as patients is essential. Even in the most advanced form, Health Telematics might not provide a blanket solution for each situation. There would be cases where human intervention is needed. It also raises concern on widening the gap between the poor and the privileged.

Based on the presentations by various resource persons, and the experiences shared between SEAR countries during the workshop, the participants appreciated the potential of Telemedicine. However, the group proposed to change the term "Telemedicine" to the broader term of "Health Telematics" in order to avoid a narrow interpretation of the scope of technology.

The participants made the following recommendations:

(1) Conduct advocacy and awareness of Health Telematics so as to gain the commitment of policy-makers, administrators, and professional groups.
(2) Incorporate Health Telematics into the renewed HFA policies/ strategies.
(3) Conduct situation analyses, and define priorities for initiating plans of action, through pilot projects on Health Telematics.
(4) Develop the national capacity, through training of human resources required to set-up and manage Health Telematics activities.
(5) Constitute national coordination committees for the development of Telematics as an integral component of social development, thus ensuring the participation of relevant sectors right from the beginning.
(6) Build Health Telematics on the available infrastructure, and choose appropriate technology based on country resources and the health needs of the people.
(7) Develop the monitoring and evaluation criteria as integral parts of the project.
(8) Develop partnerships with various stake-holders: the industry, academic institutions and research centres, and public and private sectors in support of Health Telematics.

District Health System need be strengthened to provide integrated and comprehensive health care to the people.

Notes and References

1. Eighth General Programme of Work Covering the Period 1990-93, Geneva, WHO, 1987 (Health for All Series No. 10).
2. WHO: SEARO: Health Situation in the South East Asia Region, 1994-97, New Delhi; 1999, p. 185.
3. James C. Charlesworth, Government Administration, Harpur, New York, 1951, p. 207.
4. *Ibid.*
5. WHO: Strengthening Ministeries of Health For Primary Health Care, Geneva, 1984, pp. 31-32.
6. WHO: District Health Systems, Geneva, 1995, p. 8.
7. *Ibid.*, pp. 9-10.
8. Krasae Chanawonges, Rural Development Management, Mohidol University, Thailand, 1996, p. 13.
9. WHO: *Technical Report Series*, 215, 1961, p. 4.
10. WHO: *Public Health Papers*, 46, p. 9.
11. WHO: *Public Health Papers*, 44, p. 15.
12. Dr. Montoya, Programme Technology in the Context of Health Planning, Minemographed.
13. Walter R. Sharp, Field Administration in the United Nations System, The Carnegie Endowment, London, Stevens, 1961, p. 266.
14. S.L. Goel, Advanced Public Administration, New Delhi, Sterling, 1994, p. 290.
15. *Ibid.*
16. *Ibid.*, p. 291.
17. WHO: District Health Systems, Geneva, 1995, p. 28.
18. WHO: SEARO, Report of a WHO Inter-country Meeting, Sarabayo, Indonesia, 16-20, December, 1996, New Delhi, 1996, p. 8.
19. Shalini Rajneesh, Democratic Decentralisation in Karnataka, a Ph.D. thesis, unpublished, p. 293.
20. A.P. Barnabas, Good Governance at Local Level, in *IJPA*, July-Sept., 1998, p. 453. (Special Number on Towards Good Governance).
21. Mechai Vira Vaidya, Untapped Potential, in *World Health*, March 1985, p. 4.
22. S.K. Vettivel, People's Participation in Social Development, Role of NGO's, New Delhi, Vetri Publishers, 1992, p. 5.
23. P.K. Bajpai, People's Participation in Development—A Critical Analysis, in *IJPA*, Oct.-Dec. 1998, p. 817.
24. WHO: Strenghtening Ministries of Health for Primary Health Care, Geneva, 1984, p. 39.
25. WHO: Strengthening Ministries of Health for Primary Health Care, Geneva, 1984, p. 42.
26. Documents, Action Plan for an Effective and Responsive government prepared by Department of Administrative Reforms and Public Grievances, Ministry of Personnel Public Grievances, New Delhi, Quoated in *IJPA*, Vol. XLIV, No. 3 (July-Sept. 1998) p. 637.
27. WHO: *World Health*, March 1986, p. 5.
28. George C. Salmot, 'New Problems, New Strategies, in *World Health*, January 1980, p. 15.
29. WHO: *World Health*, April 1984, p. 3.
30. R.K. Sapru, Development Administration Crises and Continuities, in *IJPA*, Oct.-Dec. 1998, p. 779.
31. The *Daily Tribune*, Dec. 27, 1988.

CHAPTER 15

BLOCK LEVEL HEALTH CARE ADMINISTRATION: COMMUNITY HEALTH CENTRES

"A health system based on primary health care cannot, and I repeat, cannot be realized, cannot be developed, cannot function, and simply cannot exist without a network of hospitals functioning in a manner I have tried to describe. But hospitals have to change their ways so that they become one of the main flag-bearers of the most daring yet the most promising health movement in the history of humanity, the movement for health for all by the year 2000."

—Dr. H. Mahler, former Director General, WHO

15

CHAPTER

Block Level Health Care Administration: Community Health Centres

INTRODUCTION

WHO defines Community Health Centre as Reference Health Centre. "The reference health centre differs from the generic health centre in that it is a functional concept that can be realized by strengthening one or more health centres to improve referral within the health system in rural areas. Thus, in addition to its generic health centre functions, it provides essential surgical, maternity and medical care, as well as carrying out preventive and promotive activities in the neighbourhood it serves. The reference health centre lightens the burden of the first referral hospital by taking over certain routine interventions, at the same time bringing appropriate care closer to the population at only a fraction of the cost of similar operations performed in local hospitals. Health centres, including reference health centres and hospitals, are components of a health care system, each playing a different but complementary role."[1]

A WHO document also mentions the role of first referral hospital as:[2,3]

> The hospital at first referral level, whether serving an urban or a rural population, is an integral part of the district health system with a key role to play in achieving health for all. It can function not only as a place to which patients with complex medical conditions are referred for diagnosis, treatment, and care, but also as a resource centre for health promotion in the district and for the planning and delivery of primary health care. This report of a WHO Study Group considers the responsibilities of the first referral hospital in its district setting, identifying its specific tasks in the provision of health care, training, and hospital support

> services, and defining its relationship both with the community and with health centres and other components of the district health system. Management principles for the first referral hospital are also discussed, in the context of the national health programme, with emphasis on decentralization, planning, and the efficient use of human and financial resources. The report concludes with recommendations for action by WHO, governments, and hospitals themselves, stressing the need for a change in approach if the first referral hospital is to fulfil its functions within a district health system based on primary health care.

The same document indicates the importance of first referral hospital in a district health set-up. To quote:[4]

> Half of the worlds people live in villages, where the organization of health services may be hampered by remoteness, adverse climate conditions, poor communications, and poverty, and perhaps by illiteracy and superstition. The first referral hospital may be very small, with a tiny staff that is limited in experience and expertise. The other half of the worlds people live in cities, some of enormous size, where poverty is again a factor and where overcrowding, pollution, and stress may be overwhelming. The problems that city hospitals must face are different from those of village hospitals, yet both types of hospitals provide essential services and it is important to see how they can be incorporated into the district health system.

In the past century medicine has grown increasingly scientific and hospitals have tended to become technological workshops for the diagnosis and treatment of disease. The trend will undoubtedly continue, but at the same time, the functional integration of hospitals into district health services is of vital importance, if they are to provide efficient, effective, affordable, and equitable services to their communities. This is not to underrate good clinical care and diagnosis, which are still the bedrock of hospital practice at the first referral level, but rather to emphasize the importance of making such care available to those most in need of it.

Within a district health system, there has to be a place to which patients with complex medical conditions can be referred for diagnosis, treatment, and care, and which can act as a resource centre for the health work of the district. This place is the first referral hospital.

CHCs are being maintained by the State Government under MNP/ BMS as on 31 March, 2001, there were 3,043 Community Health Centes while on 30.6.98, 2712 CHS were functioning in the country. As on 1.4.90 there were 1910 CHCs. Out of four Primary Health Centres, one Community Health Centre has been created with 30 beds in rural areas and 50 beds at taluk level to serve as referral hospital for the rural population. The purpose is to provide second tier referral services near their place and with better facilities so that their unnecessary approaching district hospitals may be avoided to save cost and provide better services to the rural population. Facilities required for 30 bedded/ 50 bedded hospitals have been provided in the Primary Health Centres upgraded in terms of infrastructure, personnel, equipment, etc. so that these institutions can handle cases coming to them directly or referred from Primary Health Centres.

These centres offer considerable advantages to both patients and society. From the point of view of society, hospitalization both protects the family from many of the disruptive effects of caring for the ill in the home and operates as a means of guiding the sick and injured in medically supervised institutions where their problems are less disruptive for society as a whole.[5] To quote Perry, "the success with which a hospital contributes towards meeting the patients needs can be measured by the fullness of the life he is able to lead on leaving it."[6]

A comprehensive definition of Hospital has been given by WHO which needs to be adopted by the CHCs. Hospital is an integral part of a social and medical organization, the functions of which are to provide for the complete health care of the population—both curative and preventive and whose out-patients services reach out to the family and its home environment; the hospital is also a' centre for training of health workers and for bio-social research.[7]

ORGANISATIONAL STRUCTURE (See Chart 15.1)

Personnel

The CHC is headed by Senior Medical Officer (SMO) who is generally a medical officer with 20-25 years of experience. He is the chief executive and has to ensure the smooth functioning of CHC. The other staff in CHC is as given below:

Staff for Community Health Centres

1.	Medical Officer	4
2.	Nurse Mid-Wives	7
3.	Dresser	1
4.	Pharmacist/Compounder	1
5.	Laboratory Technician	1
6.	Radiographer	2
7.	Ward Boys	1
8.	Dhobi	2
9.	Sweepers	1
10.	Mali	2
11.	Chowkidar	1

CHART 15.1

Organisational Structure of Community Health Care

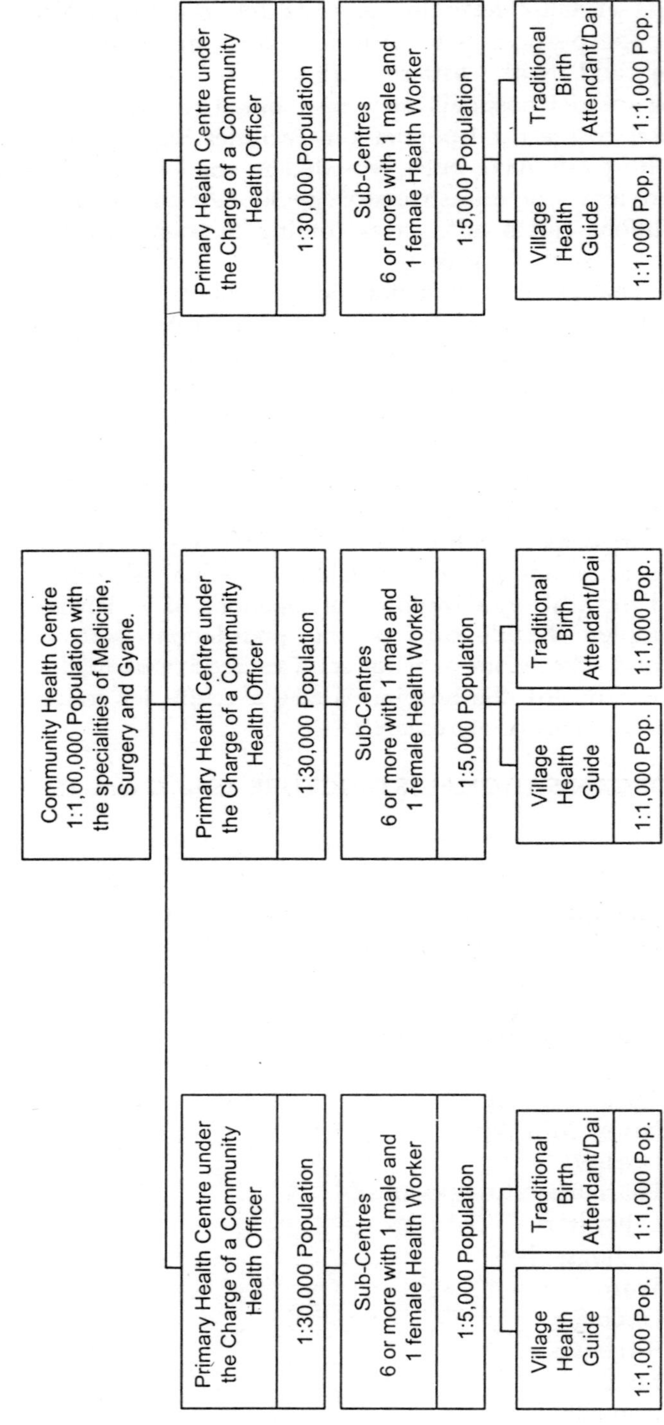

12.	Aya	1
13.	Peon	1
	Total	25

Either qualified or specially trained to work as Surgeon, Obstetrician, Physician and Paediatrician. One of the existing Medical Officers similarly should be either qualified or specially trained in Public Health.

The CHCs as per their strength require 10,848 specialists while sanctioned posts are only 6827. Out of these 6827 sanctioned posts, 3203 are lying vacant as on 30.6.98. CHCs are short of 6635 specialists. How can we expect them to provide good services? It is a very serious matter. The state governments must fill these vacant posts and sanction required additional posts.

The CHC for average population, as already mentioned, serves a population of 2.32 lakhs, an area of 115.82 sq. km., average radial distance of 1917 sq. km. and average number of villages 21,653 and 8.48 PHC per CHC.

However, we find many vacant posts at all levels affecting the efficiency of CHCs. The government should ensure that there are no vacancies. Besides, SMO should be given full support to keep the CHC in functional condition.

BUILDINGS

Firstly, there are no buildings for many CHCs. Even existing, buildings of most of the CHCs are insufficient to accommodate all the activities essential for a CHC. Many buildings are ill-maintained, unclean, and lack basic facilities. Some do not have boundary walls. The surrounding environment is not clean and full of congress grass.

EQUIPMENT

Specialists have identified the minimum essential requirements of Equipment for Community Health Centres to provide 2nd tier of health services. We may mention here the list of important categories as these would help us in assessing their availability and utilisation.

The equipment has been broadly classified under the following heads:

1. Imaging
2. Electro-medical
3. Pneumatic-hydraulic and sterilization
4. Laboratory
5. Air conditioning and refrigeration
6. Hospital utility support systems
7. Administration

8. Minor equipment and furnishings
9. Surgical instruments and packs

The equipment mentioned here is not supplied to CHC resulting to unsatisfactory services. The state health department must ensure the availability of all equipments in functional condition to the benefits of referral system.

FACILITIES

Following facilities should be provided in a CHC:

1. Radiological Investigations
2. Laboratory Investigations
3. Surgery
4. Trauma and Life Support
5. Chest
6. Surgery
7. Urogenital
8. Surgical Conditions Abscess
9. Ophthalmology
10. Gastro Enterology
11. Thoracic
12. ENT
13. Obs. and Gynaec
14. Use of drugs causing Analgesis
15. Regional Anesthesia.

NORMS OF SERVICES

Government has developed Norms of Services for CRC to avoid confusion. These norms help the health department and CRC staff to maintain standards and ensure quality health care. These norms also help in policy-making and planning for the new CHCs to be established.

The CHC staff should not restrict themselves only to the technical aspects of effectiveness but to such other aspects as well, like comparability of services and work environment, communication with patients and their relations and promotion of collective responsibility for Medicare and health of the community. The success of these norms depends upon the availability of facilities in good condition.

FUNCTIONS

1. It acts as a referral centre. All those who are referred from PHC or sub-centre are attended here with more facilities and by qualified personnel. It provides good examination facilities

or gets it done from district hospital at higher level.

2. It serves as a part of district health system, thereby getting the benefits of exchange of services.
3. It should be an integral part of the primary health care and should support all activities of primary health centres and sub-centres.
4. It should provide training to its staff to make them more and more professional and dynamic.
5. It should have intimate contact with the people, the communities and involve them in their own health promotion.

Thus, community health centre should be looked at from a wider angle and not merely from curative aspect of a higher degree. It should encompass all aspects of health care and should promote and coordinate all health activities as a part of district health system to provide better health care to the people. However, when first referral level is not competent, the case may be referred to district hospital.

Aspects of CHC Services

(i) OPD Functions

The patient either referred from below or approached directly by CRC should be received well. However, preference may be given to referred patients coming from a long distance. The patient needs the following services:

(a) Diagnosis by the specialists with the help of laboratory tests and electronic equipment supplemented by clinical sense of the doctor. This should be done thoroughly. Well begun is half done.

(b) Treatment-Diagnosis is followed by treatment which can take any of the following form:
   - (i) Sending the patient back home after prescribing treatment. This can be followed at later dates convenient to doctor and patient.
   - (ii) Treatment in the OPD.
   - (iii) Admission and treatment in a CHC ward.
   - (iv) Refer to District/Specialist hospital.
   - (v) Refer to PHC back to be followed by PHC Doctor.

The patient needs good care, courteous behaviour, prompt services and clear communication. He would judge the CHC from the care given to him and not by the technical details. However, in practice, we find that the patients feel lot of discomforts and complain of apathy of CRC staff. Let us mention some of the common problems.

Problems of OPD

(a) Lack of proper seating arrangements.
(b) Delays resulting into time wastage—It takes 2-3 hours for a patient to get his turn.
(c) Lack of punctuality—Doctors on duty are not in time resulting into rush and impatience among patients.
(d) Lack of proper examination—Patients feel that they are not properly examined and that is why they prefer private doctors resulting in the mushroom growth of Nursing homes and private practitioners.
(e) Doctors lack social conscience—Doctors do not have concern for social justice, compassion for underprivileged. There is lack of strong commitment and spirit of service, vital for the success of medical profession.
(f) Discourteous behaviour.
(g) Non-availability of medicine.
(h) Fear of hospital infection because of poor cleanliness.

Thus, there is a need of far reaching improvements in the management of OPD services to ensure optimisation of resources and satisfaction of patients. Author has rightly said that "We should not be contended merely with the availability and accessibility of health services in OPDs but rather in their acceptability and acceptance."[8]

A special out-patient clinic that sees only referred cases can be a great help to both hospital and health centre as well as achieve the objective of management by exception. Many patients can be diagnosed and treated without the need for admission when the absence of overcrowding allows the doctor to give enough time to each of them, since these patients have already been examined and their detailed history is with them. Wherever possible, medical and surgical patients should be separated. The referred note, including relevant comments and advice, should always receive a proper reply, and the patient should be referred back as soon as possible for continued treatment either at the health centre or at home to avoid confusion.

(ii) Ward

Ward is the heart of CHC where patient comes in direct and intimate contact with the staff and services of CHC. After the patient has been examined in the OPD or the emergency area, he may be advised admission in the ward. Ward management is the undivided responsibility of the ward sister concerned. Specialists visit the ward as and when necessary. A ward is that area of the hospital where all the amenities—physical, social and especially medical care—are made available to make the patients feel at home till they are discharged. In other words, a ward is a temporary home for the patients admitted there. Evidently, there is a need to ensure a healthy environment to help early recovery of the patients and to win their confidence. In each ward, there is a nursing unit to take care of the patients for all the 24 hours. The efficient planning of this unit would ensure maximum care of the patients. The broad categories of functions that should be discharged by the nursing unit are:

(a) Meeting personal needs of the patients.
(b) Efficient ward management.
(c) Proper maintenance of records of the patients.
(d) Provision of basic institutional services.
(e) Availability of diagnostic and treatment equipment.
(f) Arranging formal and informal health education of the patients and their relatives.

(iii) Specialities

CHC is provided to take care of the following specialities:

(a) Medical Care

Medical and nursing staff should make themselves available to provide services for chronic illness like asthma, diabetes, hypertension, chronic obstructive pulmonary disease, tuberculosis, heart ailment. The patient should be monitored frequently to arrive at conclusions. If controlled, patient can be referred back to primary health centres. If serious, they may be referred to specialists at higher levels.

(b) Obstetric Care

CRC must have arrangements for complicated delivery cases. CRC should provide quality maternity and child health services.

(c) Pediatric Care

There should be good arrangements for the care of children to reduce infant mortality rate. There should also be arrangement for the education of mothers who accompany the child.

(d) Surgery

Since at primary health centre, there is no arrangement for surgery, CHC must take care of minor operations. The performance of surgery requires a medical doctor with surgical background who should either be familiar with local anaesthesis techniques or work with a competent anaesthetist and trained nursing staff. It requires a suitable minor operating theatre and sterile instruments and supplies. An additional room for post-operative recovery is essential. Surgery should not be performed unless there are suitable arrangements.

Minor surgery may be performed at CRC, if the responsible surgeon considers that the person performing it has had a firm grounding in the basics of surgery and in the appropriate diagnostic and surgical techniques. All such minor surgery must be carefully monitored by the senior surgeon. There must be strict rules concerning permitted procedures and a regular and rigorous review of faults and failures. CHC should ensure good arrangements for surgical cases.

(iv) Emergency Services

The image of the CRC depends upon the type, quality and speed with which emergencies are attended to. S.K. Garg has nicely explained the need and requirements of emergency services. To quote him:[9]

> "Causality means—a patient who comes to the hospital unannounced with accidental injury and is seen and treated otherwise than at a consultative session."

Every hospital, big or small, therefore, requires to set-up a well organised emergency unit, because the image of hospital mainly depends upon the quality and type of treatment a hospital can provide to a patient suffering from any medical or surgical complications, requiring immediate care. Emergency Department of a hospital, therefore, means a section or a part of hospital to which persons injured in road accidents or those suffering from serious complications are taken for urgent treatment. The Emergency Department provides round the clock, immediate diagnosis and urgent treatment for illness of emergent nature and injuries from accidents. It is in this context that the Emergency Department of the hospital is often the point of major public impact, even more than the out-patient department, providing every important service and at the same time being the most vulnerable to criticism and censure. The department is meant to provide round the clock immediate diagnosis and best possible treatment for illness of emergency nature and injuries from accidents.[10]

To ensure that the emergencies are attended to quickly and effectively, it is necessary to have an efficient set-up well knit with other departments of the CHC with well laid out procedures and work distribution. It is to act as information centre, i.e. to reply to public queries on telephone or otherwise about first-aid, treatment of accident cases, antidotes of various poisons, etc.

- To handle medico-legal cases.
- To manage ambulance services.
- To manage a disaster.
- To carry out Research, i.e. Pathogenesis of accidents.

To achieve all this, there is a need of competent staff to manage the emergency department.

To quote C.S. Balaraman:

"The patient and his relatives accompanying are considerably excited and tense and land at the casualty office under the premise of being attended right away and given relief and solace as soon as possible. The demands on the working staff are very exacting and need to be managed in a very critical manner envisaging a competent staff pattern in the doctor, nurse and attendant to manage these problems."[11]

(v) Laboratory and X-ray Facilities

For proper diagnosis of ailments of patients it is necessary to have diagnostic laboratory facility properly manned. It is important that all laboratory investigations be adequately controlled, and useful records kept of results which should be reported without delay. The data collected should be standardized and presented in reports that can be used by health authorities and epidemiologists in health planning. Equipment should be adequately maintained. There must be an effective system for the decontamination of infected material and the safe disposal of laboratory waste. The success of medical prescription would depend upon proper laboratory diagnosis. Laboratories for routine blood, urine, microbiology, X-ray, etc., should provide round the clock service. It is desirable to locate the laboratory block and X-ray block in between the OPD and indoor area to be able to serve both the areas.

We must ensure that the technicians are really doing the job because a minor mistake on their part may ruin the life of the patients. There is a need for constant supervision over the functioning of these laboratory services.[12]

Besides, in CHC, there is reception counter, small operation theater, injection room, dental clinic, dispensary, lounge for OPD patients and office records room.

CRITICAL APPRAISAL

We present here various facts which if taken care of, can make CHCs efficient and effective.

1. Poor Quality of Service

Quality of care is very important for patient's health. Quality assurance means making sure that the services provided by the hospital are the best possible. Quality assurance is vital for the hospital's clinical support services (X-ray, laboratory, pharmacy, central sterile supplies) which have an obligation to maintain high standards. However, there is no quality care in CHC.

This indicates the carelessness of the CHC staff. The DHO must exercise his authority to ensure good quality of services if not excellent.

K.G. Aggarwal has rightly said that, "Hospital effectiveness which can be measured in terms of patient's satisfaction does not depend on the improvement of hospital services aspect alone but on the medical care aspect."[13] Goel suggests, "Effective coordination should be established between the medical services and the supportive services to ensure promptness and clarity."[14]

Kulwinder Sanga in his article relating to an excellent hospital (CHC) newly built in Punjab, "Hospital Services Poor" has found highly unsatisfactory services based on actual facts. To quote him, attendants of patients are forced to convert ordinary school exercise books purchased from the canteen from the premises into indoor patient files . . . . Most of the beds are empty. Patients complain that although antenatal check up is done, aid at delivery time is uncertain. They say doctors in the department are not available at night

Patients also complain that when an operation has to be performed doctors give a list of items, including cotton gloves to be purchased.

The area around the hospital building is full of congress grass and other wild growth."[15]

2. Quality of Behaviour

It is generally believed that many patients can be cured simply by courteous, soft and healing tongue of the CHC staff. Behaviour is an important variable though intangible in the treatment of patients. CHC staff especially the Class IV staff behaves rudely with patients as they want to extract money from patients. They forget that the patients are already in trouble. They lack the art of communication.

There is a need to inculcate among the CHC Staff the techniques of interacting with the patients who are already agitated with their sufferings. C.N. Ray in his Article, "Citizen's Charter in India: An Overview" rightly suggests the need of framing citizens' charter by CHC to maintain their dignity and honour. To quote him, "If the spirit of a charter is to prevail, the lower level officers need to be exposed and convinced of its benefits through training and orientation programmes."[16] We must ensure and encourage courteous behaviour by the medical team to patients to create good relationship.

Mary D. Shanks and D.A. Kennedy have rightly emphasized the need of human approach. To quote:

> "The hospital today is more than the combination of medical and therapeutic treatments by specialists, greater and refined medical and surgical knowledge and ever better and more effective facilities and equipment. It includes these factors as the care of its efficient operation but an additional dimension—one which is too often ignored or at least minimised—is the human and social element in the structure of the organisation."[17]

3. Quality and Availability of Medical Facilities

Quality of medical facilities is extremely poor or rather hopeless. Most of the facilities are non-functional. Medicines are not available. Infections are very high.

We must be clear that the efficiency of CHC depends not only on the competence of medical personnel but also on the availability of drugs in right quantity and quality.

4. Infrastructural Facilities Inadequate

Linen, urinals, latrines, bathrooms were extremely hopeless which is a very sad reflection on the functioning of CHCs. Cleanliness is the first and most important aspect of a CHC as it affects the organisational climate. This is more a question of attitude and not much of resources. Patients and relatives feel suffocated with stinking smell all around. CHCs must give top priority to keep the premises clean to promote both preventive and curative health care.

People are the true measure of success of policies and programmes. At the same time, people are the determinants of success. In brief, we can say that in the past, beneficiaries of CHCs were passively receiving CHC Services. A trend has emerged where in the beneficiaries and the community at large wish to participate in the programme of delivery of health services which must be kept in mind by CHCs and other staff members. All the functionaries of the CHCs must keep the importance of the patient in mind.[18]

We may also suggest that the Government must prepare a patient's charter wherein provisions should be made to compensate patients for the wrongs done by Medical Staff.

5. Referral Services not Functioning

The real purpose of creating CHCs was to provide efficient referral services within rural areas at a lower cost and with the best treatment. CHCs have failed to serve as a referral centre both up and down and thus defeating the purpose for which these were created. The state health department should review this and find out the reasons for such lapses. However, there are very few referred patients who come to CHCs because:

(a) Referral services are not known to people.
(b) There is no well defined procedure for reference.
(c) Those who come go dissatisfied.
(d) Beds remain vacant.
(e) No feed-back of the referred patients.
(f) Lack of adequate facilities as per norms mentioned earlier.

On the basis of our discussion, observation and analysis, we suggest the following to make referral system from PHC and CHC a real success:

1. Norms of services at each level to be clearly defined, i.e. primary, secondary and tertiary. The community and the providers should know about this.
2. Quality of services at each level is to be maintained in order to build and promote confidence among patients and the community. There is need to develop confidence that the patient shall be referred and promptly transferred to higher level of health care, as required.
3. Some procedures need to be designed, so that patients do not by-pass lower level of facilities.
4. Renovating and upgrading hospital buildings to provide appropriate space for services.
5. Upgrading and updating clinical skills of medical officers and staff nurses through an effective training programme.
6. Providing ambulance for transporting critical patients.
7. Installing phone, fax and paging systems in hospitals.
8. Financial powers to Senior Medical Officers in-charge of the hospitals to purchase individual items upto Rs. 5,000.
9. The user charges should be retained at the site of collection. These should be used by the Senior Medical Officer in-charge of the hospital for patient's benefit.
10. Referral and feed-back cards need to be introduced.
11. Referral guidelines that specify the 'what' and 'how' of implementing the referral system need to be provided.
12. An incentive system for patients who follow referral procedures should be envisaged
13. Linkages and communications between the first referral hospitals and primary health care facilities through regular training and out reach visits should be established.
14. Intensive information, education and communication (I.E.C.) targeted at providers and the community should be initiated.
15. District Health Committees should monitor the implementation of the referral system at district level.
16. It must be ensured that all the vacant posts are filled and mismatching is reduced to nil. All equipment should be available and be kept in working order 24 hours a day and 365 days a year.

It is expected that with these measures, there will be better functioning of the CHCs. The patients and the community will gain confidence. These CHCs will become referral points for the PHC level patients.

6. Poor Qualify of Medical Record Keeping

Medical record is a scientific, clinical, administrative and legal document relating to patient's care in which is recorded sufficient data to justify diagnosis, treatment and results.

Good record-keeping is essential. If medical records are illegible, incomplete, ambiguous, and incorrectly filled, they affect medical care. The quality of medical records is an important managerial and medical consideration. When a patient gets discharged from hospital, an accurate summary of his or her record should be made and retained and a copy sent to the source of referral for future reference.

A unit system of record-keeping should be practiced. Each patient should have a permanent number and is assigned a folder containing all relevant records, past and present, medical or surgical in-patient or out-patient indexed by a summary sheet.

- The responsibility of completing the medical records accurately and adequately should lie with the treating physician.
- Diseases should be classified (coded) according to international classification of diseases.

(a) Medical Record should be easily accessible and retrievable.

The efficiency and working of a hospital can be judged from its record maintenance quality.

Analysis of records by the author revealed the following:

(a) Medical Record-keeping is not taken seriously resulting in poor quality of health services.
(b) Decision-making by a Doctor who has not examined him in first instance becomes difficult and irrational.
(c) It causes complications in Medico-legal cases.
(d) It avoids the evaluation of medical competence of the MO/SMO concerned.
(e) It is a major hurdle in making referral system a success for which these CHCs have been created.

We, therefore, suggest that MO/SMO/CMO should be made legally and morally responsible to ensure completion of medical record sheets. They may be provided training and instructions to ensure its compliance. A column in ACR may also be made for quality of records maintained to make them realise its importance.

Storage of Medical records should be done at a place where proper conditions of temperature and circulation of air and humidity are provided. After storing the records, indexing is necessary to locate the record for retrieval.

Unfortunately this vital area has not received adequate attention. But for few exceptions, the system of medical records is very rudimentary in most of the CHCs. Trained medical record personnel are not posted in our hospitals, and it will be unrealistic to expect hospitals to make progress in this field without them in near future.

7. Nurses Involved only in Clinical Activity

The real foundation of health can be laid if nursing is properly developed for Primary Health Care. This is meant to provide preventive and promotive health education. The objective of nursing in PHC may include:

(1) health counselling to individuals, families and community groups in promoting health;
(2) provision of nursing care when necessary, and teaching and supervision of others providing nursing care;
(3) active involvement in the National Health Programmes;
(4) promotion of environmental sanitation in homes, schools, industry;
(5) case-finding related to the agency's programmes, and participation in epidemiological investigation;
(6) cooperation in community studies and other special research of the agency;
(7) participation in educational programmes for nurses, other professionals and members of the community; and
(8) educating patients in preventive health care.

Besides, we must plan the use of nurses in the promotion of primary health care.

The International Council of Nurses (ICN) representing nurses throughout the world, supports the present (WHO/UNICEF concept of Primary Health Care). In so doing, ICN affirms the commitment of nurses to effect changes in nursing education, practice and management, which are conducive to the implementation of PHC.

SUGGESTIONS

We present here the facts and suggestions to improve upon organisational structure and resources to provide decent second level health care services through CHCs.

1. SMO Lacks Administrative Skill and Competence: Need for Imparting Training

SMO is the Chief Executive of the CHC appointed on the basis of seniority in service but he lacks administrative capability for which he has to devote 50 per cent of his time. We should appoint those doctors to head the CRC who possess leadership qualities and are good at working with a team. A CRC should select dynamic and adequately qualified person and then offer them opportunities though training and work experience and self-development as professional leader who have competence in both professional and administrative field as well as high motivation. It is, therefore essential that medical personnel engaged in administration should be given training in administration so that they can become competent both in professional knowledge as well as in administrative competence.

2. Mismatching of Resources: Need for Strict Policy of Posting and Transfer

We have mentioned the need of four specialities in a CRC but in practice, we find that there is more than one consultant in one specialization while there is none in some of them. Besides about 40 per cent of the posts sanctioned are lying vacant. Even sanctioned posts fall short of target. In one of the CHCs all the four specialists were from skin. It is a very sad reflection on the State Health Department. We must ensure strict adherence in posting and transfers so that mismatching does not occur.

3. Lack of Punctuality and even Availability of Specialists in CHC: Need of Strict Supervision

Most of the Staff in CHC daily travel from the nearby city headquarters. Most of them try to absent themselves on one pretext or the other. Besides, most of the staff reach late and leave early, and that is why, they discourage the admissions of the patients in wards as they have to be otherwise present at night also to look after the admitted patients. Its indirect effect is that the utilisation of beds is not more than 30 to 40 per cent, thus incurring heavy cost and defeating the purpose for which CRCs were created. The health department must ensure the compulsory stay of the SMO and other consultants either by constructing good accommodation or by hiring good houses for them.

4. Vacant Posts: Need for Timely Appointments

Many posts of Staff Nurses, Technicians and others remain vacant affecting the services of CRC. Hospital services can't be run without the required staff. The state health department must ensure the availability of the staff to ensure optimum utilisation of CRC.

5. Equipment is Either not Available or Non-functional

A physical verification of the equipment revealed that 50 per cent of the essential equipment listed earlier has not been provided to these CHCs while a lot of equipment is out of order needing repair and maintenance. One of the SMOs told that the Staff using these instruments do not handle and maintain them properly. There is a need to inject proper culture to keep their instruments clean and in working order. The health department must also be quick in replacing them with new ones.

6. All the Services Entrusted to CHC not Available

We have listed the services which need to be provided by CHC but in practice, they are not able to meet even 50 per cent of these because of physical and financial constraints. There is a need to ensure availability of all equipment in functional form and availability of personnel through strict supervision and control. In one of the CHCs, there was a Dental Chair and other equipments but no dental surgeon but in another CHC, there was no Dental Chair but the Dental Surgeon was in position. Such glaring wastages should be curbed and supervisory personnel should be held responsible for such lapses.

We may also mention here the problems mentioned by CHC staff which need consideration and analysis:

(i) DHO and district staff do not take keen interest in removing the problems of CRC promptly.
(ii) There is always a financial constraint which affects the functioning of CRC.
(iii) Shortage of medicine continues even after reminders.
(iv) No formal linkages between PHC/CHC/Civil Hospital/ District Hospital except through DHO/District Surgeon.
(v) Lack of adequate planning and monitoring by District staff and State Health Departments.

In brief, the following actions should certainly see the system functioning more efficiently:

1. The staff members of CRC must be made aware of their responsibilities to make the Primary Health Care and district health system a success.
2. The CRC should constantly engage itself in staff development through motivation and training.
3. The CRC should ensure that its staff members should provide integrated health care and not simply remedy for diseases.
4. The CRC should continuously appraise performance particularly its quality of care in terms of humanity, effectiveness and efficiency.
5. The CHC should continuously monitor its infrastructure and health facilities to ensure that these are properly maintained.
6. The CHC should devote time and resources to action-oriented health services research.
7. The CHC should look for additional sources of funds which should be spent equitably and efficiently.
8. The CHC must design its referral system clearly.
9. CHC must engage itself constantly in improving its services and performance. Simple commitment by CRC staff is not enough. The improvement process must become basic and

continuous. If we want to safeguard the future, it is high time that all those who are serving CRC should get concerned with creativity and change—take a second look at their work system and style and evolve an appropriate work method, upholding the new criteria of promoting creativity and total change—if not a total revolution. Tarun Bahl in his article, "Truthful Living" in *The Tribune*, dated January 16, 2000, rightly says about basic values which must be cherished by CRC staff. "Truthful living is nothing but living by convictions, standing up for what one believes to be correct, taking up the cause of the downtrodden, continuing to do the right things even when one is not being watched."

10. The CRC should ensure excellent internal working environment wherein the staff feel happy in providing services.

CONCLUSION

We can conclude by saying that CHCs are not serving the purpose for which these were created to provide referral services to PHCs. CHCs have also failed to provide even basic preventive, curative and promotive health care. It is high time for the State Health Department of Government to evaluate the functioning of CHCs and revamp them to make them fit for the delivery of health care services. Otherwise, the resources invested in them would go waste as is happening at present. There is a need to provide quality health care at CRC level, which means to deliver and maintain a safe, sure and effective health care to patients.

In the new millennium, we must equip these first referral level institutions within rural set-up and ensure availability of all the specialists so that they can meet the needs of the rural people in their vicinity and at an affordable cost. In this way, we are sure to make primary health care a great success.

Notes and References

1. WHO, District Health Systems: Global and Regional Review Based on Experience in Various Countries, Geneva, 1995, p. 18.
2. H. Mahler, The Role of Hospitals in Primary Health Care, Report of a conference sponsored by the Aga Khan foundation and the World Health Organization, 22-26 Nov. 1981, Karachi, Pakistan, Geneva, Aga Khan Foundation, 1981, Part II, p. 5.
3. WHO, *Technical Report Series*, 819, Geneva, 1992 (back cover).
4. *Ibid.*, p. 11.
5. WHO, *Technical Report Series*, 395, 1968, p. 6.
6. Elen B. Perry, Ward Management, Balliere, London, 1978, p. 2.
7. WHO, *Technical Report Series*, 395, 1968, p. 1.
8. S.L. Goel & R. Kumar (Ed.), Hospital Administration and Management, New Delhi, Deep & Deep, year not mentioned, Vol. 2, p. 13.

9. S.K. Garg, Emergency Services in General Hospital in Hospital Administration & Management, S.L. Goel & R. Kumar (Ed.), New Delhi, Deep & Deep, Vol. 2, pp. 28-29.
10. S.K. Garg, *Ibid.*, pp. 28-29.
11. C.S. Balaraman, "Emergency Services in Hospitals", quoted in S.L. Goel & R. Kumar, *op. cit.*, p. 21.
12. S.L. Goel, Public Health Administration, New Delhi, Sterling, 1984, pp. 388-89.
13. K.G. Aggarwal, "Managing Patient Satisfaction in Hospitals", in *Indian Journal of Public Administration*, Vol. XXII, No. 2, April-June, 1976, p. 154.
14. S.L. Goel, Public Health Administration, New Delhi, Sterling, 1984, p. 401.
15. The *Daily Tribune*, Chandigarh, Aug. 13, 1999, p. 3.
16. C.N. Roy, "Citizens' Charters in India: An Overview", in *IJPA*, Vol. XLIV, October-December 1998, p. 814.
I7. Mary D. Shanks and Dorothy A. Kennedy, The Theory and Practice of Nursing Service Administration, McGraw Hill, London, 1965, p. 95.
18. Edy the Alexander *et al.*, Nursing Service Administration, (ed.) New York, Mosby, 1962, p. 63.

CHAPTER 16

ORGANISATION AND WORKING OF PRIMARY HEALTH CENTRES

"WHO has defined the health centre as that which covers all health facilities other than hospitals. It is usually the facility at the first contact level and has a unique potential, as well as responsibility, for increasing people's ability to solve their own problems with confidence. It provides a full range of health promotion and preventive services, as well as curative care limited mainly to ambulatory patients. It has multi-disciplinary team capable of providing the range of services mentioned above."

—Author

Organisation and Working of Primary Health Centres

PART A

RATIONALE AND PHILOSOPHY

WHO has defined the health centre as that which covers all health facilities other than hospitals. It is usually the facility at the first contact level and has a unique potential, as well as responsibility, for increasing people's ability to solve their own problems with confidence. It provides a full range of health promotion and preventive services, as well as curative care limited mainly to ambulatory patients. It has multi-disciplinary team capable of providing the range of services mentioned above.[1]

The term health centre signifies the essential facilities for the promotion and protection of the health of the people.

In the district health system, each health centre should be responsible for a defined population so that no groups or families are left without a health team to provide care. The care should include accountability for outreach for essential public health and clinical services. In most countries this population will reside in a geographically defined area. If the boundaries relate to other functions of government, it is likely that the total population will be included in planning and implementation and this increases the potential for intersectoral collaboration. A major advantage is the much greater potential for sustainability and equity.[2]

A health centre is the main institution linking the health services with the people, it has the responsibility and unique potential for providing people with the ability and confidence to solve their own problems; it provides a full range of health promotion and prevention services including mother and child care; it provides curative care primarily to ambulatory patients and those with selected conditions. It has a multi-disciplinary team providing a range of services and may or may not have a doctor.[3]

The concept of the PHC as an institution to provide both curative and preventive services can be traced to the report of the consultative council on Medical and Allied Services, held in 1920, in England, under the Chairmanship of Lord Dawson of Penn.[4] In this region, the PHC was established at Kalutura, Ceylon, in 1926 with the assistance of Rockefeller Foundation.[5] The services offered at the centre were mainly preventive health examinations of mothers and babies, immunizations, environmental sanitation, health education, and midwifery. Little attention was paid to curative medical care, on the ground that such care was the function of out-patient departments at hospitals. In addition, it was felt that the provision of curative services would so overwhelm the staff that preventive care would be neglected.

One of the fathers of the health centre movement during this period was John Grant of the Rockefeller foundation who was Professor of Public Health at the Peking Union Medical School in 1920s where he based much of the teaching and research on an Eastern Health District Centre patterned on the one in Baltimore.

Another expert of primary health care was Andrija Stampar of Yugoslavia. He was a contemporary of Grant and they worked closely together over many years. He developed a nation-wide system of health centres.

Many developing countries especially in Asia, have felt the need to provide a model for their own planning of integrated health centres. Much of the thinking current during the 1940s and 1950s can be found in a report of the WHO Expert Committee on Public Health Administration, which mentions the basic services that should be offered by rural health units, the personnel needed for local health work, the cost and financing of local health programmes, and the planning of integrated health services. Provision of Rural Health Services through Rural Health Centres was recommended by the European Conference on Rural Hygiene of Geneva, in 1931 under the Health Organisation of League of Nations. It defined the "Rural Health Centres" as:

> "An institution for the promotion of the health and welfare of the people in a given (rural) area, which seeks to achieve its purpose by grouping under one roof or coordinating in some other manner, under the direction of a health officer, all the health work of that area, together with such welfare and relief organisations as may be related to the general public health work."[6]

A working group on the role and functions of Health Centres in

District Health System met in Geneva from 12 to 16 July 1993 with participants from Dominica, Indonesia, Nigeria, Philippines and Senegal, who defined the concept as "The Generic Health Centre is a self-contained segment of the national health system guided by the district health service, of which it is a part. It comprises a variety of interrelated components that contribute to health in homes, schools, workplaces and the community including support for self-care administered at home. These components are supported by a professional staff, together with appropriate diagnostic, laboratory and logistical services and coordinate in a dedicated management structure.[7]

The concept gathered momentum in socialist countries. The Inter-governmental Conference for Eastern countries, convened at Bandung under the auspices of League of Nations recommended the integration of preventive and curative services in preference to curative services. Similar developments took place in Eastern European countries that have come under the influence of socialism.[8] This concept spread to other countries after World War II.

The underlying idea of such thinking was to give priority to preventive health care as 75 per cent of diseases are preventable and the cost of prevention is much less than the cost for curative care.

GENESIS AND GROWTH

Let us discuss in detail about the development of this concept in India. The Bhore Committee (1946) recommended that a Primary Health Centre should be set-up to serve as the focal point for providing comprehensive, curative and preventive health services in the rural areas. The report, in its long-term programme, recommended a primary health unit for a population of 20,000, a secondary unit for a population of 6,00,000 and a district headquarter's organisation for a population of three million. The committee in its short-term programme recommended a primary unit for a population of 40,000, a secondary unit for a population of one and a half million, and a district headquarter's organisation for a population of three million. To improve the operation of primary health centres, this committee recommended a reduction in the population covered by them, expansion and strengthening of district hospitals, and introduction of mobile teams of specialists to provide necessary supervisory and consultancy services to the periphery.

To cope with the family planning services required to control the rising population trend, the Government of India planned an expansion of facilities at Primary Health Centres and an increase in the number of sub-centres under each Primary Health Centre. Similarly, many health workers were provided to help in control of other endemic diseases. In this way, there was a great deal of proliferation of facilities and services. All these programmes were being run independent of each other by staff recruited under each programme. There was practically no co-ordination either at the field level or supervisory level. Such an isolated approach led to duplication, wastage of resources and poor impact on beneficiaries. This prompted the need for effective integration of services. To quote the first meeting of the executive committee of the Central Family Planning Council held on 20 September 1972: "Steps should be taken for the integration of medical, public health and family planning services at the peripheral level."[9]

The Planning Commission was also seized of the problem and in the report of the steering group on health, family planning and nutrition for the Fifth Five Year Plan, the following observations were made: "Family planning and nutrition have been in operation for a long time. These programmes are mostly vertically conceived and are being implemented at the field level by the staff deployed to implement these programmes individually, with little co-ordination or integration of the services. The steering group felt that the proper Integration of health, family planning and nutrition programmes is highly desirable as it would be more economical and effective. This could be possible only by converting unipurpose workers into multi-purpose workers. It may be appreciated that the multi-purpose health worker (who may be designated as health auxiliary for convenience of reference) would be entrusted with carrying out integrated functions and would have greater rapport with the people in rural areas who would naturally look to him for all their needs in the field of naturally reinforcing components of health, family planning and nutrition."

In pursuance of these recommendations, the Government of India appointed a committee on multi-purpose workers under the health and family planning programmes in October, 1972. The committee submitted its report in September, 1973 recommending: (i) Multi-purpose workers for the delivery of health, family planning and nutrition services to the rural community, (ii) one PHC for every 50,000 population, (iii) each PHC to be divided into 16 sub-centres each having a population of 3,000-3,500 depending on topography and means of communication; (iv) each sub-centre to have a team of one male and one female worker; (v) one male and one female supervisor to supervise the work of four sub-centres; (vi) the doctors at PHC to divide the population on a geographical basis for their field visits; (vii) for effective integration of workers engaged in vertical programmes of health and family planning, the concept of integration to be extended to the district and state levels. The committee also suggested the job responsibilities and training programme for various categories of health workers.

The Government of India accepted the recommendations of the committee except the ones in respect of one PHC for every 50,000 population and one sub-centre for 3,000 to 3,500 population; instead it was agreed to have a sub-centre for 5,000 population.

STRENGTHENING OF INFRASTRUCTURE

The rural health infrastructure was to be further strengthened in the Sixth Plan to achieve the objective of Health for All by 2000 A.D. The norms envisaged were: (i) one community health volunteer for every village for a population of 1,000 chosen by the community to form the base unit; (ii) one sub-centre for a population of 5,000 in the plains and 3,000 in the hilly and tribal areas; (iii) one PHC for 30,000 population in the plains and 20,000 in the hilly and tribal areas; and (iv) one community health centre (CHC) for a population of one lakh or one community development block.

Health infrastructure in rural areas is of prime importance for realisation of the objectives set forth in the National Health Policy and for attaining the goal of 'Health for All by the Year 2000 A.D.' Co-ordinated efforts under various Rural Health Programmes are essential to provide effective and efficient services to the people in the rural areas.

Numerous programmes and schemes are being implemented under the Minimum Needs Programme to provide Primary Health Care relevant to the actual needs of the community in the rural areas. The status of establishment of the Sub-Centres, PHCs and Community Health Centres under the Minimum Needs Programme, has been of great significance. This development is in consonance with the thrust of all plans for Rural Development.

EXTENT AND FUNCTIONS

Primary Health Centres

Primary Health Centres are established on the basis of one PHC for every 30,000 population in the plain areas and for every 20,000 population in hilly, tribal and backward areas. Number of PHCs functioning in the country was 18,981 by the end of 7th Plan (1.4.1990) which rose to 21,853 PHCs by the end of March, 1997. There was a provision of adding 1521 PHCs in Ninth Plan. Till 30.6.98, there were 22,991 PHCs functioning thereby an increase of 408 PHCs in Ninth Plan. In tribal areas there were 3306 PHCs by 30.6.98. As on 31 March 2001, 22,842 Primary Health Centres were functioned.

Out of 22,991 PHCs as on 30.6.1998, 14,288 were functioning in government buildings, 1,345 were under construction, 7,414 buildings were still required.

The average population covered by a PHC in India as on 30.6.98 is 27,345. Under these Primary Health Centres, there are 1,37,311 Sub-centres. The average rural area per PHC is 13,622 sq. km, average radial distance 658 km, average number of villages covered is 2,554.

The broad functions of a PHC are: (1) Medical Care, (2) Maternal and Child Health Services, (3) School Health Services, (4) Family Planning, (5) Control of Communicable Diseases, (6) Environmental

Sanitation, (7) Health Education, and (8) Vital Statistics. The staff to provide these services would comprise a medical officer, a woman physician, a public health nurse, a health educator, a statistical clerk, a clerk-stenographer, a mid-wife, a health inspector (Sanitarian), a laboratory technician, and several family planning field workers, with health assistant to assist the staff members. Similar range of health services has been mentioned in a "Guide to rural health centre work" issued by the Government of Burma.[10]

PHC is supposed to provide the following functions:

1. to provide preventive, promotive, curative and rehabilitative services with emphasis on preventive health care,
2. to meet local needs based on largely local resources,
3. to function as a unit for the promotion of positive health and not merely serve as a dispensary,
4. to ensure equitable and qualitative services and not merely rudimentary and traditional services,
5. to join with other sectors of socio-economic development to optimise benefit for the promotion of health services,
6. to make frequent visits to the community in order to develop sound relationships,
7. to make community surveys to locate critical areas and people needing their help,
8. to arrange exhibitions to make people aware of health development,
9. to provide training to workers in the centre,
10. to keep in constant touch with district, state and central health authorities, health research institutions to get advice and guidance,
11. to develop team work,
12. to encourage community leaders to support health development activities of health centres, and
13. health centres should empower community to take decisions with the support of PHC.

After all, moving towards greater equity is the first key principle in the PHC strategy. "PHC needs to redress the imbalance created by in-built biases in favour of high technology medicines and affluent urban-dwellers, and against the poor anywhere. Reorientation towards PHC, therefore, involves centering attention on resource allocation among different types of activity, levels of care and geographical areas."[11] Let us understand the role of Primary Health Centre *vis-a-vis* secondary and tertiary hospitals.

Primary Health Care is the first level of contact between the individual and the health system where essential health care (primary health care) is provided. A majority of prevailing health complaints and problems can be satisfactorily dealt with at this level. This level of care is closest to the people. In the Indian context, this care is provided by the primary health centres, with community participation.

Secondary Health Care deals with more complex problems. This care comprises essentially curative services and is provided by the district hospitals, sub-divisional hospitals, area hospitals, and community health centres. This level serves as the first referral level in the health system as the patients are referred to such medical institutes from the Primary Health Centre.

Tertiary Health Care offers superspecialist care. This care is provided by the regional/central hospitals, teaching hospitals and superspeciality hospitals. These institutions provide not only highly specialized care, but also planning and managerial skills and teaching for specialized staff.

There is a Need of Making Primary Health Centres functional to inject economy and efficiency in health system.

Hospitals provide a wide variety of services, from basic care to highly specialized diagnosis and treatment, depending on the technological capacity of a specific hospital. There is considerable duplication of services provided at different levels. Tertiary hospitals though equipped with highly sophisticated equipment with advanced technical capacity have to devote considerable time and resources to deliver basic secondary and even primary health care as there is lack of confidence in the system for secondary and primary health care or the people don't feel satisfied with them. Tertiary hospitals, however, are designed to treat only complicated cases, and because of their composition of skilled staff and medical equipment, the cost of treating a patient is much higher than the cost would be for the same type of patient in lower level or specialized alternative facilities. This undesirable use of the capacity of tertiary hospitals affects out-patient and in-patient services. The out-patient departments of large tertiary care hospitals often suffer from over-crowding; this situation is exacerbated by the presence of a large number of patients who require only basic curative care that could be provided in a lower cost setting such as a district hospital or health centre like sub-divisional hospitals, CHCs or other lower run medical centres. If patients requiring basic care could be shifted to medically appropriate lower-level or alternative treatment facilities, health system costs would be reduced and economic efficiency improved as the per capita cost of both outdoor and indoor patients is too high in these hospitals.

Analysis of discharge information by cause and severity of the illness or condition is needed to assess the potential for reallocation of the case load within different hospital systems. In large tertiary facilities, perhaps 75% of out-patient care and 30% to 50% of in-patient care could be easily and effectively delivered in district hospitals or at lower levels, i.e. PHCs. A comparison of the cost per out-patient visit or in-patient day between varying levels of hospital suggests that the savings could be of the order of 50% of current costs per patient. PHCs can take care of 75 per cent of diseases at their levels. Therefore, there is a need of assessment of working of Primary Health Centres to make them effective and efficient.

PART B

ORGANISATIONAL STRUCTURE OF PHC (See Chart 16.1)

(a) Organisation

The PHC functions with a Medical Officer of Health or Administrative Medical Officer as the chief of the PHC, and a Lady Medical Officer (LMO) as the second medical officer. One Block Extension Educator, one Pharmacist, a Para-Medical Worker and two Senior Health Assistants (a male and a female) function under the Medical Officer's supervision. Seven Male Multi-purpose workers are under the supervision of the Senior Health Assistant (Male) and seven Female Multi-purpose workers work under the supervision of the Senior Health Assistant (Female). Three staff members in the category of Group D (Class IV) form the lowest staff category of PHC. In the sub-centre, trained Dais (TBAs), who are not government employees, help multi-purpose worker (Female) when required.

The buildings of PHC are not adequate to meet the needs. The infrastructure generally includes a hall, 5 rooms and two in-patient wards. The hall serves as the out-patient ward, where the Administrative Medical Officer (AMO) examines the patients. The room adjacent to the right side of the hall is being used as Injection room. The room to the left of the hall is supposed to be 'Dispensary' where the pharmacist is expected to dispense medicines/drugs as per doctor's prescriptions.

In the other wing are two rooms and an in-patient ward. The first room is occupied by the Lady Medical Officer (LMO) who examines the patients there. The room adjacent to this room is the rest room as well as the staff room. Another in-patient ward is built opposite the room of the Lady Medical Officer.

Though two rooms with six beds each are provided for in-patients, due to lack of residential quarters and basic facilities, admission of in-patients is a rare phenomenon. Only emergency delivery cases and asthma cases are admitted for 2-3 days. Patients with severe weakness are admitted just for the day (working hours) to administer glucose drips and later discharged the same evening.

Let us now analyse the duties and responsibilities of important functionaries of PHC.

(b) Role of the Doctor (Administrative)

The PHC team is led by a Medical Officer (Administrative) of

CHART 16.1

Organisational Structure of Primary Health Centre

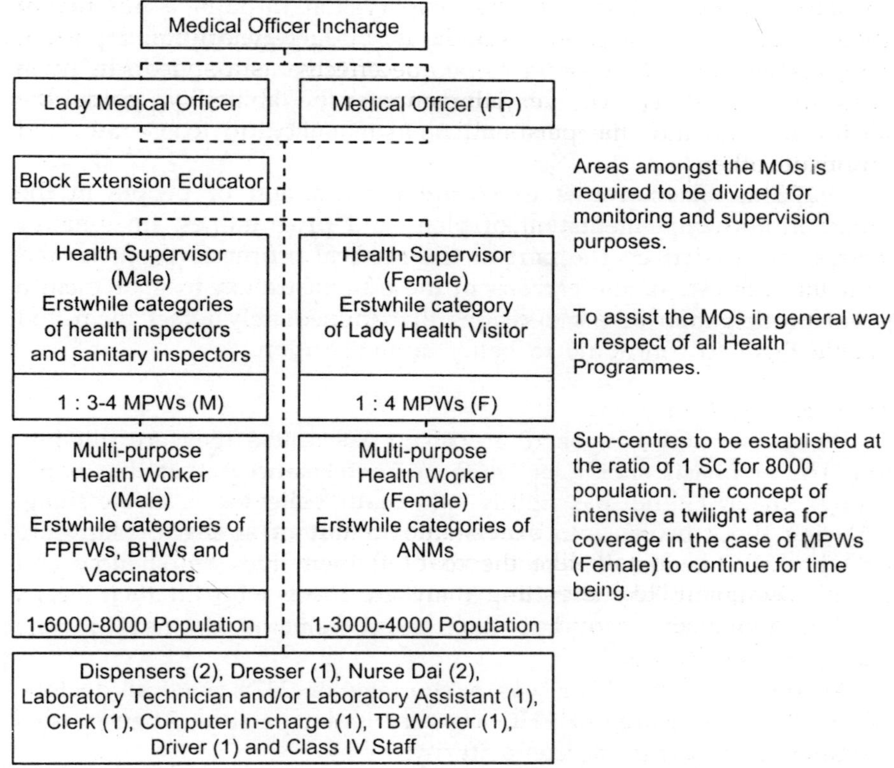

Health. Generally a lady medical officer acts as the second medical officer. While the role of the Medical Officer of Health (also called Administrative Medical Officer, AMO) includes the management of the PHC (all administrative aspects) besides attending to patients, the function of a Lady Medical Officer (LMO) is basically attending to patients alone. Only when the AMO is on leave, or is away on official work, the LMO acts as the Officer Incharge of the PHC. We now discuss the responsibilities of medical officer in-charge of the PHC.

The Medical Officer of primary health centre is responsible for providing direction and guidance in all the health activities radiating from the health centre. He keeps himself fully conversant with the area, topography, demography, community health needs and public health problems. Being the chief-executive of health of the area, he undertakes promotive, preventive and curative work in an integrated manner. For this purpose, the medical officers in the primary health centre divide the area amongst themselves on a geographical basis and are responsible for all the health programmes in their respective areas.

One of the very important tasks of the medical officer is to supervise, direct and control the performance of the sub-centres organization within the scope of law, policy and regulations already established. He can achieve effective supervision through a number of methods, viz., setting of service standards, budgetary control, reporting system, inspections, etc. In order to be effective as a supervisor, he must possess three qualities, i.e. job competence, the ability to guide the subordinates and the personal traits like ability to cooperate and motivate others.

The Chief Executive is to ensure participation of people in the formulation and implementation of plans and programmes. Imaginative measures are needed on the part of the medical officer to promote and sustain the interests of the citizens in the administration to give them a sense of participation in the decisions that immediately affect them and to enable them to contribute to better administration.

Implementation of Programmes

Words, written or spoken, are of no use unless they are put into action. The emphasis should be more on performance rather that paper planning. Khalid Gibran has rightly said that, "believing is a fine thing, but placing those beliefs into execution is a test of strength. Many are those who talk like the roar of the sea, but their lives are shallow and stagnant, like the rotting marshes. Many are those who lift their heads above the mountain tops, but their spirit remains dormant in the obscurity of the caverns."

As on 30.6.1998, there was a shortage of 2475 medical doctors. Medical officers in-charge of PHC are very junior persons. They possess no administrative experience or maturity.

It is therefore suggested that senior doctors may be posted against this post to provide leadership to manage the multi-farious activities entrusted to PHC. Besides, the vacant post must always be filled.

Walter R. Sharp has also mentioned the importance of the personnel in the organisation. He says: "Even poorly devised machinery may be made to work if it is manned with well-trained, intelligent, imaginative and devoted staff. On the other hand, the best planned organisation may produce unsatisfactory results if it is operated by mediocre or disgruntled people."[12]

Besides, the doctors must have faith in the ideals of the PHC programmes, be willing to accept hardships and be prepared to work in the spirit of service. Their ambition and enthusiasm should not be dampened by local conditions which may not provide them with the necessary facilities.

Unfortunately, the sense of dedication has been the crassest casualty of the prevailing atmosphere of cynism bred by increasing propensity towards expediency.[13]

(c) Role of Block Extension Educator[14]

The Block Extension Educator functions under the technical supervision and guidance of District Extension and Media Officer. However, he is under the immediate administrative control of the Medical Officer in-charge of PHC. One of his primary responsibilities is to promote community participation for ensuring self-reliance in the community. He is responsible for providing support to all National Health & Family Welfare Programmes in the PHC but the main function relates to the promotion of FW & MCH programmes.

As on 30.6.98, 683 posts of Block Extension Educators were lying vacant.

Health Education is based upon understanding socio-cultural factors. Block Extension Educator should understand that the most important aim of Health Education is to alter behaviour which may have directly or indirectly influenced occurrence or spread of diseases in a given cultural setting. A culturally relevant health education programme can be planned only after understanding the behaviour in all its manifestations.

Role of Senior Health Assistants

Health Assistants (Male and Female) have separate headquarters and work separately. They are not supposed to issue any instructions to the multi-purpose health workers who report weekly to the BHO/MO who in turn, issue necessary instructions to the multi-purpose health workers. In MCH clinic, ante-natal and post-natal clinics are attended by the health assistant (female) and concerned multi-purpose health worker (female). The number of such clinics under the supervision of health assistants (female) has been increased to 20 clinics in a month instead of 4 earlier. The worker (female) attends to the clinic and the pregnant and other female patients and children in the village. In the clinic, all the women in the area are to be given TT irrespective of the fact whether they are pregnant or not. The children are given immunisation against six deadly diseases, namely, diphtheria, pertussis, tatanus, tuberculosis and polo myelitis. The health assistant (female) are to supervise the Anganwadis and ensure that children are being given protected water and clean food supplements.

The number of Senior Health Assistants Male and Female in India was 25,899 and 22,661 respectively as on 31st July 1998. Out of these 3955 male and 3077 female health assistants posts were lying vacant, i.e. 15.27 per cent and 13.76 per cent respectively. There are 42 training institutes for providing in-service training to MPW (female) with an annual capacity of 2995. The training schools for male are 56 with admission capacity of 8398.

Role of Pharmacist

A pharmacist in PHC is normally appointed to: (i) dispense

medicines/drugs as per the prescriptions given by the medical officers, and (ii) maintain a record of number of out-patients treated (as also the number of in-patients, where beds are provided and in-patient treatment is given).

It was observed that the pharmacist spent very little time on dispensing drugs. He was generally found to be busy with office correspondence or certificate work. He was sent to the treasury to submit the pay bills of the PHC staff and later to collect the salary cheques. This could be attributed to the fact that PHCs have no clerical staff to perform these functions.

CRITICAL APPRAISAL

Creation of Primary Health Centres has not served its real purpose as health care activities are not being provided properly at this level, resulting in great rush at secondary and tertiary level. Besides, it is causing great hardships to rural population and urban slums as well as wastage of colossal amounts aimed at providing adequate and efficient health care. Since the success of secondary and tertiary care depends upon the soundness of Primary Health Care, therefore, it is essential to ensure its fruitful functioning.

Neither the infrastructure nor the personnel working here are satisfactory resulting in unsatisfactory functioning at this level. In most of the states, there were bitter complaints about Government-run PHCs. It was mentioned in the consolidated reports from various states that PHCs are disgustingly dirty, patients are lying on the floors, there is even lack of elementary articles like spirit and cotton sheets are drenched in blood. There were complaints about the corruption and indifference of doctors and Class IV employees. Medicines meant for free distribution are reported to be illegally sold.

Dr. M.D. Saigal, Deputy Director General of Health Services also mentioned that out of the 4,500 PHCs, 700 are without any buildings while 2,620 have no staff quarters; out of the 39,000 sub-centres functioning today, 15,000 have no buildings.[15]

We give some of the facts and suggestions which can help in improving the performance of the Primary Health Centres.

1. Lack of Coordination among the Developmental Agencies

There are a large number of developmental agencies working at block level and villages under its jurisdiction. We have already discussed that health affects and is affected by all other sectors of development. We find no coordination among these agencies. It is suggested that all the developmental agencies in a particular area must promote the problems of development simultaneously to produce sustained impact on the population inhabiting these areas.

2. Absence of Organised Structure for People's Participation

We do not find any organised structure in a block at any level to involve the beneficiaries and utilise their potential energy profitably. It is very difficult for the government to contact all the individuals/families through their paid employees. There is a need for some structure or groups of people to help themselves under the guidance of the expert advice offered by the government. We have already witnessed the failure of the Community Development Programmes as we could not associate the people with our programmes. It is suggested that the Health Department may try to set-up voluntary organisations of the people in collaboration with other developmental agencies to ensure effective communication and understanding.

3. Poor Quality of Service

Most of the people complain of very poor quality of services at PHC. A frequent question in many countries in relation to health centres is why are people bypassing them? The answer is usually to be found in the poor quality of care. Quality is a complex notion not connected merely with technical procedures, expensive drugs, and sophisticated apparatus. It has perhaps more to do with the reliability of services and with the provision of those services in a way that ensures an equitable approach, accessibility, accountability, and continuity. Understanding any concern on the part of health personnel would add sufficiently to confidence in health centres' services to make people feel secure and satisfied. Frequent staff changes, an excessive burden of tasks, and poor motivation worsen the perceived quality of services. However, the main problem more often lies in inappropriate technologies, inadequacy and unreliability of supplies, poorly trained health workers, deficient referral systems and poor organisation of work.

4. Absence of Linkages with Cultural, Social and Religious Institutions

We know that the success of health programmes depends upon their acceptance by the people. It was found that the health personnel do not try to go into the cultural, religious and social factors affecting the health of the people. These are very subtle factors which need our attention and care. The health personnel must try to enlist the cooperation of informal leaders who can help in accelerating the acceptance of these programmes. Customs and conventions of the area must be studied which can throw light on the behaviour of the people. It would be very easy to help the people provided we understand their attitude and preferences.

5. Absence of Political Will and Direction

We already know of the political crisis in the country and absence of rationality among the political leaders at the block and the lower levels. There is a need to create political will and sensitivity towards development. The Department of Health should motivate the local political leaders to associate them in the developmental tasks.

6. Absence of Missionary Spirit among the Health Personnel

The problems of public health are challenging as can be gauged from the statistics already enumerated. It is very difficult to solve these problems with bureaucratic and inhuman attitudes. It requires hard work, sympathy, and tolerance on the part of the health personnel engaged in this arduous and challenging task. Most of the people felt that the personnel working are fulfilling only their legal duties that too reluctantly. We do not need highly specialized people in these areas. We, however, require dedicated people with missionary zeal to serve the people suffering from abject poverty. We must ensure the people of their full involvement in their own welfare.

7. Non-Involvement of the Universities in the Planning and Implementation of the Programme

It is a matter of great regret that no attempt is being made to associate the faculty members of the universities and colleges to involve them with these programmes. The teachers through their knowledge and influence can help a lot in this direction if they are given due status. Some of them can take up such studies as research projects or encourage their research students to undertake such problems. Such studies can be of great use in improving the implementation and the future planning.

8. Absence of Informal Supervision through Medical Colleges/Institutes

There is no involvement of the medical colleges/institutes in the area. There must be a regular dialogue between these institutions and the persons responsible for the planning and implementation of the programme of Primary Health Care. Student doctors may be encouraged to take interest in such projects. This would ensure the quick success and the future benefits in other areas.

9. Absence of Research in the Flora and Fauna of the Area

The health department is providing allopathic medicines to the people. These medicines have side effects and are costly. No attempt is being made to encourage research in the flora and fauna of the area which can provide cheap and effective medicine without side effects. The flora and fauna of the area is full of promise. This would encourage the development of the area also indirectly. We may extract medicines from plants and animals available in the area. This would be possible only if our research in the medical colleges/institutes is relevant to the area rather than only of theoretical significance and utility.

The need for research to improve health centre function is especially acute at present because for at least two decades the role and function of health centres has been largely ignored. From the past 50 years of experience worldwide have come strong but often invalid assumptions about the functions and approaches to be used in health centres. Traditional work patterns have been solidly bureaucratized in many health systems so that one of the first issues to be confronted is the explicit need to create an intellectual climate to encourage change and improvement. The concept of primary health care, the types of interventions now available, the interactions with the rest of the health systems, and the potential for communicating with and mobilizing the community are so different from what they were when the health centres were originally set-up in developing countries that it is time for a major process of reappraisal.

The fundamental need is to encourage a spirit of problem-solving among both the health centre staff and the community. Systematic problem-solving can be organised best through applied field research. Health systems research, to systematize problem-solving, is becoming more important as health centres search for ways to improve access, utilisation, and quality of care. If health centres make community diagnoses, then the most elementary research is already a component of existing activities. Likewise, if health centres can develop adequate information systems, then simple applied research will follow naturally. Health centres should ensure that problem-solving is a routine daily activity.

FINDINGS OF THE STUDY[16]

The author conducted the research study of Primary Health Centres in Punjab. The results are as follows:

1. Inadequate PHC Buildings

All the Primary Health Centers were functioning in buildings whether Government or rented which have limited available space. Besides there is not sufficient availability of residential accommodation in remote rural areas, which is acting as a great deterrent in motivating medical officers to work in such areas.

There is an urgent need of providing adequate building accommodation in each centre to provide good environment for service. Besides, the construction of houses for the staff should be taken up as it will increase the morale and efficiency of the personnel working there.

2. Public Health Facilities

The PHCs are supposed to provide health education to the people. This would be possible only if the premises of the PHCs are clean and well equipped. It was found that most of the centres had no public health facilities, like flush latrines, piped water supply and electricity.

3. Medicines and Equipment

The supply of medicines and equipment was inadequate in most of the health centres due to the paucity of resources. Besides, there was no regular supply. The stock of medicines was inadequate in all the centres.

Steps may be taken to ensure adequate and timely supply of medicines and equipment to health centres. They should maintain adequate stock of at least life saving drugs. This will raise the confidence of the people in PHCs and the people would not rush unnecessarily to city hospitals. Medicine may not be provided according to quota system but should be given according to the needs of the people.

For efficient discharge of curative functions, the Primary Health Centres should be provided sufficient equipment like refrigerators, X-ray and laboratory facilities, oxygen cylinders, operation tables and surgical instruments. It may also be ensured that X-ray plants and laboratories remain in working condition. The existing laboratories should be suitably strengthened with equipment.

Each Primary Health Centre in the State had been provided laboratory under National Malaria Eradication Programme for the examination of malaria cases. But many of these laboratories were not equipped to handle cases for investigation of general diseases.

4. Health Education

Dissemination of health education among the masses is an important function of the health workers. It was found that health education of the people was not being done scientifically since the villagers were found ignorant about the basic health and hygienic practices.

5. Indoor Beds

Indoor beds in PHCs generally remain unutilized. It would be worthwhile if some of these beds were transferred to the nearest referral hospitals and reserved for patients referred to it by the Primary Health Centres. These beds may be utilised for other patients in case these remain unutilised. This arrangement would serve a dual purpose of reserving beds for the PHCs and also increasing the bed-strength in referral hospitals.

6. Location not Ideal

While opening a new Primary Health Center care may be taken in selecting such a site which should be easily accessible to the largest number of villages in the block as it was revealed that only those people who are within 2-3 kms. of the PHCs, are the frequent visitors to the PHC.

7. Administrative Powers of Medical Officers not Sufficient

For efficient functioning of the centres, the administrative powers should be decentralised. The Medical Officer of the PHC is supposed to be the planner, the manager, the supervisor, the coordinator as well as the Public Relation Officer, besides being a technical expert. Is he well equipped to discharge all these functions entrusted to his care? At present, all the incumbents possess no administrative competence which is essential to administer the PHC complex. It is suggested that the officers of the PHCs may be got trained in health administration either at NIHFW or some special course may be arranged for them at the State headquarters. In order to supervise and inspect sub-centres, transport facilities should be provided.

8. Linkage between Community and PHC

There are very poor linkages between the PHC staff and the community. The staff rarely find time to visit the community and diagnose its problems to ascertain its needs. The Medical Education Committee appointed by the Government of India observed that medical education should produce a basic doctor. The Committee defined, "A basic doctor is one who is well conversant with the day-to-day health problems of the rural and urban communities and who is able to play an effective role in the curative and preventive aspects of the regional and the national health problems." It is suggested that the PHC staff must visit once a week to provide health education through well arranged lectures in school building/panchayat ghars or arrange exhibitions. This would lay the foundation of health care administration.

There is a need of courteous behaviour with the patients who are already troubled with their sufferings. They can be made at ease through courteous behaviour. Tarun Bahl in his article, "Courtesy as a Habit" in the *Daily Tribune*, Oct. 10, 1999 rightly stresses the value of courtesy. To quote him, "The good thing about practising courtesy is that while it costs nothing, it can bring rich dividends. No one is too big or too busy to be courteous. It enhances others self-worth and prods them to be good in return. Many brilliant and talented people were obnoxious, pig-headed, insolent, ungrateful and ill-mannered. Their prosperity clouded their judgement and they forgot that they had to treat others with respect, dignity and humility before they can be accorded the same regard."

9. Vacant Posts Need to be Filled

Immediate steps may be taken to fill up the vacant posts of doctors and other para-medical staff to provide health care to the people. One lady doctor may be posted in each Primary Health Center, since rural women generally prefer to be examined by a lady doctor. Besides, the PHC may be put under the control of medical colleges to make the services more effective. This would also provide opportunity to under-graduate medical students to ascertain the health needs of the population.

The Fifth Plan (Approach Papers) also emphasised that the main thrust may be directed at making up the deficiencies in building staff, equipment and drugs and medicines in a coordinated way. Such studies and evaluation may be encouraged by the Health Department on institutional basis to provide clues for the effective functioning of PHCs. There is a need to invest funds to evaluate the functioning of these centres. If inadequate funds are invested, the entire effort may well be wasted whereas properly designed and supported research may yield the answer to this important question. The purpose of the study should be to ensure that PHCs and sub-centres are giving the best possible coverage in preventive and curative services within the resources available.

In the new millennium, we have to strengthen the local health system. Dr. Hiroshi Nakajima, Director-General of World Health Organisation in his Editorial "50 years of making people healthier" rightly stresses that:

> "Building up integrated health services at local level continues to be a major strategy, and has been the key to success in many areas. It has played a leading role in improving health status and increasing the life expectancy. In recent years, the Organisation has moved to broader family health approaches to provide people with a continuum of essential care at all stages of their lives and in their communities. These approaches can be traced back to the inclusive definition of health adopted in our Constitution, as well as to the primary health care strategy. But our new policy reflects a change in focus: attention now centres not so much on structures as on the people they exist to serve. In the future an even greater effort will be needed to understand users needs, expectations and potential to contribute to the definition and implementation of health priorities and interventions.
>
> This change in perspective reflects a growing awareness of the importance of developing an open and mutually respectful dialogue between health professionals and the public. Empowering people, especially women, in all cultures and segments of society with the necessary information and opportunities for health development is both an ethical and a technical imperative."

Notes and References

1. WHO: District Health System: Global and Regional Review, Based on Experience in Various Countries, Geneva, 1995, p. 18
2. WHO: The Health Centre in District Health System, Geneva, 1994, p. 5.
3. *Ibid.*
4. England and Wales, Ministry of Health, Consultative Council on Medical and Allied Services (1920), Interim Report on the Future of Medical and Allied Services, London, H.M. Stationary Office.

5. W.G. Wickremesingh, The Premier Health Unit in Ceylon, Colombo, 1951.
6. League of Nations Health Organization, European Conference on Rural Hygiene (1931), Recommendations on the Principles Governing the Organization of Medical Assistance, The Public Health Services and Sanitation in Rural Districts of Geneva.
7. WHO: District Health System: Global and Regional Review, Based on Experience in Various Countries, Geneva, 1995, p. 18 (WHO/SHS/DHS/95.1).
8. R.R. Veinerman, Social Medicine in Eastern Europe, Cambridge, Mass, Harvard University Press, 1935, p. 5, quoted in S.L. Goel, *Public Health Administration*, New Delhi, Sterling, 1984, p. 418.
9. Annual Report, Ministry of Health & Family Welfare, GOI, New Delhi, 1971-72, p. 35.
10. Government of Burma, A Guide to Rural Health Centre Work in Burma, Rangoon, Printing and Stationery.
11. WHO: Strengthening Ministries of Health for Primary Health Care, Geneva, 1984, p. 9.
12. Walter R. Sharp, Field Administrative in the UN System, London, 1961, p. 119.
13. Speech delivered by Chief Minister of J & K, at the joint meeting of the Central Council of Health and Family Planning Council on 1974-75, held at Vigyan Bhavan, New Delhi.
14. Based on the document, prepared by NIHFW, Training Management Modules for Medical Officers.
15. *Indian Express*, Chandigarh, 28 August, 1978.
16. S.L. Goel, Health Care Administration, Levels and Aspects, Sterling, 1981.

CHAPTER 17

INTERNATIONAL HEALTH CARE ADMINISTRATION: ROLE OF THE WORLD HEALTH ORGANISATION (WHO)

"The International Co-operation which is implicit in the very concept of the World Health Organisation is the alchemy which has translated the goodwill and good sense of nations into actions directed to making this world a healthier and more decent place for all mankind."

—Author

International Health Care Administration: Role of the World Health Organisation (WHO)

A. EVOLUTION AND OBJECTIVES OF THE WHO

Introduction

In the post-war period, a very significant development has been the establishment of a pivotal international organisation concerned with the problems of world peace and human welfare. This organisation is commonly known as United Nations. Since its birth, it has been playing an increasingly vital role in easing the world tensions and conflicts which can erupt into a world conflagration as well as in alleviating the widespread hunger, poverty, ignorance, want, disease and allied problems. This organisation has been supplemented by the establishment of closely allied specialized agencies which deal with each of these stupendous problems more specifically.

When the UN Charter was being framed, attention was initially focused on the problems of peace and security in the world. But at the instance of the USA, at the Yalta Conference, it was decided to create an Economic and Social Council as an integral part of the new international organisation (UN) to deal with the rapidly emerging economic and social) problems.[1] The ECOSOC is to study the problems of human and social well-being as well as to formulate appropriate policies and direct their implementation in this connection. The UN system is thus founded upon the sound idea that no peace can be stable unless it is based upon nations whose citizens are substantially free from distress, privation and frustration.[2] The realisation that removal of poverty and improvement of economic conditions all around would be potent factors for peace prompted the expansion of the UN system. The United Nations

Development System comprises the UN itself, five Regional Economic Commissions and 11 other major programmes and organs. Besides, there are 15 separate inter-governmental specialised agencies.

In this monograph, we are concerned only with the important agency influencing directly or indirectly the promotion of health. The specialised agency responsible for international health is WHO. But, there are other organs of UN (e.g., United Nations Development Programme, UNICEF, World Food Programme, etc.) and specialised agencies (e.g., FAO, ILO, etc.) which also influence the promotion of health. Thus, there is a need of coordinated effort by the UN system to produce the desired output. Coordination may be achieved through collaboration in working for the same cause, or cooperation—the sharing of a joint task by two or more parties; often it includes both modes of action. If, for instance, food shortage emerges as a top priority issue at a given time or in a particular area, the combined facilities and efforts of several agencies may be required to alleviate the distress: the technical advice and help of the FAO in increasing output, the assistance of the WHO in highlighting nutritional needs or in combating malaria and thereby releasing additional manpower for productive employment, the help of UNESCO and ILO in the field of training, the provision of emergency supply by the UNICEF, and the support of other agencies in the development of transport facilities or community organisation. In this chapter, we shall discuss the organisation and functioning of WHO with special reference to the South-East Asia Regional office.

Health and disease have no political or geographical boundaries. Disease in any part of the world is a potential danger to other parts. "Nothing on earth is more international than disease," said Paul Russel. The problems of international health is more pressing today as the world has become smaller. In his inaugural address to the 3lst Session of the South-East Regional Committee of WHO at Ulan Bator (22-28 Aug., 1978), T. Ragcha, First Vice-Chairman of the Council of Ministers, Mongolian People's Republic, said, "In our age, the age of communication boom and of increased intercourse among nations the problem of protection of human health transcends national boundaries and becomes a common concern of the international community. A failure in one country in the field of disease prevention may affect any other country. Therefore, it becomes increasingly imperative for national governments to coordinate the internal efforts in the field of health protection to develop closer cooperation between themselves and to participate actively in the work of the World Health Organisation."[3] In order to protect against the spread of the disease from one country to another many attempts were made. A brief account of those efforts which existed before the WHO came into existence is mentioned below:

1. Sanitary Conferences and Conventions

The International Public Health had its origin in the sanitary conference which opened in Paris on 23 July, 1851. Five International Sanitary Conferences were held in the 34 years after 1851. They failed to produce an agreed international sanitary convention. After this three sanitary conferences on cholera and the fourth on plague were held. They were consolidated into a single International Sanitary Convention in 1903.

2. Pan American Sanitary Bureau (PASB)

The bureau was created by the Second International Conference of American States held in Mexico city from 12 October, 1901 to 31 Jan., 1902. In 1947, the bureau became the general secretariat of an overall organisation, the Pan American Health Organisation. With the establishment of the WHO, the bureau became the WHO Regional Office for the Americas.

3. Office of International O'Hygiene Publique (OIHP/OFFICE) (1907)

It was created in 1907 to disseminate information on communicable diseases and to supervise international quarantine. The office continued to exist until 1950 when its responsibilities were taken over by the WHO.

4. The Health Organisation of the League of Nations

The creation of the League Organisation at the end of World War I called for an examination of the means for international collaboration in all fields, including health. There were many reasons for establishing a separate health organisation in addition to the already existing Paris Office (OIHP). First, since the creation of the Paris Office in 1907, other health questions beside quarantine had arisen which seemed to call for international action. Secondly, the advanced nations recognised the obligation to help improve the health of the backward nations. Finally, the menace of the typhus epidemics ranging in 1919-20 and the scale and urgency of post-war health problems loomed large. The modest resources of the office could not cope with it.

At the outbreak of World War II in 1939, international health work came almost to a standstill but was not abandoned. The League transferred its remaining functions, including those of health to the UN in April 1946. On October 16 of the same year, the functions and personnel of the League Health Organisation were formally transferred to the WHO.[4] The League of Nations Health Organisation had a great impact upon the functioning of the WHO as it left to the World Health Organisation a valuable legacy of recorded experience and in addition, certain statutory obligations for epidemiological services and publications.[5]

5. United Nations Relief and Rehabilitation Administration (UNRRA)

With the end of the Second World War emerged the urgent need to help the war devastated countries, to combat epidemics and restore their health services. It had been foreseen that no existing international health services organisation would be able to undertake this massive task. At the first session of UNRRA's council in 1943, it was agreed that health work would be one of its primary responsibilities.[6]

In June 1945, UNRRA provided 450 teams, including 380 doctors and 435 nurses, to care for the health of the millions of displaced persons who wanted to return to their countries. At the end of 1946, UNRRA, designed as a temporary organisation to deal with an emergency, terminated its official existence and its health activities were taken over by the WHO Interim Commission. It suffered from the defects associated with a large and temporary international organisation created towards the end of a World War. Nevertheless, it carried out, by far, the largest international health programme ever executed. It played a major part in the prevention of post-war epidemics and in the reconstruction of health services. Its residual funds were of immense value to its successor agencies, particularly in the health field.[7]

6. Birth of WHO

Delegates of 50 nations in the UN Conference on International Organisation held in San Francisco from 25 April to 26 June, 1945 approved a proposal put by the delegations of Brazil and China that an international conference should be held to establish an international health organisation. The constitution was drawn up at this conference in 1946. An Interim Commission was set-up to carry on the work for the new organisation which held five sessions. On 7 April, 1948, the 26 of the 61 member governments ratified the constitution and the WHO was born as a specialised agency of the United Nations. The First Health Assembly opened in Geneva on 24 June, 1948 with delegations from 50 of the 55 governments.

Thus, the creation of the WHO after World War II as a specialised agency of the United Nations marked a considerable advance in the Evolution of the International Health Organisation. It presents a culmination of efforts at international health cooperation initiated a century ago. It absorbed and unified all the existing organisations for the time being transforming it into single, worldwide inter-governmental body.

Objectives

The main objective of the WHO is "the attainment by all peoples of the highest level of health" which is set out in the Preamble of the Constitution. The Preamble of the Constitution states:

> "Health is a state of complete physical, mental and social well-being and not merely the absence of disease or infirmity. The enjoyment of the highest attainable standard of health is one of the fundamental rights of every human being without distinction of race, religion, political belief, economic and social condition. The

health of all peoples is fundamental to the attainment of peace and security and is dependent upon the fullest cooperation of individuals and states.

The achievement of any state in the promotion and protection of health is of value to all. Unequal development in different countries in the promotion of health and control of disease, especially communicable disease, is a common danger. Healthy development of the child is of basic importance; the ability to live harmoniously in a changing total environment is essential to such development.

The extension to all people of the benefits of medical, psychological and related knowledge is essential to the fullest attainment of health. Informed opinion and active cooperation on the part of the public are of the utmost importance in the improvement of the health of the people.

Governments have a responsibility for the health of their peoples which can be fulfilled only by the provision of adequate health and social measures."

Thus, WHO's work covers a wide spectrum of activities, ranging from the fight against most of the world's diseases to the award of fellowships, from the monitoring of environmental conditions detrimental to health to the collection of international statistics; from the training of health personnel to multi-lateral research endeavours.

Functions

In order to achieve its objectives, the functions of the WHO are:

(a) to act as the directing and coordinating authority on international health work;
(b) to establish and maintain effective collaboration with the United Nations, specialised agencies, governmental health administrations, professional groups, and such other organisations as may be deemed appropriate;
(c) to assist governments, upon request, in strengthening health services;
(d) to furnish appropriate technical assistance and in emergencies, necessary aid upon the request or acceptance of governments;
(e) to provide or assist in providing, upon the request of the UN Health Services and facilities to special groups, such as the peoples of Trust territories;
(f) to establish and maintain such administrative and technical services as may be required including epidemiological and statistical services;
(g) to stimulate and advance work to eradicate epidemic, endemic and other diseases;

(h) to promote, in cooperation with other specialised agencies where necessary, the prevention of accidental injuries;
(i) to promote, in cooperation with other specialised agencies where necessary, the improvement of nutrition, housing, sanitation, recreation, economic or working conditions and other aspects of environmental hygiene;
(j) to promote cooperation among scientific and professional groups which contribute to the advancement of health;
(k) to propose conventions, agreements and regulations, and make recommendations with respect to international health matters and to perform such duties as may be assigned thereby to the organisation and are consistent with its objectives;
(l) to promote maternal and child health and welfare and to foster the ability to live harmoniously in a changing total environment;
(m) to foster activities in the field of mental health, especially those affecting the harmony of human relations;
(n) to promote and conduct research in the field of health;
(o) to promote improved standards of teaching and training in the health, medical and related professions;
(p) to study and report on, in cooperation with other specialised agencies where necessary, administrative and social techniques affecting public health and medical care from preventive and curative point of view, including hospital services and social security;
(q) to provide information, counsel and assistance in the field of health;
(r) to assist in developing an informed public opinion among all peoples on matters of health;
(s) to establish and revise as necessary international nomenclatures practices;
(t) to standardise diagnostic procedures as and when necessary;
(u) to develop, establish and promote international standards with respect to food, biological, pharmaceutical and similar products; and
(v) generally to take all necessary action to attain the objective of the organisation.

Activities

The forms of assistance which may be provided include:

(a) expert personnel to provide advisory, executive and operational services;
(b) fellowships, training courses and seminars; and
(c) equipment and supplies.

The WHO-assisted projects fall in the following broad categories:

(a) Control of Communicable Disease

Control of communicable diseases (e.g., parasitic, bacterial, viral), eradication or control programmes, laboratory facilities and vaccine production.

(b) Education, Training and HRD

Education and training of professional, technical and auxiliary staff, grant of fellowships, study tours and conferences, manpower development.

(c) Coordination of Medical Research and Supporting Services

Collaborative research, reference centres, research grants for training and exchange and scientific groups.

(d) Development of Public Health Services

Public Health Administration, organisation of medical care, hospitals, laboratories and nursing services, environmental sanitation, cancer and cardiovascular diseases, drug control and vital health statistics.

(e) Development of Primary Health Care Services

We should keep in mind that WHO is in no sense of the term a World Health Service; it helps governments at their request and in accordance with the policy laid down by the Health Assembly.

B. ORGANISATIONAL STRUCTURE AND FUNCTIONS

The basic structure of the WHO comprises three organs:

(1) The World Health Assembly (Health Assembly).
(2) The Executive Board (Board).
(3) The Secretariat headed by the Director-General.

(i) Health Assembly

It is the supreme policy-making body of the Organisation. It is the only organ in which all members enjoy direct representation. As of 1 January, 1998, it consisted of 191 members and two Associate members. Each Assembly elects a President and five vice-presidents, who hold office until their successors are elected. The work of the Assembly is conducted by two main Committees: Committee A to deal predominantly with programme and budget matters, and Committee B to deal predominantly with administrative, financial and legal matters.

Decisions are taken through the adoption of resolutions, which may be tabled by any Member. There must be a two-thirds majority of the members present and voting for important questions such as the adoption of conventions or agreements and fixing the amount of the effective working budget. Decisions on other questions require a simple majority. Its functions are enumerated in the Constitution. Most important of these being:

(a) to determine the policy of the Organisation;
(b) to name the members entitled to designate a person to serve on the Board;
(c) to appoint the Director-General;
(d) to review and report activities of the Board and of the Director-General and to instruct the Board in regard to matters upon which action study, investigation or report may be considered desirable; and
(e) to supervise the financial policies of the Organisation and to review and approve the budget.

The Health Assembly has been passing resolutions affecting the health of the world as a whole. Professor E. Aujaleu (France), President of the 2lst World Health Assembly, 1968, and the Chairman of the 24th and 25th Sessions of the Executive Board, 1959-60, offered the following comments on the Assembly's role:

> The Assembly has shown considerable dignity in its discussions. It has handled extremely delicate subjects—the refugees in the Middle-East, assistance to Portugal, the health situation in Viet Nam with particular care to avoid offence and even with a certain all-round imperturbability. I believe that the Assembly has reached almost complete maturity. Its maturity will be truly complete when we refuse to divert a single hour to the raising of political problems with which we are neither competent nor qualified to deal. The moment may not be far off; at least I sincerely hope so.[8]

Most major policy decisions have been taken by the 31st Health Assembly without dissenting voices. It was remarked by Professor Julie Sulianti Saroso, President of the 25th Health Assembly that no Health Assembly has passed without decisions being taken which marked a new milestone in mankind's continual struggle against disease.

The Fifty-first Health Assembly appointed Dr. Gro Hardem Brundtland as Director-General of WHO for five years beginning 21 July, 1998 and debated on the regional allocations of the WHO Regular budget resulting in a compromise approach which was substantially more favourable to the South-East Asia Region. The Fifty-second Health Assembly reviewed and approved the programme budget for 2000-2001. It also reviewed the World Health Report, 1999, the Director Generals Report on the work of WHO and issues concerning smallpox, malaria, polio, tobacco, revised drug strategy, iodine deficiency disorders and cloning.[9]

(ii) Executive Board

It consists of 32 members technically qualified in the field of health. The Board meets at least twice a year. Its first session is generally held at the beginning of the calendar year at which it sorts out the budget and programme estimates of the Director-General. The second session follows the annual meeting of the Assembly in winter. One-third of the members retire every year. Dr. S.L. Molapo, the then Chairman of the Executive Board reviewed the role and functions of the Board. He said, "The Board has indeed performed its task efficiently, with sincerity and integrity. . . . Achievements are exacting but the faith which was the forerunner and continues to be the moving spirit of achievements is of even greater importance."[10]

The 101st session of the Executive Board considered the draft global health policy for the 21st century and WHO reforms, and reviewed the issue of regional allocations, which was further reviewed by the 102nd session. The 103rd session, *inter alia,* discussed the Drug Strategy, Tobacco Free Initiative, and Polio Eradication. It reviewed the programme budget for 2000-2001 and suggested certain adjustments. The 104th session of the Executive Board reviewed research strategies and mechanisms for cooperation as well as administration and award of foundation prizes and fellowships.[11]

(iii) The Secretariat

Secretariat is the staff of WHO headed by the Director-General who is the Chief Technical and Administrative officer of the organisation. He is assisted by Assistant Director-Generals and other staff in carrying out his duties and responsibilities. He appoints the staff in accordance with the staff regulations prescribed by the Assembly, submits the budget to the Executive Board and to the Assembly.

(iv) Regionalisation

Regionalisation connotes the geographical arrangements used by the WHO to establish decentralisation. Much of the effectiveness of the WHO has often been attributed to its decentralised structure, which enables it to come to grips as directly as possible with local and regional realities. There are six regions of the WHO, which are as follows:

	Region	*Headquarters*
1.	South East Asia	New Delhi (India)
2.	Africa	Brazzaville (Congo)
3.	The Americas	Washington D.C. (USA)
4.	Europe	Copenhagen (Denmark)
5.	Eastern Mediterranean	Alexandria (Egypt)
6.	Western Pacific	Manila (Philippines)

Each Regional Organisation consists of a deliberative organisation (Regional Committee), a Chief Executive called the Regional Director and an Administrative Office called the Regional Office.

The Fifty-first Session of the Regional Committee was preceded by WHO's 50th anniversary celebrations. Ministers of health from most SEAR countries and the Director General of WHO attended it. The Regional Committee nominated Dr. Uton Muchlar Rafei as Regional Director of the South East Region for a second term of five years with effect from 1 March 1999.[12]

Let us now discuss the structure, personnel, finances and role of the South-East Asia Regional Office of the WHO in the promotion of health among the people of this region. South-East Asia Regional Office was the first to be set-up by the WHO. It is located in New Delhi and its Regional Committee consists of eleven member-states. (See Organisational Chart 17.1, as on 30-6-2003). The names of the member-states are mentioned below (with the date of joining the Region):

	Member-state	Date of joining
1.	Bangladesh	19th May, 1972
2.	Bhutan	8th March, 1982
3.	Democratic Peoples' Republic of Korea	8th March, 1982
4.	India	12th January, 1948
5.	Indonesia	23rd May, 1950
6.	Maldive Islands	5th November, 1965
7.	Myanmar	1st July, 1948
8.	Nepal	2nd September, 1953
9.	Sri Lanka	7th July, 1948
10.	Thailand	26th September, 1947
11.	Timor-Leste	2002

The committee holds at least one session every year. The head of the Regional office is the Regional Director. He is appointed by the Board in agreement with the Regional Committee for a fixed period of five years. In the performance of his technical duties, he is assisted by Deputy Regional Director, Programme Management, WHO Programme Coordinators, Public Information Unit and a Director Support programme.

In order to further harmonize action in the Regional Office with initiatives taken at WHO headquarters, a Regional Service Appointment Review Committee was established to determine the mechanism for awarding open-ended service appointments to eligible staff members. Service appointments have no specific time limit and may be brought to an end by either party subject to certain specified conditions.

Consequent upon the global HR reform process, and in order to infuse competition and merit in recruitment, written tests and interviews are now part of the selection process for fixed-term GS and professional posts. Further streamlining of selection procedures is under way to help

CHART 17.1

Organisational Structure

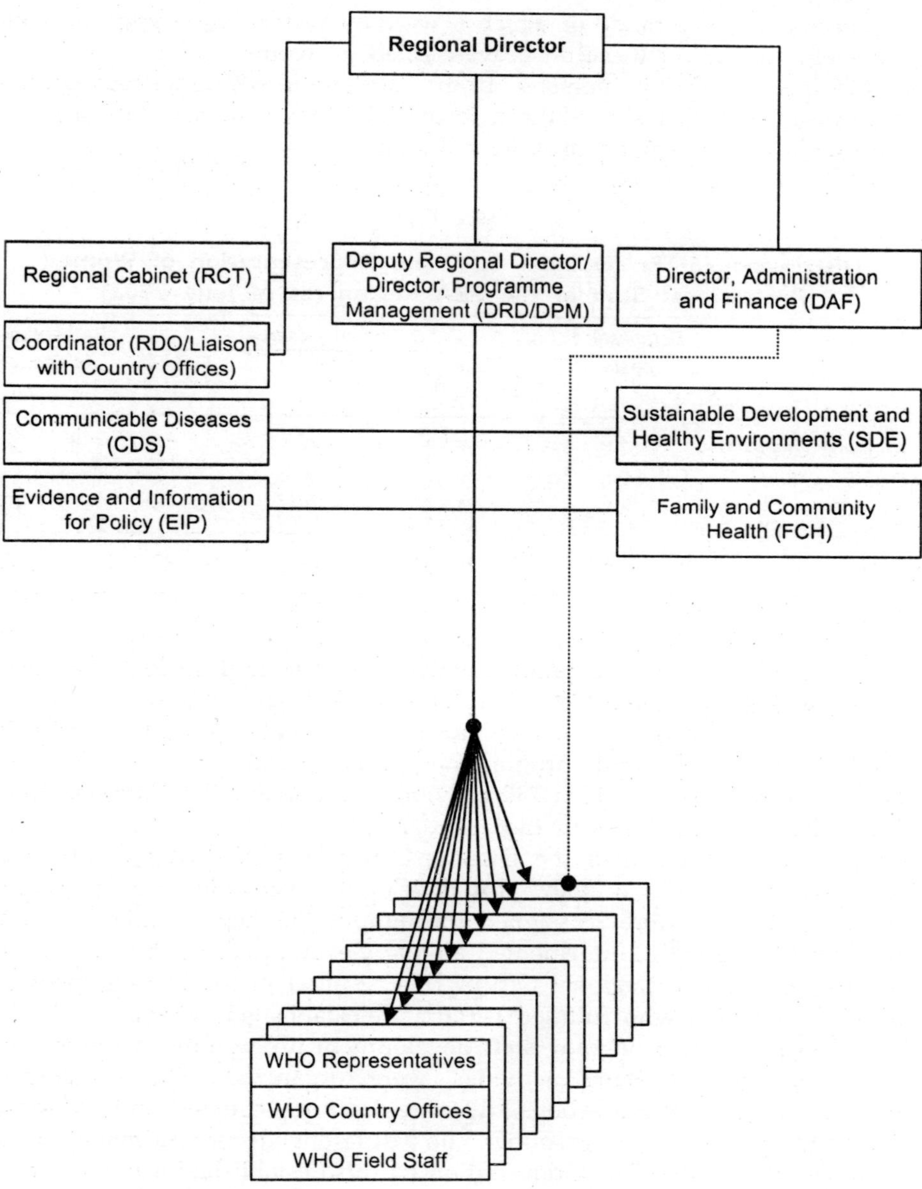

Source: The Work of WHO in the South-East Asia Region.

attract highly qualified staff and to enable fair selections.

During the reporting period, special efforts were made to recruit new appointees from unrepresented and under-represented countries, keeping in view the parallel objective of gender parity. A total of 18 appointments were made of which 6 were by way of reassignment from other regions. Six of these posts were filled by women (33 per cent) and 4 (33 per cent) by persons from unrepresented/under-represented countries. Table 17.1 shows the distribution of professional staff and the representation of women professional staff.

TABLE 17.1

Distribution of Professional Staff and Representation of Women Professional Staff in the SEA Region (as of June 2003)

Location	*Established posts*	*Staff in position*			*Percentage in female staff*
		Total	*Male*	*Female*	
Regional Office	74	54	36	18	34
Country Office	24	19	16	3	16
Field Office	41	21	13	8	43
Total	139	94	65	29	33

Source: WHO/SEARO.

As a reflection of expanded activities at the country level 24 posts of National Professional Officers (NPOs) have been established.

In the context of enhancing national capacity towards implementation of health programmes, 1083 special services agreement holders were hired of which 780 provided support for the National Polio Surveillance Programmes in India and Nepal.

In accordance with the Director-General's policy of mobility and rotation, and with a view to developing versatile careers, eight professional staff were reassigned throughout the Region. Likewise, job rotation was recently implemented among General Service staff across all departments in the Regional Office. This resulted in the reassignment of 27 staff members who fulfilled certain pre-established criteria.

As part of the ongoing staff development programme, a number of workshops and training activities were organized. These included security awareness workshops, distance learning courses and in-house briefing/orientation programmes on different technical/managerial/administrative areas. The Organization has also established a modern and well-equipped fitness centre for the Regional Office staff and their dependents.

The professional staff is recruited on the basis of international selections. The staff members belong to different nationalities. There are a number of problems in the recruitment of experts from the international market because of the adherence of the principle of geographical distribution and other procedural difficulties. The delegates to the Regional Committee wanted posts not to be allowed to remain vacant since the programme schedule would otherwise be affected adversely. To overcome the quantitative shortage relating to internationally recruited staff, the following facts and suggestions may be taken into consideration:

(a) Local talent within the region may be mobilised whenever available.
(b) A purely mathematical or quota approach based on the principle of geographical distribution would prove to be too rigid for attracting talent. A delicate compromise would therefore be advisable between overall efficiency and the principle of geographical distribution.
(c) The field staff may be given higher emoluments in order to attract first-rate health experts.
(d) A suitable balance between internal promotion and recruitment of fresh talent from outside may be worked out.
(e) Utilisation of the services of experts on a long-term basis in different regions would require greater emphasis on long-term planning and better communication between the headquarters and the regional office.

Finances

The source of income of this organisation comprises contributions received from members in accordance with a scale determined annually by the World Health Assembly. The headquarter organisation distributes the funds among the six regions of the WHO after meeting its own expenditure and the expenditure to be incurred on global and inter-regional health activities.

Most of the delegates were of the view that the region should get at least 18-20 per cent of the total regular budget of the WHO and not 12-15 as had been the practice. Though the budget appears to be large, in concrete terms it comes to virtually nothing. It is inadequate in the context of the health problems and health needs of the member-states. Anyhow, even the limited scope of the operation made possible, by the mobilisation of the finances has created a new consciousness among member-states about the health needs.

What is the role of the technical resources channelled through this office of WHO in the promotion of public health? Most of the delegates who came to attend the Regional Committee meetings were of the opinion that the resources, though very modest in relation to the total flow of external assistance into a member-state were of great value and were difficult to obtain from alternative sources. Moreover, it strengthens

TABLE 17.2

Budgetary Implementation of Activities by Country: 2002-03 Regular Budget (as of 30th June 2003)

(Expressed in US %)

Country	*Allotted*	*Dis-bursement*	*Unliquidated obligations*	*Total obligations*	*Ear-markings*	*Total committed*	*Un-committed balance*
Bangladesh	6261600	4074845 (65%)	1919087 (31%)	5993932 (96%)	211859 (3%)	6205791 (99%)	55809 (1%)
Bhutan	1382700	1149642 (83%)	232007 (17%)	1381649 (100%)	0 (0%)	1381649 (100%)	1051 (0%)
DPR Korea	2263000	1550110 (68%)	288780 (13%)	1838890 (81%)	422705 (19%)	2261595 (100%)	1405 (0%)
India	11425600	7041203 (62%)	3945127 (34%)	10986330 (96%)	419370 (4%)	11405700 (100%)	19900 (0%)
Indonesia	5071000	3792886 (75%)	1200712 (24%)	4993598 (99%)	54058 (1%)	5047656 (100%)	23344 (0%)
Maldives	957300	725997 (76%)	196026 (20%)	922023 (96%)	22201 (2%)	944224 (98%)	13076 (2%)
Myanmar	4930600	3285576 (67%)	1293951 (26%)	4579527 (93%)	350256 (7%)	4929783 (100%)	817 (0%)
Nepal	4838100	2420389 (51%)	2064507 (44%)	4484896 (95%)	212350 (4%)	4697246 (99%)	40854 (1%)
Sri Lanka	2801500	2123226 (76%)	569920 (20%)	2693146 (96%)	107500 (4%)	2800646 (100%)	854 (0%)
Thailand	3592100	1685442 (47%)	1899041 (53%)	3584483 (100%)	0 (0%)	3584483 (100%)	7617 (0%)
Timor-Leste	139000	119006 (86%)	19994 (14%)	139000 (100%)	0 (0%)	139000 (100%)	0 (0%)
Country Total	43562500	27968322 (64%)	13629152 (32%)	41597474 (96%)	1800299 (4%)	43397773 (100%)	164727 (0%)
Inter-country	6802800	4331378 (64%)	1352805 (20%)	5684183 (84%)	748399 (11%)	6432582 (95%)	370218 (5%)
SEAR Total	50365300	32299700 (64%)	14981957 (30%)	47281657 (94%)	2548698 (5%)	49830355 (99%)	534945 (1%)

Source: The Work of WHO in the South-East Asia Region.

universal cooperation in regard to developmental tasks confronting many nations. After all, it represents a partnership, not an international charity. It may, however, be emphasised here that as the technical assistance provided through this office is quantitatively small, in relative and absolute terms, its contribution should be utilised strategically within the framework of all available inputs, whether these are to be provided from

TABLE 17.3

Extra-budgetary Funds (as of 30th June 2003)

(Expressed in US %)

Country	*Allotted*	*Dis-bursement*	*Unliquidated obligations*	*Total obligations*	*Ear-markings*	*Total committed*	*Un-committed balance*
Bangladesh	8970353	4166395	1518193	5684588	199750	5884338	3086015
		(46%)	(17%)	(63%)	(2%)	(65%)	(35%)
Bhutan	162148	140458	2496	142954	0	142954	19194
		(87%)	(1%)	(88%)	(0%)	(88%)	(12%)
DPR Korea	4260469	1894746	1225570	3120316	163518	3283834	976635
		(44%)	(29%)	(73%)	(4%)	(77%)	(23%)
India	48396919	23479231	10803988	34283219	1388336	35671555	12775364
		(49%)	(22%)	(71%)	(3%)	(74%)	(26%)
Indonesia	12913590	8500721	1486622	9987343	217826	10205169	2705421
		(66%)	(11%)	(77%)	(2%)	(79%)	(21%)
Myanmar	4255860	1838196	793460	2631656	12618	2644274	1611586
		(43%)	(19%)	(62%)	(0%)	(62%)	(38%)
Nepal	10063904	4143133	1800067	5943200	602131	6545331	3518573
		(41%)	(18%)	(59%)	(6%)	(65%)	(35%)
Sri Lanka	567897	266310	150759	417069	32000	449069	418828
		(31%)	(17%)	(48%)	(4%)	(52%)	(48%)
Thailand	956326	487778	153622	641400	0	641400	314926
		(51%)	(16%)	(67%)	(0%)	(67%)	(33%)
Timor-Leste	798472	675142	57130	732272	0	732272	66200
		(85%)	(7%)	(92%)	(0%)	(92%)	(8%)
Country Total	91645938	45592110	17991907	63584017	2616179	66200196	25445742
		(50%)	(19%)	(69%)	(3%)	(72%)	(28%)
Inter-country	21598119	9609430	4083534	13692964	1001897	14694861	6903258
		(44%)	(19%)	(63%)	(5%)	(68%)	(32%)
SEAR Total	113244057	55201540	22075441	77276981	3618076	80895057	32349000
		(49%)	(19%)	(68%)	(3%)	(71%)	(29%)

Source: The Work of WHO in the South-East Asia Region.

a country's internal resources or from outside assistance including bilateral programmes. As a result, 100% implementation of the Regular Budget allocation was achieved as per Tables 17.2 and 17.3.

Working of WHO

The Regional Office has been helping the member-states in almost all fields of public health promotion. Its role continues to be of great importance. Some 50 years ago, South-East Asia had the dubious distinction of being the world's reservoir of cholera and smallpox.

Malaria claimed 100 million victims a year, with about one million deaths. Tuberculosis posed a major problem in both urban ánd rural areas. In some of the worst affected areas in Burma, Sri Lanka and India, about 80 per cent of the people suffered from filariasis; Yaws claimed about 12 million patients in Thailand and Indonesia; leprosy, Malaria and trachoma affected millions. The death rate of infants under five was as high as 50 per cent. We shall discuss the role of the Regional Office under the following heads:

1. Provision of Expertise.
2. Fellowships.
3. Equipment.
4. Headquarter Support to Regional Organisations.

I. Provision of Expertise

The Regional office attempts to provide useful know-how through experts to member-states to improve the general health conditions in most of the field

2. Fellowships

Opportunities of advanced studies abroad in the fields in which a developing country is deficient are widely recognised as an effective way of developing its human capital without which no enduring social and economic development is possible. One of the WHOs principle methods of helping governments to train technical personnel for their health services has been to provide fellowships for advanced studies abroad. The improved training thus acquired by such persons must be reflected in renewed impetus and administrative practices in the field of public health. It should be kept in mind that a WHO fellowship is awarded not primarily with a view to the personal advancement of the recipient but as a means of strengthening the health services of his country.

3. Equipment

The WHO also provides equipments and supplies. The policy of the WHO in regard to supply, that supplies are provided to meet emergency needs and the specific needs for accomplishing WHO projects, but at the same time to assist member countries to become eventually independent of foreign and even international aid wherever it is feasible.

4. Headquarter's Support to Regional Organisations

WHOs headquarters provides central technical services which form the backbone of international health work. These may be classified into 5 main heads:

(a) Epidemiological Surveillance of Communicable Diseases

Information is collected through the Weekly Epidemiological

Record, and daily telex information system.

(b) International Health Regulations

The aim of International Health Regulations is to ensure maximum security against international spread of diseases with a minimum interference with world traffic.

(c) Health Statistics

It would help to bring uniformity in the notification of diseases and causes of deaths. In this way, it would be possible to compare and define health problems more accurately.

(d) International Standardisation

To ensure and define uniform standards for the strength and purity of medical substances.

(e) Publication and Documentation

Besides the above functions, the headquarters appoints Expert Committees and scientific groups which keep the governments posted with up-to-date information on advances in the various fields of health. The experts who come together constitute a hallmark of eminence in a particular subject. Moreover, a large corpus of agreed thinking by the leading experts in any field is collected and kept up-to-date. The members of these committees did not represent their governments but acted in an entirely personal capacity. The report of these committees generally appear in the Technical Report Series.

Study groups supplement the more formal expert groups. Their functions are exploratory. The reports are also published in the Technical Report Series.

The WHO headquarter's publications of particular value to health workers are: the WHO Bulletin containing original scientific articles and monograph series. Then there are public health papers which usually contribute to the study of a particular health question. Lastly, there are Technical Report Series containing the published reports of the WHO Expert Committees and Study Groups. The WHO also publishes valuable reference books especially Health situation in the world.

Education and Training Support

WHO has been pursuing a fellowships programme for its member-countries, supporting the education and training of health professionals in various fields of medical and public health sciences. Currently, this consists of fellowships, study tours and inter-country training. A new system to train fellows through the APW mechanism has been introduced in a few countries of the Region. There has been an increasing trend of short-term training in specialized fields with greater use of regional resources. Presently, such training is in the areas of primary health care, field epidemiology, vector biology, community health care and research, malaria control and nursing. There is an upward trend in regional training as compared to extra regional fellowships. Efforts are constantly being made to assess the training needs of the countries in terms of number, duration and field of study under the WHO collaborative programmes.

During the period under review, 804 fellowship applications were received. Of these, letters of award in respect of 550 fellowships were issued. Of the 550 fellowships awarded last year, Fellowship Termination of Studies Reports in respect of 268 fellowships were received. Table 17.4 gives a broad picture of implementation of fellowships in the Region.

TABLE 17.4

Distribution of Fellowships in the SEA Region 1st July 2002 to 30th June 2003

Country	*Number of applications received*	*Number of fellowships awarded*	*Number of fellowship termination of studies report submitted*
Bangladesh	235	187	84
Bhutan	32	33	31
DPR Korea	40	74	112
India	137	67	20
Indonesia	30	30	3
Maldives	24	31	11
Myanmar	178	207	154
Nepal	56	37	15
Sri Lanka	66	96	70
Thailand	7	9	3
Timor-Leste	3	3	3
Total	808	774	506

Source: WHO/SEARO.

Further, the Region offered services to the Western Pacific (WPR) and Eastern Mediterranean (EMR) Regions in the implementation of their fellowships programme. 106 fellowships from the Western Pacific Region and 6 from the Eastern Mediterranean Region were implemented with support from SEA Regional Office.

Performance of Regionalisation

It may be pertinent here to mention that the higher executives and several delegates from the member-states have highly commended the effectiveness of the regional pattern of administration in the WHO. Dr. Candlu, Director-General of the WHO, addressed the Regional Committee of SEA in 1953. Appreciating the impact of regionalisation on the organisations functioning, he said:

> "I have worked for an almost equal time at headquarters and in one of the regions. For my part, I am convinced that but for regionalisation, most of the results for which it can be credited could not have been achieved."
>
> "To my mind regionalisation is much more than a mechanical division of assignments between headquarters and the six regional offices. . . . For me regionalisation is essentially a recognition of the fact that promotion of health on a world basis must be a truly two-way cooperation, between independent and equal partners."
>
> "In my own limited experience, I have seen many times that the mere transfer of techniques, skills and supplies from one country to another is meaningless unless it is accompanied by a thorough appreciation of the local problems. We must do everything in our power to encourage all efforts to bring about genuine cooperation between the nations of the world, however, small."[13]

Dr. P.K. Ratnasingham, Deputy Director of Health Services (PHS) Colombo, addressing the SEARO anniversary session, remarked:

> "Now after twenty years, we can say with confidence that this was a wise decision as health problems of South-East Asia have to be discussed and solutions found by the sons of the soil who feel for their own people and who will know their needs, customs and habits.[14]

Dr. Chellappah, the Ceylon representative at the First World Health Assembly in 1948 referred to the slogan of the Health Services, know your area, know your people.[15]

Dr. C. Mani, who was very active since inception of the WHO and remained as the Regional Director for 20 years remarked: For the first time in Public Health history, an International Health Organisation and the national health departments were brought together so closely and so effectively. I have no doubt that popularity and success of WHO today is in a large measure due to this effective system of decentralization. Through this system, health officials of Government and of WHO are continuously thinking together. WHO is not a far-off organisation to be approached for technical assistance through long range paper artillery. The organisation is situated on the governments very doorstep, in fact, immediately inside their doors available for consultation and assistance.[16]

Dr. L. Bernard, Assistant Director-General of the WHO stated:

The WHO has had nearly a quarter of century of practical

> experience of regionalisation. It may be fitting to acknowledge that the expenditure has been rewarding. We trust that it will enable the organisation, in the future, to contribute positively to international endeavours towards developing more rational and efficient approaches to co-operation.[17]

The same is true about other regions, for example, Dr. K. Camara, Guinea, said about the African Region: One of the happiest decisions of our agency was to set-up regional organisations. The regionalisations of WHOs activities has made it possible to establish services better adapted to their requirements in the member-states of the African region while at the same time giving more responsibility to the national health authorities with their greater awareness of local conditions.[18]

The Fifty-first Session of the Regional Committee including apart from the Director-General of WHO, Ministers of Health of Bhutan, DPR Korea, India, Indonesia, Myanmar, Nepal and Sri Lanka participated. They felicitated WHO on its achievements in the promotion of health, prevention and control of diseases and for its continued technical support and cooperation to the member-states. The Director-General Dr. Gro Herlem Brundtland, in her address, asserted WHOs continued role as the centre of excellence for providing norms and standards, supporting national capacity building and innovative approaches for health development.

C. WHO AND INDIA

A number of health projects are being implemented in India with assistance from WHO in the form of experts, and supplies and equipment.

In the field of Health and Family Welfare, India has various ongoing and purposed programmes of cooperation with international agencies like WHO, UNDP, ILO, UNICEF, UNFPA, World Bank, as also with a number of foreign agencies like SIDA (Sweden), DANIDA (Denmark), NORAD (Norway), ODA (UK) and USAID (USA), World Bank.

World Health Organisation (WHO) is collaborating with this country in providing and developing health care facilities. India makes regular annual contribution to WHO.

The WHO provides assistance to member-states on a biennium basis for supplies and equipment, training/fellowships, study tours, short-term consultants, subsidy for Group Educational Activities (Seminars/Workshops/Meetings/Conferences/Studies, etc.) and for participation of Indian experts in various symposia, workshops and seminars organised by the WHO and other international organisations in India and abroad.

D. ASSESSMENT OF THE FUNCTIONING OF THE WHO

Many member-states appear to be satisfied with the working of the Regional Office. They have made known their feeling during several sessions of the Regional Committee. To give a few examples, S.W.R.D. Bandaranaike, the then Prime Minister of Sri Lanka (erstwhile Ceylon) while addressing the 12th session of the Regional Committee said:

> "I cannot help feeling that amongst the various specialised agencies of the UN that are all, one way or another, doing useful and valuable work, the WHO takes the pre-eminent place in actual practical achievements. Various health problems of the world have been dealt with in an unobtrusive manner that does not hit the frontlines of the world press. In our region of SEA, these problems are naturally more serious and more numerous than in some other regions. But I can speak from my own personal experience of the immensely valuable work that has been done in Ceylon."[19]

Kurt Waldheim, UN Secretary General said, WHO has clearly demonstrated the catalytic role open to an international organisation with precise objectives, a clear conception of its own part and consistency in its activities, however limited the resources may be at any one time in relation to the needs. . . . The WHO has always fought for the cause of social development and can claim credit for the greater awareness which now exists for the social aspects of the development process.

Bisnuram Medhi, the then Governor of Madras while addressing the 14th Session of the Regional Committee said, "The WHO can take credit for the control of major communicable diseases and for the improvement of medical education and promotion of vital health statistics and health education in collaboration with the Government in the region with a view to improving national health services."[20]

U Nu, the former Prime Minister of Burma said, "The WHO has during the ten years of its existence amply justified its establishment. It has assisted member-countries in strengthening public health administration, in improving and developing maternal and child health and nursing services and in solving urgent health problems. . . . All this has been done without WHOs becoming a supranational health administration."[21]

K.K. Shah, the then Union Minister for Health, Family Planning, Works, Housing and Urban Development, Government of India in his address to the 23rd Session of the Regional Committee, praised the WHOs performance thus, "Suffice it to say that WHO has stood like a tower of strength in a global war against diseases and sickness."[22]

Dr. P. Dolgor, Director, Ministry of Public Health Ulan Bator, said, "WHOs activities and its achievements made in this region make us sure of the bright future ahead of this organisation."[23]

Dr. Nyom Osor, Ministry of Public Health, Mongolia said recently, "WHO has become for these decades a highly prestigious international organisation. Playing an increasingly active role in strengthening universal peace and in promoting the noble and human cause of the health cause of the health and welfare of man."[24]

Besides, most of the academic writers have been appreciating the functional role of the WHO. Stephen S. Goodspeed has said, "The work of the WHO on such problem as malaria, tuberculosis, venereal diseases and the promotion of maternal and child welfare has been outstanding. Its contribution to the welfare of mankind cannot be measured accurately enough to portray the overall usefulness of the agency, but it can be said that the work of WHO has been an unmitigated blessing."[25]

Future Assistance Policy of WHO in the South-East Asia Region

The aim of the WHO, as stated in its Constitution, is an exalted one—the attainment by all peoples of the highest possible level of health. Some striking advances have been made, but the international community still faces many health hazards and problems. The burden of preventable communicable diseases is still with us to consume a large portion of national as well as international resources. A major part of the world is still without safe water supply and minimum standards of sanitation and housing.

Hence the SEARO would have to go a long way to enable the countries of Asia to achieve the standards of health defined in the WHO Constitution. Most of these standards have already been attained by the advanced countries. It would be better if in order to become more effective, the SEARO maintains a continuous review of the scope of its programmes and its organisational capacity to implement the programme.

In order to solve these present and emerging problems, WHO's programmes must be dynamic and suited to the needs of the member-states. In a message, the Director-General of WHO, Dr. Mahler, stated:

> "Who's mission is firmly rooted in its Constitution. The constitution does not change, but, in response to new challenges, the programme based upon it must move forward in a state of perpetual evolution. This evolution is not only continual but also geared to the real needs of the countries for which WHO was created to serve.[26]

Thus, the SEARO would have to expand its operations to provide technical assistance to the member-states to find solutions to the existing and also the emerging problems of public health. This would involve much larger mobilisation of financial resources from member-states and continuous review of the administrative capacity and advance personnel and programme planning by the SEARO as well as meaningful cooperation of the member-states. We need the services of WHO more than before.

A World without WHO

Dr. Gro Harlen Brundtland, the Fifth Director-General of WHO emphatically states that the value of the World Health Organisation can be judged by looking at its achievements over the past five decades and by imagining what the world would look like today if WHO had never been born. In a world without WHO:

- there would be no global forum for reaching consensus on the sensitive health and human rights issues raised by the AIDS epidemic,
- there would be no independent honest broker to match the funding needs of developing countries in the field of health with the resources potentially available from financing agencies and donor countries,
- national health officials would not be able to count on global moral support in the battle against tobacco addiction,
- there would be no politically neutral body to monitor the health effects of radiation fallout after nuclear accidents, and
- there would be no unifying moral and technical force to galvanize, guide and support countries in achieving health for all.[27]

She further adds that over the 50 years WHO has been the torch-bearer for global health. While giant strides are being made, the new millennium will bring its own challenges. These have to be met boldly. WHO will continue to strive with its member-countries to ensure better health for all.[28]

Notes and References

1. E. Settinius, The Yalta Conference, p. 25.
2. Norman Hill, International Organisation, New York, 1952, p. 48.
3. WHO SEARO: SEA/RL31/2.
4. Report of the Interim Commission to the First World Health Assembly, Part I, p. 10.
5. WHO, The First Ten Years in the WHO, pp. 30-31.
6. WHO, SEARO, Twenty Years in South-East Asia, 1948-67, p. 13.
7. WHO, Constitution of the WHO, Art. 16.
8. WHO, *WHO Chronicle*, Vol. 22, No. 7, July 1968, p. 296.
9. WHO; SEARO, The Work of WHO in SEA Region, New Delhi, June, 1999, p. xi.
10. WHO, *WHO Chronicle*, Vol. 27, July/August, 1973, p. 283.
11. WHO, SEARO, The Work of WHO in SEA Region, New Delhi, June 1999, p. xi.
12. WHO, SEARO, The Work of WHO in SEA Region, New Delhi, June, 1999, p. xii.
13. Sixth Session of the WHO Regional Committee for South-East Asia, (New Delhi,

1953), p. 12.
14. WHO, SEARO Anniversary, Commemorative Meeting (New Delhi, October, 1968), p. 21.
15. *Ibid.*
16. *Ibid.*, p. 55.
17. 23rd Session of the WHO Regional Committee for South-East Asia (New Delhi, October, 1970), p. 64.
18. WHO, *WHO Chronicle*, Vol. 27, Nos. 7-8, p. 283.
19. 12th Session of the WHO Regional Committee for South-East Asia, (New Delhi, 1959), Min. 1, Rev. 1, Annex. 2 (Text of Address of Shri S.W.R.D. Bandaranaike, Prime Minister of Ceylon).
20. 14th Session of the WHO Regional Committee for South-East Asia (New Delhi, 1961) Min. 1, Annex. 1 (Text of Address of Shri Bisnuram, Medhi, Governor of Madras).
21. 10th Session of the WHO Regional Committee for South-East Asia, (New Delhi, 1957) Min. I, Annex. I (Text of Address of the Prime Minister of Burma).
22. 23rd Session of the WHO Regional Committee for South-East Asia (New Delhi, 1970), p. 64 (Text of Address of Mr. K.K. Shah, Union Minister for Health and Family Planning, Works, Housing and Urban Development, Government of India).
23. WHO: SEARO Anniversary (Commemorative Meeting: Sept. 27), Text of Address of P. Dolgor, Director, Department of International Affairs, Ministry of Public Health, Ulan Bator.
24. SEA/RC/31, p. 57.
25. Stephen S. Goodsspeed, The Nature and Functions of International Organisation, New York, 1967, p. 632.
26. 27th Session of the WHO Regional Committee for South-East Asia, New Delhi, October, 1974.
27. WHO: SEARO, Fifty Years of WHO in South-East Asia, New Delhi, 1999, p. 106.
28. *Ibid.*

PART V

INNOVATION IN HEALTH AND HOSPITAL SERVICES

CHAPTER 18

ADMINISTRATION OF HOSPITAL SERVICES

"Today, a hospital is a place for the definition and treatment of human ills and restoration of health and well-beings of those temporarily deprived of these. A large number of professionally and technically skilled people apply their knowledge and skill with the help of complicated equipment and appliances to produce quality care for patient. The excellence of the product—the *raison d'etre* for a hospital, therefore, depends on how well the human and material resources are applied to promote patient care."

—Author

Administration of Hospital Services

A. NATURE, CLASSIFICATION AND INDICES FOR THE MEASUREMENT OR THE EFFICIENCY OF HOSPITAL

Nature

Since many health problems require a level of medical treatment and personal care that extends beyond the range of services normally available in the patient's home or in the office of the physician, modern society has developed formal institutions for patient care intended to help meet the more complex health needs of its members. The hospital, the major social institution for the delivery of health care in the modern world, offers considerable advantages to both patient and society. From the standpoint of individual, the sick or injured person has access to centralized medical knowledge and technology so as to render treatment much more thorough and efficient. From the standpoint of society, hospitalization both protects the family from many of the disruptive effects of caring for the ill in the home and operates as a means of guiding the sick and injured into medically supervised institutions where their problems are less disruptive for society as a whole.

Functions

(a) Patient Care

The first and foremost function of a hospital is to give care to the sick and injured and restore the health of diseased persons. Ethically, this care should be given to all without discrimination of social, economic or racial nature. However, the hospitals as national investments in people's health and as centres for scientific practice of medicine, must do many more things than 'produce' medical care. The success with which a hospital contributes towards meeting the patient's need can be measured by the fullness of the life he is able to lead on leaving it.

(b) Training

The education and training of doctors and nurses have traditionally been carried out in hospitals. It is a workshop wherein the student learns by seeing what his superiors and peers do. Radiology, laboratory, radiotherapy, highly advanced surgical techniques demand a variety of skills and knowledge, all of which cannot be mastered by the doctor specialist. These activities have created the need for a large number of skilled technicians who are today the vital support to the specialist whether he is the surgeon, physician, diagnostician or therapeutist. These people are indispensable for the all-round excellence of all specialist work. To develop these technical skills, a programme should be organized by the hospital under the direction of people who have the required experience, knowledge and aptitude to teach others. The purpose of in-service education and training programme is to develop such knowledge and skills in all categories of para-medical personnel as are required to make them fit for the job they hold and keep them attuned to the growing needs of their jobs.

(c) Medical Research

The third important function of hospital is to give support to medical research. A good hospital, where the quality of professional work is excellent, is an ideal ground for medical research. As a matter of fact, excellent professional care of patients largely results from the fruits of research into new problems. An attitude of enquiry and investigation should permeate through the day-to-day care of patients. The hospital can develop facilities for research with comparative ease and speed if the staff and administration are properly motivated. True, elaborate research is expensive. There, nevertheless, remain clinical investigations of applied nature that call for little capital investment. Responsibility for creation of new knowledge is that of any enlightened profession. It is in a hospital that opportunities exist, if not abound, for organized as well as individual initiative for research.

(d) Health Education

The fourth and final object is to support and assist all activities carried out by various public health and voluntary agencies to prevent disease and promote positive health attitudes in the community through health education. Health education, immunization, social and economic rehabilitation are some of the many activities for which the hospital may provide assistance in terms of physical facilities and advisory services to staff. As a matter of fact, in the western countries, this aspect of the hospital as a community health centre is being emphasized more and more. Many ways are being devised to integrate the hospital with the activities of community health agencies.

The main function of a hospital is to promote the health of the community which it serves. Hospitals in the past were set-up primarily as charity institutions for poor and weaker sections of society. These were considered as alms houses. The only function of such institutions was the care of the sick and the poor. The hospital was considered only a shelter for the socially unfit. Hospitals are being re-oriented from just being the centres for medical care and treatment to hospitals which are supposed to provide comprehensive system of preventive and curative medicine and rehabilitation services. It has been stated in a WHO document that the hospital is an integral part of a social and medical organisation, the function of which is to provide for the population, complete health care, both curative and preventive, and whose out-patient services reach out to the family in its home environment; the hospital is also a centre for the training of health workers and for bio-social research[1] and "an institution that provides in-patient accommodation for medical and nursing care." The hospital has a noble purpose expressed in the phrase "Promotion of health and welfare of the people." Hospitals have now become indispensable to the proper care of the broad spectrum of health problems.

In the dynamic society, the hospital occupies a unique place to accommodate explosion of science into medicine and the whole galaxy of new treatment techniques, new equipment and proliferation of services which have made a profound impact on the provision of care facilities and services. Besides this, the development of socio-politico, cultural and educational systems have made the people conscious of their rights and they demand that modern and best means of medical and health care be made available to them; not only within the four walls of the hospital but at their doorstep or in the vicinity of living places. These impacts had made a hospital a complex organisation.[2]

Administration of such a complex organisation requires blending of technical and administrative competence in the right quantity, at the right time, at the right place, by the right man and in the right way or process. Each hospital is a distinct entity and as such each has to be tailored to the specific aims to be accomplished, the specific tasks to be performed, the volume of services to be rendered and the type of the community to be served. The basic purpose of the hospital is "better patient care" and return the patient back to the community as a productive unit of that community. Hospital administration is an activity to secure better output through optimum utilisation of inputs.

Classification of Hospitals

Each hospital is distinct in its characteristics as it differs in structure, functions, performance and the community it serves. However, we can classify the hospitals into different types depending upon different criteria.

According to the objectives, hospitals can be classified into three categories:

1. Teaching-cum-Research Hospitals

The main objective of these hospitals is teaching based on research and the provision of health care is secondary, e.g., All-India Institute of Medical Sciences, New Delhi, Post-Graduate Medical Education and Research Institute, Chandigarh.

2. General Hospitals

The main objective of these hospitals is to provide medical care to the people while teaching and research is secondary and incidental, e.g., district or taluka hospital, PHCs.

3. Special Hospitals

These hospitals concentrate on a particular aspect or organ of the body and provide medical care in that field e.g., Cancer, Dental, Psychiatry Hospitals, T.B. Hospitals, etc.

On the basis of ownership, hospitals can be classified into four categories:

1. Government Hospitals
2. Semi-Government Hospitals
3. Voluntary Agencies' Hospitals
4. Private/Charitable Hospitals.

According to the system of medicine we can have the following categories:

1. Allopathic Hospitals
2. Ayurvedic Hospitals
3. Homoeopathic Hospitals
4. Unani Hospitals
5. Hospitals of other systems of medicine.

Classification According to the Size

One of the major recommendations of the Health Survey and Development Committee (Bhore Committee) was the setting up of Peripheral Health Centres catering to a population of 40,000 each, which were to be linked up with secondary health centres and hospitals for purposes of referral services. In 1962, the Mudaliar Committee went further into this problem. The infrastructure for the delivery of health and medical care has closely followed the recommendations of these committees. However, the Government felt it necessary to set-up a study group on hospitals in 1966. This group submitted its report in 1968.

The group found that out of 335 districts in the country, only 125 had more than 200-bed hospitals, and out of 3,000 taluks, only 2,053 had hospitals. However, out of 5,080 primary health centres planned for the country, 4,973 were found to be established. It also found that there was unequal distribution of hospitals in various areas of the country. It recommended that the following pattern of development for hospitals be adopted:

Teaching Hospitals	500 (to be increased according to the number of students).
District Hospitals	200 (may be raised upto 300 beds depending on population).
Tehsil/Taluk Hospitals	50 (may be raised depending on population).
Primary Health Centres	6 (may be increased to 10 depending on needs).

The bed strength of 125 districts which have at least one 200-beds hospital may be raised to 300 depending on the population served. In the remaining 210 districts, hospitals having less than 200 beds, the strength should be raised to a minimum of 200 beds. Ordinarily, the distribution of these beds should be as under:

Medical	60
Surgical	40
Gynaecology and Obstetrics including Maternity	35
Paediatrics	15
Orthopaedics	5
Eye	10
ENT	10
Skin	5
Emergency	5
Isolation	10
Psychiatry	5
	200

Since the district hospital is to serve as a referral centre it should provide specialist services in Medicine, Surgery, Obstetrics, Gynaecology, Eye, ENT, Paediatrics, Dentistry, Psychiatry, VD, T.B. Clinic, etc.

The staff norms as fixed by the Government for the different kinds of hospitals in India are as under:[3]

Sr. No.	*Name of the Post*	*No. of Posts (norms)*
	50-BED HOSPITAL	
1.	Medical Officer PCMS I	1
2.	Medical Officer PCMS II (including one Female)	2
3.	PJMS	—
4.	Dental Surgeon	1

5. Pharmacists	3
6. Nursing Sister	1
7. Staff Nurses/ANMS	8
8. Lab. Technician (Grade I), Lab. Technician (Grade II)	1
9. Radiographer	1
10. Clerk-*cum*-Storekeeper	1
11. Cooks	2
12. Mali	1
13. Dhobi	2
14. Class IV including Sweepers	17

100-BED HOSPITAL

1. Medical Officer PCMS I	1
2. Medical Officer PCMS II	3
3. Dental Surgeon	1
4. Anaesthetist	1
5. Radiologist	1
6. Pathologist	1
7. Casualty Medical Officers	3
8. House Surgeons	5
9. Matron	1
10. Nursing Sisters	4
11. Staff Nurses	20
12. Pharmacists	5
13. Storekeepers	2
14. Clerks	4
15. Accountant	1
16. Lab. Technician Grade I	2
17. Lab. Technician Grade II	
18. Lab. Attendant	1
19. Cooks	2
20. Helper	2
21. Radiographer	1
22. Carpenter/Painter	1
23. Chowkidar	3
24. Class IV including Sweepers	50
25. Biochemist	—
26. Operation Room Asstt.	2
27. Cashier	1
28. Head Clerk	1
29. Electrician	1
30. Plumber	1

200-BED HOSPITAL

Post	Number
1. Medical Officer PCMS I	2
2. Medical Officer PCMS II	4
3. Anaesthetist	1
4. Pathologist	1
5. Radiologist	1
6. Biochemist	1
7. Dental Surgeon	1
8. Casualty Medical Officers	3
9. House Surgeons	10
10. Matron	1
11. Nursing Sisters	10
12. Staff Nurses	32
13. Radiographer	1
14. Pharmacists	5
15. Lab. Asstt. Grade I	4
16. Lab. Asstt. Grade II	
17. Lab. Attendants	2
18. Dietician	1
19. Cooks	4
20. Head Cook	1
21. Stenographer	1
22. Accountant	1
23. Storekeepers	2
24. Clerks	2
25. Dental Mechanic	1
26. Carpenter/Painter	1
27. Caretaker/Steward	1
28. Chowkidar	3
29. Mali	2
30. Other Class IV posts including Sweepers	81
31. Registrar	—
32. Hawaldar	—
33. Assistant Matron	1
34. Cashier	1
35. Head Clerk	1
36. Operation Room Assistants	2
37. Electrician	1
38. Barber	—
39. Plumber	1

Indices for Measuring the Efficiency of a Hospital

It is very difficult to measure the efficiency of a hospital because of the complex nature of problems that it entails. There are many indices which can help us in evaluation of its quantitative performance. But, what about quality? It can be ascertained only through specially designed surveys. These surveys may be conducted both by persons inside the organisation and outside the organisation to locate the problems and suggest remedies for its future performance. Very few studies are available which have been conducted in this field. The studies carried out by NIHFW on different aspects of hospital administration throw light on various issues. Besides, the Committees of Parliament have done a useful work in analysing the performance of the All-India Institute of Medical Sciences and the three hospitals of Delhi. Research institutions and the universities should take interest and help the hospital management to their services. We mention below some of the indices which are commonly used to measure the efficiency of hospitals:

1. $$\text{Bed occupancy ratio} = \frac{\text{Number of patient-days' during the year} \times 100}{\text{Number of bed-days during the year}}$$

This ratio tells us to how far the available bed capacity has been utilised.

2. $$\text{Average duration of illness} = \frac{\text{The Number of patient-days' during the year}}{\text{Total number of in-patient admissions during the year}}$$

The index is complementary to the other index 'average turn-over interval'. This is more useful if computed for individual diseases.

3. $$\text{Turn-over interval} = \frac{\text{The total vacant bed-days during the year}}{\text{The number of in-patients' admission during the year}}$$

The index indicates the number of days on an average per patient for which a bed has been remained unused.

4. $$\text{The average out-patient admission} = \frac{\text{The total number of out-patients during the year}}{\text{The total number of out-patients admissions during the year}}$$

5. $$\text{Average daily out-patient admissions} = \frac{\text{The total number of out-patients during the year}}{\text{The total number of new out-patients admissions during the year}}$$

The index tells the average workload on OPD.

6. $$\text{Cost of daily diet} = \frac{\text{Total expenditure on diet during the year}}{\text{Total number of in-patient days}}$$

$$7.\ \text{Average cost of medicine} = \frac{\text{Total cost of medicines for in-patients for the year}}{\text{Total number of in-patients' admissions}}$$

$$8.\ \text{Fatality rate} = \frac{\text{No. of in-patients' deaths during the specified period} \times 100}{\text{No. of discharges during the same period}}$$

$$9.\ \text{Autopsy rate} = \frac{\text{No. of autopsies performed} \times 100}{\text{No. of in-patients' deaths}}$$

Staff Services and Auxiliary Services

These are explained with the help of a Chart (Fig. 18.1). Let us discuss some of these services to understand the mechanics of hospital administration.

B. ASPECTS OF HOSPITAL SERVICES

The services provided in a hospital differ from one hospital to another. It is very difficult to discuss all these services here. We can classify these services into three categories e.g., Line services, Supporting Services and Auxiliary Services.

Line Services

(a) Emergency Services (Casualty Services)

The casualty department provides round-the-clock, immediate diagnosis and treatment for illness of an urgent nature and injuries from accidents. Simple cases after administering preliminary treatment are discharged with instructions to attend OPD as a follow-up measure. Cases of serious nature are admitted in emergency wards to provide immediate medical care. Such patients are either discharged after 2-3 days or are transferred to permanent in-patient wards. Emergency service is acquiring increasing importance due to modern problems arising out of urbanisation and mechanisation. The best services must be provided to the patients in the Emergency wards as the patients and their relatives are under emotional strain and surcharged with suspense and anxiety about the consequences of the disease or calamity that has come up suddenly. Such an approach would alleviate a large part of sufferings born out of fear and suspicion of the unknown. The Public Accounts Committee (1977-78) suggested that—

> In order that the emergencies are attended to quickly and effectively, it is necessary to have an efficient set-up, well-knit with other departments of the hospitals with well laid-out procedure and work distribution.

FIG. 18.1

Procedure in an Emergency Service

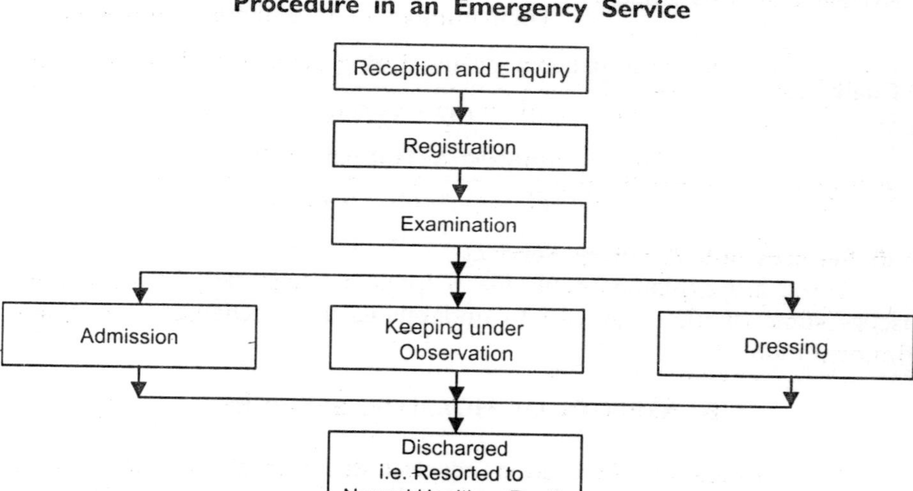

(b) Out-Patient Services

The out-patient department is one of the most important department. All the patients suffering from diseases of minor, serious, acute and chronic nature are examined. It should be designed to provide services to one per cent of the population of the area. It should be large enough to avoid congestion. The functions of the out-patient services are—provision of diagnostic, curative, preventive and rehabilitative services on an ambulatory basis. We can explain the whole process with the help of a flow diagram (Fig. 18.2).

Out-patient department should be so planned that the building is separate from the indoor area. It should be well connected to the laboratories, X-ray department and other supportive services. It should have enough accommodation to avoid congestion. Depending upon the size of the hospital and resources available separate areas of examination for the specialists should be provided.

(c) In-Patient Services (Wards)

After the patient has been examined in the OPD or the emergency area, he may be advised admission in the wards. Wards are of different types—open general wards (rows of beds in a big ward area), 4-5 bed units, and private wards for paying patients. Each ward has generally a doctor's duty room, dressing room, central Nursing Staff Station and other essential items needed for patient care. The departments to which direct patient access should be provided are the operating theatre suite, X-ray and physical medicine departments. The pharmacy and pathology departments should also be readily accessible from the wards for the convenience of the staff.

FIG. 18.2

Procedure of an OPD

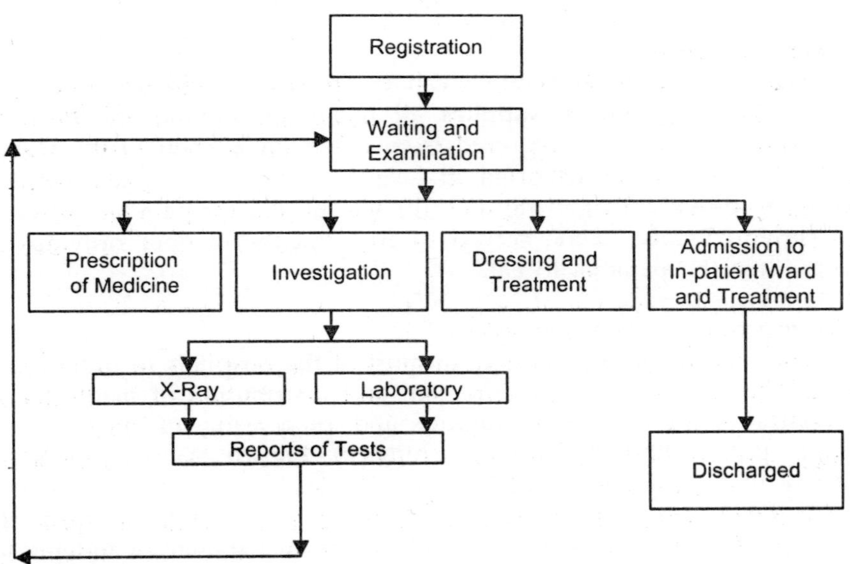

(d) Intensive-Care Unit

Some of the patients admitted to hospitals require acute, multi-disciplinary and intensive observation and treatment, e.g., patients of shock, coma, heart attack, lung, kidney, brain diseases, etc. It is desirable to have an intensive-care unit for such patients. Like the emergency services, this requires much better staffing pattern—one nurse for 1½ beds per shift. The staff needs to be specially trained to work in this area. This is very costly and should be set-up only at the apex-hospitals.

(e) Operation Theatres

Each operating room set should have a pre-anaesthesia room and sterilisation room and a scrub room for nurses and doctors. There is a trend to provide simple laboratory facilities within the operating area to serve the purpose during emergency.

Supportive Services

(a) Central Sterile Supply Services Management

The Central Sterile Supply Department is supposed to store, sterilise, maintain and issue those instruments, materials and garments which are required to be sterile. This requirement may steadily decrease as the use of disposable items becomes more economical. The Central Sterile Supply Department should have direct lines of communication with all wards, operation threatres, out-patient and casualty departments, and to a lesser extent, with X-ray and pathology departments. Air control in this department is essential to check contamination through air. Proper control with indicators for sterilisation procedures is essential.

(b) Diet Management

The catering department, which comprises the kitchen, bulk-food stores and dining rooms, supplies all meals throughout the hospital. Direct and easy access is required from the main kitchen to the wards. The food should be transported in heated trolleys. This department is required to provide: (i) general diet, (b) special diet for patients suffering from certain diseases. Food served in an attractive manner provides an incentive for the patients to eat.

(c) Pharmaceutical Services Management

The pharmaceutical services in most of the hospitals in India today represent the functions of procurement and distribution of medicaments by medical store and compounding and dispensing of medicine on doctor's prescription by persons hitherto known as compounders, generally under the control of Medical Officers.

In OPD, drugs are distributed on prescription while in wards the drugs are sent either on indents collecting for all patients; or indents for individual patient. Besides, every good hospital has a manufacturing section for various formulations and intravenous fluids.

(d) Laundry

There is a need for an efficient mechanical laundry to ensure the availability of bacteria-free washed linen. The small hospitals may get the cleaning done from washermen with due care and supervision. The aim is to make available to the patients clean and disinfected linen.

(e) Laboratory and X-Ray Facilities

For proper diagnosis of ailments of patients it is necessary to have diagnostic laboratory facility properly manned. The success of medical prescription depend upon proper laboratory diagnosis. Laboratories for routine blood, urine, microbiology, X-ray, etc., should provide round-the-clock service. It is desirable to locate the laboratory block and X-ray block in between the OPD and indoor area to be able to serve both the areas.

We must ensure that the technicians are really doing the job because a minor mistake on their part may ruin the life of the patients. There is a need for constant supervision over the functioning of these laboratory services.

(f) Nursing Services

Nursing services should be managed by a matron who is assisted by a sister in-charge of the wards and staff nurses. Nursing sisters control the ward and arrange the leave day off of nurses. The accepted norms by Indian Nursing Council for a general ward is one staff nurse per live beds. This norm is never achieved in practice resulting in poor service. Besides, nurses are engaged in non-nursing activities which results in poor service to the patients. The Public Accounts Committee was critical of Nursing Services in three hospitals of Delhi. The Committee remarked:

> In view of the fact that the nurse-patient ratio excluding the specialised departments, is 1:33 in the Safdarjung Hospital and 1:19 in the Willingdon Hospital as against the ideal ratio of 1:5, the Committee feels that there is considerable shortage of nurses for manning the emergency and casualty services in the three hospitals.

The same situation prevails in most of the hospitals.

Auxiliary Services

(a) Registration and Indoor Case Records

Registration is a must for a hospital to enrol new patients with proper entry in OPD cards and keep track of the revisits of the patients. Medical records help in regulating admission of patients. It helps in codifying the record according to internal disease index. It also collects statistics of hospital stay of patients, i.e., admission, discharge, average stay, etc., for future planning and management. According to Calender:

> The hospital's admission procedure should be such that the patient is made to feel welcome and secure. Every employee who comes in contact with the patient should make him feel that each one is genuinely interested in his welfare. This experience is the patient's first introduction to the hospital and should be a pleasant one.[4]

(b) Stores

The Central Store receives, stores and issues bulk items which can, with advantage, be stored centrally. Stores are of different types—Pharmacy Stores, Chemical Stores, Linen Stores, Surgical Stores, Glassware Stores. Stock policy should be devised in such a way that vital and essential items are always available. It should be managed by a competent stores officer.

(c) Transport

Transport requirements for the carriage of supplies and patients are:

(a) Trolleys;
(b) Stretchers; and
(c) Wheel chairs.

FIG. 18.3

Aspects of Hospital Services

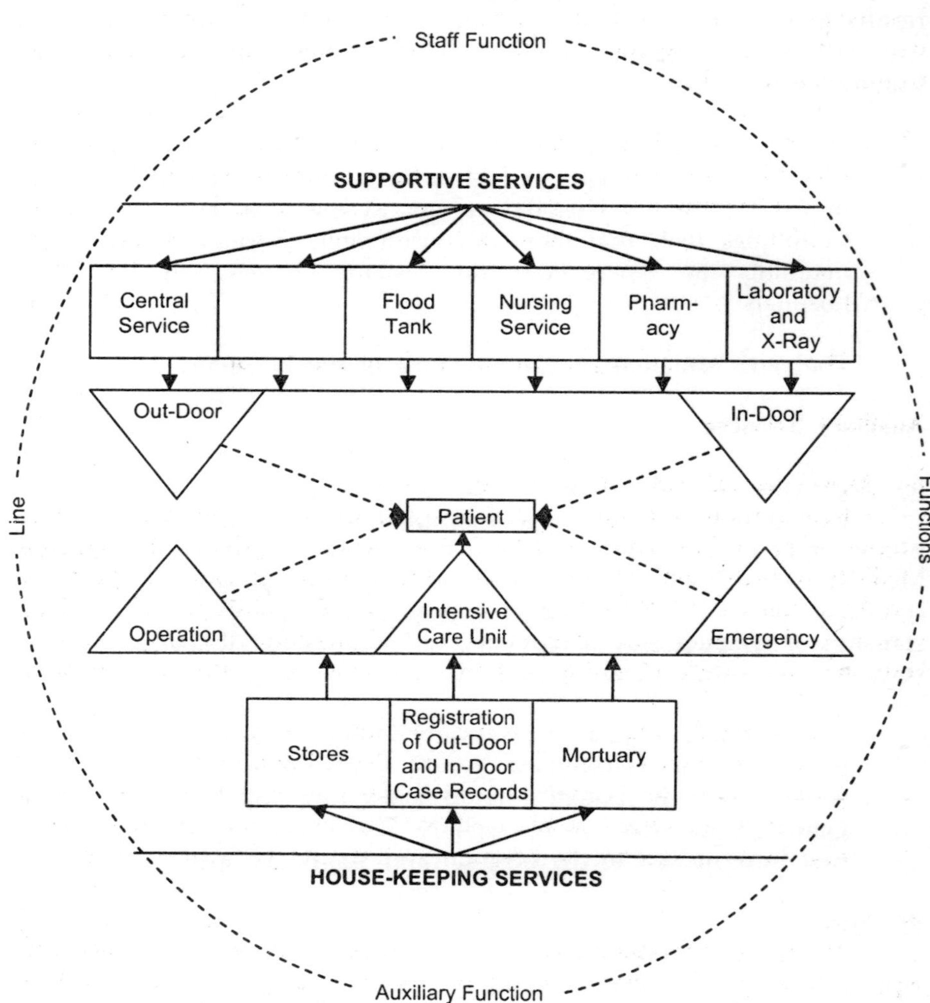

It is preferable to have a central transport gang to shift the patients. Supplies should also be distributed to all wards by the central areas.

(d) Mortuary

Each hospital should have a cold storage area or mortuary where dead bodies are kept before they are claimed by the relations. Sometimes post-mortems need to be done for medico-legal reasons. Unclaimed bodies should be disposed-off according to rules.

C. BRIEF DESCRIPTIONS OF SOME HOSPITALS OF DIFFERENT KINDS AND SYSTEMS

(i) Teaching-cum-Research Hospitals

Every teaching institution has an attached hospital which provides clinical material for teaching and training of the students. Such hospitals also provide facilities for research both for the teachers and the taught.

The method of treating a patient in a teaching-*cum*-research hospital varies from that available in a general hospital. In the case of the former, apart from treatment, the patient is used for teaching and research. Here the patient is first handled by a trainee who examines him thoroughly, records his detailed history and suggests the diagnosis and treatment. The case is then presented by the trainee to the teacher (called consultant) who goes through the history recorded by the trainee and also examines the patient. The treatment is prescribed only by the consultant. In this way the patient, besides receiving treatment also acts as 'material' for teaching. He is used for research by the teachers and the taught. It has to be accepted that the treatment in a teaching-*cum*-research institute takes more time than in a general hospital.

Let us describe briefly Post-Graduate Institute of Medical Education and Research, Chandigarh, to understand the organisation and working of such hospitals.

The Post-Graduate Institute of Medical Education and Research, Chandigarh, was established by the Government of Punjab in 1962. It was declared an institution of national importance by an Act of Parliament with effect from April 1967.

The PGIMER, Chandigarh offers 68 different courses leading to the award of degrees of B.Sc., M.Sc., M.D., M.S., M.Ch., D.M., M.D.S. and Ph.D., etc. As on 31 March 1982, a total of 1,671 residents completed their training and obtained their post-graduate qualifications. The Nehru Hospital attached to the institute has a bed strength of 774. During the year 1981-82, the registration of in-patients and out-patients was 25,403 and 5,67,726 respectively.

The administration of the institute including the Nehru Hospital is under the control of a Director, who is assisted by the Dean (for teaching purposes) and the Medical Superintendent (administrative purposes).

(ii) General Hospital

The main function of the general hospital is to provide treatment to the patient. No detailed history of the illness of the patient is recorded. Here the medical officer hears a verbal account of the illness of the patient, examines him and prescribes the treatment. The treatment is quick and less time-consuming. The only disadvantage of this system of treatment is that sometimes the serious illness may go undiagnosed properly.

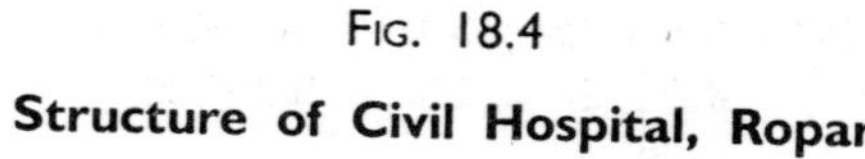

FIG. 18.4

Structure of Civil Hospital, Ropar

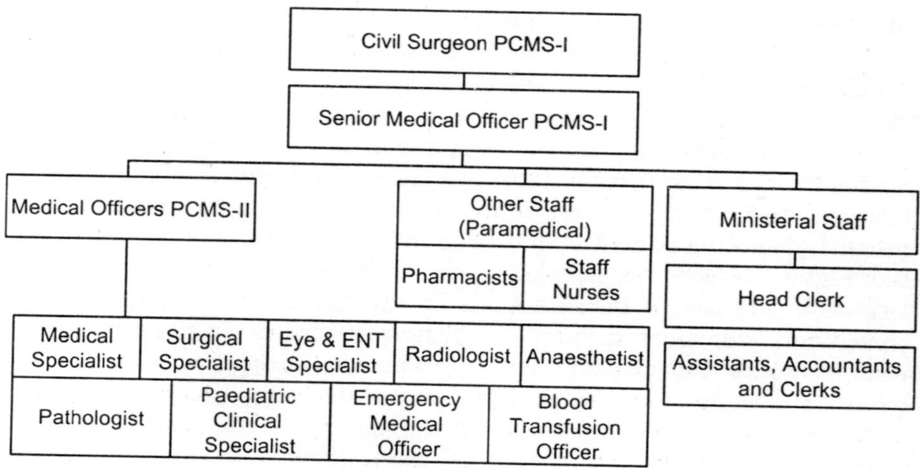

Let us describe a Government General Hospital with reference to Civil Hospital, Ropar (Punjab). It is a 100-bed hospital (56 male and 44 female) with a provision for 10 extra beds. It provides the following special services:

Speciality	*Bed Strength*
Medical	30
Surgery	30
Eye	10
Paediatrics	10
Obstetrics and Gynaecology	20

It has been provided with all the facilities which can serve the patients.

The affairs of the hospital are managed by the Chief Medical Officer (PCMS Class I); who has under him 12 Doctors, 5 Pharmacists, Radiographer/X-ray Assistant, 4 Laboratory Technicians, 1 Matron, 2 Nursing sisters, 10 staff nurses. Besides, there are 10 members belonging to ministerial staff, 53 belonging to Class IV, one carpenter, one driver, one plumber and one electrician.

We shall explain in the next chapter the working of Primary Health Centres in detail which are like mini-general hospitals.

(iii) Working of the Special Hospitals

We shall explain this with the help of Chest Diseases Hospital, Patiala and the Punjab Mental Hospital, Amritsar.

Chest Diseases Hospital at Patiala

The hospital was started with the name, T.B. Clinic, in 1949, with ten beds only. It has been named as Chest Diseases Hospital. It has been serving as Training and Demonstration Centre as well since 1962. The hospital is under the control of Director of Research and Medical Education, Punjab. The day-to-day affairs of the hospital are looked after by the Deputy Medical Superintendent. The details can be seen from the Organisational Chart (Fig. 18.5).

Services

The hospital provides patient care—out-door as well as in-door. It also provides community health services at all levels, i.e., (a) Primary prevention, (b) Secondary prevention, (c) Tertiary prevention.

(a) BCG Vaccination is given to each child immediately after birth.
(b) The hospital has got mobile team, mobile X-ray plant and they move to places where they can detect cases. Such as at fairs where the public is gathered, at factories, industries, camps, schools, etc., through survey and screening of all the population.
(c) For this rehabilitation services are available. Rehabilitation includes everything that is done for the patient.

It also serves as educational centre and provides:

(i) Integration of tuberculosis course. In the general nursing 'A' Grade Diploma Programme.
(ii) Tuberculosis course for the medical students.
(iii) House job facilities for medical group.
(iv) T.B. health visitors' training.
(v) Multi-purpose worker's training.

(iv) Punjab Mental Hospital at Amritsar (See Fig. 18.6)

The Punjab Mental Hospital, Amritsar, was set-up in 1949 with 50 beds. The present strength is 811 (512 male and 299 female). Treatment facilities are available at three levels in this hospital as given below:

(a) The in-doors: Certified patients are admitted at the in-doors of this hospital from the states of Punjab, Haryana, Himachal Pradesh and the Union Territory of Chandigarh.
(b) The Out-Patient Department: Consultation facilities for the patients coming from Punjab, Haryana, Himachal Pradesh, Union Territory of Chandigarh and adjoining areas of Uttar Pradesh and Rajasthan are provided at the out-patient department.

FIG. 18.5

Organisation of the Chest Disease Institute, Patiala

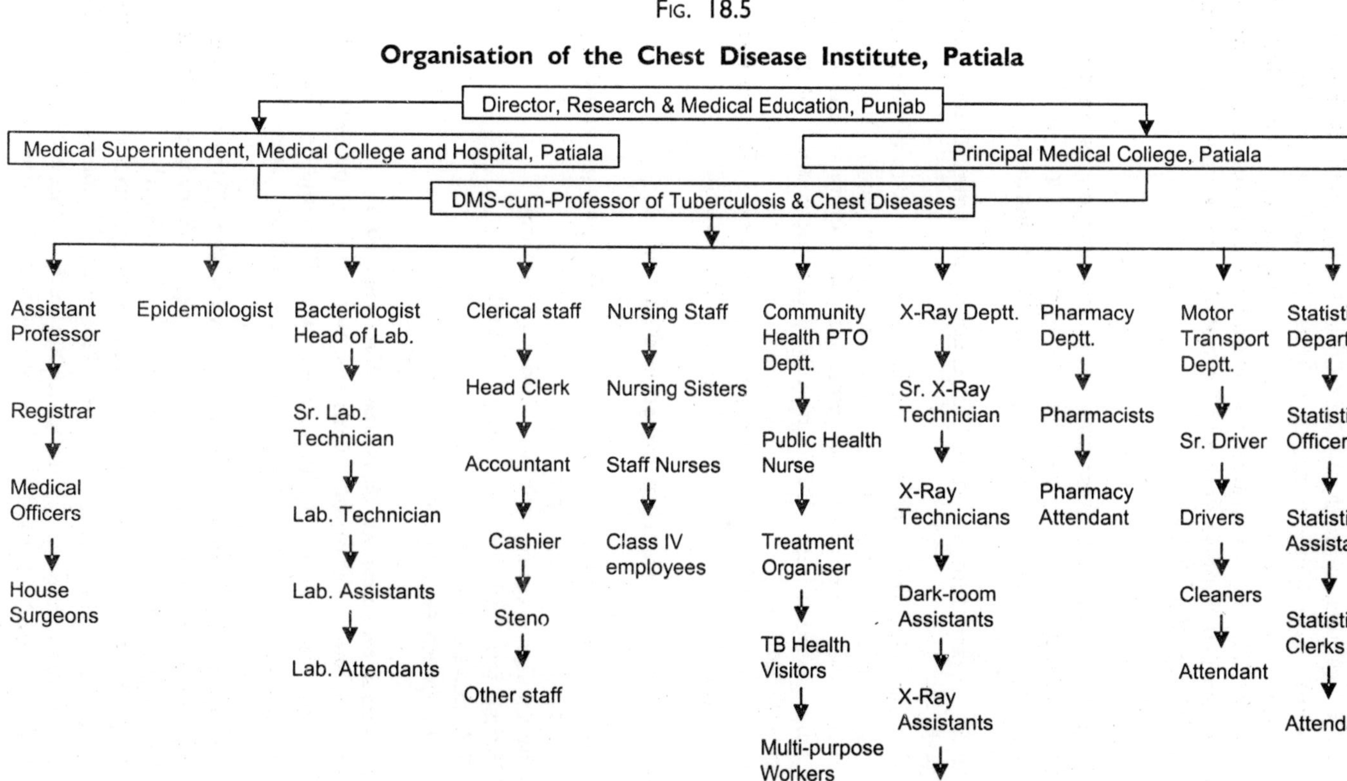

Fig. 18.6

Structure of Punjab Mental Hospital, Amritsar

Medical Superintendent PCMS-I
Deputy Medical Superintendent PCMS-I
Senior Medical Superintendent PCMS-I
Assistant Medical Superintendent PCMS-II
Senior Registrar Administrative Wing PCMS-II
Head Clerk
Assistant Store Keeper and Clerks
1. Overseers Sub-overseers and Warden Overseers
2. Ward Supervisors
3. Physical Training Instructors
4. Weavers, Tailors and Blacksmith
5. Teachers: Art, Craft & Music
Medical Wing PCMS-II
Medical Officer
Psychiatry Wing
Psychiatric Social Worker
Psychology Wing
Clinical Psychologist
Occupational Therapy Wing
Chief Occupational Therapists, Occupational Therapists and Junior Occupational Therapists
Other Paramedical Staff
Pharmacists Staff Nurses, Male Nurses, Sanitary Inspector

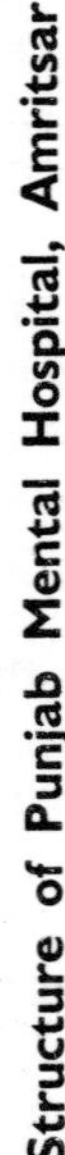

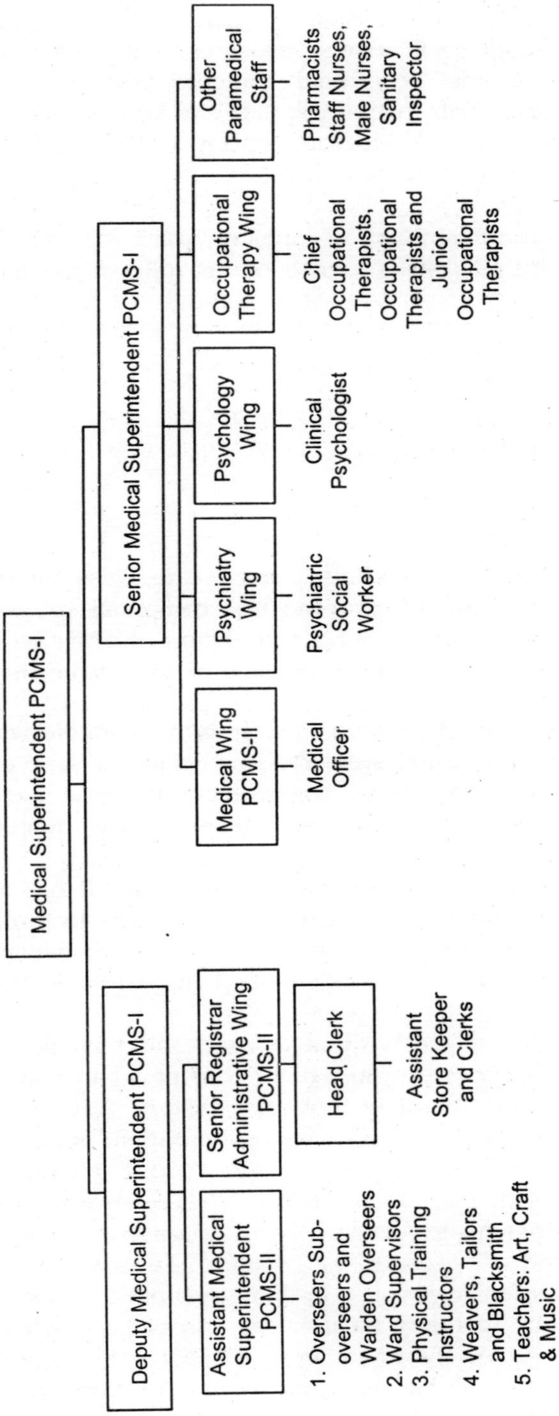

(c) The Family Care Unit: This unit consisting of 70 ward-beds and 30 single-seat rooms provides intensive psychiatric treatment to the uncertified patients who need a short duration admission in the hospital. The unit is managed by a team consisting of 1 Medical Officer, 1 Clinical Psychologist and a Psychiatric Trained Nurse.

The hospital administration is looked after by the Medical Superintendent. The hospital staff consists of the following categories of employees:

Category of staff	*Sanctioned Posts*
Class I	6
Class II	8
Class III	83
Class IV	141
Wardens	332

The hospital besides providing patient care, also serves as a training centre for medical and para-medical personnel in psychiatry, clinical psychology, psychiatric nursing and mental health. Besides, the faculty carries out research on various aspects of mental health

(v) Working of a Hospital (Homoeopathic System of Medicine)

Hospitals in the traditional system of medicine are simple as they do not require costly equipments to diagnose the ailments. Let us now describe the working of a teaching-*cum*-patient care homoeopathic institution located at Chandigarh.

It was set-up in 1974 under private management. It has a faculty consisting of 13 staff members—1 principal, 9 whole-time lecturers and 3 part-time lecturers belonging to the western system of medicine. The intake capacity of the college is 50 students and the course is of 4 years' duration.

The college serves as the hospital as well and provides both in-patient and out-patient services. The patient first of all is registered by the registration clerk who maintains the case history (backbone of the system) of the patients. After the registration, the patient is examined by the doctors/faculty members on duty. It takes about half an hour to record the case history of the patient. There is no referral system, since every doctor is competent to deal with all diseases as there is no classification of individual diseases, e.g., Cancer, Tuberculosis, etc. The chronic cases are admitted to provide in-door treatment. It has a simple laboratory structure and operation theatre. There is no para-medical staff.

The hospital is visited by about 35 to 80 new patients and 100 to 150 old patients per day. It has 25 beds located in three rooms. The patients are administered medicine through a dispensary. Besides, there is a pharmacy section for the formulation of medicine.

The cost of such a hospital is negligible compared to that of hospitals based on the western system of medicine The setting up of such hospitals would lower the cost of medical care and would supplement the efforts of allopathic system of medicine.

(vi) Working of an Ayurvedic Hospital/Dispensary

The Ayurvedic system of medicine is also very simple. After the registration, the patients are examined by the doctor on duty. The patients are treated on the philosophy of *vayu*, *pitta* and *kapha*. We discuss now the working of an Ayurvedic dispensary located in Sector 37, Chandigarh, under the control of the government.

It has 2 doctors—one male and one female. Both are qualified. They have G.A.M.S./B.A.M.S. degrees. The patients are first of all registered by the Registration clerk and, thereafter, examined by one of the two doctors. It takes about 3-5 minutes to examine the patient. The doctors are taking the help of the stethoscope, manometer, etc. After the examination the medicines are prescribed. The patient gets free available medicines from the dispensary while he has to buy the rest from the market. There is no surgery and referral system. About 60 to 90 new patients and 150 to 200 old patients visit the hospital daily.

The big Ayurvedic hospitals have in-door facilities as well, e.g., the hospital at Patiala has 100 beds.

These hospitals are very easy to operate and involve negligible expenditure. The government should encourage such hospitals to reduce the rising cost of medical care.

D. WORKING OF HOSPITALS

Hospitals are providing medical care only to those who approach them. Hospitals are not serving as the centres of total health care—preventive, curative, promotive and rehabilitative. Hospitals have poor linkages with the community and the family. They are providing expensive medical care and not comprehensive health care. The hospital has been described by Dorothea Sick as a "Self-chosen ghetto of the medical profession" and modern doctors as "Professional Cripples" useless without a hospital. Physicians in developing countries become estranged from their own people in the course of their training. The ablest men and women are not tackling the most acute and difficult problems.[5] Besides, the faith of the people in the efficiency of hospital system is decreasing because of the negligence and indifference on the part of hospital authorities. Lawrence J. Sakarai is very critical of the role of most of the doctors in a hospital. He feels, barring some dedicated doctors, most of them are ruthless and says:

He (Doctor) exploits the gullible, conspires against the sick and

> cares little for medicine unless it makes him money . . . He could murder you through indifference, drugs or just sheer inefficiency all by masquerading under the garb of an ancient oath rendered superfluous in the business of our times.[6]

Dr. W.V. Rajan in his article, 'Men, Medicine and Misadventure' in *The Tribune* (Nov. 25, 1979), rightly mentioned that,

> "It is an unedifying fact, that we have no accurate recorded data on the occurrence and incidence of misadventures in drug administration, diagnostic procedures and surgical operation in hospitals . . . . In a complex hospital, negligence becomes error, scientific detachment and incompetence becomes a lack of specialised equipments . . . . Medicine is still not an exact science in spite of the great advances in bio-chemical sciences. It is imperative for doctors, nurses and para-medical personnel to exhibit utmost precaution, care, judgement and skill in dealing with and treating patients, balancing the relative risk of the disease with the risk involved in the use of drugs, surgery or diagnostic procedures, apart from the cost-benefit consideration."

What can be done to prevent the erosion of the values among the medical professions? What can we do to maintain the confidence of the people in the hospital services? How can we improve the functioning of the hospital system? How can we coordinate the functioning of hospitals? How can we check the rising costs of hospital services? These questions are being raised even in the context of the developed world. The 1968 report of the Secretary's Advisory Committee on hospital effectiveness, US Department of Health, Education and Welfare, Washington, D.C., emphasised the need to improve the internal efficiency of the hospital as a functioning mechanism to provide decent health care to all. We shall discuss in the following pages the answers to these questions. The analysis is based upon the already published documents especially the reports of the Parliamentary Committee and the personal discussion of the author with the health experts, general administrators and the beneficiaries of the hospital services.

Improving Patient-Satisfaction and Harmonious Relationship between the Patients/Relatives and Hospital Authorities

Hospitals should try to establish cordial, equitable and, therefore, mutually profitable relations between the hospitals and their beneficiaries. The patients mostly complain of discourteous behaviour of hospital staff especially at the lower level . . . This irritates the patients and their relatives. The test of the efficiency of a hospital is the satisfaction of the beneficiaries. The sympathetic and courteous behaviour of hospital staff would have a soothing and lasting effect on the patients and their relatives. It is suggested that all hospital personnel must inspire confidence and put the nervous patients and their relatives at ease.

> The hospital today is more than the combination of medical and therapeutic treatment by specialists, greater and refined medical and surgical knowledge and ever better and more effective facilities and equipment. It includes these factors as the core of its efficient operation but an additional dimension—one which is too often ignored or at least minimised—is the human and social element in the structure of the organisation.[7]

The ideal of service must be encouraged among the personnel responsible for health care. It is the responsibility of the hospital authorities to set the pattern for the philosophy of patient care. It was rightly mentioned by Gardner that,

> No society can reach heights of greatness unless in all fields critical to its growth and creativity there is an ample supply of dedicated men and women.[8]

Most of the patients complained of a great distance between the doctors and the patients. This gap between the doctors and the patients must be bridged through personal attention given by the doctors to the patients. According to K.G. Agarwal, "Hospital effectiveness which can be measured in terms of patient satisfaction does not depend on the improvement of hospital service aspect alone but on the medical care aspect. Hospital effectiveness has a positive association with the hospital social system. The hospital social system is almost the measure of its organisational health . . . some element of democracy must be introduced in the hospitals. This might take care of the alienation of hospital staff that we see all around these."[9] K.K. Kaul, Professor and Head, Smt. Patel Paediatric Centre, Government Medical College, Jabalpur (M.P.), has rightly said,

> To restore their reputation, hospitals need to develop a strong system of public relations and intimate involvement with the community they serve.[10]

Besides these, there are other areas which must be attended to by hospital authorities to build the image of the hospitals. The most irritating factor for the dissatisfaction of the patients is that they have to wait for a long time in the out-patient departments because of the poor planning and management of hospitals. Most of the studies conducted in this regard found the time to be excessive and intolerable, i.e., varying between 2 to 3 hours per patient. The Public Accounts Committee remarked that,

> Although certain delays are inherent in the situation and thus are inevitable, yet to a certain extent these can be overcome by rationalising the existing procedures and strengthening the organisations where necessary.

The patients also complain of the preferential treatment being given to VIPs and influential people. Some of the patients were of the view that these big hospitals are meant only to serve the VIPs. B.L. Agnihotri, in a letter to *The Tribune*, mentioned about the unsatisfactory conditions in hospitals in Himachal Pradesh. He mentioned that,

> After waiting for two hours we were told by some interns that senior doctors were not concerned about the general public and only attended to VIPs and persons with recommendations from the secretariat. The majority of the doctors agree that conditions in these hospitals are bad but they feel helpless in the matter.[11]

The patients also complained of the lack of coordination between supportive services and the medical services. Most of the patients complained of the non-availability either of their X-ray report or other laboratory reports. They go on wasting their time in tracing their reports. Besides, many patients complained that preferential treatment is given to friends and relatives of the hospital staff. Many patients complained of the non-availability of medicines. Besides, patients are referred to other departments which results in great delays for the treatment to be given to them because of unsatisfactory coordination among the various departments of the hospital. In order to improve this relationship, the Public Accounts Committee suggested the following:

(1) To encourage polite and courteous behaviour of the staff towards the patients, orientation and in-serve training opportunities should be provided to the staff.
(2) Out-patients should be properly guided by the doctors issuing prescriptions regarding the procedure to be followed to get their blood, urine, stool, etc., samples tested.
(3) Laboratories may be modernised and out-dated equipment replaced as early as possible to improve the accuracy of the test results because these tests form the basis of the medical treatment which the patients are to be imparted.

Further, it is suggested on the basis of the observations by the author that the patients may be issued the slips on arrival on which may be indicated the probable time of his examination by the doctor.

The following steps could also be taken to improve matters:

(a) Effective coordination should be established between the medical services and the supportive services to ensure promptness and clarity.

(b) Effective coordination and cooperation must be ensured among the various departments of the hospital to help the patients in diagnosing their ailments. It is suggested that a medical board may meet once a week where all the specialities may be represented and the patients needing the attention of more than one speciality may be asked to attend the board.

(c) A receptionist well versed with the functioning of hospital system may be appointed to guide the patients to approach the hospital properly.

(d) There is a need of playcards and signboards to guide the patients and their relatives.

(e) Provision of cheap and quality goods to be used by the patients or their relatives.

(f) Arrangement of stay of the relatives in Dharamsalas specially constructed for the purpose.

(g) Hospital beds may be given to patients according to the severity of the disease rather than other trifle considerations like obliging the VIPs.

In brief, the functioning of the hospital should be organised and re-organised to serve the patients most efficiently. All the personnel engaged in patient care must keep the following definitions of the "patient" in their minds:[12]

The patient is the most important in the Hospital.
The patient is not dependent upon us—we are dependent on him.
The patient is not an interruption of our work—he is the purpose of it.
The patient is not an outsider to our business—he is our business.
The patient is a person and not a statistic. He has feelings, emotions, biases and wants.
It is our business to satisfy him.

The participation of people in the formulation and administration of local and national plans and programmes that affect their well-being is particularly important at a time when developing countries like India are rapidly widening the scope of public services and adopting technological advances for improving their administration. Both developments could make public administration increasingly complex and more difficult for the mass of citizens to understand. Imaginative measures are needed to promote and sustain the interest of citizens in the hospital administration to give them a sense of participation in the decisions of hospitals that immediately affect them and to enable them to contribute to better administration. Citizen participation in hospital administration is also an important safeguard against the abuse of administrative authority. It is a method for tapping human and material resources for development that might otherwise remain inert. It is a means for communicating to people the results of hospital action in fields that are of interest to them. To quote Pt. Jawaharlal Nehru, "Administration not only has to be good but also to be felt to be good by the people."

Administration is manned by and meant for human beings. Administration does not exist for itself but for the citizens. Jawaharlal Nehru while delivering the inaugural address at the Indian Institute of Public Administration said, "Administration like most things is, in the final analysis, a human problem to deal with human beings, not with some statistical data . . . there is the danger that pure administrators at the top (not so much at the bottom, because they come into contact with human beings) may come to regard human beings as mere abstractions . . . the administrator may think in abstract of the people he deals with, come to conclusions which are justifiable apparently, but which miss the human element. After all, whatever department of Government you deal with, it is ultimately a problem of human beings and the moment we forget them, we are driven away from reality."

Thus, Hospital Administration is not to exist in some kind of ivory tower. The true test of Hospital Administration is the welfare of the people visiting the hospitals. The Administrative Reforms Commission has also observed in this very connection that, "If, in the prosperity of the people, lies the strength of a Government, it is in their contentment that lie the security and stability of democracy." In the words of Sir Harold Scot: "If a wide general knowledge is useful, even more valuable is a knowledge of people. It is very important that the young administrator should not retire into his cell when he leaves his office, but should mix with all kinds and conditions of people. From them, he will learn things that are not in his files.

It, therefore, follows that all the citizens have a right to participate in administration at all levels and they should in the interest of efficient functioning of administration in a democracy exercise this right.

It would be improper to describe this participation as hindrance nuisance, interference or obstacle to efficient administration. Citizen participation, on the other hand, is an important part of the unfolding democratic process and not only should it be understood and welcomed but the sooner we all learn to use it, the better it would be for us all.

In the past, the beneficiaries of hospital services were passively receiving hospital services. In modern times, there is a trend wherein the beneficiaries and the community at large wish to participate in the programmes of delivery of hospital and related community services. The hospital authorities must be alive to this emerging change and develop their hospital service plans accordingly.

We must set-up the Patient Complaint Enquiry Committee for all hospitals on the pattern of Patient Complaint Enquiry Committee set-up in the Directorate-General of Health Services to look into the public complaints regarding the services in government and other hospitals in the Union Territory of Delhi.

Lack of Managerial Training on the Part of the Hospital Administrators

Hospital Administration is a science as well as an art. The hospital administration has become complex and requires administrative capability to solve its managerial problems to provide the optimum care to the patients. It is, therefore, necessary that the persons charged with the efficient running of the hospitals are trained in the managerial techniques and tools which may be applied by them for getting the best out of the resources available. A Diploma in Health and Hospital Administration was started by the PGI in collaboration with the Punjab University (Department of Public Administration). It continued for two years—1975-76 and 1976-77, and was discontinued later on. Similarly, refresher courses are arranged twice a year by the NIHFW. What has been the impact of this training? Such a training could not make much impact as the trainers were acquainting them with the problems of management without their applicability in the Indian context. It is suggested that,

(a) All the Governments, Union and the States, must ensure that the top officers are appointed in the hospitals after giving them managerial training. What happens is that the persons on promotion become hospital administrators, without any management background.
(b) The trainers in the art of hospital administration must be given intensive training before they start imparting instruction. They should not bewilder the participants, with glamorous managerial techniques applicable in advanced countries but should provide them with simple tools, useful and applicable in the Indian context.
(c) A model hospital run on the modern lines may be set-up. The participants may be taken to this hospital to let them observe the application of techniques being taught to them.
(d) Training may be restricted only to those who are to shoulder this responsibility at present or in the immediate future.
(e) A regular follow-up of the training programme must be taken up to ensure the utility of training.

The hospital administrators should not be taught merely the art and science of managing formal organisation which would add to the efficiency of hospitals. Rensis Likert, in his article, "Motivational Approach to Management Development in *Harvard Business Review* (pp. 37-77, July-August 1959) has mentioned a number of such principles which when taught intensively to the administrators would add to the performance of an organisation. These factors are as follows:

(i) Extent of loyalty to the institution and identification with it and its objectives.
(ii) Extent to which the goals of units and individuals facilitate the achievement of the organisation's objectives.
(iii) Level of motivation among members of the organisation with regard to such variables as:
    (a) Performance including both quality and quantity of work done.
    (b) Concern for elimination of waste and reduction of costs.
    (c) Concern for improving the product.
    (d) Concern for improving processes.
(iv) Degree of confidence and trust among members of the organisation in each other and in the different hierarchical levels.
(v) Amount and quality of the teamwork in units and between units of the organisation.
(vi) Extent to which people feel that delegation is effective.
(vii) Extent to which the members feel that their ideas, information, knowledge of processes, and experiences are being used in the decision-making processes of the organisation.
(viii) Upward, downward, and sideward efficiency and adequacy of the communication process.
(ix) Leadership skills and abilities of supervisors and managers, including their basic philosophies of management and orientation towards leadership processes.
(x) Hospital Services Consultancy Corporation: We may mention here the recent development in India to improve hospital efficiency. The government have set-up a company in the public sector under the Ministry of Health and Family Welfare, called "Hospital Services Consultancy Corporation (India) Limited" with an equity investment of Rs. 50 lakhs to provide comprehensive consultancy services both within the country and in developing countries on all aspects of establishment and management of hospital facilities. It is to provide the following services:
    (i) carry out analysis of the requests for hospital services, conduct feasibility studies and prepare initial project reports,
    (ii) undertake preparation of architectural designs for hospitals,
    (iii) undertake hospital construction on turn-key basis,

(iv) undertake supply of equipments needed for running the hospital services,
(v) prepare and supply medical as well as para-medical manpower needed for the management of such hospitals,
(vi) undertake administration of the hospital for a period of time on contractual basis, and
(vii) provide consultancy services in building up low cost primary health services, family planning services, etc., in developing countries.

Hospitals should make use of this Corporation to improve efficiency.

Medical Audit not a Regular Feature in most of the Hospitals

The purpose of Medical Audit is to evaluate impinging on patient care. All the deaths in a hospital where cause of death are not certain are investigated by the Mortality Review Committee. This improves the knowledge of the medical personnel and enhances their capability of handling such cases in future. The Health Survey and Planning Committee (1959-61) recommended the use of medical audit in all hospitals. The Delhi Hospital Review headed by Dr. K.N. Rao (1968) also recommended the appointment of a Medical Audit Committee in each hospital. Such committee will ensure specific checks on the quality of work performed in the hospitals. We have found the following drawbacks in some of the hospitals where such committees are functioning:

(1) Poor recording of a case history.
(2) Sketchy documentation.
(3) Operation notes not properly recorded.
(4) Lack of inter-departmental coordination.
(5) Incomplete case-notes.
(6) Not proper follow-up by the senior faculty members.

Either mortality committees have not been set-up in hospitals or function irregularly. The Public Accounts Committee also mentioned that,

> "Although the recommendations of the review committee to carry out hospital mortality review periodically was accepted by the Government in February 1970, it was only after a lapse of six years (May 1976) that the mortality review committee started functioning in Willingdon Hospital (Rammanohar Lohia Hospital)."

The conditions are worse in hospitals under the control of State Governments in this regard. Thus, there is a need to set-up such committees to ensure efficient and effective medical audit.

Unsatisfactory System of Drugs and Medical Supplies

The efficiency of hospital services depends not only on the competence of medical personnel but also on the availability of drugs in right quantity and quality. We are witnessing a number of problems in regard to the drugs management in hospitals. Some of the important problems are:[13]

(a) Pilferage of drugs.
(b) Purchase of drugs at higher prices from the open market because of lack of advance planning.
(c) Use of adulterated drugs.
(d) Shortage of essential drugs.
(e) Corruption among the authorities in a hospital.
(f) Qualified persons not responsible for drug management.
(g) Absence of regular inspections to check the drug stores.
(h) Use of expired drugs.

The Committee on pilferage of drugs observed,

> "Some government hospital authorities were in league with drug suppliers. By manipulating records and accounts, hospital stores returned part of their stocks to suppliers for a financial consideration, or sold them to chemists at rock bottom prices. Often drugs obtained under the Central Government Health Scheme or the Employees' States Insurance Scheme were found to be falsely indented and sold to chemists."[14]

The Public Accounts Committee in its (1977-78) report was very critical of the drug management in the Central Government in Delhi. The Committee remarked:

> "Certain medicines consumed by patients in the hospitals were sub-standard . . . There have been periodical reports of shortage of certain medicines and it appears that no effective machinery exists to take notice of such shortage in time for remedial action in a coordinated manner."[15]

We give here some suggestions to remove these defects:

(a) Different colours and designs of medicines may be specially manufactured for the distribution through hospitals like the service stamps used in the Government offices.
(b) The machinery to ensure quality drugs in the States needs to be strengthened.
(c) Advance planning of the requirements of the drugs should be done to ensure regular supply.

(d) Cheap drugs may be manufactured by the Government and all multi-national drug companies may be either wound up or asked to manufacture cheap drugs.
(e) The working of medical depots under the Ministry of Health and Family Welfare needs to be streamlined so that the hospitals may not get the opportunity to purchase drugs from the open market.
(f) *Ad hoc* purchases may not be encouraged except under serious circumstances.
(g) The hospital authorities should ensure that only genuine and fully tested medicines are provided to the patients. Time-barred medicines may not be used. Timely action may be taken to ensure that medicines may not become time-barred through the exchange of such medicines from the firms.
(h) Drug stores should be under the control of qualified pharmacists and not semi-skilled compounders

Less Emphasis on Human Side of Medicine

Many people visiting the hospitals constantly turn to doctors without showing any sign of physical disorder. Most of the doctors do not bother to diagnose their problems and administer them sleep inducing drugs which are ultimately harmful. Tranquillizers and barbiturates are being dispensed on a large scale. "It is because medicine has become so accustomed to searching for technical answers to its dilemmas that quests for answers on the behavioural side continue to be deferred."

What can be done to make the doctors understand all this? The situation can be improved by providing courses in anthropology, sociology, and psychology to the doctors. According to Maureen A. Bailey,

> "In the face of a virtual epidemic of behavioural disorders, modern health care must place a new emphasis on solving the human side of medicine."[16]

Absence of Cost Consciousness among Hospital Authorities and Staff

The budgets of hospitals are increasing beyond proportions over the years which is beyond the capacity of poor countries like India. The whole of the health budget is spent in maintaining few hospitals neglecting the vast population needing health and medical care. According to H.A. Goddard,

> "In the management or administration of any enterprise, the quality, quantity, timing, and cost of the work necessary to reach the objectives of the enterprise are inter-related factors which must be given constant attention. If the resources for health work, in

trained persons and in finances, were unlimited the need for constant attention to these factors would not be so great. But the limitation in the number of trained personnel and the lack of adequate financial resources are major obstacles to greatly improved health in the world today. We must, therefore, husband our resources carefully to accomplish as much as possible with what we have available."[17]

A serious problem in health care administration is the absence of cost-consciousness among the staff of public health administrations. All over the world, health service staff—even of the highest professional cadre—are taught little about the economics of health services and know little about the costs of the equipment and supplies they use. Doctors tend to employ what is new without regard to cost. It is a fashion to prescribe costly drugs. They are also subjected to considerable sales pressure from manufacturing firms. A cheaper drug or cheaper equipment may give just as good a result for the vast majority of patients. Cost-consciousness is not just a matter for central administrators or planners but should be inculcated in all those working in health care. More people can be provided with services if no service cost more than what is a must to provide the necessary level of care. The price paid for high-cost technology for a few is no technology at all for the many.

Another aspect of this problem is the use of hospital non-judiciously. In the more developed countries, the majority of secondary care is generally given in hospitals, and increasingly the hospitals in which it is provided tend to be large, i.e., 500 beds or more. The larger hospital offers the opportunity for a high degree or specialisation and for achieving the fullest use of expensive specialised equipment. The larger the hospital and the more specialised its work, the larger catchment area it needs to serve. The higher average transport costs for staff and patients may be justified by the quality of service that a large hospital should be able to provide.

In the developing countries like India where the bulk of the population live in rural areas with limited public or private facilities for long distance travel, such transport is costly, except for the few patients who can be transported to hospital in vehicles travelling for other purposes. Moreover, in-patient care must be provided much more selectively if it is not to absorb an excessive share of the health budget. It must be confined to those with a high probability of deriving clear and lasting benefit from it. The emphasis should be on ambulatory services.

For these reasons, hospitals should on average be smaller in developing countries than in more developed countries and they should not be used to provide the most sophisticated technology. Costs can be saved if limited number of relatives accompany the patient and take responsibility for preparing food and providing basic patient care. But many developing countries have followed the example of more developed countries and concentrated on a high proportion of their health service expenditure on large urban hospitals, many of them teaching hospitals, equipped to provide tertiary care with high technology. These hospitals have been set-up before smaller district hospitals have been developed and as transport is not normally developed they tend to be used to provide secondary care to the urban population. Moreover, they are mainly used for patients who do not need their special facilities, e.g., the chronically disabled, children suffering from malnutrition, and patients with minor illness who could be treated in a much simpler hospital or at home. In some countries, the out-patient department of a regional hospital is even used to provide primary care as there is no referral system and time of super-specialists is wasted on minor problems which could be dealt elsewhere. It is suggested that the referral system must be made statutory to screen the patients.

Absence of Proper Space Planning

A large number of hospitals in the country have come to be established and housed in buildings which were not originally designed for the present needs and technology. The new hospitals have also to undergo changes as new facilities are provided to the community. The planning of hospital facilities in such a changing situation within the constraints of the existing space availability is one of the biggest problems that any hospital faces.

> "Moreover, hospital development is often designed in an *ad hoc* way or based on 'type plans', with the result defects are repeated in new hospital construction and remains unremedied in the existing ones.[18]

There is also lack of coordination between the hospital authorities and transport authorities resulting in the poor transport facilities available to the patients. The buildings and equipment are not maintained properly. It is suggested that—

(a) Hospital Engineering section must be set-up in all big hospitals to take care of the building and equipment.
(b) Hospitals may be located at places wherefrom transport facilities are easily available so that the patients can reach back home the same day.
(c) Proper maintenance of hospital equipment should be ensured otherwise these would tell upon the efficiency of the hospitals.
(d) Hospital planning and administration should receive greater attention.
(e) Operational studies on such aspects as the utilisation of

hospitals, over-crowding and referral system would help to define requirements realistically and bring improvements and economy in hospital design.

Poor Management of Dietary Services

The dietary unit stands as the second major department of a hospital from the point of view of expenditure. It needs careful analysis and control. Most of the patients always complain of poor and costly diets served in the hospitals. There is a problem of excess diets issued as compared to the number of patients resulting in huge expenditure. Besides, many of the patients do not consume all that is served to them. Patients generally prefer food from their houses as they do not like hospital food. The Public Accounts Committee (1977-78) has mentioned in this connection:

> "The Committee are constrained to note that whereas economy on expenditure on diet is being thought of by reducing quantum of diet, other measures to effect economy without diminishing the quality and quantity of diet such as plugging leakages of diet, have not been given the attention they deserve. In the opinion of the committee the leakage of diets may be possibly one of the reasons for issue of excess diets over the census figure. Therefore, it is necessary that institutional arrangements are made to watch that leakages of diet and dietary materials do not take place."

It is suggested that the efficient management of dietary services may be done to achieve economy and quality. The hospital authorities must compare the cost of dietary services with other hospital dietary services and thus try to locate the defects and remedy them.

Non-Availability and Non-Judicious Utilisation of Blood

There is a lot of resentment among the patients and their regarding the availability of blood required for certain ailments. Most of the patients complain about the prevalence of corruption in the supply of blood to patients. Besides, it is mentioned that only high ups in the Government can get the required supply of blood while the poor people are denied this right. It is suggested that the supply of blood must be made according to the needs of the patients rather than on the basis of their status. This would motivate the general public to donate blood for saving the lives of the people—a noble cause. The present author was entrusted with the task of arranging a camp to donate blood. The people when approached were very critical about the use of blood taken from voluntary workers. This feeling prevents most of the potential donors of blood to contribute to this noble cause. It is necessary to manage the blood banks in the hospitals judiciously to inspire confidence among the people in general—donors as well as consumers of the service.

Absence of Effective Personnel and Materials Planning

In most of the hospitals, there is no personnel planning, resulting in the under-utilisation of resources. Expenditure on personnel is mounting high and care must be taken to ensure optimum utilisation of resources. After the personnel, materials constitute about 50 per cent of the total expenditure of an organisation. Optimum utilisation of these resources must be ensured to achieve high productivity. There have been many cases where articles lying in bulk quantities in one department were purchased by the other and sometimes in emergency at exorbitant prices. The situation can be improved by designing a proper system of purchase, storage and utilisation. The hospital authorities must ensure whether the existing staff in the various departments has been deployed consistent with the work-load and are accordingly to prescribed norms. Besides, they are to ensure economy by avoiding wastage, duplication through inventory control. A study may be carried out in every hospital after three years in the following areas to ensure optimum utilisation:

1. Corporate Planning.
2. Manpower Utilisation.
3. Materials Management Drugs Control.
4. Management Information System.
5. Organisational Planning and Development.

Thus, periodic studies of the functioning of hospitals are needed to enable the administrators to manage them efficiently.

Absence of Planned Regionalisation to Ensure Graded Patient Care

At present, all hospitals whether at the state, district or local levels are working in isolation and their services are not provided in a coordinated manner. Most of the patients visit all these hospitals and are examined afresh by all of them resulting in wastage of efforts and resources. The medical staff prescribe medicines to patients without having a proper awareness of his previous treatment.

Recently Mrs Indira Gandhi, Prime Minister of India, while presiding over a function at Lady Hardinge Medical College at Delhi, rightly mentioned (quoted by Dr. P.N. Chhuttani, Ex-Director, PGI, in his article "Decentralisation Needed" published in Medical View Point column of *The Tribune*, dated 4-5-1980) that "The referral system has entirely failed in almost all our larger towns and cities. Consequently, there is growing overcrowding at our major hospitals whose services stand diluted. In the larger cities there is the multiplicity of the controlling authorities—The Government, the Municipal Corporation, the Municipal Committee, Voluntary Organisations, Private Hospitals, etc." She further stated that "there is no common meeting ground and hospital services have become almost totally unregulated. Consequently, the conditions in our capital city are chaotic. The poor and the needy flock towards the larger, better known hospitals in the hope of better treatment and care only to find that they have to wait for days to be examined, much less to find a place to stay. Patients wander from hospital to hospital. Besides, facing considerable inconvenience, their efforts to seek relief cause duplication of work and expenditure. It is thus necessary that every big city must have an apex body, perhaps called the hospital board, to establish referral hospitals for every zone."

Referral System

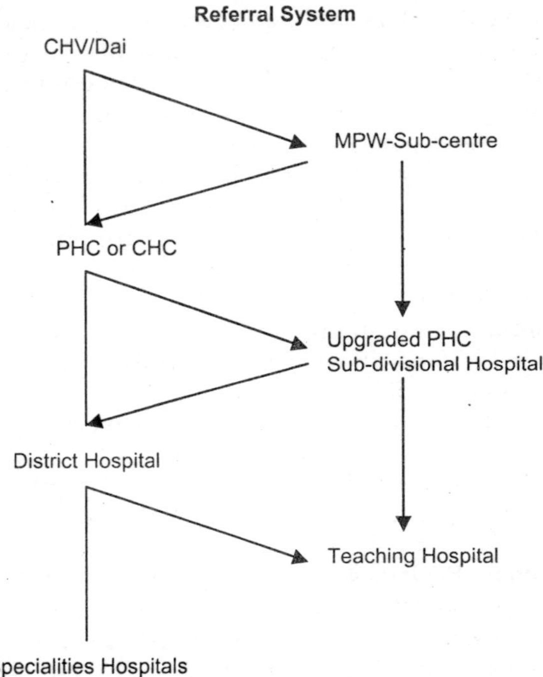

How can we get out of this chaos to design a system of patient care? The answer is—introduction of Regionalisation. Regionalisation connotes the development of graded patient care within a defined geographical or functional area from lower to higher levels adapting the health services to the characteristics and needs of the area and, thus, ensure the optimum utilisation of resources. The essential characteristics of regionalisation are:[19]

(a) Two-way flow of patients,
(b) Two-way flow of records,
(c) Two-way flow of services,
(d) Two-way flow of personnel,
(e) Mobile units,
(f) Centralised administration and decentralised execution,
(g) Coordinating education programme for the region,

(h) Communication and transport between components, and
(i) Coordination with other community health services.

Thus, regionalisation would ensure the best utilisation of time of the specialists and provision of comprehensive health care to the patients nearer their homes with all the benefits of specialities. The regional area should neither be too large nor too small but should be such as to ensure adequate span of attention. It would also automatically develop referral system scientifically.

The referral system presents the following five aspects:[20]

(a) It has to be built into the organisational structure of the medical services of a country. The rule should be that only when one unit cannot provide what a patient needs should the patient be referred to the next higher unit in the chain.
(b) The referral system has to be organised both internally and externally. 'Internally' means that patients in the hospital have to be referred from the in-patients to the out-patients department just as soon as their health situation permits. The 'externally' referred system exists among the several institutions on different levels of the hierarchy.
(c) The referral system must be established for the purpose of diagnosis and treatment and used for both in-patients and out-patients.
(d) It is a two-way system. Patients should be referred to higher level institutions for diagnosis and treatment when necessary, but they should also be referred back to the referring institution as soon as possible.
(e) The referral system concerns not only patients and diagnostic facilities but also the personnel of the medical services.

This is also a two-way system, so that human knowledge and skills are utilised fully and are continually developed through consultations and the interchange of ideas and experience.

The specialists from the regional hospital must come to the District hospital and the specialist from the District hospital to the health centre on a regular basis as consultants, to hold specialist clinics and give guidance; the medical and para-medical personnel should go to the higher level institution regularly for in-service training.

Absence of any Legislation for the Organisation and Functioning of Hospitals

At present there is no comprehensive legislation to guide the organisation and management of hospitals. There is need of a hospital legislation to ensure maintenance of standards, to define rights and duties of the hospital staff and to ensure the efficient functioning of

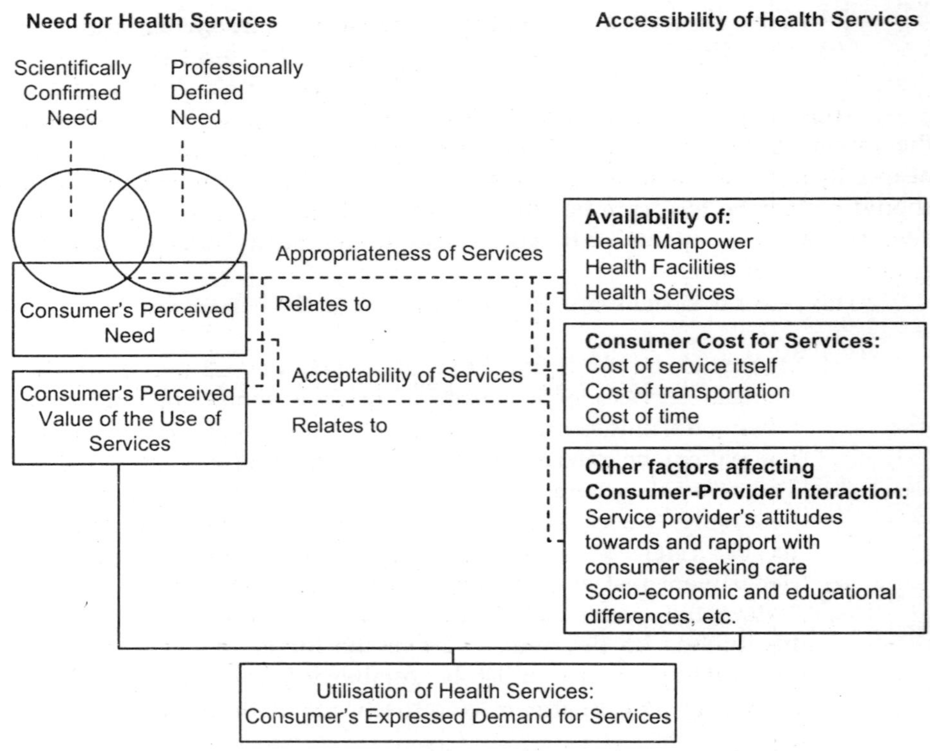

hospitals. It is suggested that the Government of India may set-up a body Development Council for Hospitals with its branches in the States like the Medical Council of India, to lay down policies to ensure that the hospitals have requisite facilities and provide efficient services to the patients. It has become a common practice to set-up nursing homes in the private sector. These so-called 'nursing homes' are often huge money-making projects devised by the specialists in league with one another. All these nursing homes must be under the control of the proposed council. It should be the duty of the council to see that the specialities like the private industry do not fleece the people and provide medical care of right quality and at a reasonable price. Besides, the proposed council may attend to the complaints of the patients to ensure smooth relations between the hospital authorities and the beneficiaries and thus help in the building of a Welfare State, a cherished ideal in the constitutions of most of the states in the world.

We must attend to all these problems to ensure efficiency of the hospitals. These problems also emanate from a number of constraints on hospital authorities, e.g., shortage of staff at all levels, absence of proper accommodation to provide space to the ever increasing number of patients, shortage of funds, shortage of medicine, shortage of equipment, political and administrative inference, etc., which need to be attended to by the governments at the Union and State level to provide satisfactory hospital services. Besides, the patients and their relatives must cooperate with the hospital authorities to make the best use of the available resources. Thus, we shall have to have a three-pronged attack—increasing internal efficiency, mobilising government support and enlisting people's cooperation to ensure the reputation, prestige, credibility and viability of the hospital services.

Notes and References

1. WHO, *Technical Report Series*, 1968, 395, p. 6.
2. WHO, *Technical Report Series*, 1957, 122, p. 4.
3. Punjab Government Memo. No. 118754-BI-66/30459, dated 25.10.1977 (from the Secretary to Government of Punjab, Medical and Health Deptt. to the Director, Health Services, Punjab).
4. Tiny M. Calender, *Unit Administration*, W.B. Saunders Co., London, 1962, p. 66.
5. V. Ramalingaswami, "Medicine, Health and Human Development" in *Health and Basic Services: Key to Development by UNICEF*, New Delhi, p. 10.
6. Lawrence J. Sakarai, "The Hippocratic Oath: License to Kill" in *Sunday Standard*, Chandigarh, 12 August, 1979 (Sunday Magazine, p. 1).
7. Mary D. Shanks and Dorothy A. Kennedy, The Theory and Practice of Nursing Service Administration, McGraw-Hill, London, 1965, p. 95.
8. John W. Gardner, Excellence, New York, 1961, Harper and Brothers, p. 154.
9. K.G. Agarwal, "Managing Patient Satisfaction in Hospitals" in the *Indian Journal of Public Administration*, Vol. XXII, No. 2, April-June 1976, p. 277.
10. K.K. Kaul, "Hospitalisation of Children", *Health and Population—Perspective and Issues*, 2(1): 49-53, 1979.
11. *The Tribune*, Chandigarh, November 1, 1979.
12. Edythe Alexander *et al.*, Nursing Service Administration (ed.), New York, C.V. Mosby Co., 1962, p. 63.
13. Based upon personal discussion with hospital staff at Chandigarh.
14. *Indian Journal of Hospital Pharmacy*, Vol. VII, No. 3-4/70.
15. Lok Sabha Secretariat, Public Accounts Committee, Forty-ninth Report, Sixth Lok Sabha, December 1977, p. 142.
16. Maureen A. Bailey, "The Human Side" in *World Health*, December 1975, p. 4.
17. H.A. Goddard, Principles of Administration applied to Nursing Service, World Health Organisation, Geneva, 1958, p. 84.
18. WHO, SEA/RC/21/2, p. VIII.
19. Timmappaya Regionalisation of Health Care (Mimeographed).
20. WHO, SEARO; SEA/RC 23/1, pp. 39-40.

CHAPTER 19

HEALTH EDUCATION AND HEALTH DEVELOPMENT

"The aim of health education is to help people achieve health by their own actions and efforts. Health education begins therefore with the interest of people in improving their condition of living, and aims at developing a sense of responsibility for their own health betterment as individuals and as members of families, communities or government."

—World Health Organisation

Health Education and Health Development

Health Education is the sum of experiences which favourably influence habits, attitudes and knowledge relating to individual, community and racial health.

Health Education has been an integral part of the functions of health personnel since time immemorial to educate the people pertaining to factors which influence their health. We have been engaged in the 20th century in finding out new technology and medicines to tackle the problems of health. That is why super speciality hospitals have come up in a big way. However, we have ignored the role of health education in preventing killer diseases resulting from faulty life style, use of alcohol, smoking, drugs, etc. Let us analyse these health hazards which are causing great misery to individual, families and society.

(I) (i) Defective Life Styles

Muhammad Al-Khrateeb[1] in his Article, "New Life Styles' New Diseases" rightly remarks that Recent Social Development—such as bigger incomes and greater availability of a wide variety of commodities—have led to changes in life styles that threaten health. Coronary diseases are on the increase because of changes in diets; people are eating more fats, carbohydrates and animal proteins; fast-food restaurants offer hamburgers, hot dogs and fried chicken; the intake of salt from canned food is rapidly increasing; access to transport facilities reduce physical exercise; and stress is common in their daily life.

(ii) Non-availability of Balanced Diet

On the other hand, there is a large population in the developing countries especially India which is suffering from a number of diseases caused by malnutrition and under-nutrition. Some of the diseases are protein-energy malnutrition-related diseases e.g., low birth weights,

Iodine deficiency disorders, Vitamin A deficiency disorders, iron deficiency, Anaemia, etc. These diseases do not require super specialists' interventions but timely Primary health care and education of mother and simple medicinal interventions.

The International Conference on Nutrition (ICN) in 1992 enunciated the following goals: (1) reduce severe and moderate malnutrition among children under five years of age by half of the 1990 levels, (2) increase the percentage of newborns having an adequate birth weight (2500 grams or more) to 90%, (3) reduce to less than 10% and possibly eliminate iodine deficiency disorders, (4) eliminate Vitamin A deficiency and its consequences including blindness, and (5) reduce iron deficiency anaemia.

Drawing up an integrated national strategy for the prevention of non-communicable diseases is both advisable and economically justifiable. But prevention of such diseases cannot be achieved through the efforts of health officials alone. Health education has to be made accessible to the entire population and non-health institutions and various mass media should be mobilized to this end. Research data yielded by national as well as international studies show that early intervention can make the prevention of diseases possible.[2]

(2) Use of Excessive Alcohol, Smoking and Drugs

World Health, July-August 1995 has published figures about prevalence of alcohol, tobacco and drugs which are quite alarmings.[3] In developed countries, typically 70-90% of adults consume alcohol. Studies in a number of industrialized countries suggest that 5-10% of drinkers are dependent on alcohol.

For several diseases, including cancers of the mouth, Oesophagus and pharynx, as well as for many forms of injury including motor vehicle accidents, industrial accidents, drowning, falls, suicide and homicide, the contribution of alcohol is well known, the risk increasing steadily with the amount consumed.

World-wide, there are about 1100 million smokers with 800 million in developing countries and 300 million in developed countries. About 6000 million cigarettes are smoked every year. In developed countries, about 41% of men and 21% of women regularly smoke cigarettes. In developing countries, about 50% of men but only about 8% of women smoke.

Tobacco causes about 3 million deaths a year now, with about one-third of them in developing countries. If current smoking trends persist, tobacco is likely to kill approximately 10 million people a year in 30-40 years time, with about 70% of them in developing countries.

If current smoking trends persist, about 500 million people currently alive (about 9% of the world's population) will eventually be killed by tobacco, and half of them will be in middle age when they die, losing about 20-25 years of life.

In many developing countries heroin and cocaine use is becoming more common and increasingly problematic. In several countries heroin use is increasingly replacing traditional patterns of substance use including opium smoking.

In many developing countries drug injecting is becoming increasingly common, and in these countries injecting often means the sharing of injecting equipment, with the risk of HIV, hepatitis and other infections.

One crude estimate suggests that, world-wide, between 160,000 and 210,000 deaths every year are associated with drug injecting.

Norman Sartorius in his Article, "Putting a Higher Value on Health" in *World Health,* June 1986 has cautioned about the negative effects of the use of these horrible drinks in excess. To quote:[4]

> "The abuse of psychoactive substances including alcohol, tobacco and narcotic and psychotropic drugs causes enormous damage to the health and productivity of nations. It undermines the quality of life of individuals and their families, and threatens the welfare of communities. The health consequences of abuse are also grave, and range from violence and delinquency to liver cirrhosis, brain damage and lung cancer.

Dr. H. Mahler, Former Director General of World Health Organisation in his Article, "Smoking or Health: The Choice is Yours" rightly stated,[5] "Smoking increases the risk of lung cancer, heart disease and respiratory infections of all kinds. In fact, many of the diseases associated with smoking have become current only in the last few generations, when the habit of smoking factory made cigarettes became widespread."

The latest report of South-East Asia Region on Health situation in 1994-97 has clearly brought out the consequences of the use of these substances. A major problem with the use of alcohol is its impact on the health and well-being of the family. A study carried out in India in 1996 reported that drinking families from lower income groups spend from 15% to 45% of their income on alcohol. A high proportion of hospital beds are occupied by the physically and mentally damaged victims of alcohol dependence. Many beds occupied by accidents affected patients are because of alcohol.

The causal relationship between tobacco use and diseases such as cancers, cardiovascular diseases, and chronic respiratory disorders is increasingly being studied in most countries of the Region. In India, the number of avoidable cases of chronic heart and obstructive lung diseases has been estimated at 12 million per year. Cancer incidence data reveal that almost 50% and 25% of cancers in men and women respectively are related to tobacco use. The incidence of oral cancer caused by chewing tobacco is estimated to be one of the world's highest, at about one-third of all cancer cases. Annually, tobacco-related conditions are reported to cause 635,000 deaths in India.[6]

The basic question is how to tackle these non-communicable diseases? How to motivate the people using these substances not to do so? What can be done by health experts? The only answer to these questions is the need of strengthening Health Education intensively. Muhammad Al-Khateeb[7] suggests that drawing upon integrated national strategy for the prevention of non-communicable diseases is both advisable and economically justifiable. But prevention of such diseases cannot be achieved through the efforts of health officials alone. Health education has to be made accessible to the entire population, and non-health institutions and various mass media should be mobilised to this end. Research data yielded by national as well as international studies show that early intervention can make the prevention of disease possible.

Achieving 'Health for All' requires much more than just setting up a health centre in every district and providing a high standard of medical care within easy reach of everyone.

A key element in the primary health care approach to Health for All is health education, which seeks to bring about a change in behaviour patterns by making essential health information available to all people in a simple, direct and effective manner. It is hoped that people will thus be motivated to evaluate their habits and practices, and will modify them according to the requirements of health protection and promotion.

Behavioural change, however, is too complex a process to be initiated simply by providing a set of facts. The motivation to break a habit must be much stronger than the force of habits or the pleasure derived from a certain practice. The spiritual dimension can be highly influential in this process of behavioural change.[8]

In spite of overwhelming evidence linking tobacco consumption and various diseases, including cancer, the consumption of cigarettes in nearly all countries of the world is increasing. The rise in tobacco consumption is especially seen among women and the youth. Non-smoking campaigns over the past years have been less than successful. This is mainly because of the aggressive advertisements and counter-attacks by the tobacco industry and the fact that nicotine is addictive. Moreover, most governments are reluctant to take a strong stand on this issue considering that tobacco is a source of revenue and of foreign exchange.

The need for heightened global advocacy for tobacco control has been stressed by Dr. Gro Harlem Brundtland, WHO Director-General, in her statement to the Fifty-first World Health Assembly in May 1998. To quote her:

> "I am a doctor, I believe in science and evidence . . . Tobacco is a killer, Tobacco should not be advertised, subsidized or glamorized."

Of late there is a move to ban Tobacco companies from sponsoring Sports events in India leading to a major debate as to whether it would be at the cost of the Sports activity and so on.

MEANING, NATURE AND SCOPE OF HEALTH EDUCATION

The most important aim of Health Education is to alter behaviour which may have directly or indirectly influenced occurrence of spread of diseases in a given cultural setting. A culturally relevant health education programme can be planned only after understanding the behaviour in all its manifestations. One of the best definitions of Health Education was offered by Wood in 1926: "Health Education is the sum of experiences which favourably influences habits, attitudes and knowledge relating to individual, community, and racial health."[9]

Different authorities have differently viewed the aims of health education. According to one source:[10]

> "The aim of health education is to help people achieve health by their own actions and efforts. Health education begins therefore with the interest of people in improving their condition of living, and aims at developing a sense of responsibility for their own health betterment as individuals and as members of families, communities or government."

Another source[11] highlights that, "Health education aims at promoting the greater possible fulfilment of inherited powers of the body and the mind and the happy adjustment of individual to society. It is the educational approach to health problem and as such is concerned with practical measures for the promotion of health and the control and treatment of disease."

Unfortunately, the experts and development planners have failed to improve the lives of the people as they do not understand properly the science to communicate effectively with each other or with the people are trying to help. Most of the people in authority today, who are guiding the people in this field, have not realised the urgency of such education and the benefit it can generate; consequently governments have not taken any substantial steps in this direction.

Health education does not mean merely removal of ignorance. On the contrary, it involves four important things:

(i) It provides a person with appropriate knowledge to enjoy decent health and also the knowledge about the occurrence and spread of disease thus enabling him to adopt relevant preventive measures;
(ii) It creates in him an interest in his own health and well-being;
(iii) It even creates in him an interest for the health of others

members of his family as well as of those living in his surrounding; and

(iv) It creates in him a desire to support health education programmes in his area.

Besides, Health Education should make the people understand the benefits that they can derive from modern medicine. K.S. Sanjive, Professor of Medicine has said:

> "It will not be an exaggeration to say that the paramount step in the effort to take modern medicine to every corner of the country and every citizen is health education. Health education in its widest sense of getting every one to understand what modern medicine can do to diminish disease and death and to be properly motivated to utilise this knowledge in their daily lives, requires the simple quality of sincerity more than highly specialised techniques."[12]

Neglect of health education is one of the main reasons why scientific medicine is not taking root in the country and people are steeped in ignorance and superstition.

ESSENTIALS OF HEALTH EDUCATION

Health education would be possible only if the health educator and the receiver are in constant dialogue with each other. It is not wholly correct that the purpose of health education is to manipulate the receiver. What might be more appropriate is a circular diagram in which the parties to the "Communication Contract" as it is sometimes called, function dually as senders and receivers.

This model would avoid the possibilities of misinterpretation. We know that even well-planned campaigns can end in failures if there is no

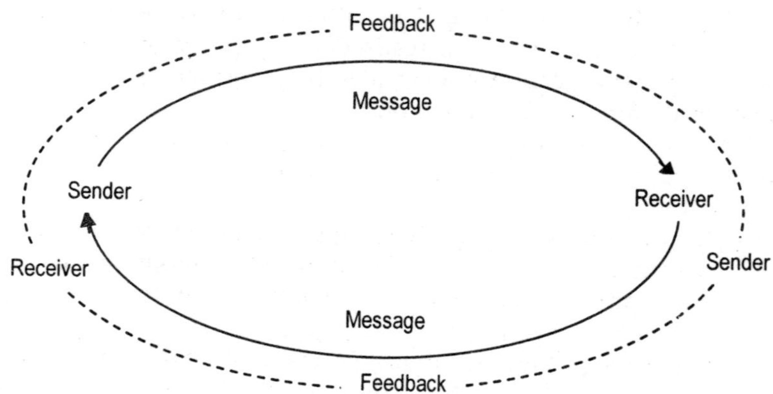

proper monitoring or feed-back to make sure that the wrong effect is not being created by the communicator, however innocently.

In a democratic society, the dynamic power which impels governments to action is the voice and enlightenment of the people. People can only pressurise their executive or legislative machinery to undertake suitable health measures when they themselves are aware of the means of warding off disease and promotion of positive health. This knowledge (Health Education) is therefore a pre-condition and prerequisite to creating the demand for health and setting the pace of implementation of environmental sanitation and the total health policy.

FUNCTIONS OF HEALTH EDUCATION PROGRAMME (See Chart 19.1)

No health education programme can function in isolation. A health education programme has to be an integral part of various other development programmes. Functionally, a health education programme should aim at bringing about the following changes:

CHART 19.1

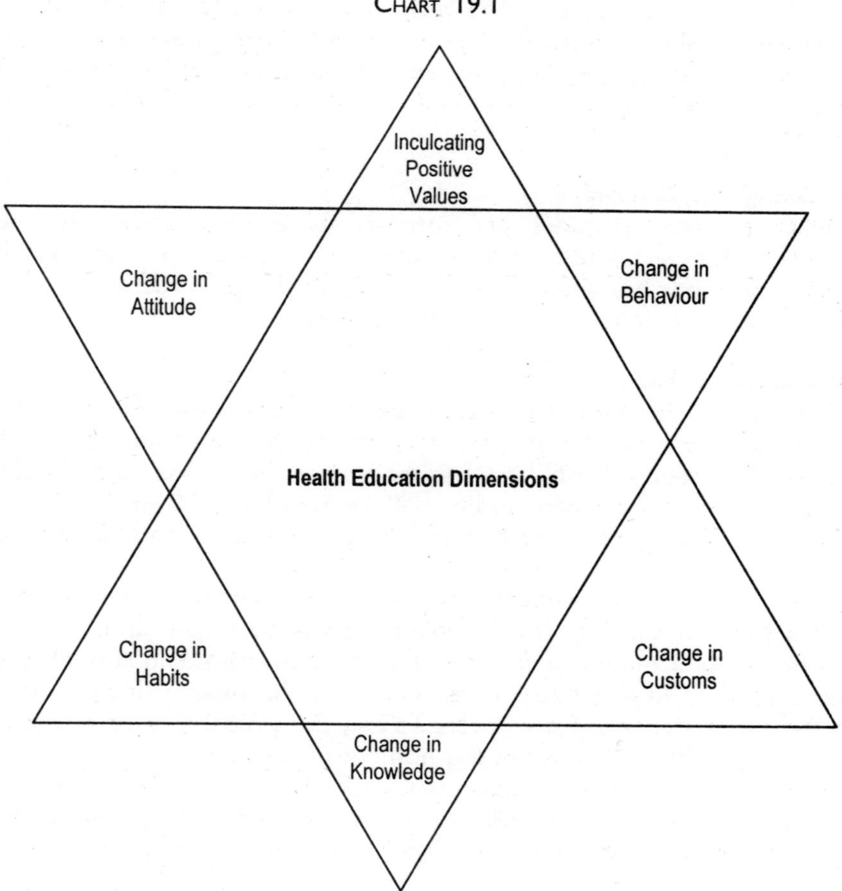

(1) A Change in Knowledge

The most important need which health education programme can serve is to provide appropriate knowledge about health and diseases to the people. This knowledge should be provided in such a way that the recipients do not find it hard to accept it. How to provide this knowledge in an acceptable way? This is the first challenge faced by a health educator. Meaningful responses are relatively easier to learn than the meaningless ones. The health educator can do a lot better by making his demands on the response of receivers which are meaningful. For instance, the health educator who gives a big lecture to the mother on the value of practising family planning without indicating its benefits to her as an individual would be showing inadequate understanding of this principle, for she has to look into her own benefits first. Vigorous efforts would be required to proliferate suggestions that are realistic and meaningful.

(2) A Change in Attitude

A change in attitude is possible only when the new knowledge that is offered is acceptable to the recipients. Its utility should also be well known to them. Normally, provision of appropriate knowledge should lead to formation of positive attitudes not only towards a person's own health but also towards the health of other members of the community.

(3) A Change in Behaviour

Once positive attitudes are formed, these must reflect in the behaviour of the recipients. They should not only become mindful of their past behaviour but should also avoid doing things which can in any way influence occurrence or spread of diseases.

(4) A Change in Habit

The change in the behaviour of the recipients must lead to habit formation. A habit can be formed only when the behaviour becomes repetitive. If proper habits are formed, not only the individuals concerned but the whole community will be benefited. Habit formation, however, is a slow process and it has been well said, that 'habits die hard'.

The persuasive communicator or health educator should be interested both in the long range effects of his messages and in their initial effects. As a matter of fact, he should be interested in turning the learned responses into habitual ones. What are the other principles that guide the establishment of a response? First, the probability of response will increase with the increase in the number of rewarded repetitions. As long as the stimulus with reinforcement following each correct response is not adequately repeated, it will not become a habitual response. Many messages are short-lived because of lack of reinforcement and are likely to become extinct. Second, in order to establish habit patterns, it would be necessary to have a shorter interval between response and reward. Third, habit formation is easier when stimuli are presented in isolation. A nutrition message when unaccompanied by another message such as sanitation message facilitates habit formation. Fourthly, timely increase in reinforcement will further strengthen habit formation. Fifth, receiver's original level of motivation will also influence her habit formation. The mother having a better level of motivation from the beginning will find habit formation much easier. Sixth, providing timely information about receiver performance would lead to further improvement in performance. Providing selective information to a mother on the positive aspects of her performance will also improve her performance. Thus, communication of health ideas can yield the desired result if the above principles are followed religiously.

(5) A Change in Customs

Acquisition of positive attitudes leading to appropriate habit formation must sooner or later, evolve into customs. Only when a substantial number of people in a given cultural setting start behaving in a customary manner, one can say that behaviour has become a part of their customs.

Don Palmer in his article, "Social Health: A True Story, Culture and Tradition as Medicine" in the *Daily Tribune* dated 26th January 2000, rightly stresses "the need of health education. Modern urban life, devoid of the goodness of social health, can be particularly tough for young indigenous inhabitants of developed countries. Some kill themselves, while many more drift into drugs, alcohol and crime. Now a prison programme is helping in rehabilitation of aboriginal offenders by reintroducing them to their cultural traditions."

It needs to be re-emphasised that health education is a slow process and that it proceeds gradually—a part of the process may get established without any problem but additional efforts may be required to complete the whole process. This process may be directed towards the following important programmes: (See Chart 19.2)

(a) Personal hygiene.
(b) Knowledge of modern medicine i.e., use of health services.
(c) Nutrition.
(d) Mental health.
(e) Prevention of communicable diseases.
(f) Care of children.
(g) Environmental sanitation.
(h) Human physiology.
(i) Lifestyle diseases.
(j) Education about Alcohol and drugs.

CHART 19.2

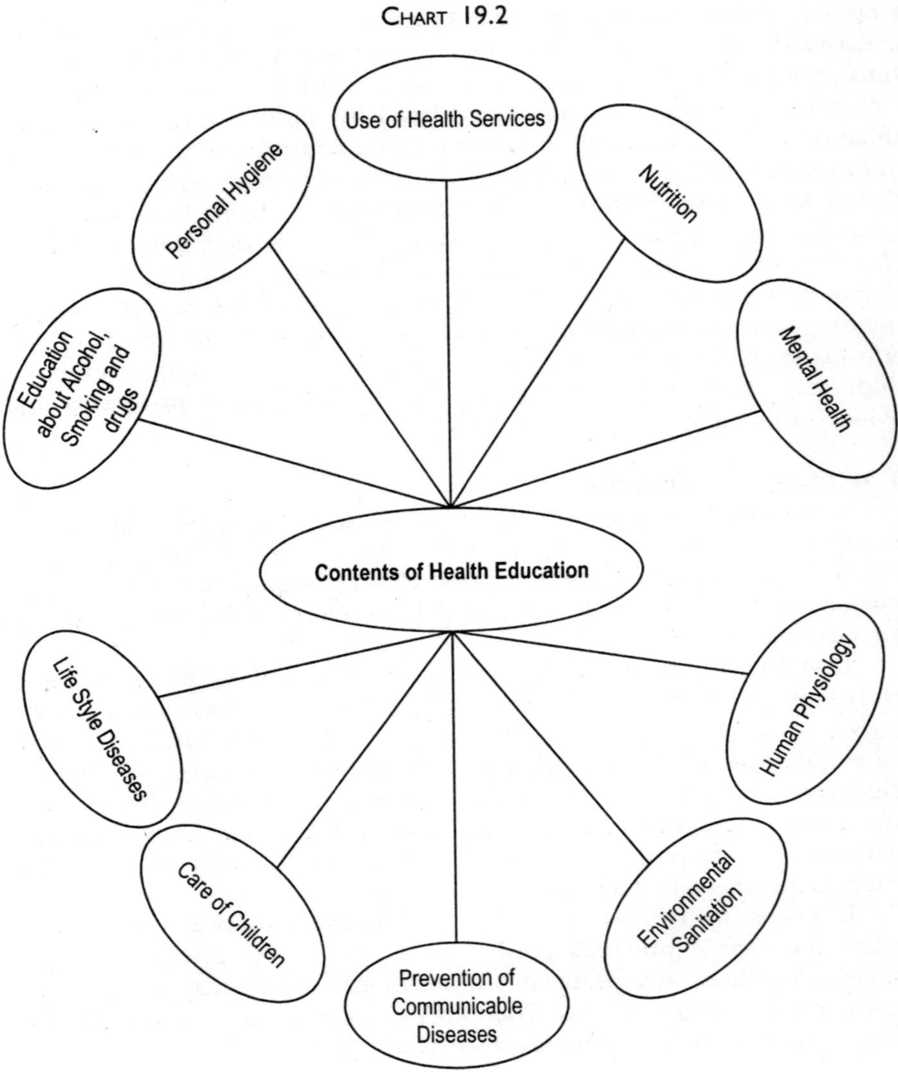

Health education must be imparted keeping in mind latest developments in the field of health. Life is changing fast and the individuals must be educated in the new technology—its role and limitations. Mr. V. Tatochenko, a member of the WHO Expert Panel on Maternal and Child Health in his Article on "Education for Health" said, "Rapid changes in life styles and the evolution of views on health and disease call for new departures in health education. A quick glance of health education material of even one generation ago will show how fast it tends to get out of date. Medical facts, it has been estimated, get outdated within a decade or so. Effective health education, therefore, requires a continuous stream of knowledge, development of the people's ability to absorb it, and decisions taken on the basis of a constantly changing body of information.[13]

METHODS OF HEALTH EDUCATION

Health organisations are set-up to promote positive health. A good health organisation must establish environmental linkages—points of interactions with the environment. These can be classified into four categories: enabling, functional, normative and diffused. The enabling linkage ensures and protects the organisational authority to operate its access to resources and its power to achieve results. Functional linkage is to link the programme with the task environment. Normative linkages try to modify the behaviour of the people into the existing value system of the society. Diffused linkages imply reaching the clients through public relation (health education).

Sociologists have categorised diffusion process which leads to a widespread acceptance of the programme into five critical stages awareness (the individuals first introduction to a new idea or practice), interest (the stage at which he actively seeks further information and background data), evaluation (the stage of assessment on critical grounds), trial (a limited phase of experiment), and finally acceptance or adoption. These processes have been occurring for centuries. The need of the present day health administration is to accelerate adoption of the health programmes and to control diffusion process in a short span of time to achieve effective implementation of health programmes.

Changes in knowledge, attitudes, behaviour, habits and customs can be brought about by 'personal' as well as 'impersonal' methods of health education. These methods have certain advantages and disadvantages. While personal methods involve face-to-face interaction, the impersonal methods do not require such a close personal contact. Personal methods are indeed more convincing and generally more successful. However, the success of personal methods greatly depends on the establishment of a good rapport between the health educator and his recipients. The impersonal methods are relatively simpler and even less time-consuming. The radio, the newspapers, the posters, and the pamphlets, etc. can all play an important role in imparting health education. Experience with personal and impersonal methods of health education have revealed that if both the methods are used simultaneously one can obtain better results than simply using one or the other method. The most important aspect in the adoption of the programme is the use of inter-personal relationships. Alastair Metheson, Deputy Director of UNICEF's division remarks on the basis of his research that:

"To get people to act in ways that conform to new values almost always requires that mass communications to be reinforced by personal influence."[14]

Thus, we see that communication, i.e., dissemination of information is only an important element in health education. The adoption or acceptance may not take place simply by communicating health information. A study conducted by United States Public Health Services has revealed that, "Unfortunately knowledge alone does not motivate a person to act in accordance with it. He may well know the correct answers to questions without really believing and accepting such information as the basis for his own action."

Dr. Gisela Gastrin, a Finnish physician mentions in his article "How Education Helps"; "People can be motivated to adjust their outlook towards health and disease, but before this can happen their negative attitudes have to be countered with factual information."

Education needs to be a part of a comprehensive programme in which responsibilities involving the health authorities and others are clearly delineated and resources allocated."[15]

For effective health education, people's involvement is essential. Eric R. Ram[16] in his article, "Information is Power" in *World Health,* rightly says that making people aware of their rights and responsibilities helps them to determine their own health priorities and take part in solving their own health problems, a step so essential in the process of empowerment of the people. We have to employ all credible channels of communication, including the traditional methods of story-telling and drama, in order to reach all people. Films, radio and television whenever available can be useful, but we have to recognize their limitations; they are useful in creating awareness among people in their communities, but to bring about a real change in health practices, people have to decide for themselves and take responsibility for their own health.

It was mentioned by Dr. E. Berthat in his article, "A New Role for Teachers" that besides information and motivation, action is indispensable. He said that "Information and motivation are not enough; it remains for governments to ensure that a good health infrastructure is available to all the people. Health education has to convince the men and women who are responsible for taking decisions that health is a basic raw-material for their country's eventual social and economic development.[17]

A health educator, as a persuasive communicator can make the best possible use of the personal methods of health education. But he has to see that the messages which he is delivering get mentally registered with his recipients. Actually, he can present his message and then wait until he gets the requisite response from his recipients. D.F. Skinner has distinguished between two types of approaches to the learning situation, as 'operant behaviour' and 'respondent behaviour'. The two situations have also been described as involving instrumental learning and conditional learning. In 'instrumental learning situations', which involves 'operant behaviour', the health educator will present his message and then wait for the receiver to make a correct response. When the receiver makes this response, the health educator will attempt to fix the response by the appropriate award or reinforcement. On the other hand in 'conditional learning situation' which involves 'respondent behaviour', the health educator presents his message in such a way that he elicits the response that he wants from his recipients and thus the stimulus that originally served to elicit the response becomes the reinforcing or rewarding element in conditioning. Undoubtedly, conditioning is much more efficient than instrumental learning. It is, however, necessary for the health educator to be aware of both kinds of situations since the condition for using 'respondent behaviour' may not be present in the persuasive situation. The health educator has to be aware that the recipients of his messages differ in the ways in which they learn a given response. They may give different responses essentially in the same situation because of certain specific reasons.

TRAINING OF PERSONNEL FOR HEALTH EDUCATION

We can divide the personnel for health education in two categories, i.e., Health Workers like teachers, social workers, physicians, nurses, etc., and Specialists, i.e., the persons specially trained for this function.

Objectives of training for Health Workers are:

(1) To create an awareness and understanding of the health education aspects of health work and of the principles and procedures to be considered in achieving these purposes;
(2) To foster an interest in health education in all health personnel;
(3) To teach the right way to communicate with individual families, community groups, and the general public;
(4) To stress the importance of team work for the realisation of effective health education; and
(5) To strengthen the aspects of health education in the curriculum of medical education.

The main objectives of training health education Specialists are:

(a) To establish professional standards to secure public confidence. It is essential that such specialists possess an ethical code and technical competence which govern their behaviour and standards of performance.
(b) To prepare specialists to encompass health education planning, organisation, coordination, dissemination, training, studies and research.

The health education Specialist should acquire through his basic education and post-graduate training the following qualities:

(a) A high degree of competence involving a thorough understanding of the importance and implication of cultural, economic and social influences in relation to health.
(b) Special competence in planning, organisation, administration, evaluation, etc., of health education aspects of health programmes.
(c) The ability to give technical leadership in planning and conduct of health education, training for health workers and workers in closely related fields (content, methods, planning, etc.).
(d) Skill in giving technical guidance and consultation on planning, preparation, pre-testing, production, and use of visual materials.
(e) The ability to assume technical leadership in cooperation with others in planning and execution of studies and research on major health education problems.
(f) Thorough knowledge of educational principles and methods involved in planning and arranging of seminars, conferences, meetings, courses, teaching units, etc.
(g) They should acquire latest information from research in teaching and learning relevant to health education.

THE ROLE OF UNION AND STATE GOVERNMENT IN THE PROMOTION OF HEALTH EDUCATION IN INDIA

Imparting of health education is the responsibility of all professions, i.e. teachers, community leaders and parents. Central and the State Health Departments have instituted a separate bureau or division or section to provide expertise to health education programmes and assist in the training of health workers at various levels of health administration. There is also one premier institute—All India Institute of Hygiene and Public Health, Calcutta to provide training in the field of Health Education. Health Education forms part of all types of training courses in public health subjects.

CENTRAL HEALTH EDUCATION BUREAU (CHEB)

On the recommendation of the Planning Commission, the Government of India set-up a Central Health Education Bureau in the Directorate-General of Health Services under the Ministry of Health and Family Welfare, New Delhi, in 1956. It was entrusted with the following functions:

(1) To interpret the plans, programmes, and achievements of Health Ministry.
(2) To train key health and community welfare workers in health education and research methods and to evolve effective methodology and tools of training.
(3) To design, guide, coordinate and conduct researches in health behaviour, health education and aids.
(4) To prepare and distribute 'typed' health education materials to states and other agencies.
(5) To render technical and other assistance to official and non-official agencies engaged in health education work and to coordinate their programmes.
(6) To cooperate and collaborate with international agencies in promoting health education activities.

The Central Health Education Bureau—an apex Institute in Health Education—imparts in-service training to all categories of personnel in health and related sectors at the state and district levels. They in turn disseminate the message of health education in the community at large. The Bureau, also continues to provide up-to-date information on current issues and development in health education, besides communication and training. The Bureau achieves its objectives through eight technical divisions, namely, Training, Media, Editorial, Health Education Services, Research and Evaluation, Field Study and Demonstration, Centre and Health-Related Vocational Courses. The Training Division runs a post-graduate Diploma Course in Health Education of two years' duration at the University of Delhi; Media personnel training course of eight weeks' duration; Certificate courses in Health Education for para-medical professionals, medical officers, teachers and key trainers; district-level medical officers' course, etc. Besides, about 25 orientation courses of one-day duration are held for Nursing, para-medical professionals and international visitors.

The Media Division is the Information, Education and Communication unit of the Bureau. The Editorial Division brings out three periodicals, namely, *Swasth Hind* (English monthly), *Arogya Sandesh* (Hindi monthly) and *Swasth Siksha Samachar* devoted to important public health problems, plans and policies of the Ministry of Health and Family Welfare. It also prepares and produces printed materials like folders, pamphlets, etc., on important public health subjects. The School Health Division promotes health education in the school system. The Health Education Services Division renders technical guidance to State Health Education Bureau and assists government and non-government agencies in promoting health education in the country. It also co-ordinates with international and national agencies.

The CHEB is a nodal agency for promoting Health-Related Vocational Courses (HRVCs) at the stage of education in the country in collaboration with the Department of Education. The HRVC Division develops curricula and textbooks for various HRVCs and persuades the States/UTs to start these courses. The Research Division conducts Behavioural Studies on various aspects of health problems that serve as a basis for launching health education campaigns. It also conducts Social Science Research Methods Courses. The Field Study and Demonstration Centres of the Bureau are field laboratories to test and evaluate methods and the media of health education which can be adopted elsewhere.

It may not be an exaggeration to say that all these contributions of CHEB have failed to produce the desired impact on the health status of the people. It is unfortunate that some of the 'good' workers who were earlier associated with the CHEB left it in favour of highly remunerative assignments with the World Health Organisation. If the CHEB has to prove its utility in a meaningful manner then it has to have suitably trained persons on its staff. Otherwise, the CHEB, without technically qualified people, is likely to become a rehabilitation centre for the relatives and friends of highups in the Government.

The state of Health Education Bureaus in different States of India is no better. Most of the literature produced by them lacks the necessary appeal for the rural masses. It has little or no relevance to the realities of the health situation. Many a time the authorities of these bureaus derive a sense of satisfaction by merely distributing pamphlets to the people. No effort is made to evaluate its impact on the health behaviour of the people. It is common knowledge that a substantial part of this literature goes to the junk shop where its value is judged only in terms of its weight. Unless, those responsible for producing the health education material also become seriously involved in knowing how it is used, very little is likely to be known about utility to the people for whom it is meant. A visit to a District Hospital in North India will show how irrelevant is the health education material which gets displayed on the walls of the ward or in the OPD in the hospital. While one may find an excess of posters on a disease like smallpox, which is no longer a problem, one may not see any poster on common problems as measles and diarrhoea.

Thus, a lot depends on how the Central and State Ministries of Health plan and implement their health education programmes. Actually, planning and implementation of health education programme at the Centre, State and District levels also depends on the available financial resources. Health education programmes for the hospital and for the health centers do not have any separate funding. In practice, the money allocated for health education either lapses at the Head office or is not made available at these places. It is necessary for a developing country like India to attach the highest importance to health education. Without planning appropriate health education programmes, one can hardly hope to bring about a positive change in the existing health condition. "Planning of health education should be an integral part of the overall national health planning."[18]

HEALTH EDUCATION IN HOSPITALS

Gone are those days when people used to feel frightened at the thought of going to a hospital. Hospitals were considered as sordid places where people waited for death. Today, the image of hospitals has vastly changed. People expect hospitals to be well organised so that all the services offered by them are well received by the clients. Somehow, the modern hospitals, both teaching and non-teaching, continue to attach the highest importance to providing curative services. The teaching hospitals, in particular, assign a great prestige and value to medical education and research activities. Thus, the medical scientists remain 'wedded to curative medicine rather than to preventive medicine.' A developed country, like the United States of America, had a couple of decades back, recognised the need of combining curative aspects of diseases with preventive aspects. Such a recognition had led to the opening of some of the best schools of hygiene and public health in the world in some of the prestigious American Universities like the Harvard, John Hopkins, North Carolina and California. Thus, for a developing country like India, there is not only a need for combining curative services with preventive services but there is also the need for introducing effective health education programmes in the teaching as well as non-teaching hospitals.

In February 1977, India organised a national workshop with WHO's collaboration on health education in hospitals which was attended by sixty hospital and health administrators and health educators. This is going to be extended to cover other hospitals in the country. The efforts of Sri Lanka are noteworthy in this direction. Most of the country's larger hospitals have accepted health education as one of their functions. Each of these hospitals has been equipped and the staff have been trained in health education. Educational work is undertaken in wards, clinics and out-patient departments. These activities are coordinated with those in the communities.

The functions, which the teaching and non-teaching hospitals can perform in the modern times need to be defined properly. At present, no effort has been made to study the functions of these hospitals in relation to the needs of the people. Even among the staff members of these hospitals there is a great deal of confusion about individual's role, perception, role expectation and role performance. The health administrators have differently perceived the roles of the different members of the teaching hospitals. These hospitals, no doubt, can play a significant role in imparting health education to the patients because they have certain basic facilities available to them in the form of staff members like physicians, nurses, social workers, photographers and artists and they also have various audio-visual aids.

The object of health education, as defined by WHO is to help people attain not just freedom from disease or infirmity but a state of complete mental, physical and social well-being. If this object is followed seriously then the hospitals cannot escape the responsibility of organising relevant health education programmes with the help of experts in the field of health education. The hospitals provide an extraordinary opportunity to the medical staff to communicate modern concepts and ideas about health not only to the patients but also to their relatives who accompany them to the clinic for moral support. In fact, health education can be provided at the out-patient departments in the special clinics, in the wards and even at the registration counter. The Departments of Obstetrics and Gynaecology and Pediatrics can play a special role in organising suitable health education programmes for their clients when they come to them for ante-natal and post-natal care. Actually, the immunization activities can also be combined with certain well-planned health education activities. At the Primary Health Centre level too, there is a great scope for imparting health education to the patients and their attendants, but unfortunately, the medical staff there rarely uses this opportunity to educate them by providing certain basic knowledge about prevention of diseases. Similarly, the in-patients provide a tremendous opportunity to the medical staff to talk to them about various health protective, preventive and promotive measures. If these situations were utilized properly to educate people who come to the hospitals for seeking medical care, the general health of the Indian people would have been much better than what it is today. As long as the specialists and the super-specialists working in the teaching hospitals will not realize that they themselves have to become health educators rather than leave this task to the paramedical only, one can hardly hope for a positive change in the health status of the Indian people in the near future. The specialists like the general surgeons, orthopedic surgeons, obstetricians, pediatric surgeons, eye surgeons, dental surgeons, plastic surgeons and the like can all, in their own distinct ways, play an exceedingly important role of providing specific disease-related health education to the patients when they come to them for treatment. No one can deny that a person involved in an automobile accident can understand the value of wearing a helmet much more quickly if he is told about it by an orthopedic or plastic surgeon to whom he has approached for the treatment of his head injury. Similarly, a pediatrician, treating a case of neo-natorum tetanus can use this opportunity of educating the mother about the devastating effect of the traditional practice of applying cowdung on the umbilical cord.

The kind of value and respect which the patients attach to the word of a medical specialist is virtually beyond the domain of a para-medical like the present day community health workers who just have a three-month training at a health centre. Unfortunately, not many teaching hospitals provide good examples of working in teams. The specialists succumb to a certain tendency of working in their own closed compartments. Thus, the higher the specialisation, the greater the possibility of compartmentalisation. Health education can have its impact only when it becomes the responsibility of the entire team of specialists. If all of them equally realise the importance of health education, they can create a desirable preventive atmosphere in the hospitals. The most frequent complaint against the hospital administration are lack of sympathy and courtesy on the part of medical and administrative staff. This is particularly the case in the OPD's and Emergency Ward as the patients and their attendants are already in a state of agony and tension. It is suggested that the medical and administrative staff must spare some time to console the patients and their relatives. This would provide a great psychological and moral satisfaction to patients. The hospital authorities must foster goodwill, trust and understanding among the patients and their relatives. This would operate genuine climate and real situation where health education can be imparted to the people. In this way the functioning of the hospital would not be limited to its four walls but would infiltrate in the whole community served by the hospital. This would create a good relationship between the hospital and the community it serves.

CONCLUSIONS AND RECOMMENDATIONS

Without evaluating the impact of health education programmes on the bulk of the people, one cannot possibly identify positive as well as negative aspects of the programme. An objective evaluation of the health education programme alone can help one improve the guidelines for future action. 'Cost-benefit' analysis should be an integral part of this evaluation, so that one may assess how available resources have been utilized. Through objective evaluation; one may also be able to curtail mass production of ritualistic health education material as produced by various health education bureaus. The amount thus saved can be effectively utilised for a more purposeful and meaningful health education programme.

Health education is the most difficult task as habits, usages and customs are deeply entrenched. But health administration would fail in its purpose if it could not produce social change through health education. That is why it has been said that "it is easier to destroy mountains than to change our customs."[19] Professional training helps the health experts to deal with the health changes effectively. Their pharmacopoeia in both fields must be strong in order to translate the findings of biological investigations into social application. So over and above each technical act; there is a corresponding education function which doubles the value of the act, increases its efficiency and endows it with real human and social value.[20] G. Borkar in his book, "Health in Independent India" writes that all progress in public health depends ultimately on the willing assent and cooperation of the people and their active participation in measures intended for individual and community health protection, considering how much of illness is the result of ignorance of simple hygienic laws or indifference to their application. In practice, no single measure is productive of greater returns to outlay than health education.[21] Thus, health education can influence the lives of people for many generations. WHO conducted an interview of a Mongolian Feldsher. He stated that "conducting continuous health education is my first duty, prevention is our basic principle. Every effort is made to raise the health knowledge of the people. Child care, correct feeding and vaccinations are among the most important topics for health education.[22]

In order to improve the functioning of the administration of health education at the Union and State levels in India, the following facts and suggestions may be taken into consideration:[23]

1. Effective Role for Hospitals in Health Education as Patients are Amenable to their Advice

Hospitals within the country are not serving as agencies of health education. Health education can be imparted to mothers when they come to hospitals with their babies. During their stay in the hospital, mothers can be taught how to care for their children during sickness and how to feed them correctly. The mental field is also full of promise. Hospital physicians can do much in this direction by their own attitude to patients, give them simple instructions and, above all, treat them as persons rather than cases.

2. Modernise Health Education Institutes

Those very institutions responsible for imparting health education courses are lacking in standards for sanitary facilities. It is difficult to see how the concepts of sanitation can be effectively imparted among trainees, under such conditions. The curricula and contents of health education need careful planning. The educational methods for health education used in a country or community should be regularly evaluated and revised in line with socio-economic development. Health education should be oriented to health consciousness and not disease consciousness.

3. Constant Research and Evaluation

There is the necessity of research in behavioural sciences for the improvement of health education. Dr. B.S. Sehgal, Director, CHEB, New Delhi, said, "It was essential to conduct research on the behavioural sciences, in order to build-up a body of knowledge for meeting the challenges posed by the health programmes."[24]

4. Special Attention to Training of Trainers

Training for trainers needs re-orientation and re-examination. We should supplement classroom-based academically oriented training strategy in health education with the actual practice based on models of social change. The emphasis should be on learning by doing and nor by listening alone. To quote a UNICEF/WHO study:

> "Efforts in health education have often been limited to giving information dogmatically, as if this alone would bring about a transformation. Inevitably, the outcome has been disappointing. The pattern of existing resources—economic, human and cultural—has been forgotten and this too has contributed to health education's failure."[25]

5. Creation of Womens' Club as in Democratic Republic of Korea (DRK)

Women can be effectively approached only by women workers. The experiment of mother's club has been sufficiently rewarding and useful in the People's Democratic Republic of Korea as agencies of socio-economic development. The process of social and economic development is a process of human development for people is the target as well as essential variable in development. Communication being a two-way process, provides for participation at whatever stage of enlightenment the individuals composing a society find themselves. Mother clubs if established in India in right earnest can be the key factors in both the communication and development process since they can be the instruments for getting facts to the people upon which decisions can be based.[26]

6. Understand Local Social-cultural Issues

Before launching any programme of health education, the health educator must assess the local problems and possess the knowledge about the beliefs, conceptions and misconceptions which the people have formed about diseases, their causation and cure. This is possible provided the multi-disciplinary studies of rural communities are encouraged. Such studies would throw light about the cultural background of the people. He can arrange his programmes accordingly and this will save him from antagonism and hostility.

7. Create Good Relations with Mass Media

There is less coordination between health education and the means of mass media communication which needs strengthening on positive lines.

It needs to be recognised that most of our health education programmes and activities are so ritualistic in nature that they rarely correspond to the realities of the situation. In most situations the health educator's knowledge of the cultural content of health education programme is often so deficient that they find it hard to deliver the health education messages in a culturally acceptable manner. It needs to be stressed that the cultural aspect of health education programme is of the greatest importance in the Indian situation. Anthropological and sociological studies in the area of health education are so few in our country that health educators find it extremely hard to understand the many changing aspects of the communities they deal with. There is, thus, an urgent need to study the social and cultural context of health and disease, and to design health services in such a way as will gain the acceptance and support of the people involved. The social scientists can help the health educator in the following ways:

(1) to understand the role of socio-cultural factors in health, including people's beliefs about etiology, diagnosis and therapy of prevalent diseases;
(2) to understand the food culture including people's belief regarding consumption or rejection of various foods on socio-cultural considerations;
(3) to understand people's attitudes towards acceptance or rejection of health education programmes; and
(4) to help them plan and develop culturally relevant health education programmes.

South-East Regional Office of WHO has also expressed its dissatisfaction over the lack of importance to health education in its report, "Health Situation in the South-East Asian Region, 1994-97", (p. 72).

Despite these achievements, health education and promotion practices are faced with major constraints—the low priority accorded to health education at the policy level, high illiteracy levels, inadequate resources, poor social status of women, and limited capacity for health promotion research are but only a few examples. To overcome such constraints, new thinking and innovative approaches are required. As we move into the 21st century, the challenges for health promotion go beyond the wider articulation of the concept of health promotion, to building infrastructure and achieving adequate levels of resources both technical and financial, in order to respond effectively to the increasing demands for health promotion in the Region. "Settings for health" represent the organizational base of the infrastructure required for health promotion.

Partnerships which effectively respond to the health needs of specific population groups, such as workers, women and school children, need to be more vigorously pursued. Healthy public policies need to be developed to ensure supportive environments for individual and community health action, and to protect people from lifestyle-related problems such as those due to tobacco and alcohol. Documentation and dissemination of health promotion outcomes are also critical to the legitimization of the cause of health promotion in the Region.

New health challenges mean that new and diverse networks need to be created to achieve intersectoral collaboration. Such network should provide mutual assistance within and among countries, and facilitate the exchange of information about which strategies have proved effective. All countries need to develop the appropriate political, legal, educational, social and economic environments required to support health promotion. In this venture of health education, mass-media if properly used can help solve the problems.

Health promoters and educators need to be convinced that the mass-media can operate in the public interest and should play a critical role in social affairs, including health issues. The health concerns of readers, listeners and viewers are very much the concerns of the print and broadcast journalists. The basis of the relationship between the health and media sectors should therefore be one of partnership, not one of user-helper.

Health and media are not naturally inclined to work in unison. Historically, medical scientists trained in the methodical and meticulous search for knowledge have been somewhat skeptical of any effort at popularizing their work. Some doctors even view the media with suspicion and ambivalence. Media people, on the other hand, need to have their source material in language understandable to the layman; they have motive to dwell on technical details and often lose patience with lengthy scientific nappers.

Yet media and health in a close partnership have much to contribute to the public's welfare. Without the involvement of the media, the health sector cannot hope to inform the public on health issues or to help stimulate a community's involvement, which is critical to the success of any health effort. Without the technical input of the health sector the media cannot fulfil their obligations to serve the interest of the public and these public interests certainly include health.

The complexity of the media, with their obsession for meeting dead lines and their own technical constraints, is little appreciated or understood by health professionals. Those in health who work in partnership with the media need to acquire a rudimentary knowledge of how media works—not in order to become media specialists but to be more empathetic in their dealings with the journalists and broadcasters. This in turn will call for a good hard look at the core curriculum of the training of health promoters and educators.

Whether the health professionals can play their rightful role in battling successfully against lifestyle-related illness—including AIDS and whether health education and promotion practitioners will enter the 21st century adequately prepared for the communication challenges, will depend on the actions that health authorities take now.[27]

In the new millennium, we need to harness all the resources especially the mass-media in a planned manner. This would require active collaboration between media and health specialists. Jack Ling[28] in his article, "Health and the Media" has rightly stressed that the health sector should focus on making technical subjects digestible and understandable to the layman. In particular, the health professionals should identify existing, credible channels of communication, including traditional ones, in order to reach the public. The media offers the public health community more than just access to air-time and newspaper space; they are also a source of communications expertise that is needed to ensure the success of large-scale health promotion campaigns and transmit technical information about health to a mass audience.

What is more useful is the follow-up of media-transmitted message that can be effected by village health workers. For instance, primary health care workers can be an effective channel of communication by delivering in person the same messages that have been delivered to a target audience in print or over the radio, thus increasing the overall impact of the educational drive.

A dialogue has to be initiated between decision-makers in media and in public health. The object of that dialogue should be to heighten awareness among the media personnel about the important responsibility they hold for the health and well-being of their people, and equally to alert health professionals to their own responsibility for ensuring that their health initiatives reach all people. Without this whole-hearted backing from the media in conveying health messages to the greatest number of people, we risk having only Health for Some and not Health for All.

However, the success of health education would depend in the long-run upon the shoulders of the providers of health care to the people. They should be motivated to do this job as a part of their medical duties. S.S. Sooch in his Article, "Revamping Health Care" in the *Daily Tribune* (26 January, 2000) rightly remarks that there is a general feeling that most of the health care providers in the government-run hospitals are indifferent, apathetic and insensitive and a few even outrightly arrogant in their behaviour. A sense of compassion and human touch is simply missing. A series of crash courses should be arranged to expose the entire staff to the art of public relations.

Health Education is vital to provide health to all in 21st century.

This is the cheapest and most effective tool of health care. The success of Primary Health Care in 21st Century depends upon the identification of community needs through community needs assessment surveys and later on providing health education to the community so that they can solve their health problems themselves.

Notes and References

1. Muhammad Al-Khateeb, 'New Lifestyles, New Disease" in *World Health*, July 1989, p. 23.
2. *Ibid.*
3. WHO, *World Health*, July-August 1995, p. 16.
4. *World Health*, June 1986, p. 2.

5. *World Health,* Feb.-March 1980, p. 1.
6. WHO, SEARO: Health Situation in the South-East Asia Region, 1994-97, New Delhi, 1999, pp. 149-51.
7. *World Health,* July 1989, p. 23.
8. Abdulmoneim Aly: Health Education Through Religion, in *World Health,* July 1989, p. 27.
9. John J. Hanlon, Principles of Public Health Administration, St. Louis, 1960, p. 402.
10. WHO, *Technical Report Series,* No. 89, p. 4.
11. WHO, *Ibid.,* No. 156, p. 3.
12. K.S. Sanjiva, Planning India's Health, Orient Longman, New Delhi, 1971, p. 64.
13. WHO, *World Health,* Feb.-March 1979, p. 24.
14. UNICEF, UNICEF News, "Communication: A Tool for Development", Issue 84/1975/12, p. 18.
15. WHO, *World Health,* Nov. 1975, p. 14.
16. *World Health,* Jan.-Feb. 1989, p. 9.
17. *World Health,* May 1979, p. 25.
18. WHO: *Technical Report Series,* No. 89, 1954.
19. Bosnian proverb.
20. WHO: *Technical Report Series,* 1954.
21. Borkar, Health in Independent India, p. 217.
22. WHO, *World Health,* April 1977, p. 20.
23. Based on personal discussion and interview.
24. WHO, SEARO: SEA/RC 23, p. 88.
25. UNICEF, Health and Basic Services, Keys to Development, *op. cit.,* p. 46.
26. For further details refer to author's article, "Role of Communication in Family Planning Setting up of Mother's Club in PEN, Family Planning Association of India, Haryana Branch, May 1977.
27. Jack C.S. Ling, "The Media its Role," in *World Health,* January-Feb. 1989, p. 25.
28. Jack Ling, "Health and Media" in *World Health,* March 1986, p. 15.

CHAPTER 20

MODERNISING HEALTH AND HOSPITAL ADMINISTRATION

Administration of health services needs constant review and research to ensure availability, accessibility and utilisation.
We cannot continue doing what we have always done
Tomorrow cannot be just more of yesterdays
We need flexibility and progmation as much as innovation
But the stress must invariably be on education.

—Author

Modernising Health and Hospital Administration

A. NEED AND NATURE OF MANAGEMENT IMPROVEMENT

People of advanced countries get their health services as much for granted as the essential utility services like water, electricity, public transport, etc. Despite the magic bullets of the modern medicine, the health services in the developing countries are far from satisfactory. The people living in the developing world, and especially 70 per cent of them living in rural areas, have little or no access to modern medical and health care resulting in high rates of morbidity and mortality from diseases which are preventable. If we want to reach the objective of providing decent quality health care to all by the first quarter of 21st century. We will have to introduce innovations in technical and administrative fields. It has been recognized by health experts in all the countries that the difficulties in meeting the health needs of the community are largely dependent upon the capabilities to design and manage the health care delivery system. The management of health care system can help in the greater achievement of goals through the optimum utilization of resources available—men, money and material. Indian ranks in Human Development index is 128 as per Human Development Report, 2000. To quote Dr. Chi-Yuen Wu of UNDP:

> "To create administrative capabilities, commensurate with requirements, developing countries must be able among other things, to use modern management techniques more effectively than in the case of the industrially advanced countries."

Joginder Singh in his article, "Reducing Government Flab—Time to Drain the Swamp" in *The Tribune*, March 16, 2000 righly observes that it is amazing that the government is always emphasising on its employees to function with full coordination and assist the citizens with the quickest possible response. Notwithstanding all the instructions/orders of the government, the position on the ground remains anything but people-oriented. The responsiveness of the administration to the people who matter is individual-oriented. There is hardly any response where the common good matters, unless powerful interests back it.

The need of the hour for our country, burdened with poverty, illiteracy, backwardness and rampant corruption, is effective and dynamic governance. Good governance and effective management can provide the panacea for all the ills and stumbling blocks in the system. Transformation of the country is possible only when the necessary changes are brought about. We need a revolution of a different kind led by the right-thinking and right-acting leaders, who should not only prepare but also implement a blueprint for future development in a fixed time schedule.

Unfortunately, present management systems are not functioning well as these are managed by untrained personnel. This is the common management challenge faced by those in charge of the health services. To quote a recently published book: [1]

> "In the field of health, we rarely have consciously trained executives. . . . We have expected a vast army of professional care givers to fill individual human needs, mainly on a *laissez faire* basis, mostly without planning without coordination, without sufficient for (those) who either do not look for care, cannot afford it or cannot get to it."
>
> "With little or no formal training, administrators. . . . have arisen from our midst willy-nilly, too few through natural ability, too many by viture of their staying—power on particular job, lack of available competition, or the administrator's uncritical need for power and control. . . ."
>
> "In health administration, there are few theoreticians, few training centres, few books, and an almost absolute dearth of strict scientific investigations."

Thus, there is a great need to improve the functioning of health care management with the help of modern management techniques. A modern management system is one which is designed to make the existing health care delivery process effective and efficient. Modern management methods and techniques are in reality, only techniques for improving this process by making it more accurate and reliable, by making the process respond faster, or by giving the health-manager the ability and capability to manage better.

Health administration in a country is a part of the total administration and thus influences and is influenced by this general administrative culture. Let us have a look at the general administrative apparatus prevailing in developing countries. In India, for instance, the administrative machinery has not been adequate to handle the tasks of economic and social development. The administrative inadequacies in a national government has a retarding influence on economic and social development. This lack of efficiency in administration equally holds good for the health organizations as well. The widespread feeling of inefficiency of the administrative machinery was rightly sensed and expressed by Mrs. Gandhi in a broadcast to the nation shortly after assuming the high office of the Prime Minister. She said:

> "In economic development as in other fields of national activity, there is a disconcerting gap between intention and action. To bridge this gap, we should boldly adopt whatever far-reaching changes in administration may be found necessary. We must introduce new organizational patterns and modern tools and techniques of management and administration. We shall instill into the government machinery greater efficiency and sense of urgency and make it more responsive to the needs of the people."[2]

In the health sector, it was emphasized that "better management of health services is essential if higher standards of health care are to be achieved. . . . that progress. . . .today is to a higher extent dependent on education and development of the management, than it is on medical research and increase of material resources."[3]

The development of public administration remains an essential prerequisite for successful economic development of the country. Therefore, far-reaching improvements in public administration are required if the objectives of planned socio-economic development are to be realised.

Before we analyse the meaning, nature, scope and application of management techniques for administrative improvements and reforms, let us be clear about the concept of administrative improvement first.

Administrative improvement means the act or the process of improving the administration. As stated in a United Nations Report:

> "Management improvement comprised the planning, implementation and evaluation of various measures conducive to the increase of organizational effectiveness and efficiency."[4]

Administrative reform is still widely regarded as a special type of improvement activity, even when it is often closely connected with other activities. The concept of the "administrative reform", as it is applied in practice, also has its weakness. In a report by the Secretariat of the United Nations Programme in Public Administration for the period from 1950 to 1966, it is stated that:

"Efforts at administrative reform too often stop with the preparation of reports or promulgation of law."[5]

In a number of countries the word 'reform' has also a close relationship to political concepts and attitudes, which makes it less suited for general use than the broader concept of 'improvement' or 'effectiveness'.

Public administration in any country cannot remain static over a period of time. There are always scientific, economic, political social, cultural and other changes taking place in a country. Health organizations like other organizations, must adjust themselves to these changes in order to be effective and responsive to the needs of the people. Peter Drucker, an expert in the field of management has said: "Social awareness is organizational self-interest. The needs of the society, is left unfilled, turn into social diseases. No institution whether business or hospital or University or Government agency is likely to survive in a diseased society."

The design of an administrative system is a basic aid to the achievement of its primary objectives; if the design is unsound, the achievement of objectives is likely to fall short of expectations. Therefore, there is a great need to improve the structure and functioning of the administrative organizations.

Most of the economic and social progress in the developing countries is halted because the administrative apparatus in these countries is not upto the mark. Therefore, there is an urgent need of administrative improvement in these countries. H. Paul Appleby has rightly remarked that the full success of the plan, therefore, turns rather exclusively on administrative reform to make the Government as an organism equal to its identified goals.

The administrative capability of a Government and the manner in which the development programmes are likely to be carried out are intimately related. On the other hand, administrative inadequacies in a national Government have a retarding influence on economic and social development. These deficiencies prevent the vast flood of money, talent and material from achieving their objectives. As early as 1950, the Secretary-General of the United Nations pointed out that, "Any systematic effort towards economic development must be preceded by or coupled with efforts to make more effective the functioning of Government machinery."[6]

During the last few decades, phenomenal changes are taking place at a fast rate in the field of science and technology as well as administration also, which today, has to shoulder multifarious task designed to fulfil the rising aspirations of the people. In the words of Prof. Waldo, Public Administration is, "a part of the cultural complex, and it not only is acted upon, it acts." It is a great creative force. There is an urgent need to re-orient (improve) the system of public administration to cope with changes in technology and social behaviour and maximise opportunities for raising productivity, and thus the standard of living of the people.

According to Sir Isaiah Berlin, "It is certainly a reasonable hypothesis that one of the principal causes of confusion, misery and fear is blind adherence to outworn notions, pathological suspicion of any form of critical examination, frantic efforts to prevent any degree of rational analysis of what we believe, we live by and for."

Thus, public administration including health administration must be recreated, renewed and revitalised to produce the predesigned changes and output in the modernization of societies. This necessitates a different trend and magnitude of administrative culture and capability.

Scope of Management Improvement

If the need for change and effectiveness is to be fulfilled, management improvement must be considered to be an organization-wide continuous activity. This important function must embrace the total needs based on the objectives and goals of the public administration and the resources available. The improvement efforts must be regarded as a whole involving a spectrum of different types and levels of activity. There is, in principle, no reason why 'administrative reform' and 'organization and methods' should be set-up as separate and isolated activities. These and other new activities should rather be merged and coordinated into a total, carefully planned and organized "management improvement programme" involving the whole organization. The needs require centrally planned improvement programme, and for coordination purposes decentralized programmes in different ministries and institutions. Each agency or institution of importance should be responsible for its own programme, planned in cooperation with the central authorities.

As the implementation of significant changes in organizational structure and behaviour is complex and time consuming task and is closely related to the long-term development planning of the country, improvement programme must be planned on long-term (from ten to fifteen years), medium-term (from four to five years) and short-term (yearly) basis.

Strategies and Policies in Administrative Improvement

As stated in a UN publication, the following strategies and policies are necessary to bring about administrative improvement:

(a) Improvement work must be a systematically planned organised activity with specific work programmes, a continuous activity, and it should be based on long-term planning and development.
(b) Classification of objectives and goals is necessary to be able to

measure or evaluate the effectiveness and manage the improvement work.

(c) Improvement work must be recognised as a responsibility of the management; and in planning and organising improvement projects, participation and involvement of management in the organizations affected by possible changes are of great importance.

(d) Special resources must be allocated to the improvement projects including the support of professional staff of high quality with special qualifications in the management fields.

(e) Improvement work must be based on the concept or the organization as a socio-technical system where human and social factors are of primary importance.

(f) Training and development of the members of organizations — both management and staff, usually constitute one of the most important parts of improvement work.

(g) Improvement projects should from the beginning be oriented towards implementation and change, step by step, and not only towards writing reports and giving recommendations. Such projects should include specific implementation plans.

(h) As a rule, there is need for both centralised and decentralised (though coordinated) improvement programmes. It is advisable first to build-up a strong, central activity.

(i) An improvement work programme should be formalised as an obligation for the public administration institutions and tied with long-term development plans, and budgeting and accounting control procedures.

(j) The improvement project organization should be flexible. A task force, under a responsible project leader and a Steering Committee, is often a usual type of organization.

(k) In larger projects, pilot studies of the implementation of new organizational structures in a limited part of the administration are often necessary and useful to demonstrate effects and results.

(l) Improvement projects must be planned in terms of activities, time and resources. The setting of deadlines or time-limits in the work programmes has frequently proved most helpful in the effort to obtain a high level activity and results.[7]

After explaining the concept of administrative improvements, let us discuss the need, type and utility of management techniques as an instrument of administrative improvements and reforms.

B. NEED FOR MANAGEMENT TECHNIQUES

In a developing country, such as ours, there is a great haste to achieve maximum growth and progress in the shortest time possible. It is felt that the scope of experimentation is a costly and slow process. As such, we need to learn from the experience of others and use their results to help achieve our goals. A word of caution at this point is in order. Nothing succeeds like success. So too is the case of the glamorous instances of technology and management techniques and their tall claims of progress and development. Such a philosophy has done more harm than good. A few years before, modern management techniques were thought to be a panacea for all problems. Some problems did get solved while a host of others took birth as a result; many of the over popular techniques have found their graveyards whilst a lot of organizations which should have gone to the graveyards for not putting into use the 'over popular' techniques, have passed the test of time and resistance. In this context, Ernest Dale and L.C. Michelon observes that:

> "Today's manager lives in a world of rapid change, and yet the rate of change is likely to increase in the years ahead. Unless, he can keep up with this change, he is likely to find himself obsolete — perhaps unpromotable or even unemployable."[8]

Thus, there is a great need to enhance the administrative capability of health administrators so that they can use these techniques profitably. Administrative capability is an important means of converting or processing programme inputs into outputs such as goods and services. It has been mentioned by Gabriel that, "What makes the leadership variable so crucial in implementation process, is its dynamic, not passive quality, i.e., its capability to act and react on these critical inputs. It is this manipulative and transferring quality of leadership that could significantly determine the administrative capability of implementing organisation."[9]

Administrative capability is "the capacity to obtain intended results through organizations."[10]

Katz says:

> "Administrative capability for development involves the ability to mobilize, allocate and combine the actions that are technically needed to achieve development objectives."[11]

Organizations are not simply structures but action-oriented system and the success and failure of the organizations are to be measured in terms of this action system. Action system is a structured device in which resources are mobilized and transformed by use of certain skill and technology to produce pre-designed output all taking place by the influence of administrative capability within an environmental context.

Health administrators should facilitate the accomplishment of desired objectives with the least friction and the most satisfaction to those for whom the task is done and those engaged in the enterprise. Thus, there is a need to understand and portray the management techniques in all its various facets.

Management techniques are of added significance for the health sector as this sector deals with preventive, promotive, and curative and rehabilitative aspects of health care activities and uses the services of Government, private and voluntary agencies. Most of the practitioners, academicians and political elite are not happy with the performance of this sector as the majority of people in the developing world do not have access even to rudimentary health care. After personal discussions with some of the health experts and top management of health personnel at Chandigarh, it was revealed that the present administration was in a bad state and needed radical reforms. It was confirmed by personal visits to some of the health institutions and their field establishments, as also by the health and medical personnel at District and Block levels. This is resulting in huge wastage of resources. There have been a large number of administrative problems which account for the unsatisfactory working of the health administration. These problems have already been examined in the earlier chapters. Some of the specific problems which need immediate solutions can be mentioned as:

(a) Absence of effective health policy to meet the need of the people.
(b) Absence of coordination between the health and socio-economic sector; between Western and indigenous system of medicine and among Government, Private and Voluntary administration.
(c) Lack of effective planning, monitoring, implementation and evaluation machinery.
(d) Lack of an effective manpower planning resulting in the concentration of health services in the urban sectors.
(e) Absence of people's participation in the health care delivery operations.
(f) Absence of decentralisation resulting in inefficiency of operations.
(g) Disproportionate investments for secondary and tertiary health care.
(h) Top heavy administrative set-up.
(i) Defective organisations and procedure—an obstacle in the way of efficient services.
(j) Lack of interest to improve administrative structure and procedure, i.e., absence of innovative leadership.

In reviewing the management of health services, the delegates who came to attend the 25th Regional Committee meeting of the South-East Asia Region of WHO, noted the following considerations and constraints:[12]

(a) lack of a clear development policy and clear objectives for health services in relation to socio-economic development;
(b) inadequate understanding of health problems and the problem of tackling it from the viewpoint of consumers and provides of health care;
(c) poor utilisation of existing resources and inadequate harnessing of potential resources, human and other for health;
(d) inadequate coordination and integration between different authorities and organizations providing health services in the same geographical areas;
(e) inadequate or no integration of preventive, curative and family planning services;
(f) the increasing cost of health services and their inequitable distribution, with the result that the basic health needs of all the people were not being met;
(g) the participation of communities in the promotion of their own health and in contributing to health services policy-making, financing and decision-making;
(h) the need to find ways of developing new types of health manpower, including local multi-purpose health workers, and of employing them on a wider scale;
(i) the need to develop an organization in the countries of the region for improved delivery of health services within the existing constraints—both financial and manpower—for the masses in rural areas, which alone constitutes about 80 per cent of the population; and
(j) meager allocation of fund (3 to 5 per cent) for health in the overall socio-economic development plans in most countries of the Region.

C. NATURE AND CLASSIFICATION OF MANAGEMENT TECHNIQUES

Nature

In order to understand the meaning of 'management techniques' we must be clear about the two concepts, namely, 'management' and 'techniques'. In simple words, management is the handling of tools and techniques to achieve a desired goal. In other words, management infers planning, organising and controlling of human and other resources to achieve specified goals. A technique is a set of procedural steps which may be loosely or rigorously stated, which embody a multiple idea content and which are concerned with doing work to achieve an objective.

In other words, we can say that management technique is a set of procedural steps which may be loosely stated, embodying a multiple-idea content and which are either concerned with decision-making in general or with decision relating to planning, organising or controlling of human and/or other resources with a view to achieving the specified objectives. Management techniques make positive efforts to analyse the situation in a systematic and scientific manner and provide a rational basis for decisions. Adoption of these techniques would encourage greater professionalism in administrative activities. If a new administrative culture is also developed side by side, it would be possible to make optimum use of available and potential resources. According to one of the ILO publications, management techniques are systematic procedures of investigating, planning, controlling and supervising which can be applied to management problems.[13] Thus, modern management techniques, in actuality, are the techniques for improving the management process by making it more accurate, by making the process respond faster, or by giving the manager greater control. From the above discussion, we can say that management techniques have the following features:

1. They are a set of procedural or formal steps. This is basic for any management technique. Procedural or formal steps lead to 'systematic' approach which has been the highlight of any scientific method, the root of all sound modern management theory. They take us from the known facts to the unknown parts of the problem.
2. They have a multiple-idea content. They do not have a single idea, but a number of them though related ones.
3. They help in decision-making in general or with decisions relating either to planning, organising or controlling or to any combination of these three processes of planning, organising and controlling of human and/or other resources with a view to achieving certain specified objectives.
4. They give the idea of efficiency which, according to Clay, can further be broken into five components:
   (a) economy of efforts in terms of money and other resources;
   (b) speed;
   (c) quality;
   (d) stability; and
   (e) aesthetic or rhythmical approach.
5. They are consistent in their results.

Functional Classification of Management Techniques

Management techniques can be classified in different ways. For example, they can be grouped according to the outlet and the department in which they are applied as, for example, preventive techniques, promotive techniques and curative techniques. This does not, however, cover all techniques. For example, where would we place the techniques of brain-storming or critical examination? An alternative can be classification according to parent discipline. But it is more an historical approach than a current use, because many of the techniques are developed in one field but later on used in a number of fields. Clay gives a classification which is based on the objective of the technique, i.e., what does the technique hope to achieve? He mentions the following eight objectives which various management techniques attempt to achieve.[14]

1. Detection (To find out or discover something e.g., what is happening or what is wrong?)

We can include such technique here as input-output Analysis, Attitude Survey, Production Study, Activity Sampling, Critical Examination, Break-even Analysis.

2. Evaluation (To measure or estimate the value of an item)

We can include such techniques here as Job Evaluation, Work Measurement, Work Estimation, Performance Appraisal, Cost-Benefit Analysis.

3. Improvement (To improve performance)

We can include such techniques here as Management by Objectives, Method Study, Value Analysis, etc.

4. Optimization (To optimise performance)

We can include such techniques here as Linear Programming, Ergonomics, Operations Research, etc.

5. Specification (To specify a desired value or situation or action)

Here we can include such technique as Layout Planning for Offices and Plants layout, designing, etc.

6. Control

Here we can include such techniques as Cost Control, Credit Control, Labour Control, Inventory Control, Production Control, Budget Control, etc.

7. Communication (To communicate information)

Here we can include such techniques as Visual Aids, Suggestion Schemes, Report Writing, Communication Theory, Information Theory, Management Information, etc.

8. Demonstration (To demonstrate something)

Here we can include such technique as Programmed Learning, Job Instruction, Management Development and Training, etc.

This achievement criteria tells us that these techniques can help us in discovering or finding something in evaluating the performance, in improving the performance, in optimizing the performance, in specifying a desired value or a situation, in controlling a variable, in communication or in demonstration.

The management techniques can also be classified in terms of various resources employed in an organization, viz., human material, machinery and equipment, money and time. As such, some of the techniques which can be applied to bring about increased managerial capability, efficiency, effectiveness and productivity can be categorized as under:

Sr. No.	*Source*	*Management Techniques*
1.	Human Resources	1. Organizational analysis 2. Job Evaluation 3. Training 4. Incentive Schemes 5. Suggestion Schemes 6. Method Study 7. Work Measurement
2.	Material	1. Inventory Control 2. Value Analysis 3. Material Handling 4. Standardisation 5. ABC/VED
3.	Machinery and Equipment	1. Method Study 2. Value Analysis
4.	Space and Building	1. Labour Planning 2. Method Study
5.	Money	1. Cost Benefit Analysis 2. Budgetary Control 3. Performance Budgeting 4. Management Accounting
6.	Time	1. Method Study 2. Work Measurement 3. Network Analysis (PERT/CPM)

Before we proceed to discuss the systematic applicability of management techniques according to the level of activities of management, let us discuss in brief the meaning and utility of some of the important techniques.

O & M

It is generally used to describe the activities of groups of people in

Government or other public bodies or in private institutions who are asked to advise health administrators or managers on the question of Organization and Method so as to increase the efficiency of work for which they are responsible, either by providing a better service, or a cheaper one or both.

PERSONNEL ADMINISTRATION

Participative Management and Organizational Development (OD)

The health of an organization is measured in terms of its capability to adjust with internal and external environmental challenges. We find now-a-days that in big health organizations like hospitals, there is a lot of friction amongst the experts and other staff generating an atmosphere of frustration and low morale, resulting in the overall inefficiency. We can introduce the technique of OD in such large hospitals to maintain the healthy atmosphere of work. A comprehensive definition of OD has been given by Backhard. According to him:

"Organizational Development is an effort:
(1) Planned;
(2) Organization-wide;
(3) Managed from the top to;
(4) Increase organization effectiveness and health through; and
(5) Planned interventions in the organizations' 'Process' using behavioural science knowledge."[15]

OD depends upon the purely internal initiative of the employees of an organization. The present emphasis in health administration is only on structural changes but structural changes without personnel dedication and capabilities would be of no avail. It is high time that we introduce OD in all our big health institutions to ward-off the bureaucratic attitudes which result in low output and stagnation. We have also the other technique to achieve this objective, e.g. Management by Objectives, Participative Management. We must try to integrate all these techniques for optimizing the efficiency of personnel in an organization.

The most important task of Personnel Department must be to give abundant evidence of its belief that personnel in an organization are key to development. This requires proper motivation of the employees. Motivation is of utmost importance as it constitutes the base for the management functions of planning and organising. It has been noticed that the performance of the personnel either as individuals or members of a group is less as compared to their capabilities in terms of skills, abilities and capacities. Finer, for example, states that demonstrated performance generally never exceeds more than fifty per cent of the individual's ability to perform.[16] Most individuals tend to balance their efforts around an assessment of relative costs (time and energy) and benefits.[17] A climate of creativity must be developed and maintained by management. Maier and Hayes say that the optimal climate for creativity. . . .in whatever human conditions is optimal for individual freedom and self-expression in social setting.[18]

It is the duty of the officers of such units to make the employees feel that their work and their association with a given organisation represent a vehicle which will accelerate the achievement of personal goals as well as the achievement of goals of the organisation. This would require the active participation of the employees in the decision-making process of the organisation.

> "Participation is . . . an individual's mental and emotional involvement in a group situation that encourages him to contribute to group goals and to share responsibility for them."[19]

Management Information System

The significance of information for administration can be compared to what Napoleon said about the army: "an army marches on its stomach," — any administration marches on information. As the universe is saturated with information, health administration must select pertinent information for their programmes otherwise it is difficult to make any rational policy or decision. This technique is tailored to provide such information to the decision-makers which is most relevant, accurate, complete, concise, timely, economic, reliable and efficient.[20] A good information system provides data for monitoring and evaluating the programmes and gives the requisite feedback to the administrators and planners at all levels.[21]

The development of a suitable technique for a health information system would improve the capacity of health administrators to make appropriate policy-decisions. The information system may not serve the purpose if the health administrators are not committed to use the information constructively. The health administrators should use the available information sensibly and logically rather than construct complex information system which may not be used. We can show with the help of the diagram the functions of information for policy formulation.

ABC Analysis

It is a technique which would enable a busy executive to chase those activities ardently which would quicken the wheels of administrative machinery. By arranging his work into an order of priorities, he can decide on which items to concentrate first, which others to deal later, and yet which others to delegate to his assistants. When done more systematically and in quantitative terms, this system of building up priorities of work is called the ABC Analysis. ABC Analysis can be of great use in dealing with materials management in hospitals. Forty to sixty per cent of the total expenditure of an organization is generally spent on materials. The other form of ABC Analysis is VED, i.e., arranging the activities in the orders of Vital, Essential and Desirable.

Network Analysis (PERT/CPM)

Both the Critical Path Method (CPM) and Programme Evaluation and Review Technique (PERT) emphasize efficient performance and temporal dimensions of a project. In the simplest form of PERT, a project is viewed as a total system and consists of setting up of schedule of dates for various stages and exercise of management control, mainly through project status reports, on its progress. The CPM is basically a technique to reduce the time required to implement a project. By breaking the project into activities that must be undertaken for its implementation and by determining their time sequence, it is possible to isolate the most critical activities in the project and to compute the critical path schedule for their implementation. Network planning provides the basis for both CPM and PERT.[22]

Moder and Philips enlist the following key advantages of using PERT:

1. It encourages logical discipline in planning, scheduling and control of projects.
2. It encourages more long-range and detailed project planning.
3. It provides a standard method of documenting and communicating Project Plans, Schedules and Time and Cost Performance.
4. It identifies the most critical elements in the Plan, thus focusing management attention on the 10-20 per cent of the project that is most constraining on the schedule.
5. It illustrates the effects of technical and procedural changes on overall schedules.[23]

The application of PERT/CPM can be profitably utilised in the Programmes and Projects of Health, e.g., construction of Hospitals, Eradication of Communicable Diseases, Family Planning Programmes, Administration of Environmental Programmes, etc. Care should be taken that the cost of the PERT/CPM should not take away large resources of the Project.

Cost-Benefit Analysis

This technique is designed to consider the social costs and benefits attributable to the project. The benefits are expressed in monetary terms to determine whether a given programme is economically sound, and to select the best out of several programmes. Its advantage lies not in making decision-making simpler, but in its possibilities for systematic examination of each part of a problem in hand, for putting diverse decision on a para and following logical sequence.[24]

Cost-Benefit Analysis is an aid to systematic thought and helps the planners to decide as to what should be done — on the relative merits of different programmes. How far, for example, should resources be devoted to health education or maternal and child health services or immunization against particular disease? Any given budget for health may be distributed between programmes by including, first, those with the highest ratio of benefits to cost, then those with the next larger and so on, until the budget is fully allocated. The limitation of this method in the field of health administration is that it is difficult to express the benefits in monetary terms. We must encounter this limitation by making our tools of research methodology perfect.

Cost-Effective Analysis

Cost effectiveness methods are those that search for the least costly way of achieving a defined result. Cost effectiveness analysis are easier to make as the aim is clear. It helps the health administrator in managing his health resources at the local level. The problem is to find the way of achieving the objective at lowest cost, e.g., to find effective ways of treating patients without sending them to hospital. Linear Programming can help in this direction.

Systems Approach

A system is an integrated assembly of interacting elements, designed to carry out cooperatively a pre-determined function. There are five major elements in a system approach — selecting objectives, designing alternatives, building models, weighing cost against effectiveness and the application of suitable criterion.

The application of systems analysis is useful in health management in that it provides for:[25]

1. consideration of all variables, over and above the biological and technical, that affect health intervention programmes;
2. a planning approach that relates input to output;
3. an emphasis on quantification;
4. rigour in analytical methods;
5. orientation towards health problems rather than towards categories of service;
6. communication with key governmental decision-making centres that utilised comparable methods;
7. early attention to planning and priority setting;
8. improved inter-disciplinary collaboration; and
9. the use of wide range of analytical models and methods of considerable power.

Application of Management Techniques for Administrative Improvement and Administrative Reforms

Having discussed the importance and utility of some of the important Management Techniques, we shall explain the application of the management techniques at different levels of management and to situations covering time horizons.

It reveals that one technique or the other is applied in one form or the other at all the three levels of management. Because the lowest level has to perform operational functions, management techniques like World Study, Network Analysis, Capacity Utilisation Studies are adopted. At the middle level, where the policy is executed, some more important techniques like Manpower Planning, Cost Benefit Analysis, Statistics and Forecasting, etc., are applied to effect improvements. The top managements uses more strategic techniques like Technological Forecasting, Performance Budgeting, Operational Research Studies, etc.

UTILITY AND LIMITATIONS

Utility

Let us explain the use of these techniques in improving the health services with some examples:

1. In a case study, a 750-bedded hospital (Medical Institute) was facing acute shortage of nursing personnel. The study of the utilisation of nursing personnel in this hospital revealed that 33 per cent time of the nurses was being spent on non-nursing duties. Besides, there was 25 per cent turnover of the nurses. There was a great delay in appointing the new incumbents. The study suggested that if the nurses are not given non-nursing duties, a saving of rupees three lakhs can take place. This was studied with the help of the techniques of organizational analysis.
2. A study was conducted by the writer of a University Health Centre where there was a problem of pilferage of drugs. The Chief Medical Officer of the Centre was finding it very difficult to plug this loop-hole as he himself was busy in examining the patients for all the duty time. It was suggested that the whole stock of the medicine may be classified on the basis on the cost with the help of the technique of ABC analysis. It was suggested to the Chief Medical Officer to keep 'A' category of drugs under lock and key to be issued only under his signature. He could check for other drugs once a month concentrating only on A and B categories. This helped the Centre to save about Rs. 25,000 annually.
3. A study was carried out by C.R. Prasad on the 'Application of Quantitative methods in Hospital Management'. He studied

the problems of patients who were wasting a lot of their time to get the prescriptions (to pay the cash and to receive the medicine). The patients had to stand in line for about 45 minutes. Prasad applied Sampling Techniques and used Simulation Procedures. He was able to suggest a model by which the average time of waiting could be reduced to 16 minutes from 45 minutes.[26]

The examples of the use of other techniques would be taken up in the relevant chapters.

Thus, we find that there is an ever-increasing array of methods and ιechniques available to assist the management for the acceleration of socio-economic development, with stated policies, objectives and priorities. Further, the impact of interdependence of the management techniques solely depend upon the development of improved management. But it is generally acknowledged that the availability and application of modern management skills do not meet the needs that are felt to exist.

Shortage and difficulties for the greater development and application of management skills are always encountered. Some of them are as under:

1. Shortage of experts in management techniques, and especially of those with knowledge and experience of the special problems of the health sector;
2. Difficulty in recruiting staff to specialise in health management and managerial technologies because of working conditions or lack of career prospects for personnel other than physicians;
3. Shortage of general management capability, together with lack of appreciation of 'systems thinking' and orientation to modern management on the part of doctors and health administrators;
4. Insufficient ability to identify situations in which the available consultants and other sources of expertise could best be used;
5. Lack of a form of organization that can fully utilize the available management skills;
6. Shortage of staff of various kinds (not just those with specific management skills);
7. Shortage of teachers in management for medical schools etc; and
8. Insufficient development of management methods for dealing with such difficulties, characteristic of health services as: defining objectives, public participation, coordination, motivation and supervision.

From the above, it is inferred that there is a room for improvement to make simultaneous progress on several fronts by:

(a) spreading the determination to overcome the difficulties mentioned and establishing confidence in using techniques;
(b) general management training and experience for health professionals;
(c) production of management specialists of various kinds, especially those with a broad experience in addition to their specialist skill;
(d) organisational changes necessary to utilise management skills and provide appropriate career and working conditions for their practitioners; and
(e) research and development to adapt management techniques to the health needs.[27]

No doubt, the theory of management techniques in the context of administrative improvement and administrative reforms can be learned in a classroom, from a text-book or through correspondence, but, these cannot replace the practical experience, only through which one acquires the skill of the technique.

Critical Appraisal of Management Techniques

Although the needs for modern management technology differ from country to country and from situation to situation, it is not to be expected that these differences will always be accurately interpreted, or that the most appropriate techniques will automatically be invoked. In fact, techniques like most other things, are susceptible to the influences of fashion. Their value depends on the circumstances in which they are applied. In other words, the use of management techniques, just as the exploitation of any other resources, have to be subject to continuous feedback and review.

There have been many instances when in a hurry to borrow from West, we blindly adopt the management techniques/technology in the 'as-it-is' form without even taking into consideration their limitations. John Argenti in one of his papers observes that "after all, many of the sophisticated techniques have not been employed by a great number of organizations in U.K.—we should not blindly employ the technique. We should be sure of its potentialities and also skilled in its use." This means that suitable technology has to be devised to provide for decent health care to the people much more economically than the affluent and advanced countries. Thus, there is a need to evolve appropriate management techniques and technology to suit our environment.

Modernizing Health Administration requires outstanding leadership. Eminent Industrialist, Mr. Rahul Bajaj, Chairman and Managing Director, Bajaj Auto Limited and President, CII, delivered the

Convocation Address at the 49th Annual Convocation of the SNDT Women's University, Mumbai. He said, "To realize our goals and aspirations, we need outstanding leadership in every field and at every level. Leadership means that there is no field at every level. Leadership means that there is no substitute for excellence, no tolerance of mediocrity and no compromise with integrity. Leadership is not just charisma, not public relations, not showmanship. Leadership is performance, consistent behaviour and trust-worthiness"

We are in a hurry; we wish to achieve much; we cannot afford the luxury of wasting our resources for experimentation. What is, therefore, needed is a proper identification of opportunities, setting out of priority areas and accordingly, continually devising technology and techniques appropriate to our set-up, our value system and technologies that are compatible. The call is, therefore, to stress on the 'know-why' rather than just on the 'know-how' of techniques and technology. This can materialize only when we bear in mind the following motto:

THE RIGHT TECHNIQUE/TECHNOLOGY
AT THE RIGHT PLACE
AT THE RIGHT TIME
AT THE RIGHT COST
BY THE RIGHT METHODS/MEANS
BY THE RIGHT PERSONNEL

Notes and References

1. Milton Greenbelt, Myron Sharaf R. and Evelyn Stone M., Dynamics of Institutional Change, Pittsburgh, University of Pittsburgh Press, 1971, pp. 239-40.
2. All India Radio Broadcast, June 26, 1966; Selected Speeches of Mrs. Indira Gandhi, January 1966 to Aug. 1969, Publication Division, March 1971.
3. WHO: *Public Health Papers*, 55, p. 68.
4. UN: "Inter-regional Seminar on Administration of Management Improvement Services", Vol. I, Copenhagen, Denmark, Oct. 1970, p. 24.
5. UN: United Nations Programmes in Public Administration (E/4296-ST/TAO/M/38), pp. 11-12.
6. UN: Official Record of the Economic and Social Council (E.1708), Agenda Item No. 10, p. 3.
7. UN: Inter-Regional Seminar on Administration of Management Improvement Services.
8. Earnest Dale and L.C. Michelon: "Modern Management Techniques", Penguin Books, 1974, p. 9.
9. Legisias V. Gabriel: College of Public Administration, University of Philippines, "Administrative capability as a neglected dimension in the implementation of development programme and projects", Seventieth General Assembly and Conference of EROPA on Implementation, the Problem Achieving Results", 24-31 October, 1973, Vol. III, pp. 3-14.
10. Saul M. Katz: "A Methodological note on Appraising Administrative Capability for Development" (UN Publication, Sales No. E-69 II. 4-2), p. 8.
11. *Ibid.*, pp. 99-100.

12. World Health Organisation, Regional Office of South-East Asia, New Delhi (SEA/RC/26, pp. 31-32).
13. ILO: "Introduction to Work Study", Geneva, 1969, p. 26.
14. M.J. Clay, General Theory of Management Techniques, Part I, in *Work Study and Management Services*, London.
15. R. Bechhard, Organisation Development: Strategies and Models, Addison-Wesley, 1969, p. 9.
16. H. Finer, Theory and Practice of Modern Government, p. 106.
17. Eli Ginzberg, "Perspectives on Work Motivation", *Personnel*, Vol. 31, No. (July), 1959, pp. 48-49.
18. Norman Mair, R.F. and Hayes John, J., Creative Management (New York: John Wiley & Sons, Inc. 1962), p. 36.
19. Davis Keith, "The Case for Participative Management", *Business Horizon*, Vol. 6, No. 3 (1963), p. 141.
20. Walters, Albert F., "Management and Motivation: Releasing Human Potential", *Personnel*, Vol. 39, No. 2 (March-April, 1962), pp. 8-16 as reprinted in Harold Koontz and Cyrill O'Donnel, *Management: A Book of Readings* (New York: McGraw-Hill Book Company, 1964), pp. 382-83.
21. For details refers: Information Systems for Modern Management by Murdicks Robert G. and Ross, Joel E., Prentice-Hall of India (P) Ltd., Delhi, 1977.
22. For details see: PERT & CPM—Principles and Applications by Srinath, L.S., Affiliated East-West Press, Delhi, 1975.
23. J. Joseph, Moder and Cecil, Phillips R., "Project Management with CPM and PERT, (New York: Reinhold, 1964), pp. 5-6.
24. For details see: Cost-Benefit Analysis in Administration by Trevor Newton, George Allen & Unwin, London, 1972 and Weisbrod, B.A., "Concepts of Costs and Benefits," in Chanse, S.B. (ed.) *Problems in Public Expenditure Analysis*, Washington, D.C., Brookings, 1968, pp. 257-62; and Williams, A., "The Cost-Benefit Approach", *British Medical Bulletin*, 30, 252-56 (1974).
25. *WHO Technical Report Series*, 596, "Application of System Analysis and Health Management", 1976, pp. 7-8.
26. *World Health*, Paper 55, *op. cit.*, p. 61.
27. William Newman, H. *et. al.*, The Process of Management, (Englewood Cliffs, N.J., Prentice-Hall, 1976), pp. 338-45.

APPENDIX I

NATIONAL HEALTH POLICY

Introductory

1. The Constitution of India envisages the establishment of a new social order based on equality, freedom, justice and the dignity of the individual. It aims at the elimination of poverty, ignorance and ill-health and directs the state to regard the raising of the level of nutrition and the standard of living of its people and the improvement of public health as among its primary duties, securing the health and strength of workers, men and women, specially ensuring that children are given opportunities and facilities to develop in a healthy manner.

1.1. Since the inception of the planning process in the country, the successive Five Year Plans have been providing the framework within which the States may develop their health services infrastructure, facilities for medical education, research, etc. Similar guidance has sought to be provided through the discussions and conclusion arrived at in the Joint Conferences of the Central Councils of Health and Family Welfare and the National Development Council. Besides, central legislation has been enacted to regulate standards of medical education, prevention of food adulteration, maintenance of standards in the manufacture and sale of certified drugs, etc.

1.2. While the broad approaches contained in the successive Plan documents and discussions in the forums referred to in para 1.1 may have generally served the needs of the situation in the past, it is felt that an integrated, comprehensive approach towards the future development of medical education, research and health services requires to be established to serve the actual health needs and priorities of the country. It is in this context that the need has been felt to evolve a National Health Policy.

Our Heritage

2. Indian has, a rich, centuries-old heritage of medical and health sciences. The Philosophy of Ayurveda and the skills enunciated by Charaka and Shushruta bear testimony to our ancient tradition in the scientific health care of our people. The approach of our ancient medical systems was of a holistic nature, which took into account all aspects of human health and disease. Over the centuries, with the intrusion of

foreign influences and mingling of cultures, various systems of medicine evolved and have continued to be practised widely. However, the allopathic system of medicine has, in a relatively short period of time, made a major impact on the entire approach to health care and pattern of development of the health services infrastructure in the country.

Progress Achieved

3. During the last three decades and more, since the attainment of independence, considerable progress has been achieved in the promotion of the health status of our people. Smallpox has been eliminated; plague is no longer a problem; mortality from cholera and related diseases has decreased and malaria brought under control to a considerable extent. The mortality rate per thousand of population has been reduced from 27.4 to 14.8 and the life expectancy at birth has increased from 32.7 to over 52. A fairly extensive network of dispensaries, hospitals and institutions providing specialised curative care has developed and a large stock of medical and health personnel, of various levels, has become available. Significant indigenous capacity has been established for the production of drugs and pharmaceutical vaccines, sera, hospital equipment, etc.

The Existing Picture

4. In spite of such impressive progress, the demographic and health picture of the country still constitutes a cause for serious and urgent concern. The high rate of population growth continues to have an adverse effect on the health of our people and the quality of their lives. The mortality rates for women and children are still distressingly high; almost one-third of the total deaths occur among children below the age of 5 years, infant mortality is around 129 per thousand live births. Efforts at the nutritional levels of our people have still to bear fruit and the extent and severity of malnutrition continues to be exceptionally high. Communicable and non-communicable diseases have still to be brought under effective control and eradicated. Blindness, Leprosy and TB continue to have a high incidence. Only 31 per cent of the rural population has access to potable water supply and 0.5 per cent enjoys basic sanitation.

4.1. High incidence of diarrhoeal diseases and other preventive and infectious diseases, specially amongst infants and children, lack of safe drinking water and poor environmental sanitation, poverty and ignorance are among the major contributory causes of the high incidence of diseases and mortality.

4.2. The existing situation has been largely engendered by the almost wholesale adoption of health manpower development policies and the establishment of curative centres based on the western models, which are inappropriate and irrelevant to real needs of our people and the socio-economic conditions obtaining in the country. The hospital-based disease, and cure-oriented approach towards the establishment of medical services has provided benefits to the upper crusts of society, specially those residing in the urban areas. The proliferation of this approach has been at the cost of providing comprehensive primary health care services to the entire population, whether residing in the urban or the rural areas. Furthermore, the continued high emphasis on the curative approach has led to the neglect of the preventive, promotive, public health and rehabilitative aspects of health care. The existing approach, instead of improving awareness and building up self-reliance, has tended to enhance dependency and weaken the community's capacity to cope with its problems. The prevailing policies in regard to the education and training of medical and health personnel, at various levels, has resulted in the development of a cultural gap between the people and the personnel providing care. The various health programmes have, by and large, failed to involve individuals and families in establishing a self-reliant community. Also, over the years, the planning process has become largely oblivious of the fact that the ultimate goal of achieving a satisfactory health status for all our people cannot be secured without involving the community in the identification of their health needs and priorities as well as in the implementation and management of the various health and related programmes.

Need for Evolving a Health Policy—the Revised 20-Point Programme

5. India is committed to attaining the goal of "Health for All by the Year 2000 A.D." through the universal provision of comprehensive primary health care services. The attainment of this goal requires a thorough overhaul of the existing approaches to the education and training of medical and health personnel and the reorganisation of the health services infrastructure. Furthermore, considering the large variety of inputs into health, it is necessary to secure the overall national socio-economic development process, specially in the more closely health-related sectors, e.g., drugs and pharmaceuticals, agriculture and food production, rural development, education and social welfare, housing, water supply and sanitation, prevention of food adulteration, maintenance of prescribed standards in the manufacture and sale of drugs and the conservation of the environment. In sum, the contours of the National Health Policy have to be evolved within a fully integrated planning framework which seeks to provide universal, comprehensive primary health care services, relevant to the actual needs and priorities of the community at a cost which the people can afford, ensuring that the planning and implementation of the various health programmes is through the organised involvement and participation of the community, adequately utilising the services being rendered by private voluntary organisations active in the health sector.

5.1. It is also necessary to ensure that the pattern of development of the health services infrastructure in the future fully takes into account the revised 20-Point Programme. The said Programme attributes very high priority to the promotion of family planning as a people's programme, on a voluntary basis; substantial augmentation and provision of primary health care facilities on a universal basis; control of Leprosy, TB and Blindness; acceleration of welfare programmes for women and children; nutrition programmes for pregnant women, nursing mothers and children, especially in the tribal, hilly and backward areas. The Programme also places high emphasis on the supply of drinking water to all problem villages, improvements in the housing and environment of the weaker sections of society; increased production of essential food items; integrated rural development; spread of universal elementary education; expansion of the public distribution system, etc.

Population Stabilisation

6. Irrespective of the changes, no matter how fundamental that may be, brought about in the overall approach to health care and the restructuring of the health services, not much headway is likely to be achieved in improving the health status of the people unless success is achieved in securing the small family norm, through voluntary efforts, and moving towards the goal of population stabilisation. In view of the vital importance of securing the balanced growth of the population, it is necessary to enunciate, separately, a National Population Policy.

Medical and Health Education

7. It is also necessary to appreciate that the effective delivery of health care services would depend very largely on the nature of education, training and appropriate orientation towards community health of all categories of medical and health personnel and their capacity to function as an integrated team, each of its members performing given tasks within a coordinated action programme. It is, therefore, of crucial importance that the entire basis and approach towards medical and health education, at all levels, is reviewed in terms of national needs and priorities and the curricular programmes restructured to produce personnel of various grades of skill and competence, who are professionally equipped and socially motivated to effectively deal with day-to-day problems, within the existing constraints. Towards this end, it is necessary to formulate, separately, a National Medical and Health Education Policy which (i) sets out the changes required to be brought about in the curricular contents and training programme of medical and health personnel, at various levels of functioning; (ii) takes into account the need for establishing the extremely essential inter-relations between functionaries of various grades; (iii) provides guidelines for the production of health personnel on the basis of realistically assessed manpower requirements; (iv) seeks to resolve the existing sharp regional imbalances in their availability; and (v) ensures that personnel at all levels are socially motivated towards the rendering of community health services.

Need for Providing Primary Health Care with Special Emphasis on the Preventive, Promotive and Rehabilitative Aspects

8. Presently, despite the constraints of resources, there is disproportionate emphasis on the establishment of curative centres—dispensaries, hospitals, institutions for specialist treatment—the large majority of which are located in the urban areas of the country. The vast majority of those seeking medical relief have to travel long distance to the nearest curative centre, seeking relief for ailments which could have been readily and effectively handled at community level. Also, for want of a well-established referral system, those seeking curative care have the tendency to visit various specialist centres, thus further contributing to congestions, duplication of efforts and consequential waste of resources. To put an end to the existing all-round unsatisfactory situation, it is urgently necessary to restructure the health services within the following broad approach:

1. To provide, within a phased, time-bound programme, a well-dispersed network of comprehensive primary health care services, integrally linked within the extension and health education approach which takes into account the fact that a large majority of health functions can be effectively handled and resolved by the people themselves, with the organised support of volunteers, auxilliaries, paramedicos and adequately trained multi-purpose workers of various grades of skill and competence, of both sexes. There are a large number of private, voluntary organisations active in the health field all over the country. Their services and support would require to be utilised and intermixed with the governmental efforts in an integrated manner.
2. To be effective, the establishment of the primary health care approach would involve large scale transfer of knowledge, simple skills and technologies to Health Volunteers, selected by the communities and enjoying their confidence. The functioning of the front-line workers, selected by the community would require to be related to definitive action plans for the translation of medical and health knowledge into practical action, involving the use of simple and inexpensive interventions which can be readily implemented by persons who have undergone short periods of training. The quality of training of these health guides/workers would be of crucial importance to the success of this approach.
3. The success of the decentralised primary health care system would depend vitally on the organised building-up of individual self-reliance and effective community participation, on the provision of organised, back-up support of the secondary and tertiary levels of the health care services,

providing adequate logistical and technical assistance.

4. The decentralisation of services would require the establishment of a well worked out referral system to provide adequate expertise at the various levels of the organisational set-up nearest to the community, depending upon the actual needs and problems of the area, and thus ensure against the continuation of the existing rush towards the curative centres in the urban areas. The effective establishment of the referral system would also ensure the optimal utilisation of expertise at the higher levels of the hierarchical structure. This approach would not only lead to the progressive improvement of comprehensive health care services at the primary level but also provide for timely attention being available to those in need of urgent specialist care, whether they live in the rural or the urban areas.
5. To ensure that the approach to health care does not merely constitute a collection of disparate health interventions but consists of an integrated package of services seeking to tackle the entire range of poor health conditions, on a broad front, it is necessary to establish a nation-wide chain of sanitary-cum-epidemiological stations. The location and functioning of these stations may be between the primary and secondary levels of the hierarchical structure, depending upon the local situations and other relevant consideration. Each such station would require to have suitably trained staff equipped to identify, plan and provide preventive, promotive and mental health care services. It would be beneficial, depending upon the local situations, to establish such stations at the Primary Health Centres. The district health organisation should have, as an integral part of its set-up, a well organised epidemiological unit to coordinate and superintend the functioning of the field stations. These stations would participate in the integrated action plans to eradicate and control diseases, besides tackling specific local environmental health problems. In the urban agglomerations, the municipal and local authorities should be equipped to perform similar functions, being supported with adequate resources and expertise, to effectively deal with local preventable public health problems. The aforesaid approach should be implemented and extended through community participation and contributions, in whatever form possible, to achieve meaningful results within a time-bound programme.
6. The location of curative centres should be related to the populations they serve, keeping in view the densities of population, distances, topography, transport connections. These centres should function within the recommended referral system, the gamut of general specialities required to

deal with the local disease patterns being provided as near to the community as possible, at the secondary level of the hierarchical organisation. The concept of domiciliary care and the field-camps approach should be utilised to the fullest extent, to reduce the pressures on these centres, socially in efforts relating to the control and eradication of blindness, tuberculosis, leprosy, etc. To maximise the unilisation of available resources, new and additional curative centres should be established only in exceptional cases, the basic attempt being towards the upgradation of existing facilities, at selected locations, the guiding principle being to provide specialists services as near to the beneficiaries as may be possible, within a well-planned network. Expenditure should be reduced through the fullest possible use of cheap locally available building materials, resort to appropriate architectural designs and engineering concepts and by economical investment in the purchase of machineries and equipment, ensuring against avoidable duplication of such acquisitions. It is also necessary to devise effective mechanisms for the repair, maintenance and proper upkeep of all bio-medical equipments to secure their maximum utilisation.

7. With a view to reducing governmental expenditure and fully utilising untapped resources, planned programmes may be devised related to the local requirements and potentials, to encourage the establishment of practice by professional, increased investment by non-governmental agencies in establishing curative centres and by offering organised logistical, financial and technical support to voluntary agencies active in the health field.
8. While the major focus of attention in restructuring the existing governmental health organisations would relate to establishing comprehensive primary health care and public health services, within an integrated referral system, planned attention would also require to be devoted to the establishment of centres equipped to provide speciality and super-speciality services, through a well dispersed network of centres, to ensure that the present and future requirements of specialist treatment are adequately available within the country. To reduce governmental expenditures involved in the establishment of such centres, planned efforts should be made to encourage private investments in such fields so that the majority of such centres, within the governmental set-up, can provide adequate care and treatment to those entitled to free care, the affluent sectors being looked after by the paying clinics. Care would also require to be taken to ensure the appropriate dispersal of such centres, to remove the existing regional imbalances and

to provide services within the reach of all, whether residing in the rural or the urban areas.

9. Special, well-coordinated programmes should be launched to provide mental health care as well as medical care and the physical and social rehabilitation of those who are mentally retarded, deaf, dumb, blind, physically disabled, infirm and the aged. Also, suitably organised programmes would require to be launched to ensure against the prevention of various disabilities.
10. In the establishment of the re-organised services, the first priority should be accorded to provide services to those residing in the tribal, hilly and backward areas as well as to endemic disease affected populations and the vulnerable sections of the society.
11. In the re-organised health service scheme, efforts should be made to ensure adequate mobility of personnel, at all levels of functioning.
12. In the various approaches, set out in (1) to (11) above, organised efforts would require to be made to fully utilise and assist in the enlargement of the services being provided by private voluntary organisations active in the health field. In this context, planning, encouragement and support would also require to be afforded to fresh voluntary efforts, specially those which seek to serve the needs of the rural areas and the urban slums.

Re-orientation of the Existing Health Personnel

9. A dynamic process of change and innovation is required to be brought about in the entire approach to health manpower development, ensuring the emergence of fully integrated bands of workers functioning within the "Health Team" approach.

Private Practice by Governmental Functionaries

10. It is desirable for the States to take steps to phase out the system of private practice by medical personnel in government service, providing at the same time for payment of appropriate compensatory non-practising allowance. The States would require to carefully review the existing situation, with special reference to the availability and dispersal of private practitioners, and take timely decisions in regard to this vital issue.

Practitioners of Indigenous and other Systems of Medicine and their Role in Health Care

11. The country has a large stock of health manpower comprising of private practitioners in various systems, for example, Ayurveda, Unani, Siddha, Homoeopathy, Yoga, Naturopathy, etc. This resource has

not so far been adequately utilised. The practitioners of these various systems enjoy high local acceptance and respect and consequently exert considerable influence on health beliefs and practices. It is, therefore, necessary to initiate organised measures to enable each of these various systems of medicine and health care to develop in accordance with its genius. Simultaneously, planned efforts should be made to dovetail the functioning of the practitioners of these various systems and integrate their services, at the appropriate levels, within specified areas of responsibility and functioning, in the overall health care delivery system, specially in regard to the preventive, promotive and public health objectives. Well considered steps would also require to be launched to move towards a meaningful phased integration of the indigenous and the modern systems.

Problems Requiring Urgent Attention

12. Besides the recommended restructuring of the health services infrastructure, reorientation of the medical and health manpower, community involvement and exploitation of the services of private medical practitioners, specially those of the traditional and other systems, involvement and utilisation of the services of the voluntary agencies active in the health field, etc., it would be necessary to devote planned, time-bound attention to some of the more important inputs required for improved health care. Of these, priority attention would require to be devoted to:

(i) *Nutrition*: National and regional strategies should be evolved and implemented, on a time-bound basis, to ensure adequate nutrition for all segments of the population through a well-developed distribution system, specially in the rural areas and urban slums. Food of acceptable quality must be available to every person in accordance with his physical needs. Low cost, processed and ready-to-eat foods should be produced and made readily available. The overall strategy would necessarily involve organised efforts at improving the purchasing power of the poorer sections of the society. Schemes like employment guarantee scheme, to which the government is committed could yield optimal results if these are suitably linked to the objective of providing adequate nutrition and health cover to the rural and urban poor. The achievement of this objective is dependent on integrated socio-economic development leading to the generation of productive employment for all those constituting the labour force. Employment guarantee scheme and similar efforts would require to be specially enforced to provide social security for identified vulnerable sections of the society. Measures aimed at improving eating habits, inculcation of desirable nutritional practices, improved and scientific utilisation of available food materials and effective popularisation of improved cooking practices would require to be implemented. Besides, a nation-wide programme to promote breast-feeding of infants and eradication of various social taboos detrimental to the promotion of health would need to be initiated. Simultaneously, the problems of communities afflicted by chronic nutritional disorders should be tackled through special schemes including the organisation of supplementary feeding programmes directed to the vulnerable section of the population. The force and effect of such programmes should be ensured by delivering them within the setting of fully integrated health care activities, to ensure the inculcation of the educational aspects, in the over-all strategy.

(ii) *Prevention of food adulteration and maintenance of the quality of drugs*: Stringent measures are required to be taken to check and prevent the adulteration and contamination of foods at the various stages of their production, processing, storage, transport, distribution, etc. To ensure uniformity of approach, the existing laws would require to be reviewed and effective legislation enacted by the Centre. Similarly, the most urgent measures required to be taken to ensure against the manufacture and sale of spurious and sub-standard drugs.

(iii) *Water supply and Sanitation*: The provision of safe drinking water and the sanitary disposal of waters, human and animal wastes, both in urban and rural areas, must constitute an integrated package. The enormous backlog in the provision of these services to the rural population and in the urban agglomerations must be made up on the most urgent basis. The provision of water supply and basic sanitation facilities would not automatically improve health. The availability of such facilities should be accompanied by intensive health education campaigns for the improvement of personal hygiene, the economical use of water and the sanitary disposal of waste in a manner that will improve individual and community health. All water supply schemes must be fully integrated with efforts at proper water management, including the drainage and disposal of waste waters. To reduce expenditure and for achieving a quick headway it would be necessary to devise appropriate technologies in the planning and management of the delivery systems. Besides, the involvement of the community in the implementation and management of the systems would be of crucial importance, both for reducing costs as well as to see that the beneficiaries value and protect the services provided to them.

(iv) *Environmental Protection*: While preventive, promotive, public health services are established and the curative services reorganised to prevent, control and treat diseases, it would be equally necessary to ensure against the haphazard exploitation of resources which cause ecological disturbances leading to fresh health hazards. It is, therefore, necessary that economic development plans, in the various sectors, are devised in adequate consultation with the Central and the State health authorities. It is also vitally essential to ensure that the present and future industrial and urban development plans are centrally reviewed to ensure against congestions, the unchecked release of noxious emissions and the pollution of air and water. In this context, it is vital to ensure that the siting and location of all manufacturing units is strictly regulated through legal measures, if necessary. Central and State health authorities must necessarily be consulted in establishing locational development and urbanisation programmes. Environmental appraisal procedures must be developed and strictly applied in according clearance to the various developmental projects.

(v) *Immunisation Programme*: It is necessary to launch an organised, nationwide immunisation programme, aimed at cent per cent coverage of targeted population groups with vaccines against preventable and communicable diseases. Such an approach would not only prevent and reduce disease and disability but also bring down the existing high infant and child mortality rate.

(vi) *Maternal and Child Health Services*: A vicious relationship exists between high birth rates and high infant mortality, contributing to the desire for more children. The highest priority would, therefore, require to be devoted to efforts at launching special programmes for the improvement of maternal and child health, with a special focus on the less-privileged sections of society. Such programmes would require to be decentralised to the maximum possible extent, their delivery being at the primary level, nearest to the doorsteps of the beneficiaries. While efforts should continue at providing refresher training and orientation to the traditional birth attendants, schemes and programmes should be launched to ensure that progressively all deliveries are conducted by competently trained persons so that complicated cases receive timely and expert attention, within a comprehensive programme providing ante-natal, intra-natal and post-natal care.

(vii) *School Health Programme*: Organised school health services, integrally linked with the general, preventive and curative services would require to be established within a time-limited programme.

(viii) *Occupational Health Services*: There is urgent need for launching well-considered schemes to prevent and treat diseases and injuries arising from occupational hazards, not only in the various industries but also in the comparatively un-organised sectors like agriculture. For this purpose, the coverage of the Employees State Insurance Act, 1948, may be suitably extended ensuring adequate coordination of efforts with the general health services. In their respective spheres of responsibility, the Centre and the States must introduce organised occupational health services to reduce morbidity, disabilities and mortality and thus promote better health and increased welfare and productivity on all fronts.

Health Education

13. The recommended efforts, on various fronts, would bear only marginal results unless nation-wide health education programmes, backed by appropriate communication strategies are launched to provide health information in easily understandable form, to motivate the development of an attitude for healthy living. The public health education programmes should be supplemented by health, nutrition and population education programmes in ill educational institutions, at various levels. Simultaneously, efforts would require to be made to promote universal education, specially adult and family education, without which the various efforts to organise preventive and promotive health activities, family planning and improved maternal and child health cannot bear fruit.

Management Information System

14. Appropriate decision-making and programme planning in the health and related field is not possible without establishing an effective health information system. A nation-wide organisational set-up should be established to procure essential health information. Such information is required not only for assisting in planning and decision-making but also to provide timely warnings about emerging health problems and for reviewing, monitoring and evaluating the various on-going health programmes. The building up of a well conceived health information system is also necessary for assessing medical and health manpower requirements and taking timely decisions, on a continuing basis, regarding the manpower requirements in the future.

Medical Industry

15. The country has built-up sound technological and manufacturing capability in the field of drugs, vaccines, bio-medical equipment, etc. The available knowhow requires to be adequately exploited to increase the production of essential and life saving drugs

and vaccines of proven quality to fully meet the national requirements, specially in regard to the national programmes to combat Malaria, TB, Leprosy, Blindness, Diarrhoeal diseases, etc. The production of the essential, life-saving drugs under their generic names and the adoption of economical packaging practices would considerably reduce the unit cost of medicines bringing them within the poorer sections of society, besides significantly reducing the expenditure being incurred by the governmental organisation on the purchase of drugs. In view of the low cost of indigenous and herbal gardens, producing drugs of certified quality and making them easily available.

15.1. The practitioners of the modern medical system rely heavily on diagnostic aids involving extensive use of costly, sophisticated bio-medical equipment. Effective mechanisms should be established to identify essential equipment required for extensive use and to promote and enlarge their indigenous manufacture, for such devices being readily available, at reasonable prices, for use at the health care centres.

Health Insurance

16. Besides mobilising the community resources, through its active participation in the implementation and management of national health and related programmes, it would be necessary to devise well considered health insurance schemes, on a State-wise basis, for mobilising additional resources for health promotion and ensuring that the community shares the cost of the services, in keeping with its paying capacity.

Health Legislation

17. It is necessary to urgently review all existing legislation and work towards a unified, comprehensive legislation in the health field, enforceable all over the country.

Medical Research

18. The frontiers of the medical sciences are expanding at a phenomenal pace. To maintain the country's lead in this field as well as to ensure self-sufficiency and generation of the requisite competence in the future, it is necessary to have an organised programme for the building up and extension of fundamental and basic research in the field of bio-medical and allied sciences. Priority attention would require to be devoted to the resolution of problems relating to the containment and eradication of the existing, widely prevalent diseases as well as to deal with emerging health problems. The basic objective of medical research and the ultimate test of its utility would involve the translation of available knowhow into simple, low-cost, easily applicable appropriate technologies, devices and interventions suiting local conditions, thus placing the latest technological achievements, within the reach of health personnel, and to the front line health workers, in the remotest corners of the country. Therefore, besides devotion to basic, fundamental

research, high priority should be accorded to applied, operational research including action research for continuously improving the cost effective delivery of health services. Priorities would require to be identified and laid down in collaboration with social scientists, planners and decision-makers and the public. Basic research efforts should devote high priority to the discovery and development of more effective treatment and preventive procedures in regard to communicable and tropical diseases—Blindness, Leprosy, TB. etc. Very high priority would also have to be devoted to contraception research to urgently improve the effectiveness and acceptability of existing methods as well as to discover more effective and acceptable devices. Equally high attention would require to be devoted to nutrition research, to improve the health status of the community. The overall effort should aim at the balanced development of basic, clinical and problem-oriented operational research.

Inter-sectoral Cooperation

19. All health and human development must ultimately constitute an integral component of the overall socio-economic developmental process in the country. It is thus of vital importance to ensure effective coordination between the health and its more intimately related sectors. It is, therefore, necessary to set-up standing mechanisms, at the Centre and in the States, for securing inter-sectoral coordination of the various efforts in the fields of health and family planning, medical education and research, drugs and pharmaceuticals, agriculture and food, water supply and drainage, housing, education and social welfare and rural development. The coordination and review committees, to be set-up, should review progress, resolve bottlenecks and bring about such shifts in the contents and priorities of programmes as may appear necessary, to achieve the overall objectives. At the community level, it would be desirable to devise arrangements for health and all other developmental activities being coordinated under an integrated programme of rural development.

Monitoring and Review of Progress

20. It would be of crucial importance to monitor and periodically review the success of the efforts made and the results achieved. For this purpose, it is necessary to urgently identify the base line situation and to evolve a phased programme for the achievement of short and long-term objectives in the various sectors of activity. Towards this end, the current level of achievement as well as the broad indicators for the achievement of certain basic health and family welfare goals are set out in the annexed tabular statement. These goals, as well as other allied objectives, would require to be further worked upon and specific targets for achievement established by the Central and the State Governments in regard to the various areas of functioning.

Goals for Health and Family Welfare Programmes

Sl. No.	Indicator		Current Level	Goals 1985	Goals 1990	Goals 2000
(1)	(2)		(3)	(4)	(5)	(6)
1.	Infant mortality rate	Rural	136 (1978)	122	—	—
		Urban	70 (1978)	60	—	—
		Total	125 (1978)	106	87	below 60
	Pre-natal mortality		67 (1976)		—	30-35
2.	Crude death rate	Around	14	12	10.4	9.0
3.	Pre-school child (1-5 yrs.) mortality		24 (1976-77)	20-24	15.20	10
4.	Maternal mortality rate		4-5 (976)	3-4	2-3	below 2
5.	Life expectancy at birth (yrs.)	Male	52.6 (1976-81)	55.1	57.6	64
		Female	51.6 (1976-81)	54.3	57.1	64
6.	Babies with birth weight below 2,500 gms. (percentage)		30	25	18	10
7.	Crude birth rate	Around	35	31	27.0	21.0
8.	Effective couple protection (percentage)		23.6 (March 1982)	37.0	42.0	60.0
9.	Net Reproduction Rate (NRR)		1.48 (1981)	1.34	1.17	1.00
10.	Growth rate (Annual)		2.24 (1971-81)	1.90	1.66	1.20
11.	Family size		4.4 (1975)	3.8		2.3
12.	Pregnant mothers receiving ante-natal care (%)		40-50	50-60	60-75	100
13.	Deliveries by trained birth attendants (%)		30-35	50	80	100
14.	Immunisation status (% coverage)					
	TT (for pregnant women)		20	60	100	100
	TT (for school children)					
	10 years			40	100	100
	16 years		20	60	100	100

DPT (children below 3 years)	25	70	85	85
Polio (infants)	5	50	70	85
BCG (infants)	65	70	80	85
DT (new school entrants 5-6 years)	20	80	85	85
Typhoid (new school entrants 5-6 years)	2	70	85	85
15. Leprosy—percentage of disease-arrested cases out of those detected	20	40	60	80
16. TB—percentage of disease-arrested cases out of those detected	50	60	75	90
17. Blindness—incidence of (%)	1.4	1	0.7	0.3

APPENDIX II

DRAFT HEALTH POLICY

The approach adopted by the Working Group was as follows:

(i) to consider introductory chapter with a view to suggest gaps that need to be filled;
(ii) clause by clause consideration of the Draft Policy; and
(iii) need to augment goals set out at the end of the Health Policy.

The Working Group deliberated the National Health Policy at great length and made the following critical observations and suggestions

(1) The policy right at the outset must indicate its strong commitment to Health for all and give an indication of the linkage with the last policy.
The approach must stress on decentralization for ensuring sustainability, higher accountability and inter-sectoral integration at the grass-root level. Decentralization needs to be achieved by relying on the provisions of the 73rd and 74th Amendments so as to provide a more pro-active role to the people and the people's representatives.

The following points must be included more strongly:

(2) Establishing a workable referral system.
(3) Quality of care.
(4) A strong system of surveillance with emphasis on public health.
(5) Involvement of the community and local bodies. For such a process, decentralization must focus upon developing capacity of the people's representatives and communities at large in matters related to health planning goals, etc.
(6) The National Health Policy should have flexibility with the States and address local needs through the adoption of strategies like mobile clinics which have been found useful in some parts of the North-East.
(7) Utilization of information technology in enhancing the understanding of the people as well as providers.

(8) Demystify medicine and develop in every State a cadre of persons capable of addressing the first line of community health/public health needs at the primary level.

(9) Manpower development in general and specialization in particular, should be need-based. The policy of production of doctors, giving weightage to only some specialities, needs to be reviewed in order to ensure availability of all disciplines in equal measure. It was observed that in some states there were a surfeit of gynaecologists but very few anaesthetists.

(10) Need to reassess the issues related to the deployment of manpower in primary health care institutions. While absenteeism of doctors in rural areas continues to be a problem, despite several incentives having been provided, there is need to have properly trained para medics or medical personnel for traditional systems of medicine.

(11) There is also need to focus more on strengthening communication facilities at PHCs' by way of telephones and transport for immediate referral of needy patients.

(12) The Working Group felt that greater focus and importance should be given to the increasing role of traditional systems of medicine, particularly Ayurveda. To give a fillip to ISM and integrate it as an alternative system of medicine, it was felt that following initiatives, in specific terms, need to be considered:

- Traditional/Indian medicines to be integrated in the National Health System and not to be used as 'alternative'.
- Provide for practitioners of traditional systems of medicines in all PHCs/CHCs. This will help overcome to some extent the difficulty being felt on account of absenteeism of doctors.
- Formulate a policy on medical plants to ensure that they are not patented by Multi-national Companies and also growing/packaging them for export. It was felt that this comparative advantage that we were enjoying in this sector was, unlike in China, not being fully exploited due to low importance being accorded to it within the country. Therefore, to begin with, we need to increase the budgetary allocation to ISM preferably upto 20% of Health budget and also give it great priority and role in our National Health System.
- It would be necessary to improve the job opportunities and working conditions of not only the practitioners of ISM but also other para professionals such as Pharmacists, Nurses, Technicians, etc. in order to attract people to take up study of alternative systems of medicines.

- Finally, laying down of guidelines for the type and level of care that a practitioner of ISM can be permitted to provide while handling trauma or accident cases.

(13) Issues related to ethics in Medical Research and organ transplant also need to be clearly brought out.

(14) There was discussion regarding the efficacy of single doctor PHCs where absenteeism was highest due to and resulting in low patient turnover. It was suggested that the structure should be examined to arrive at the appropriate level/ population for placing a fully qualified and trained allopathy doctor.

(15) It was unanimously felt that not only should greater stress be laid on exploiting information technology for health education but more importantly strengthen and evolve a format for a multi-sectoral approach making the linkages between health and non-health sectors stronger. In fact, it was felt that in view of the critical importance of non-health sectors on health outcomes the issues related to multi-sectoral linkages should be indicated under a separate heading.

(16) It was felt that while there was need for increasing the health budgets as a proportion to the total budget and redefining priorities so as to provide for a referral system, there was also a case for better targeting of Government services to the poor and needy. Even if the percentage of GDP or SDP to be assigned to health cannot be spelt out, the need to move towards a reasonable bench mark should be recognized in the Policy.

(17) It was observed that in several State Governments' doctors were being permitted private practice, having adverse impact on patient care. It was, therefore, felt that the National Health Policy should be a clear mention of this issue, though it was a State subject. In addition to banning such practice, it was felt that priority be accorded for Hospital Advisory Committees to be constituted consisting of all stake-holders as this could be one effective means of closely supervising the doctors and other health functionaries and ensuring better accountability.

(18) There was need to sharply focus on the two issues that continue to plague the country's health system, urban bias and gender bias, making it quite inequitous. It was observed that in the collection and monitoring of programmes, coverage of women be ensured. Besides, there is also need to consider sensitizing and changing the mindset and orientation of health workers at all levels, to specific problems of women.

(19) There was much discussion on the current system of drug procurement by Government of India creating enormous

problems at State levels. Decentralization of drug procurement or constitution of a Committee at the Central Ministry level to monitor the supply of drugs and equipment for filling up gaps and taking corrective action for timely supply could be some solutions that the National Health Policy could consider spelling out.

(20) Other observations made pertained to drafting, as well as specific programmative interventions such as need for according higher focus on blood separation of components; involvement of community in the Malaria programme, greater stress for home and community-based palliative care for cancer patients; broadening the immunization programme to include Hepatitis B and MMR; focussing on establishing day care centres for the mentally ill, greater attention to nutrition which could be detailed under a separate heading; an integrated drug policy, etc.

(21) Overall, it was observed that a stronger justification for a new National Health Policy, sustainability of delivery system, the persistence of regional imbalances, burgeoning private sector necessitating regulation and co-option so as to achieve the HFA goals etc. need to be brought more clearly, alongside spelling out the primary goals and aim of the Health Policy—equity and efficiency—i.e., is more being spent wisely and is it equitable.

(22) It was also observed that the National Health Policy be set within the contextual framework of wide socio-eonomic disparities prevailing in the country and increasingly widening. Such a framework would enable a more cost effective system of care using time tested, relevant and need-based technology and not driven by costly technologies which may not be relevant and instead contribute to pushing up the cost of care.

(23) Over reliance on expensive diagnostics is unaffordable for most people. While dependence on such expensive diagnostic techniques must be controlled and time tested techniques which have worked should not be abandoned.

(24) There should be special mention of population.

(25) There should be emphasis on re-training of Government doctors who are to rise in the profession so that they are equipped to handle multifarious public health, financial administrative issues and are certainly not exposed to work that they are not familiar with.

(26) Portion of Nutrition should form a separate heading.

(27) Portion of Dental Health should be linked with non-communicable diseases.

(28) Health Insurance and Health Finance should be clubbed.

(29) Need to collect data of access by women and treatment of women should be emphasized.

(30) Regional imbalances and intra-State disparities must be brought out more strongly with some strategies on how to reduce the disparity.

(31) The need to identify proper technology for hospital waste management (incinerators, etc.) should be recognized.

(32) There should be District Level Planning Bodies to plan for the Health of the District along with their plan for economic and social development.

(33) Decentralized local bodies should get support and guidance from the respective Health Departments and their performance reviewed by them from time to time.

(34) The financial responsibility indicated in Para 11.2 should develop on all levels of the Government, not on the State only.

(35) Issues relating to old aged people need to be focussed. Specific steps for geriatric groups need elaboration.

(36) IPP VI—Research in Andhra Pradesh—80% expenditure on health in private sector.

(37) On disabled persons one chapter to be incorporated. Recommendations of the Sub-Committee on disabled persons to be incorporated.

Appendix III

NATIONAL POPULATION POLICY, 2000
ACTION PLAN

OPERATIONAL STRATEGIES

(i) & (ii) Converge Service Delivery at Village Levels

1. Utilise village self-help groups to organise and provide basic services for reproductive and child health care, combined with the ongoing Integrated Child Development Scheme (ICDS). Village self-help groups are in existence through centrally sponsored schemes of: (a) Department of Women and Child Development, Ministry of HRD, (b) Ministry of Rural Development, and (c) Ministry of Environment and Forests. Organise neighbourhood acceptor groups, and provide them with a revolving fund that may be accessed for income generation activities. The groups may establish rules of eligibility, interest rates, and accountability for which capital may be advanced, usually to be repaid in instalments within two years. The repayments may be used to fund another acceptor group in a nearby community, who would exert pressure to ensure timely repayments. Two trained birth attendants and the anganwadi worker (AWW) should be members of this group.
2. Implement at village levels a one-stop integrated and coordinated service delivery package for basic health care, family planning and maternal and child health-related services, provided by the community and for the community. Train and motivate the village self-help acceptor groups to become the primary contact at household levels. Once every fortnight, these acceptor groups will meet, and provide at one place 6 different services for: (i) registration of births, deaths, marriage and pregnancy; (ii) weighing of children under 5 years, and recording the weight on a standard growth chart; (iii) counselling and advocacy for contraception, plus free supply of contraceptives; (iv) preventive care, with availability of basic medicines for common ailments; antipyretics for fevers, antibiotic ointments for infections,

ORT/ORS[1] for childhood diarrhoeas, together with standardised indigenous medication and homeopathic cures; (v) nutrition supplements; and (vi) advocacy and encouragement for the continued enrolment of children in school up to age 14. One health staff, appointed by the panchayat, will be suitably trained to provide guidance. Clustering services for women and children at one place and time at village levels will promote positive interactions in health benefits and reduce service delivery costs.

3. Wherever these village self-help groups have not developed for any reason, community midwives, practitioners of ISMH, retired school teachers and ex-defence personnel may be organised into neighbourhood groups to perform similar functions.
4. At village levels, the anganwadi centre may become the pivot of basic health care activities, contraceptive counselling and supply, nutrition education and supplementation, as well as pre-school activities. The anganwadi centres can also function as depots for ORS/basic medicines and contraceptives.
5. A maternity hut should be established in each village to be used as the village delivery room, with storage space for supplies and medicines. It should be adequately equipped with kits for midwifery, ante-natal care, and delivery; basic medication for obstetric emergency aid; contraceptives, drugs and medicines for common ailments; and indigenous medicines/supplies for maternal and new-born care. The panchayat may appoint a competent and mature mid-wife, to look after this village maternity hut. She may be assisted by volunteers.
6. Trained birth attendants as well as the vast pool of traditional dais should be made familiar with emergency and referral procedures. This will greatly assist the Auxiliary Nurse Midwife (ANM) at the sub-centres to monitor and respond to maternal morbidity/emergencies at village levels.
7. Each village may maintain a list of community mid-wives, village health guides, panchayat sewa sahayaks, trained birth attendants, practitioners of indigenous systems of medicine, primary school teachers and other relevant persons, as well as the nearest institutional health care facilities that may be accessed for integrated service delivery. These persons may also be helpful in involving civil society in monitoring availability, quality and accessibility of reproductive and child health services; in disseminating education and

1. Oral Rehydration Therapy/Oral Rehydration Salts.

communication on the benefits of smaller and healthier families, with emphasis on education of the girl child; and female participation in the work force.

8. Provide a wider basket of choices in contraception, through innovative social marketing schemes to reach household levels.

   Comment: Meaningful decentralisation will result only if the convergence of the national family welfare programme with the ICDS programme is strengthened. The focus of the ICDS programme on nutrition improvement at village levels and on pre-school activities must be widened to include maternal and child health care services. Convergence of several related activities at service delivery levels with, in particular, the ICDS programme, is critical for extending outreach and increasing access to services. Intersectoral coordination with appropriate training and sensitisation among field functionaries will facilitate dissemination of integrated reproductive and child health services to village and household levels. People will willingly cooperate in the registration of births, deaths, marriages and pregnancies if they perceive some benefit. At the village level, this community meeting every fortnight, may become their most convenient access to basic health care, both for maternal and child health, as well as for common ailments. Households may participate to receive integrated service delivery, alongwith information about ongoing micro-credit and thrift schemes. Government and non-government functionaries will be expected to function in harmony to ensure integrated service delivery. The panchayat will promote this coordination and exercise effective supervision.

(iii) Empowering Women for Improved Health and Nutrition

1. Create an enabling environment for women and children to benefit from products and services disseminated under the reproductive and child health programme. Cluster services for women and children at the same place and time. This promotes positive interactions in health benefits and reduces service delivery costs.
2. As a measure to empower women, open more child care centres in rural areas and in urban slums, where a woman worker may leave her children in responsible hands. This will encourage female participation in paid employment, reduce school drop-out rates, particularly for the girl child, and promote school enrolment as well. The anganwadis provide a partial solution.

3. To empower women, pursue programmes of social afforestation to facilitate access to fuelwood and fodder. Similarly, pursue drinking water schemes for increasing access to portable water. This will reduce long absences from home, and the need for large number of children to perform such tasks.
4. In any reward scheme intended for household levels, priority may be given to energy saving devices such as solar cookers, or provision of sanitation facilities, or extension of telephone lines. This will empower households, in particular women.
5. Improve district, sub-district and panchayat-level health management with coordination and collaboration between district health officer, sub-district health officer and the panchayat for planning and implementation activities. There is need to—
   - Strengthen the referral network between the district health office, district hospital and the community health centres, the primary health centres and the sub-centres in management of obstetric and neo-natal complications.
   - Strengthen community health centres to provide comprehensive emergency obstetric and neo-natal care. These may function as clinical training centres as well. Strengthen primary health centres to provide essential obstetric and neo-natal care. Strengthen sub-centres to provide a comprehensive range of services, with delivery rooms, counselling for contraception, supplies of free contraceptives, ORS and basic medicines, together with facilities for immunisation.
   - Establish rigorous problem identification mechanisms through maternal and peri-natal audit, from village level upwards.
6. Ensure adequate transportation at village levels, sub-centre levels, zila parishads, primary health centres and at community health centres. Identifying women at risk is meaningful only if women with complications can reach emergency care in time.
7. Improve the accessibility and quality of maternal and child health services through—
   - Deployment of community mid-wives and additional health providers at village levels; cluster services for women and children at the same place and time, from village level upwards, e.g. ante-natal and post-partum care, monitoring infant growth, availability of contraceptives and medicine kits; and routinised immunisations at sub-centre levels.
   - Strengthen the capacity of primary health centres to

provide basic emergency obstetric and neo-natal health care.

- Involve professional agencies in developing and disseminating training modules for standard procedures in the management of obstetric and neo-natal cases. The aim should be to routinise these procedures at all appropriate levels.
- Improve supervision by developing guidance and supervision checklists.

8. Monitor performance of maternal and child healths services at each level by using the maternal and child health local area monitoring system, which includes monitoring the incidence and coverage of ante-natal visits, deliveries assisted by trained health care personnel and post-natal visits, among other indicators. The ANM at the sub-centre should be responsible and accountable for registering every pregnancy and child birth in her jurisdiction, and for providing universal ante-natal and post-natal services.
9. Improve technical skills of maternal and child health care providers by:
   - Strengthening skills of health personnel and health providers through classroom and on-the-job training in the management of obstetric and neo-natal emergencies. This should include training of birth attendants and community midwives at district-level hospitals in life-saving skills, such as management of asphyxia and hypothermia.
   - Training on integrated management of childhood illnesses for infants (1 week-2 months).
10. Support community activities such as dissemination of JEC material, including leaflets and posters, and promotion of folk jatras, songs and dances to promote healthy mother and healthy baby messages, along with good management practices to ensure safe motherhood, including early recognition of danger signs.
11. Programme development comprising—
    - Partnership in family health and nutrition. The anganwadi worker will identify women and children in the villages who suffer from malnutrition and/or micro-nutritional deficiencies, including iron, vitamin A, and iodine deficiency; provide nutritional supplements and monitor nutritional status.
    - Convergence, strengthening and universalisation of the nutritional programmes of the Department of Family Welfare and the ICDS run by the Department of Women and Child Development, ensuring training and timely

supply of food supplements and medicines.

- Include STD/RTI and HIV/AIDS prevention, screening and management, in maternal and child health services.
- Provide quality care in family planning, including information, increased contraceptive choices for both spacing and terminal methods, increase access to good quality and affordable contraceptive supplies and services at diverse delivery points, counselling about the safety, efficacy and possible side effects of each method, and appropriate follow-up.

12. Develop a health package for adolescents.
13. Expand the availability of safe abortion care. Abortion is legal, but there are barriers limiting women's access to safe abortion services. Some operational strategies are:
    - Community-level education campaigns should target women, household decision-makers and adolescents about the availability of safe abortion services and the dangers of unsafe abortion.
    - Make safe and legal abortion services more attractive to women and household decision-makers by: (i) increasing geographic spread; (ii) enhancing affordability; (iii) ensuring confidentiality; and (iv) providing compassionate abortion care, including post-abortion counselling.
    - Adopt updated and simple technologies that are safe and easy, e.g. manual vacuum extraction not necessarily dependent upon anaesthesia, or non-surgical techniques which are non-invasive.
    - Promote collaborative arrangements with private sector health professionals, NGOs and the public sector, to increase the availability and coverage of safe abortion services, including training of mid-level providers.
    - Eliminate the current cumbersome procedures for registration of abortion clinics. Simplify and facilitate the establishment of additional training centres for safe abortions in the public, private, and NGO sectors. Train these health care providers in provision of clinical services for safe abortions.
    - Formulate and notify standards for abortion services. Strengthen enforcement mechanisms at district and sub-district levels to ensure that these norms are followed.
    - Follow norms-based registration of service provision centres, and thereby switch the onus of meticulous observance of standards onto the provider.
    - Provide competent post-abortion care, including management of complications and identification of other health needs of post-abortion patients, and linking with

appropriate services. As part of post-abortion care, physicians may be trained to provide family planning counselling and services such as sterilisation and reversible modern methods such as IUDs, as well as oral contraceptives and condoms.

- Modify syllabus and curricula for medical graduates, as well as for continuing education and in-house learning, to provide for practical training in the newer procedures.
- Ensure services for termination of pregnancy at primary health centres and at community health centres.

14. Develop maternity hospitals at sub-district levels and at community health centres to function as FRUs for complicated and life-threatening deliveries.
15. Formulate and enforce standards for clinical services in the public, private, and NGO sectors.
16. Focus on distribution of non-clinical methods of contraception (condoms and oral contraceptive pills) through free supply, social marketing as well as commercial sales.
17. Create a national network consisting of public, private and NGO centres, identified by a common logo, for delivering reproductive and child health services free to any client. The provider will be compensated for the service provided, on the basis of a coupon, duly counter-signed by the beneficiary, and paid for by a system to be devised. The compensation will be identical to providers across all sectors. The end-user will choose the provider of the service. A group of management experts will devise checks and balances to prevent misuse.

(iv) Child Health and Survival

1. Support community activities, from village level upwards to monitor early and adequate ante-natal, natal and post-natal care. Focus attention on neo-natal health care and nutrition.
2. Set-up a National Technical Committee on neo-natal care, to align programme and project interventions with newly emerging technologies in neo-natal and peri-natal care.
3. Pursue compulsory registration of births in coordination with the ICDS Programme.
4. After the birth of a child, provide counselling and advocacy about contraception, to encourage adoption of a reversible or a terminal method. This will also contribute to the health and well-being of both mother and child.
5. Improve capacities at health centres in basic midwifery services, essential neo-natal care, including the management of sick neo-nates outside the hospital.
6. Sensitise and train health personnel in the integrated

management of childhood illnesses. Standard case management of diarrhoea and acute respiratory infections must be provided at sub-centres and primary health centres, with appropriate training, and adequate equipment. Besides, training in this sector may be imparted to health care providers at village levels, especially in indigenous systems.

7. Strengthen critical interventions aimed at bringing about reductions in maternal malnutrition, morbidity and mortality, by ensuring availability of supplies and equipment at village levels, and at sub-centres.
8. Pursue rigorously the pulse polio campaign to eradicate polio.
9. Ensure 100 per cent routine immunisation for all vaccine preventable diseases, in particular tetanus and measles.
10. As a child survival initiative, explore promotional and motivational measures for couples below the poverty line who marry after the legal age of marriage, to have the first child after the mother reaches the age of 21, and adopt a terminal method of contraception after the birth of the second child.
11. Children form a vulnerable group and certain sub-groups merit focused attention and intervention, such as street children and child labourers. Encourage voluntary groups as well as NGOs to formulate and implement special schemes for these groups of children.
12. Explore the feasibility of a national health insurance covering hospitalisation costs for children below 5 years, whose parents have adopted the small norm, and opted for a terminal method of contraception after the birth of the second child.
13. Expand the ICDS to include children between 6-9 years of age, specifically to promote and ensure 100 per cent school enrolment, particularly for girls. Promote primary education with the help of anganwadi workers, and encourage retention in school till age 14. Education promotes awareness, late marriages, small family size and higher child survival rates.
14. Provide vocational training for girls. This will enhance perception of the immediate utility of educating girls, and gradually raise the average age of marriage. It will also increase enrolment and retention of girls at primary school, and likely also at secondary school levels. Involve NGOs, the voluntary sector and the private sector, as necessary, to target employment opportunities.

(v) Meeting the Unmet Needs for Family Welfare Services

1. Strengthen, energise and make publicly accountable the cutting edge of health infrastructure at the village, sub-centre and primary health centre levels.

2. Address on priority the different unmet needs detailed in Appendix IV, in particular, an increase in rural infrastructure, deployment of sanctioned and appropriately trained health personnel, and provisioning of essential equipment and drugs.
3. Formulate and implement innovative social marketing schemes to provide subsidised products and services in areas where the existing coverage of the public, private and NGO sectors is insufficient in order to increase outreach and coverage.
4. Improve facilities for referral transportation at panchayat, zilla parishad and primary health centre levels. At sub-centres, provide ANMs with soft loans for purchase of mopeds, to enhance their mobility. This will increase coverage of ante-natal and post-natal check-ups, which, in turn, and will bring about reductions in maternal and infant mortality.
5. Encourage local entrepreneurs at village and block levels to start ambulance services through special schemes, with appropriate vehicles to facilitate transportation of persons requiring emergency as well as essential medical attention.
6. Provide special loan schemes and make site allotments at village levels to facilitate the starting of chemist shops for basic medicines and provision for medical first aid.

(vi) Under-Served Population Groups

(a) Urban Slums

1. Finalise a comprehensive urban health care strategy.
2. Facilitate service delivery centres in urban slums to provide comprehensive basic health, reproductive and child health services by NGOs and private sector organisations, including corporate houses.
3. Promote networks of retired government doctors and para-medical and non-medical personnel who may function as health care providers for clinical and non-clinical services on remunerative terms.
4. Strengthen social marketing programmes for non-clinical family planning products and services in urban slums.
5. Initiate specially targeted information, education and communication campaigns for urban slums on family planning, immunization, ante-natal, natal and post-natal check-ups and other reproductive health care services. Integrate aggressive health education programmes with health and medical care programmes, with emphasis on environmental health, personal hygiene and healthy habits, nutrition education and population education.

6. Promote inter-sectoral coordination between departments/ municipal bodies dealing with water and sanitation, industry and pollution, housing, transport, education and nutrition, and women and child development, to deal with unplanned and uncoordinated settlements.
7. Streamline the referral systems and linkages between the primary, secondary and tertiary levels of health care in the urban areas.
8. Link the provision of continued facilities to urban slum-dwellers with their observance of the small family norm.

(b) Tribal Communities, Hill Area Populations and Displaced and Migrant Populations

1. Many tribal communities are dwindling in numbers, and may not need fertility regulation. Instead, they may need information and counselling in respect of infertility.
2. The NGO sector may be encouraged to formulate and implement a system of preventive and curative health care that responds to seasonal variations in the availability of work, income and food for tribal and hill area communities and migrant and displaced populations. To begin with, mobile clinics may provide some degree of regular coverage and outreach.
3. Many tribal communities are dependent upon indigenous systems of medicine which necessitates a regular supply of local flora, fauna and minerals, or of standardised medication derived from these. Husbandry of such local resources and of preparation and distribution of standardised formulations should be encouraged.
4. Health care providers in the public, private and NGO sectors should be sensitised to adopt a "burden of disease" approach to meet the special needs of tribal and hill area communities.

(c) Adolescents

1. Ensure for adolescents access to information, counselling and services, including reproductive health services, that are affordable and accessible. Strengthen primary health centres and sub-centres, to provide counselling, both to adolescents and also to newly weds (who may also be adolescents). Emphasise proper spacing of children.
2. Provide for adolescents the package of nutritional services available under the ICDS programme.
   Comment: Improvements in health status of adolescent girls has an inter-generational impact. It reduces the risk of low

birth weight and minimizes neo-natal mortality. Malnutrition is a problem that seriously impairs the health of adolescent and adult women and has its roots in early childhood. The causal linkages between anaemia and low birth weight, prematurity, peri-natal mortality, and maternal mortality has been extensively studied and established.

3. Enforce the Child Marriage Restraint Act, 1976, to reduce the incidence of teenage pregnancies. Preventing the marriage of girls below the legally permissible age of 18 should become a national concern.
   Comment: It will promote higher retention of girls at schools, and is also likely to encourage their participation in the paid work force.
4. Provide integrated intervention in pockets with unmet needs in the urban slums, remote rural areas, border districts and among tribal populations.

(d) Increased Participation of Men in Planned Parenthood

1. Focus attention on men in the information and education campaigns to promote the small family norm, and to raise awareness by emphasising the significant benefits of fewer children, better spacing, better health and nutrition, and better education.
2. Currently, over 97 per cent of the sterilizations are tubectomies. Repopularise vasectomies, in particular the no-scalpel vasectomy, as a safe, simple, painless procedure, more convenient and acceptable to men.
3. In the continuing education and training at all levels, there is need to ensure that the no-scalpel vasectomy, and all such emerging techniques and skills are included in the syllabi, together with abundant practical training. Medical graduates, and all those participating in "in-service" continuing education and training, will be equipped to handle this intervention.

(vii) Diverse Health Care Providers

1. At district and sub-district levels, maintain block-wise data base of private medical practitioners whose credentials may be certified by the Indian Medical Association (IMA). Explore the possibility of accrediting these private practitioners for a year at a time, and assign to each a satellite population, not exceeding 5,000 (depending upon distances and spread), for whom they may provide reproductive and child health services. The private practitioners would be compensated for

the services rendered through designated agencies. Renewal of contracts after one year may be guided by client satisfaction. This will serve as an incentive to expand the coverage and outreach of high quality health care. Appropriate checks and balances will safeguard misuse.

2. Revive the earlier system of the licensed medical practitioners who, after appropriate certification from the IMA, may participate in the provision of clinical services.
3. Involve the non-medical fraternity in couselling and advocacy so as to demystify the national family welfare effort, such as retired defence personnel, retired school teachers and other persons who are active and willing to get involved.
4. Modify the under/post-graduate medical, nursing, and paramedical professional course syllabi and curricula, in consultation with the Medical Council of India, the Councils of ISMH, and the Indian Nursing Council, in order to reflect the concepts and implementation strategies of the reproductive and child health programme and the national population policy. This will also be applied to all in-service training and educational curricula.
5. Ensure the efficient functioning of the First Referral Units, i.e. 30-bed hospitals at block levels which provide emergency obstetric and child health care, to bring about reductions in Maternal Mortality Ratio (MMR) and Infant Mortality Rate (IMR). In many states, these FRUs are not operational on account of an acute shortage of specialists, i.e. gynaecologist/ obstetrician, anaesthetist and pediatrician. Augment the availability of specialists in these three disciplines, by increasing seats in medical institutions, and simultaneously enable and facilitate the acquisition of in-service post-graduate qualifications through the National Board of Medical Examination and open universities like IGNOU in larger numbers. As an incentive, seats will be reserved for those in-service medical graduates who are willing to abide by a bond to serve for 5 years at First Referral Units after completion of the course. States would need to sanction posts of Specialists at the FRUs. Further, these specialists should be provided with clear promotion channels.

(viii) *(a) Collaboration with and Commitments from the Non-Government Sector*

1. There remain innumerable hurdles that inhibit genuine long-term collaboration between the government and non-government sectors. A forum of representatives from government, the non-government organisations and the private sector may identify these hurdles and prepare

guidelines that will facilitate and promote collaborative arrangements.

2. Collaboration with and commitments from NGOs to augment advocacy, counselling and clinical services, while accessing village levels. This will require increased clinic outlets as well as mobile clinics.
3. Collaboration between the voluntary sector and the NGOs will facilitate dissemination of efficient service delivery to village levels. The guidelines could articulate the role and responsibility of each sector.
4. Encourage the voluntary sector to motivate village-level self-help groups to participate in community activities.
5. Specific collaboration with the non-government sector in the social marketing of contraceptives to reach village levels will be encouraged.

(viii) *(b) Collaboration with the Commitments from Industry*

1. The corporate sector and industry could, for instance, take on the challenge of strengthening the management information systems in the seven most deficient states, at primary health centre and sub-centre levels. Introduce electronic data entry machines to lighten the tedious work load of ANMs and the multi-purpose workers at sub-centres and the doctors at the primary health centres, while enabling wider coverage and outreach.
2. Collaboration with non-government sectors in running professionally sound advertisement and marketing campaigns for products and services, targeting all segments of the population, from village level upwards, in other words, strengthen advocacy and IEC, including social marketing of contraceptives.
3. Provide markets to sustain the income-generating activities from village levels upwards. In turn, this will ensure consistent motivation among the community for pursuing health and education-related community activities.
4. Help promote transportation to remote and inaccessible areas up to village levels. This will greatly assist the coverage and outreach of social marketing of products and services.
5. The social responsibility of the corporate sector in industry must, at the very minimum, extend to providing preventive reproductive and child health care for its own employees (if > 100 workers are engaged).
6. Create a national network consisting of voluntary, public, private and non-government health centres, identified by a common logo, for delivering reproductive and child health

services, free to any client. The provider will be compensated for the service provided, on the basis of a coupon system, duly counter-signed by the beneficiary and paid for by a system that will be fully articulated. The compensation will be identical to providers, across all sectors. The end user exercises choices in the source of service delivery. A committee of management experts will be set-up to devise ways of ensuring that this system is not abused.

7. Form a consortium of the voluntary sector the non-government sector and the private corporate sector to aid government in the provision and outreach of basic reproductive and child health care and basic education.
8. In the area of basic education, set-up privately run/managed primary schools for children up to age 14-15. Alternately, if the schools are set-up/managed by the panchayat, the private corporate sector could provide the mid-day meals, the text-books and/or the uniforms.

(ix) Mainstreaming Indian Systems of Medicine and Homeopathy

1. Provide appropriate training and orientation in respect of the RCH programme for the institutionally qualified ISMH medical practitioners (already educated in midwifery, obstetrics and gynaecology over 5½ years), and utilise their services to fill in gaps in manpower at appropriate levels in the health infrastructure, and at sub-centres and primary health centres, as necessary.
2. Utilise the ISMH institutions, dispensaries and hospitals for health and population-related programmes.
3. Disseminate the tried and tested concepts and practices of the indigenous systems of medicine, together with ISMH medication at village maternity huts and at household levels for ante-natal and post-natal care, besides nurture of the newborn.
4. Utilise the services of ISMH 'barefoot doctors' after appropriate training and orientation towards providing advocacy and counselling for disseminating supplies and equipment, and as depot-holders at village levels.

(x) Contraceptive Technology and Research on RCH

1. Government will encourage, support and advance the pursuit of medical and social science research on reproductive and child health, in consultation with ICMR and the network of academic and research institutions.
2. The international Institute of Population Sciences and the

Population Research Centres will continue to review programme and monitoring indicators to ensure their continued relevance to strategic goals.

3. Government will restructure the Population Research Centres, if necessary.
4. Standards for clinical and non-clinical interventions will be issued and regularly reviewed.
5. A constant review and evaluation of the community needs assessment approach will be pursued to align programme delivery with good management practices and with newly emerging technologies.
6. A committee of international and Indian experts, voluntary and non-government organisations and government may be set-up to regularly review and recommend specific incorporation of the advances in contraceptive technology and,. in particular, the newly emerging techniques, into programme development.

(xi) Providing for the Older Population

1. Sensitize, train and equip rural and urban health centres and hospitals towards providing geriatric health care.
2. Encourage NGOs and voluntary organizations to formulate and strengthen a series of formal and informal avenues that make the elderly economically self-reliant.
3. Tax benefits could be explored as an encouragement for children to look after their aged parents.

(xii) Information Education and Communication

1. Converge IEC efforts across the social sectors. The two sectors of Family Welfare and Education have coordinated a mutually supportive IEC strategy. The Zila Saksharta Samitis design and deliver joint IEC campaigns in the local idiom, promoting the cause of literacy as well as family welfare. Optimal use of folk media has served to successfully mobilize local populations. The state of Tamil Nadu made exemplary use of the IEC strategy by spreading the message through every possible media, including public transport, on mile stones on national highways as well as through advertisement and hoardings on roadsides, along city/rural roads, on billboards, and through processions, films, school dramas, public meetings, local theatre and folk songs.
2. Involve departments of rural development, social welfare, transport, cooperatives, education with special reference to schools, to improve clarity and focus of the IEC effort, and to

extend coverage and outreach. Health and population education must be inculcated from the school levels.

3. Fund the nagarpalikas, panchayats, NGOs and community organizations for interactive and participatory IEC activities.
4. Demonstration of support by elected leaders, opinion-makers, and religious leaders with close involvement in the reproductive and child health programme greatly influences the behaviour and response patterns of individuals and communities. This serves to enthuse communities to be attentive towards the quality and coverage of maternal and child health services, including referral care. Public leaders and film stars could spread widely the messages of the small family norm, female literacy, delayed marriages for women, fewer babies, healthier babies, child immunization and so on. The involvement and enthusiastic participation of elected leaders will ensure dedicated involvement of administrators at district and sub-district levels. Demonstration of strong support to the small family norm, as well as personal example, by political, community, business, professional, and religious leaders, media and film stars, sports personalities and opinion-makers, will enhance its acceptance throughout society.
5. Utilise radio and television as the most powerful media for disseminating relevant socio-demographic messages. Government could explore the feasibility of appropriate regulations, and even legislation, if necessary, to mandate the broadcast of social messages during prime time.
6. Utilise dairy cooperatives, the public distribution systems, other established networks like the LIC at district and sub-district levels for IEG and for distribution of contraceptives and basic medicines to target infant/childhood diarrhoeas, anaemia and malnutrition among adolescent girls and pregnant mothers. This will widen outreach and coverage.
7. Sensitise the field level functionaries across diverse sectors (education, rural development, forest and environment, women and child development, drinking water mission, cooperatives) to the strategies, goals and objectives of the population stabilisation programmes.
8. Involve civil society for disseminating information, counselling and spreading education about the small family norm, the need for fewer but healthier babies, higher female literacy and later marriages for women. Civil society could also be of assistance in monitoring the availability of contraceptives, vaccines and drugs in rural areas and in urban slums.

APPENDIX IV

HEALTH RESOURCES INDICATORS

Indicator	*Year*	*Bangla-desh*	*Bhutan*	*DPR Korea*	*India*	*Indo-nesia*	*Maldives*	*Myanmar*	*Nepal*	*Sri Lanka*	*Thailand*	*Timor-Leste*
Total expenditure on health (as % of GDP)	2000	3.8	4.1	2.1	4.9	2.7	7.6	2.2	5.4	3.6	3.7	9.4
Public share to total health expenditure (%)	2000	36.4	90.6	77.3	17.8	23.7	83.4	17.1	29.3	49.0	57.4	N/a
Per capita total health expenditure (International dollars)	2000	47	64	33	71	84	254	24	66	120	237	N/a
Physicians per 10,000 population	2001	2.51	1.6	29.7	5.2	1.1	8.4	3.0	0.54	4.1	3.0	N/a
Hospital beds per 10,000 population	2001	3.36	16.0	136.1	6.9	6.03	17.4	6.3	1.5	29	22.3	N/a

Source: WHO : Health Situation in South-East Asia, Basic Indicators, 2002.

Primary Health Care Coverage Indicators

Indicator		*Year*	*Bangla-desh*	*Bhutan*	*DPR Korea*	*India*	*Indo-nesia*	*Maldives*	*Myanmar*	*Nepal*	*Sri Lanka*	*Thailand*	*Timor-Leste*
Infants immunized (%)	DPT3	2001	70.2	88	37.4	52.1	95	98	89	80	88	94.6	58
	OPV3	2001	69.1	89	76.5	59.2	88.4	98	93	80	88	94.8	84
	BCG	2001	90	93	63.9	69.1	93.1	99.5	95	95	100	100	n/a
	Measles	2001	62.1	79	34.4	41.7	86.8	99	90	75	81	88.1	n/a
Pregnant women immunized with tetanus toxoid (%)		2001	63.7	73	4.6	66.8	73.4	94	77	24.2	90	76.3	n/a
Attended by trained personnel: (% of live births)	Pregnant women	2001	33.7	72	100	65.1	71.9	93	60.1	35	98	83.4	n/a
	Deliveries	2001	21.8	23.7	98.6	42.3	62.3	97	77.5	13,5	97	94.5	n/a
Women of child bearing age using contraceptives (%)		2001	53.8	30.7	67	48.2	66.4	42	55.1	38.9	71	72.2	N/a
Population with access to safe water (%)	Total	2001	97.3	77.8	99.9	77.9	N/a	76.5	71.5	59	75.4	92.7	N/a
	Urban	2001	99.2	97.5	n/a	92.6	88.2	n/a	89.2	61	96	n/a	n/a
	Rural	2001	96.7	73.2	n/a	72.3	71.9	n/a	65.8	59	74.6	n/a	n/a
Population with access to adequate sanitation (%)	Total	2001	54.1	88	99.2	36	N/a	85	63.1	23	72.6	97.7	n/a
	Urban	2001	74.6	n/a	n/a	80.7	86.9	n/a	83.6	74	87	n/a	n/a
	Rural	2001	49.3	n/a	n/a	18.9	54.2	n/a	56.5	18	68.3	n/a	n/a

Source: WHO : Health Situation in South-East Asia, Basic Indicators, 2002.

Health Status Indicators

Indicator		Year	Bangla-desh	Bhutan	DPR Korea	India	Indo-nesia	Maldives	Myanmar	Nepal	Sri Lanka	Thailand	Timor-Leste
Life expectancy at Birth (years)	Total	2002	62.6	61.3	65.8	61	66.4	64.6	62.3	60.1	70.3	69.3	57.5
	Male	2002	62.6	60.2	64.4	60.1	64.9	64.5	60.7	59.9	67.2	66	54.8
	Female	2002	62.6	62.4	67.1	62	67.9	65	63.9	60.2	74.3	72.7	60.5
Healthy life Expectancy (HALE)	Total	2002	54.3	52.9	58.9	53.4	58.2	56.8	51.6	51.8	61.3	60	49.7
at birth (years)	Male	2002	53.3	52.9	58	53.3	57.4	57.4	49.9	52.5	59.2	57.7	47.9
	Female	2002	53.3	52.9	59.7	53.6	58.9	56.3	53.5	51.1	64	62.5	51.8
Infant mortality rate (per 1000 live births)		2001	51	60.5	21.8	68	41.4	21	59.8	64.2	15.4	21.5	70-95
Under-five mortality	Male	2002	71	93	56	87	45	38	78	81	20	32	142
rate (per 1000 live births)	Female	2002	73	92	54	95	36	43	78	87	16	26	108
Total fertility rate (per woman)		2001	3.6	5.2	2.1	3.1	2.4	5.5	3	4.6	2.1	2	N/a
Maternal mortality ratio (per 100,000 live births)		2000	230	258	105	407	373	100	100/180	415	59.6	13.2	800
Low birth weight newborns (%)		2000	19.5	15.1	9	23	7.7	17.6	15	23.2	16.7	8.1	N/a
Children with low weight for age (%)		2000	47.7	18.7	60.6	47	20.3	30	35.5	47.1	29.4	11.3	45

Source: WHO : Health Situation in South-East Asia, Basic Indicators, 2002.

Gender Equity Indicators

Indicator	*Year*	*Bangla-desh*	*Bhutan*	*DPR Korea*	*India*	*Indo-nesia*	*Maldives*	*Myanmar*	*Nepal*	*Sri Lanka*	*Thailand*	*Timor-Leste*
Life expectancy at birth ratio (females as a % of males)	2001	99.7	103.6	106.7	102.8	104.7	100.8	105.3	98.8	111.3	109.9	N/a
Gender-related development index (GDI)	2001	0.495	N/a	N/a	0.574	0.677	N/a	N/a	0.479	0.726	0.766	N/a
Gender empowerment measure (GEM)	2001	0.218	N/a	N/a	N/a	N/a	N/a	N/a	N/a	0.272	0.457	N/a
Ratio of earned income (females as % of males)	2001	56	N/a	N/a	N/a	N/a	N/a	N/a	N/a	50	61	N/a
Seats held in parliament (% women)	2001	2	9.3	N/a	9.3	8	6	N/a	7.9	4.4	9.6	N/a
Professional and technical workers (% women)	2001	25	N/a	N/a	N/a	Na/	40	N/a	N/a	49	55	N/a
Adult literacy ratio (females as a % of males)	2000	61.1	55	100	66.4	89.2	99.8	90.6	40.4	94.3	96.7	N/a
Primary school enrolment ratio (females as a % of males)	1999/2000	97.2	75.6	93.5	84.9	96.6	100.8	99	79.8	97.2	95.3	N/a
Secondary school enrolment ratio (females as a % of males)	1999/2000	108.1	28.6	N/a	68.3	95.1	106.8	99.7	72.1	106.6	102.3	N/a

Source: WHO : Health Situation in South-East Asia, Basic Indicators, 2002.

Health-related Millennium Development Goals

Indicator	Year	Bangla-desh	Bhutan	DPR Korea	India	Indo-nesia	Maldives	Myanmar	Nepal	Sri Lanka	Thailand	Timor-Leste
Goal (G) Target (T) Indicator (I)												
Goal 1 : READICATE EXTREME POVERTY AND HUNGER												
Target 2 : Halve, between 1990 and 2015, the proportion of people who suffer from hunger												
G1.T2.I4 – Prevalence of underweight children (under-five years of age)	1990	54	39.7	5	53.4	41.7	N/a	32.4	46.9	37.6	20.8	N/a
	2001	47.7	18.7	27.9	47	24.6	30	35.5	48.3	29.4	11.3	45
G1.T2.I4 – Proportion (%) of population below minimum level of dietary energy consumption	1991	35	N/a	18	25	9	N/a	10	19	29	28	N/a
	1999	35	N/a	34	24	6	N/a	6	19	23	18	N/a
Goal 4 : REDUCE CHILD MORTALITY												
Target 5 : Reduce by two-thirds, between 1990 and 2015, the under-five mortality rate												
G4.T5.I13 – Under-five mortality rate (probability of dying between birth and age 5)	1990	136	96.9	23	112	84	48	130	165	22.6	42	N/a
	2002	72.3	84	90	90.9	51.4	30	78	91	18.3	31.4	125
G4.T5.I14 – Infant mortality rate	1990	92	70.7	14.1	80	60	34	100	102	19.3	32.8	N/a
	2000	51	60.5	21.8	68	40.9	21	59.8	64.2	15.4	21.5	70-95
4.T5.I15 – Proportion (%) of 1 year-old children immunized for measles	1990	53	69	99.7	32.7	90.3	85	71	65	86	58.1	N/a
	2001	76	78	34	56	93.9	99	73	71	99	94	N/a
Goal 5: IMPROVE MATERNAL HEALTH												
Target 6 : Reduce by three-quarters, between 1990 and 2015, the maternal mortality ratio												
G5.T6.I16 – Maternal mortality ratio	1990	470	380	N/a	420	425	500	100/190	850	42	36	N/a
	2001	230	355	105	407	373	100	255	415	59.6	13.2	800
G5.T6.I17 – Proportion (%) of births attended by skilled health personnel	1990	14	15.1	N/a	89/36	31.7	95	N/a	9	85.2	84.8	N/a
	2001	21.8	23.7	98.6	42.3	64.8	97	77.5	10.9	97	94.5	N/a

Health-related Millennium Development Goals

Indicator	Year	Bangladesh	Bhutan	DPR Korea	India	Indonesia	Maldives	Myanmar	Nepai	Sri Lanka	Thailand	Timor-Leste
Goal 6 : COMBAT HIV/AIDS, MALARIA AND OTHER DISEASES												
Target 7 : Have halted by 2015, and begun to reverse, the spread of HIV/AIDS												
G6.T7.I18 – HIV prevalence among young people	1990	N/a	N/a	N/a	N/a	N/a	N/a	N/a	N/a	N/a	N/a	N/a
15-24 years age group	2001(M)	0.01	N/a	N/a	0.22	0.05	N/a	N/a	0.02	0.02	0.88	N/a
15-49 years age group	2001 (F)	0.01	N/a	N/a	0.46	0.05	N/a	N/a	0.03	0.03	1.32	N/a
	2001	<0.1	<0.1	0.8	0.8	0.1	·0.1	1.3	<0.1	<0.1	1.7	N/a
G6.T7.I19 – Condom use in high risk population	1990	N/a	N/a	N/a	N/a	N/a	N/a	N/a	N/a	N/a	N/a	N/a
	2001(M)	N/a	N/a	N/a	51.2	N/a	N/a	N/a	N/a	44.4	N/a	N/a
	2001(F)	N/a	N/a	N/a	39.8	N/a	N/a	N/a	N/a	N/a	N/a	N/a
G6.T7..I20 – Ratio of children orphaned/	1990	N/a	N/a	N/a	N/a	Na/	N/a	N/a	N/a	N/a	N/a	N/a
non-orphaned in schools	2001	2,100	N/a	N/a	N/a	18,000	N/a	N/a	13,000	2,000	290,000	N/a
Target 8 : Have halted by 2015, and begun to reverse the incidence of malaria and other major diseases												
G6.T8.I21 – Malaria death rate per 100,000 in children	1990	N/a	N/a	N/a	N/a	N/a	N/a	N/a	N/a	N/a	N/a	N/a
(0-4 years of age)	2000	1	8	0	6	0	N/a	3	11	4	9	N/a
G6.T8.I21 – Malaria death rate per 100,000 (all ages)	1990	N/a	N/a	N/a	N/a	N/a	N/a	N/a	N/a	N/a	N/a	N/a
	2002	7.5	11.4	2.9	3.2	N/a	14.6	17.7	5.5	6.4	6.4	3.8
G6.T8.I21 –Malaria prevalence rate per 100,000	1990	N/a	N/a	N/a	N/a	N/a	N/a	N/a	N/a	N/a	N/a	N/a
	2002	34	44	19	14	15	N/a	22	78	57	49	22

Health-related Millennium Development Goals

Indicator	Year	Bangla-desh	Bhutan	DPR Korea	India	Indo-nesia	Maldives	Myanmar	Nepal	Sri Lanka	Thailand	Timor-Leste
Target 8 (continued)												
G6.T8.I22 – Proportion (%) of population under age 5 in malaria risk areas using insecticide-treated bed nets	1990	N/a	N/a	N/a	N/a	N/a	N/a	N/a	N/a	N/a	N/a	N/a
	2000	N/a	N/a	N/a	N/a	0.1	N/a	N/a	N/a	N/a	N/a	N/a
G6.T8.I22 – Proportion (%) of population under age 5 with fever being treated with anti-malarial drugs	1990	N/a	N/a	N/a	N/a	N/a	N/a	N/a	N/a	N/a	N/a	N/a
	2000	N/a	N/a	N/a	N/a	4	N/a	N/a	N/a	N/a	N/a	N/a
G6.T8.I23 – Tuberculosis death rate per 100,000	1990	N/a	N/a	N/a	N/a	N/a	N/a	N/a	N/a	N/a	N/a	N/a
	2002	54.4	23	31.8	40.4	66.1	3.5	33.2	26.4	11.4	18.5	54.6
G6.T8.I23 – Tuberculosis prevalence rate per 100,000	1990	N/a	N/a	N/a	N/a	N/a	N/a	N/a	N/a	N/a	N/a	N/a
	2000	471	215	343	426	739	48	268	300	116	241	779
G6.T8.I24 – Proportion (%) of Smear Positive Pulmonary Tuberculosis cases detected and put under directly observed treatment shot course (DOTS)	1990	N/a	N/a	N/a	N/a	N/a	N/a	N/a	N/a	N/a	N/a	N/a
	2001	83	90	91	84	87	95	82	86	77	69	N/a

Health-related Millennium Development Goals

Indicator	Year	Bangladesh	Bhutan	DPR Korea	India	Indonesia	Maldives	Myanmar	Nepal	Sri Lanka	Thailand	Timor-Leste
Goal 7 : ENSURE ENVIRONMENT SUSTAINABILITY												
Target 9: Integrate the principles of sustainable development into country policies and programmes and reverse the loss of environmental resources												
G7.T9.I29 – Proportion (%) of population using biomass fuels	1990	N/a	N/a	N/a	N/a	N/a	N/a	N/a	N/a	N/a	N/a	N/a
	2000	96	N/a	N/a	81	63	N/a	100	97	89	72	N/a
Target 10 : Halve, by 2015, the proportion of people without sustainable access to safe drinking water												
G7.T10.I30 – Proportion (%) of population with sustainable access to an improved water source, rural	1990	93	N/a	N/a	61	62	N/a	N/a	64	62	78	N/a
	2000	97	60	100	79	69	100	66	87	70	81	N/a
G7.T10.I30 – Propotion (%) of population with sustainable access to an improved water source, urban	1990	99	N/a	N/a	88	92	N/a	N/a	93	91	87	N/a
	2000	99	86	100	95	90	100	89	94	98	95	N/a
Target 11 : By 2020 to have achieved a significant improvement in the lives of at least 100 million slum dwellers												
G7.T11.I31 – Proportion (%) of urban population with access to improved sanitation	1990	81	N/a	N/a	44	66	N/a	N/a	69	94	95	N/a
	2000	71	65	99	61	69	100	84	73	97	96	N/a
Goal 8: Develop Global Partnership for Development												
Target 17: In cooperation with pharmaceutical companies, provide access to affordable, essential drugs in developing countries												
G8.T17.I46 – Proportion (%) of population with access to affordable essential drugs on a sustainable basis	1990	N/a	N/a	N/a	N/a	N/a	N/a	N/a	N/a	N/a	N/a	N/a
	1997	80	80	50	80	80	80	50	50	95	80	N/a

Demographic Indicators

Indicator	*Year*	*Bangla-desh*	*Bhutan*	*DPR Korea*	*India*	*Indo-nesia*	*Maldives*	*Myanmar*	*Nepal*	*Sri Lanka*	*Thailand*	*Timor-Leste*
Total population (thousands)	2002	143364	805	22586	1041144	217534	309	48956	24153	19287	64344	850
Surface area (thousands of sq.km)	2000	144	47	121	3287	1905	0.3	677	147	66	513	15
Population density (per sq.km)	2002	996	17	187	317	114	1030	72	164	292	125	58
Population growth rate (%0	2000-2005	2.09	2.55	0.68	1.52	1.21	1.96	1.16	2.32	0.94	1.14	3.93
Crude birth rate (per 1000 population)	2000-2005	29.9	34.09	16.7	23.8	20	20	23.2	34	17.3	17.8	25.4
Crude deajth rate (per 1000 population)	2000-2005	8.7	8.64	9.9	8.4	7.1	4	11.6	9.9	6.3	6.2	13.2
Urban population (%)	2000	24.5	14.5	60.2	28.4	40.9	27.4	27.7	11.9	23.6	21.6	15
Average annual growth rate of the urban population (%)	2000-2005	3.98	5.95	1.62	2.81	3.57	3.52	2.86	5.07	2.84	2.67	2.21

Socio-economic Indicators

Indicator		Year	Bangla-desh	Bhutan	DPR Korea	India	Indo-nesia	Maldives	Myanmar	Nepal	Sri Lanka	Thailand	Timor-Leste
Gross national income (GNI) per capita (US$)		2001	370	640	N/a	460	6.80	2040	N/a	250	830	1970	478
Gross domestic product (GDP) per capita growth rate (%)		2000-2001	3.3	4	N/a	2.7	1.8	4.5	N/a	3.4	1	0.9	N/a
Average annual change in consumer rice index (%)		2000-2001	1.1	N/a	N/a	3.7	11.5	0.6	21.1	2.8	14.2	1.7	N/a
Human Development Index (HDI)		2001	0.502	0.511	N/a	0.90	0.682	0.751	0.549	0.499	0.73	0.768	N/a
Dependency	Total	2000	72	89	48	62	55	89	61	81	48	47	84
ratio	Old-age (65+)	2000	5	8	9	8	7	7	7	7	9	8	5
	Young (0-14)	2000	67	81	39	54	48	83	53	74	39	39	79
Adult literacy rate (%)	Total	2000	40	47.3	100	57.2	86.8	96.9	84.7	41.7	91.6	95.5	N/a
	Male	2000	49.4	61.1	100	68.4	91.8	97	88.9	59.4	94.4	97.1	N/a
	Female	2000	30.2	33.6	100	45.4	81.9	96.8	80.5	24	89	93.9	N/a
Gross primary	Total	1999/2000	106.11	N/a	N/a	100.93	107.89	133.71	90.95	126.38	105.91	93.50	N/a
school enrolment	Male	1999/2000	107.57	82	108	108.88	109.71	133.22	91.39	140	107.39	95.72	N/a
ratio (%)	Female	1999/2000	104.57	62	101	92.39	106	134.23	90.51	111.74	104.38	91.24	N/a
Gross secondary	Total	1999/2000	53.73	N/a	N/a	49.92	54.88	42.75	34.87	53.90	72.12	78.95	N/a
School enrolment	Male	1999/2000	51.7	7	N/a	58.91	56.23	41.36	34.92	62.26	69.85	78.06	N/a
ratio (%)	Female	1999/2000	55.90	2	N/a	40.22	53.50	44.17	34.81	74.86	74.47	79.85	N/a

Sources:
1. UN, *World Population Prospects*, The 2000 Revision, Volume I: Comprehensive Tables, New York, 2001.
2. UN, *2000 Demographic Yearbook*, New York, 2002.
3. UN, *World Urbanization Prospects, The 1999 Revision*, New York, 2001.
4. World Bank, *World Development Report*, 2003, Oxford University Press, New York, 2003.
5. UNDP, *Human Development Report 2003*, Oxford University Press, New York, 2003.
6. UNESCO, <http://www>. unesco.org.Junly 2002 assessment.
7. UNESCO, *Statistical Yearbook*, 1999.
8. WHO, Regional Office for South-East Asia, Routine and *Ad hoc* reports from countries to the EHP Unit, New Delhi, 2002.
9. UNICEF, *The State of the World's Children*, 2003, Oxford University Press, New York, 2003.
10. Timor-Leste, *Health Profile*, Dilli, 26, August, 2002.

11. Bhutan, Ministry of Health and Education, *Report on National Health Survey,* 2000.
12. Maldives, *Statistical Health Report,* 2002, Geneva, 2002.
13. WHO, Regional Office for South-East Asia, Health Situation in the South-East Asia Region, 1998-2000, New Delhi, 2002.
14. WHO, Regional Office for South-East Asia, country reported HFA data set 1997.
15. http//millenniumidicators,un.org/unsed, FAO estimates (3690), July 2003.
16. <http://millenniumindicators>. un.org.unsed. WHO (29996), July 2003.
17. WHO, Geneva, The World Health Report, 2002 (draft) Annex tables and MDG data set (draft), June 2003.
18. Myammar, Health in Myanmar, 2002.
19. Nepal, Demographic and Health Survey, 2001.
20. Country Presentation at the Consultative Meeting on MDG Dataset, June 2003, WHO/SEARO, New Delhi.
21. WHO, Genveva, Global Tuberculosis Control, *WHO Report,* 2003.

APPENDIX V

NATIONAL HEALTH POLICY, 2002

I. Introductory

1.1 A National Health Policy was last formulated in 1983, and since then there have been marked changes in the determinant factors relating to the heath sector. Some of the policy initiatives outlined in the NHP-1983 have yielded results, while, in several other areas, the outcome has not been as expected

1.2 The NHP-1983 gave a general exposition of the policies which required recommendation in the circumstances then prevailing in the health sector. The noteworthy initiatives under that policy were:

(i) A phased, time-bound programme for setting up a well-dispersed network of comprehensive primary health care services, linked with extension and health education, designed in the context of the ground reality that elementary health problems can be resolved by the people themselves;
(ii) Intermediation through Health Volunteers' having appropriate knowledge, simple skills and requisite technologies;
(iii) Establishment of a well-worked out referral system to ensure that patient load at the higher levels of the hierarchy is not needlessly burdened by those who can be treated at the decentralized level; and
(iv) An integrated net-work of evenly spread speciality and super-speciality services; encouragement of such facilities through private investments for patients who can pay, so that the draw on the Government's facilities is limited to those entitled to free use.

1.3 Government initiatives in the pubic health sector have recorded some noteworthy successes over time. Smallpox and Guinea Worm Disease have been eradicated from the country; Polio is on the verge of being eradicated, Leprosy, Kala Azar, and Filariasis can be expected to be eliminated in the foreseeable future. There has been a substantial drop in the Total Fertility Rate and Infant Mortality Rate. The success of the initiatives taken in the public health field are reflected in the progressive improvement of many demographic/epidemiological/infrastructural

Box I

Achievements through the Years—1951-2000

Indicator	*1951*	*1981*	*2000*
Demographic Changes			
Life Expectancy	36.7	54	64.6 (RGI)
Crude Birth Rate	40.8	33.9 (SRS)	26.1 (99-SRS)
Crude Death Rate	25	12.5 (SRS)	8.7 (99-SRS)
IMR	146	110	70 (99-SRS)
Epidemiological Shifts			
Malaria (cases in million)	75	2.7	2.2
Leprosy cases per 10,000 population	38.1	57.3	3.74
Small Pox (no. of cases)	>44,887	Eradicated	
Guineaworm (no. of cases)		>39,792	Eradicated
Polio		29709	265
Infrastructure			
SC/PHC/CHC	725	57,363	1,63,181 (99-RHS)
Dispensaries & Hospitals (all)	9209	23,555	43,322 (95-96-CBHI)
Beds (Pvt & Public)	117,198	569,495	8,70,161 (95-96-CBHI)
Doctors (Allopathy)	61,800	2,68,700	5,03,900 (98-99-MCI)
Nursing Personnel	18,054	1,43,887	7,37,000 (99-INC)

indicators over time (Box I).

1.4 While noting that the public health initiatives over the years have contributed significantly to the improvement of these health indicators, it is to be acknowledged that public health indicators/disease-burden statistics are the outcome of several complementary initiatives under the wider umbrella of the developmental sector, covering Rural Development, Agriculture, Food Production, Sanitation, Drinking Water Supply, Education, etc. Despite the impressive public health gains as revealed in the statistics in Box-I, there is no gainsaying the fact that the morbidity and mortality levels in the country are still unacceptably high. These unsatisfactory health indices are, in turn, an indication of the limited success of the public health system in meeting the preventive and curative requirements of the general population.

1.5 Out of the communicable diseases which have persisted over time, the incidence of Malaria staged a resurgence in the 1980s before stabilising at a fairly high prevalence level during the 1990s. Over the years, an increasing level of insecticide-resistance has developed in the malarial vectors in many parts of the country, while the incidence of the more deadly P-Falciparum Malaria has risen to about 50 percent in the country as a whole. In respect of TB, the public health scenario has not shown any significant decline in the pool of infection amongst the community, and there has been a distressing trend in the increase of drug resistance to the type of infection prevailing in the country. A new and extremely virulent communicable disease—HIV/AIDS—has emerged on the health scene since the declaration of the NHP-1983. As there is no existing therapeutic cure or vaccine for this infection, the disease constitutes a serious threat, not merely to public health but to economic development in the country. The common water-borne infections—Gastroenteritis, Cholera, and some forms of Hepatitis—continue to contribute to a high level of morbidity in the population, even though the mortality rate may have been somewhat moderated.

1.6 The period after the announcement of NHP-83 has also seen an increase in mortality through 'life-style' diseases—diabetes, cancer and cardiovascular diseases. The increase in life expectancy has increased the requirement for geriatric care. Similarly, the increasing burden of trauma cases is also a significant public health problem.

1.7 Another area of grave concern in the public health domain is the persistent incidence of macro and micro-nutrient deficiencies, especially among women and children. In the vulnerable sub-category of women and the girl child, this has the multiplier effect through the birth of low birth weight babies and serious ramifications of the consequential mental and physical retarded growth.

1.8 NHP-1983, in a spirit of optimistic empathy for the health needs of the people, particularly the poor and under-privileged, had hoped to provide 'Health for All by the year 2000 AD', through the universal provision of comprehensive primary health care services. In retrospect, it is observed that the financial resources and public health administrative capacity which it was possible to marshal, was far short of that necessary to achieve such an ambitious and holistic goal. Against this backdrop, it is felt that it would be appropriate to pitch NHP-2002 at a level consistent with our realistic expectations about financial resources, and about the likely increase in Public Health administrative capacity. The recommendations of NHP-2002 will, therefore, attempt to maximize the broad-based availability of health services to the citizenry of the country on the basis of realistic considerations of capacity. The changed circumstances relating to the health sector of the country since 1983 have generated a situation in which it is now necessary to review the field, and to formulate a new policy framework as the National Health Policy-2002. NHP-2002 will attempt to set out a new policy framework for the accelerated achievement of Public health goals in the socio-economic circumstances currently prevailing in the country.

2. Current Scenario

2.1 Financial Resources

2.1.1 The public health investment in the country over the years has been comparatively low, and as a percentage of GDP has declined from 1.3 percent in 1990 to 0.9 percent in 1999. The aggregate expenditure in the Health sector is 5.2 percent of the GDP. Out of this, about 17 percent of the aggregate expenditure is public health spending, the balance being out-of-pocket expenditure. The central budgetary allocation for health over this period, as a percentage of the total Central Budget, has been stagnant at 1.3 percent, while that in the States has declined from 7.0 percent to 5.5 percent. The current annual per capita public health expenditure in the country is no more than Rs. 200. Given these statistics, it is no surprise that the reach and quality of public health services has been below the desirable standard. Under the constitutional structure, public health is the responsibility of the States. In this framework, it has been the expectation that the principal contribution for the funding of public health services will be from the resources of the States, with some supplementary input from Central resources. In this backdrop, the contribution of Central resources to the overall public health funding has been limited to about 15 percent. The fiscal resources of the State Governments are known to be very inelastic. This is reflected in the declining percentage of State resources allocated to the health sector out of the State Budget. If the decentralized public health services in the country are to improve significantly, there is a need for the injection of substantial resources into the health sector from the Central Government Budget. This approach is a necessity—despite the formal Constitutional provision in regard to public health,—if the State public health services, which are a major component of the initiatives in the social sector, are not to become entirely moribund. The NHP-2002 has been formulated taking into consideration these ground realities in regard to the availability of resources.

2.2 Equity

2.2.1 In the period when centralized planning was accepted as a key instrument of development in the country, the attainment of an equitable regional distribution was considered one of its major objectives. Despite this conscious focus in the development process, the statistics given in Box-II clearly indicate that the attainment of health indices has been very uneven across the rural-urban divide.

Also, the statistics bring out the wide differences between the attainments of health goals in the better perfuming States as compared to the low-performing States. It is clear that national averages of health Indices hide wide disparities in public health facilities and health standards in different parts of the country. Given a situation in which

Box II

Differentials in Health Status among States

Sector	*Population BPL (%)*	*IMR/ Per 1000 Live Births (1999-SRS)*	*<5 Mortality per 1000 (NFHS-II)*	*Weight for Age % of Children under 3 years (<-2SD)*	*MMR/ Lakh (Annual Report 2000)*	*Leprosy cases per 10000 population*	*Malaria +ve cases in year 2000 (in thous-ands)*
India	**26.1**	**70**	**94.9**	**47**	**408**	**3.7**	**2200**
Rural	27.09	75	103.7	49.6	—	—	—
Urban	23.62	44	63.1	38.4	—	—	—
Better Performing States							
Kerala	12.72	14	18.8	27	87	0.9	5.1
Maharashtra	25.02	48	58.1	50	135	3.1	138
Tamil Nadu	21.12	52	63.3	37	79	4.1	56
Low Performing States							
Orissa	47.15	97	104.4	54	498	7.05	483
Bihar	42.60	63	105.1	54	707	11.83	132
Rajasthan	15.28	81	114.9	51	607	0.8	53
Uttar Pradesh	31.15	84	122.5	52	707	4.3	99
Madhya Pradesh	37.43	90	137.6	55	498	3.83	528

national averages in respect of most indices are themselves at unacceptably low levels, the wide inter-State disparity implies that, for vulnerable sections of society in several States, access to public health services is nominal and health standards are grossly inadequate. Despite a thrust in the NHP-1983 for making good the unmet needs of public health services by establishing more public health institutions at a decentralized level, a large gap in facilities still persists. Applying current norms to the population projected for the year 2000, it is estimated that the shortfall in the number of SCs/PHCs/CHCs is of the order of 16 percent. However, this shortage is as high as 58 percent when disaggregated for CHCs only. The NHP-2002 will need to address itself to making good these deficiencies so as to narrow the gap between the various States, as also the gap across the rural-urban divide.

2.2.2 Access to, and benefits from, the public health system have been very uneven between the better-endowed and the more vulnerable sections of society. This is particularly true for women, children and the socially disadvantaged sections of society. The statistics given in Box-III highlight the handicap suffered in the health sector on account of socio-economic inequity.

2.2.3 It is a principal objective of NHP-2002 to evolve a policy structure which reduces these inequities and allows the disadvantaged

Box III

Differentials in Health Status Among Socio-Economic Groups

Indicator	*Infant Mortality/1000*	*Under 5 Mortality/1000*	*% Children Underweight*
India	70	94.9	47
Social Inequity			
Scheduled Castes	83	119.3	53.5
Scheduled Tribes	84.2	126.6	55.9
Other Disadvantaged	76	103.1	47.3
Others	61.8	82.6	41.1

sections of society a fairer access to public health services.

2.3 Delivery of National Public Health Programmes

2.3.1 It is self-evident that in a country as large as India, which has a wide variety of socio-economic settings, national health programmes have to be designed with enough flexibility to permit the State public health administrations to craft their own programme package according to their needs. Also, the implementation of the national health programme can only be carried out through the State Governments decentralized public health machinery. Since, for-various reasons, the responsibility of the Central Government in funding additional public health services will continue over a period of time, the role of the Central Government in designing broad-based public health initiatives will inevitably continue. Moreover, it has been observed that the technical and managerial expertise for designing large-span public health programmes exists with the Central Government in a considerable degree; this expertise can be gainfully utilized in designing national health programmes for implementation in varying socio-economic settings in the States. With this background, the NHP-2002 attempts to define the role of the Central Government and the State Governments in the public health sector of the country.

2.3.2.1 Over the last decade or so, the Government has relied upon a 'vertical' implementational structure for the major disease control programmes. Through this, the system has been able to make a substantial dent in reducing the burden of specific diseases. However, such an organizational structure, which requires independent manpower for each disease programme, is extremely expensive and difficult to sustain. Over a long time-range, 'vertical' structures may only be affordable for those diseases which offer a reasonable possibility of elimination or eradication in a foreseeable time-span.

2.3.2.2 It is a widespread perception that, over the last decade and a half, the rural health staff has become a vertical structure exclusively for the implementation of family welfare activities. As a result, for those public health programmes where there is no separate vertical structure, there is no identifiable service delivery system at all. The Policy will address this distortion in the public health system.

2.4 The State of Public Health Infrastructure

2.4.1 The delineation of NHP-2002 would be required to be based on an objective assessment of the quality and efficiency of the existing public health machinery in the field. It would detract from the quality of the exercise if, while framing a new policy, it were not acknowledged that the existing public health infrastructure is far from satisfactory. For the outdoor medical facilities in existence, funding is generally insufficient; the presence of medical and para-medical personnel is often much less than that required by prescribed norms; the availability of consumables is frequently negligible; the equipment in many public hospitals is often obsolescent and unusable; and, the buildings are in a dilapidated state. In the indoor treatment facilities, again, the equipment is often obsolescent; the availability of essential drugs is minimal; the capacity of the facilities is grossly inadequate, which leads to over-crowding, and consequentially to a steep deterioration in the quality of the services. As a result of such inadequate public health facilities, it has been estimated that less than 20 percent of the population, which seek OPD services, and less than 45 percent of that which seek indoor treatment, avail of such services in public hospitals. This is despite the fact that most of these patients do not have the means to make out-of-pocket payments for private health services except at the cost of other essential expenditure for items such as basic nutrition.

2.5 Extending Public Health Services

2.5.1 While there is a general shortage of medical personnel in the country, this shortfall is disproportionately impacted on the less-developed and rural areas. No incentive system attempted so far, has induced private medical personnel to go to such areas; and, even in the public health sector, the effort to deploy medical personnel in such under-served areas, has usually been a losing battle. In such a situation, the possibility needs to be examined of entrusting some limited public health functions to nurses, paramedics and other personnel from the extended health sector after imparting adequate training to them.

2.5.2 India has a vast reservoir of practitioners in the Indian Systems of Medicine and Homoeopathy, who have undergone formal training in their own disciplines. The possibility of using such practitioners in the implementation of State/Central Government public health programmes, in order to increase the reach of basic health care in the country, is addressed in the NHP-2002.

2.6 Role of Local Self-Government Institutions

2.6.1 Some States have adopted a policy of devolving programmes and funds in the health sector through different levels of the Panchayati Raj Institutions. Generally, the experience has been an encouraging one. The adoption of such an organisational structure has enabled need-based allocation of resources and closer supervision through the elected representatives. The Policy examines the need for a wider adoption of this mode of delivery of health services, in rural as well as urban areas, in other parts of the country.

2.7 Norms for Health Care Personnel

2.7.1 It is observed that the deployment of doctors and nurses, in both public and private institutions, is *ad-hoc* and significantly short of the requirement for minimal standards of patient care. This policy will make a specific recommendation in regard to this deficiency.

2.8 Education of Health Care Professionals

2.8.1 Medical and Dental Colleges are not evenly spread across various parts of the country. Apart from the uneven geographical distribution of medical institutions, the quality of education is highly uneven and in several instances even sub-standard. It is a common perception that the syllabus is excessively theoretical, making it difficult for the fresh graduate to effectively meet even the primary health care needs of the population. There is a general reluctance on the part of graduate doctors to serve in areas distant from their native place. NHP-2002 will suggest policy initiatives to rectify the resultant disparities.

2.8.2.1 Certain medical disciplines, such as molecular biology and gene-manipulation, have become relevant in the period after the formulation of the previous National Health Policy. The components of medical research in recent years have changed radically. In the foreseeable future such research will rely increasingly on the new disciplines. It is observed that the current under-graduate medical syllabus does not cover such emerging subjects. The Policy will make appropriate recommendations in respect of such deficiencies.

2.8.2.2 Also, certain speciality disciplines—Anesthesiology, Radiology and Forensic Medicine—are currently very scarce, resulting in critical deficiencies in the package of available public health services. This Policy will recommend some measures to alleviate such critical shortages.

2.9 Need for Specialists in 'Public Health' and 'Family Medicine'

2.9.1 In any developing country with inadequate availability of health services, the requirement of expertise in the areas of 'public health' and 'family medicine' is markedly more than the expertise required for other clinical specialities. In India, the situation is that public health expertise is non-existent in the private health sector, and far short of requirement in the public health sector. Also, the current curriculum in the graduate/post-graduate courses is outdated and unrelated to contemporary community needs. In respect of 'family medicine', it needs to be noted that the more talented medical graduates generally seek specialization in clinical disciplines, while the remaining go into general practice. While the availability of post-graduate educational facilities is 50 percent of the total number of qualifying graduates each year, and can be considered adequate, the distribution of the disciplines in the post-graduate training facilities is overwhelmingly in favour of clinical specializations. NHP-2002 examines the possible means for ensuring adequate availability of personnel with specialization in the 'public health' and 'family medicine' disciplines, to discharge the public health responsibilities in the country.

2.10 Nursing Personnel

2.10.1 The ratio of nursing personnel in the country *vis-a-vis* doctors/beds is very low according to professionally accepted norms. There is also an acute shortage of nurses trained in super-epeciality disciplines for deployment in tertiary care facilities. NHP-2002 addresses these problems.

2.11 Use of Generic Drugs and Vaccines

2.11.1 India enjoys a relatively low-cost health care system because of the widespread availability of indigenously manufactured generic drugs and vaccines. There is an apprehension that globalization will lead to an increase in the costs of drugs, thereby leading to rising trends in overall health costs. This Policy recommends measures to ensure the future Health Security of the country.

2.12 Urban Health

2.12.1.1 In most urban areas, public health services are very meagre. To the extent that such services exist, there is no uniform organizational structure. The urban population in the country is presently as high as 30 percent and is likely to go up to around 33 percent by 2010. The bulk of the increase is likely to take place through migration, resulting in slums without any infrastructure support. Even the meagre public health services which are available do not percolate to such unplanned habitations, forcing people to avail of private health care through out-of-pocket expenditure.

2.12.1.2 The rising vehicle density in large urban agglomerations has also led to an increased number of serious accidents requiring treatment in well-equipped trauma centres. NHP-2002 will address itself to the need for providing this unserved urban population a minimum standard of broad-based health care facilities.

2.13 Mental Health

2.13.1 Mental health disorders are actually much more prevalent than is apparent on the surface. While such disorders do not contribute significantly to mortality, they have a serious beating on the quality of life of the affected persons and their families. Sometimes, based on religious faith, mental disorders are treated as spiritual affliction. This has led to the establishment of unlicensed mental institutions as an adjunct to religious institutions where reliance is placed on faith cure. Serious conditions of mental disorder require hospitalization and treatment under trained supervision. Mental health institutions are woefully deficient in physical infrastructure and trained manpower. NHP-2002 will address itself to these deficiencies in the public health sector.

2.14 Information, Education and Communication

2.14.1 A substantial component of primary health care consists of initiatives for disseminating to the citizenry, public health-related information. IEC initiatives are adopted not only for disseminating curative guidelines (for the TB, Malaria, Leprosy, Cataract Blindness Programmes), but also as part of the effort to bring about a behavioural change to prevent HIV/AIDS and other life-style diseases. Public health programmes, particularly, need high visibility at the decentralized level in order to have an impact. This task is difficult as 35 percent of our country's population is illiterate. The present IEC strategy is too fragmented, relies too heavily on the mass media and does not address the needs of this segment of the population. It is often felt that the effectiveness of IEO programme is difficult to judge; and consequently it is often asserted that accountability, in regard to the productive use of such funds is doubtful. The Policy, while projecting an IEC strategy, will fully address the inherent problems encountered in any IEC programme designed for improving awareness and bringing about a behavioural change in the general population.

2.14.2 It is widely accepted that school and college students are the most impressionable targets for imparting information relating to the basic principles of preventive health care. The policy will attempt to target this group to improve the general level of awareness in regard to 'health-promoting' behaviour.

2.15 Health Research

2.15.1 Over the years, health research activity in the country has been very limited. In the Government sector, such research has been confined to the research institutions under the Indian Council of Medical Research, and other institutions funded by the States/Central Government. Research in the private sector has assumed some significance only in the last decade. In our country, where the aggregate annual health expenditure is of the order of Rs. 80,000 crores, the expenditure in 1998-99 on research, both public and private sectors, was only of the order of Rs. 1150 crores. It would be reasonable to infer that with such low research expenditure, it is virtually impossible to make any dramatic break-through within the country, by way of new molecules and vaccines; also, without a minimal back-up of applied and operational research, it would be difficult to assess whether the health expenditure in the country is being incurred through optimal applications and appropriate public health strategies. Medical Research in the country needs to be focused on therapeutic drugs/vaccines for tropical diseases, which are normally neglected by international pharmaceutical companies on account of their limited profitability potential. The thrust will need to be in the newly-emerging frontier areas of research based on genetics, genome-based drug and vaccine development, molecular biology, etc. NHP-2002 will address these inadequacies and spell out a minimal quantum of expenditure for the coming decade, looking to the national needs and the capacity of the research institutions to absorb the funds.

2.16 Role of the Private Sector

2.16.1 Considering the economic restructuring under way in the country, and over the globe, in the last decade, the changing role of the private sector in providing health care will also have to be addressed in this Policy. Currently, the contribution of private health care is principally through independent practitioners. Also, the private sector contributes significantly to secondary-level care and some tertiary care. It is a widespread perception that private health services are very uneven in quality, sometimes even sub-standard. Private health services are also perceived to be financially exploitative, and the observance of professional ethics is noted only as an exception. With the increasing role of private health care, the implementation of statutory regulation, and the monitoring of minimum standards of diagnostic centres/medical institutions becomes imperative. The Policy will address the issues regarding the establishment of a comprehensive information system, and based on that the establishment of a regulatory mechanism to ensure the maintaining of adequate standards by diagnostic centres/medical institutions, as well as the proper conduct of clinical practice and delivery of medical services.

2.16.2 Currently, non-Govemmental service providers are treating a large number of patients at the primary level for major diseases. However, the treatment regimens followed are diverse and not scientifically optimal, leading to an increase in the incidence of drug resistance. This policy will address itself to recommending arrangements which will eliminate the risks arising from inappropriate treatment.

2.16.3 The increasing spread of information technology raises the possibility of its adoption in the health sector. NHP-2002 will examine this possibility.

2.17 The Role of Civil Society

2.17.1 Historically, it has been the practice to implement major national disease control programmes through the public health machinery of the State/Central Governments. It has become increasingly apparent that certain components of such programmes cannot be efficiently implemented merely through government functionaries. A considerable change in the mode of implementation has come about in the last two decades, with the increasing involvement of NGOs and other institutions of civil society. It is to be recognized that widespread debate on various public health issues has, in fact, been initiated and sustained by NGOs and other members of the civil society. Also, an increasing contribution is being made by such institutions in the delivery of different components of public health services. Certain disease control programmes require close inter-action with the beneficiaries for regular administration of drugs; periodic carrying out of pathological tests; dissemination of information regarding disease control and other general health information. NHP-2002 will address such issues and suggest policy instruments for the implementation of public health programmes through individuals and institutions of civil society.

2.18 National Disease Surveillance Network

2.18.1 The technical network available in the country for disease surveillance is extremely rudimentary and to the extent that the system exists, it extends only up to the district level. Disease statistics are not flowing through an integrated network from the decentralized public health facilities to the State/Central Government health administration. Such an arrangement only provides belated information, which, at best, serves a limited statistical purpose. The absence of an efficient disease surveillance network is a major handicap in providing a prompt and cost-effective health care system. The efficient disease surveillance network set-up for Polio and HIV/AIDS has demonstrated the enormous value of such a public health instrument. Real-time information on focal outbreaks of common communicable diseases—Malaria, GE, Cholera and JE—and the seasonal trends of diseases, would enable timely intervention, resulting in the containment of the thrust of epidemics. In order to be able to use an integrated disease surveillance network for operational purposes, real-time information is necessary at all levels of the health administration. The Policy would address itself to this major systemic shortcoming in the administration.

2.19 Health Statistics

2.19.1 The absence of a systematic and scientific health statistics data-base is a major deficiency in the current scenario. The health statistics collected are not the product of a rigorous methodology. Statistics available from different parts of the country, in respect of major diseases, are often not obtained in a manner which make aggregation possible or meaningful.

2.19.2.1 Further, the absence of proper and systematic documentation of the various financial resources used in the health sector is another lacuna in the existing health information scenario. This makes it difficult to understand trends and levels of health spending by private and public providers of health care in the country, and, consequently, to address related policy issues and to formulate future investment policies.

2.19.2.2 NHP-2002 will address itself to the programme for putting in place a modern and scientific health statistics database as well as a system of national health accounts.

2.20 Women's Health

2.20.1 Social, cultural and economic factors continue to inhibit women from gaining adequate access even to the existing public health facilities. This handicap does not merely affect women as individuals; it also has an adverse impact on the health, general well-being and development of the entire family, particularly children. This policy recognises the catalytic role of empowered women in improving the overall health standards of the community.

2.21 Medical Ethics

2.21.1 Professional medical ethics in the health sector is an area which has not received much attention. Professional practices are perceived to be grossly commercial and the medical profession has lost its elevated position as a provider of basic services to fellow human beings. In the past, medical research has been conducted within the ethical guidelines notified by the Indian Council of Medical Research. The first document containing these guidelines was released in 1960, and was comprehensively revised in 2001. With the rapid developments in the approach to medical research, a periodic revision will no doubt be more frequently required in future. Also, the new frontier areas of research—involving gene manipulation, organ/human cloning and stem cell research—impinge on visceral issues relating to the sanctity of human life and the moral dilemma of human intervention in the designing of life forms. Besides this, in the emerging areas of research, there is the uncharted risk of creating new life forms, which may irreversibly damage the environment as it exists today. NHP-2002 recognises that this moral and religious dilemma, which was not relevant even two years ago, now pervades mainstream health sector issues.

2.22 Enforcement of Quality Standards for Food and Drugs

2.22.1 There is an increasing expectation and need of the citizenry for efficient enforcement of reasonable quality standards for food and drugs. Recognizing this, the Policy will make an appropriate policy recommendation on this issue.

2.23 Regulation of Standards in Para Medical Disciplines

2.23.1 It has been observed that a large number of training institutions have mushroomed, particularly in the private sector, for para medical personnel with various skills—Lab Technicians, Radio Diagnosis Technicians, Physiotherapists, etc. Currently, there is no regulation/ monitoring, either of the curriculae of these institutions, or of the performance of the practitioners in these disciplines. This Policy will make recommendations to ensure the standardization of such training and the monitoring of actual performance.

2.24 Environmental and Occupational Health

2.24.1 The ambient environmental conditions are a significant determinant of the health risks to which a community is exposed. Unsafe drinking water, unhygienic sanitation and air pollution significantly contribute to the burden of disease, particularly in urban settings. The initiatives in respect of these environmental factors are conventionally undertaken by the participants, whether private or public, in the other development sectors. In this backdrop, the Policy initiatives, and the efficient implementation of the linked programmes in the health sector, would succeed only to the extent that they are complemented by appropriate policies and programmes in the other environment-related sectors.

2.24.2 Work conditions in several sectors of employment in the country are sub-standard. As a result, workers engaged in such employment become particularly vulnerable to occupation-linked ailments. The long-term risk of chronic morbidity is particularly marked in the case of child labour. NHP-2002 will address the risk faced by this particularly vulnerable section of society.

2.25 Providing Medical Facilities to Users from Overseas

2.25.1 The secondary and tertiary facilities available in the country are of good quality and cost-effective compared to international medical facilities. This is true not only of facilities in the allopathic disciplines, but also of those belonging to the alternative systems of medicine, particularly Ayurveda. The Policy will assess the possibilities of encouraging the development of paid treatment-packages for patients from overseas.

2.26 The Impact of Globalisation on the Health Sector

2.26.1 There are some apprehensions about the possible adverse impact of economic globalisation on the health sector. Pharmaceutical drugs and other health services have always been available in the country at extremely inexpensive prices. India has established a reputation around the globe for the innovative development of original process patents for the manufacture of a wide-range of drugs and vaccines within the ambit of the existing patent laws. With the adoption of Trade Related Intellectual Property Rights (TRIPs), and the subsequent alignment of domestic patent laws consistent with the commitments under TRIPs, there will be a significant shift in the scope of the parameters regulating the manufacture of new drugs/vaccines. Global experience has shown that the introduction of a TRIPs-consistent patent regime for drugs in a developing country results in an across-the-board increase in the cost of drugs and medical services. NHP-2002 will address itself to the future imperatives of health security in the country, in the post-TRIPs era.

2.27 Inter-Sectoral Contribution to Health

2.27.1 It is well recognized that the overall well-being of the citizenry depends on the synergistic functioning of the various sectors in the socio-economy. The health status of the citizenry would, *inter alia*, be dependent on adequate nutrition, safe drinking water, basic sanitation, a clean environment and primary education, especially for the girl child. The policies and the mode of functioning in these independent areas would necessarily overlap each other to contribute to the health status of the community. From the policy perspective, it is therefore imperative that the independent policies of each of these inter-connected sectors, be in tandem, and that the interface between the policies of the two connected sectors, be smooth.

2.27.2 Sectoral policy documents are meant to serve as a guide to action for institutions and individual participants operating in that sector. Consistent with this role, NHP-2002 limits itself to making recommendations for the participants operating within the health sector. The policy aspects relating to inter-connected sectors, which, while crucial, fall outside the domain of the health sector, will not be covered by specific recommendations in this Policy document. Needless to say, the future attainment of the various goals set out in this policy assumes a reasonable complementary performance in these inter-connected sectors.

2.28 Population Growth and Health Standards

2.28.1 Efforts made over the years for improving health standards have been partially neutralized by the rapid growth of the population. It is well recognized that population stabilization measures and general health initiatives, when effectively synchronized, synergistically maximize the socio-economic well-being of the people. Government has separately announced the 'National Population Policy-2000'. The principal common features covered under the National Population Policy-2000 and NHP-

2002, relate to the prevention and control of communicable diseases; giving priority to the containment of HIV/AIDS infection; the universal immunization of children against all major preventable diseases; addressing the unmet needs for basic and reproductive health services, and supplementation of infrastructure. The synchronized implementation of these two Policies—National Population Policy-2000 and National Health Policy-2002—will be the very cornerstone of any national structural plan to improve the health standards in the country.

2.29 Alternative Systems of Medicine

2.29.1 Under the overarching umbrella of the national health framework, the alternative systems of medicine—Ayurveda, Unani, Siddha and Homoeopathy—have a substantial role. Because of inherent advantages, such as diversity, modest cost, low level of technological input and the growing popularity of natural plant-based products, these systems are attractive, particularly in the underserved, remote and tribal areas. The alternative systems will draw upon the substantial untapped potential of India as one of the eight important global centers for plant diversity in medicinal and aromatic plants. The Policy focuses on building up credibility for the alternative systems, by encouraging evidence-based research to determine their efficacy, safety and dosage, and also encourages certification and quality-marking of products to enable a wider popular acceptance of these systems of medicine. The Policy also envisages the consolidation of documentary knowledge contained in these systems to protect it against attack from foreign commercial entities by way of malafide action under patent laws in other countries. The main components of NHP-2002 apply equally to the alternative systems of medicines. However, the Policy features specific to the alternative systems of medicine will be presented as a separate document.

3. Objectives

3.1 The main objective of this policy is to achieve an acceptable standard of good health amongst the general population of the country. The approach would be to increase access to the decentralized public health system by establishing new infrastructure in deficient areas, and by upgrading the infrastructure in the existing institutions. Overriding importance would be given to ensuring a more equitable access to health services across the social and geographical expanse of the country. Emphasis will be given to increasing the aggregate public health investment through a substantially increased contribution by the Central Government. It is expected that this initiative will strengthen the capacity of the public health administration at the State level to render effective service delivery. The contribution of the private sector in providing health services would be much enhanced, particularly for the population

Box IV

Goals to be Achieved by 2000-2015

Goal	Year
Eradicate Polio and Yaws	2005
Eliminate Leprosy	2005
Eliminate Kala Azar	2010
Eliminate Lymphatic Filariasis	2015
Achieve Zero level growth of HIV/AIDS	2007
Reduce Mortality by 50% on account of TB, Malaria and Other Vector and Water Borne diseases	2010
Reduce Prevalence of Blindness to 0.5%	2010
Reduce IMR to 30/1000 and MMR to 100/Lakh	2010
Increase utilization of public health facilities from current level of <20 to >75%	2010
Establish an integrated system of surveillance, National Health Accounts and Health Statistics	2005
Increase health expenditure by Government as a % of GDP from the existing 0.9% to 2.0%	2010
Increase share of Central grants to Constitute at least 25% of total health spending	2010
Increase State Sector Health spending from 5.5% to 7% of the budget	2005
Further increase to 8%	2010

group which can afford to pay for services. Primacy will be given to preventive and first-line curative initiatives at the primary health level through increased sectoral share of allocation. Emphasis will be laid on rational use of drugs within the allopathic system. Increased access to tried and tested systems of traditional medicine will be ensured. Within these broad objectives, NHP-2002 will endeavour to achieve the time-bound goals mentioned in Box-IV.

4. NHP-2002—Policy Prescriptions

4.1 Financial Resources

4.1.1 The paucity of public health investment is a stark reality. Given the extremely difficult fiscal position of the State Governments, the Central Government will have to play a key role in augmenting public health investments.

Taking into account the gap in health care facilities, it is planned, under the policy to increase health sector expenditure to 6 percent of GDP, with 2 percent of GDP being contributed as public health investment, by the year 2010. The State Governments would also need to increase the commitment to the health sector. In the first phase, by 2005, they would be expected to increase the commitment of their resources to 7 percent of the Budget; and, in the second phase, by 2010, to increase it to 8 percent of the Budget. With the stepping up of the public health investment, the Central Government's contribution would rise to 25 percent from the existing 15 percent by 2010. The provisioning of higher public health investments will also be contingent upon the increase in the absorptive capacity of the public health administration so as to utilize the funds gainfully.

4.2 Equity

4.2.1 To meet the objective of reducing various types of inequities and imbalances—inter-regional; across the rural-urban divide; and between economic classes—the most cost-effective method would be to increase the sectoral outlay in the primary health sector. Such outlets afford access to a vast number of individuals, and also facilitate preventive and early stage curative initiative, which are cost effective. In recognition of this public health principle, NHP-2002 sets out an increased allocation of 55 percent of the total public health investment for the primary health sector; the secondary and tertiary health sectors being targeted for 35 percent and 10 percent respectively. The Policy projects that the increased aggregate outlays for the primary health sector will be utilized for strengthening existing facilities and opening additional public health service outlets, consistent with the norms for such facilities.

4.3 Delivery of National Public Health Programmes

4.3.1.1 This policy envisages a key role for the Central Government in designing national programmes with the active participation of the State Governments. Also, the Policy ensures the provisioning of financial resources, in addition to technical support, monitoring and evaluation at the national level by the Centre. However, to optimize the utilization of the public health infrastructure at the primary level, NHP-2002 envisages the gradual convergence of all health programmes under a single field administration. Vertical programmes for control of major diseases like TB, Malaria, HIV/AIDS, as also the RCH and Universal Immunization Programmes, would need to be continued till moderate levels of prevalence are reached. The integration of the programmes will bring about a desirable optimisation of outcomes through a convergence of all public health inputs. The Policy also envisages that programme implementation be effected through autonomous bodies at State and district levels. The interventions of State Health Departments may be limited to the overall monitoring of the achievement of programme targets and other technical aspects. The relative distancing of the programme implementation from the State Health Departments will give the project team greater operational flexibility. Also, the presence of State Government officials, social activists, private health professionals and MLAs/MPs on the management boards of the autonomous bodies will facilitate well-informed decision-making.

4.3.1.2 The Policy also highlights the need for developing the capacity within the State Public Health administration for scientific designing of public health projects, suited to the local situation.

4.3.2 The Policy envisages that apart from the exclusive staff in a vertical structure for the disease control programmes, all rural health staff should be available for the entire gamut of public health activities at the decentralized level, irrespective of whether these activities relate to national programmes or other public health initiatives. It would be for the Head of the District Health administration to allocate the time of the rural health staff between the various programmes, depending on the local need. NHP-2002 recognizes that to implement such a change, not only would the public health administrators be required to change their mindset, but the rural health staff would need to be trained and reoriented.

4.4 The State of Public Health Infrastructure

4.4.1.1 As has been highlighted in the earlier part of the Policy, the decentralized Public health service outlets have become practically dysfunctional over large parts of the country. On account of resource constraints, the supply of drugs by the State Governments is grossly inadequate. The patients at the decentralized level have little use for diagnostic services, which in any case would still require them to purchase therapeutic drugs privately. In a situation in which the patient is not getting any therapeutic drugs, there is little incentive for the potential beneficiaries to seek the advice of the medical professionals in the public health system. This results in there being no demand for medical services, so medical professionals and paramedics often absent themselves from their place of duty. It is also observed that the functioning of the public health service outlets in some States like the four Southern States—Kerala, Andhra Pradesh, Tamil Nadu and Karnataka—is relatively better, because some quantum of drugs is distributed through the primary health system network, and the patients have a stake in approaching the Public Health facilities. In this backdrop, the Policy envisages kick-starting the revival of the Primary Health System by providing some essential drugs under Central Government funding through the decentralized health system. It is expected that the provisioning of essential drugs at the public health service centres will create a demand for other professional services from the local population, which, in turn, will boost the general revival of activities in these service centres. In sum, this initiative under NHP-2002 is launched in the belief that the creation of a beneficiary interest in the public health system, will ensure a more effective supervision of the public health personnel through community monitoring, than has been achieved through the regular administrative line of control.

4.4.1.2 This Policy recognizes the need for more frequent in-service training of public health medical personnel, at the level of medical

Box V

Public Health Spending in Select Countries

Indicator	*% Population with income of <$1 day*	*Infant Mortality Rate/1000*	*% Health Expenditure to GDP*	*% Public Expenditure on Health to Total Health Expenditure*
India	44.2	70	5.2	17.3
China	18.5	31	2.7	24.9
Sri Lanka	6.6	16	3	45.4
UK	—	6	5.8	96.9
USA	—	7	13.7	44.1

officers as well as paramedics. Such training would help to update the personnel on recent advancements in science, and would also equip them for their new assignments, when they are moved from one discipline of public health administration to another.

4.4.1.3 Global experience has shown that the quality of public health services, as reflected in the attainment of improved public health indices, is closely linked to the quantum and quality of investment through public funding in the primary health sector. Box-V gives statistics which clearly show that standards of health are more a function of the accurate targeting of expenditure on the decentralised primary sector (as observed in China and Sri Lanka), than a function of the aggregate health expenditure.

Therefore the Policy, while committing additional aggregate financial resources, places great reliance on the strengthening of the primary health structure for the attaining of improved public health outcomes on an equitable basis. Further, it also recognizes the practical need for levying reasonable user-charges for certain secondary and tertiary public health care services, for those who can afford to pay.

4.5 Extending Public Health Services

4.5.1.1 This policy envisages that, in the context of the availability and spread of allopathic graduates in their jurisdiction, State Governments would consider the need for expanding the pool of medical practitioners to include a cadre of licentiates of medical practice, as also practitioners of Indian Systems of Medicine and Homoeopathy. Simple services/procedures can be provided by such practitioners even outside their disciplines, as part of the basic primary health services in under-served areas. Also, NHP-2002 envisages that the scope of the use of paramedical manpower of allopathic disciplines, in a prescribed functional area adjunct to their current functions, would also be examined for meeting simple public health requirements. This would be on the lines of the services rendered by nurse practitioners in several developed countries. These extended areas of functioning of different categories of medical manpower can be permitted, after adequate training, and subject to the monitoring of their performance through professional councils.

4.5.1.2 NHP-2002 also recognizes the need for States to simplify the recruitment procedures and rules for contract employment in order to provide trained medical manpower in under-served arm. State Governments could also rigorously enforce a mandatory two-year rural posting before the awarding of the graduate degree. This would not only make trained medical manpower available in the underserved areas, but would offer valuable clinical experience to the graduating doctors.

4.6 Role of Local Self-Government Institutions

4.6.1 NHP-2002 lays great emphasis upon the implementation of public health programmes through local self-government institutions. The structure of the national disease control programmes will have specific components for implementation through such entities. The Policy urges all State Governments to consider decentralizing the implementation of the programmes to such Institutions by 2005. In order to achieve this, financial incentives, over and above the resources normatively allocated for disease control programmes, will be provided by the Central Government.

4.7 Norms for Health Care Personnel

4.7.1 Minimal statutory norms for the deployment of doctors and nurses in medical institutions need to be introduced urgently under the provisions of the Indian Medical Council Act and Indian Nursing Council Act, respectively. These norms can be progressively reviewed and made more stringent as the medical institutions improve their capacity for meeting better normative standards.

4.8 Education of Health Care Professionals

4.8.1.1 In order to ameliorate the problems being faced on account of the uneven spread of medical and dental colleges in various parts of the country, this policy envisages the setting up of a Medical Grants Commission for funding new Government Medical and Dental Colleges in different parts of the country. Also, it is envisaged that the Medical Grants Commission will fund the upgradation of the infrastructure of the existing Government Medical and Dental Colleges of the country, so as to ensure an improved standard of medical education

4.8.1.2 To enable fresh graduates to contribute effectively to the providing of primary health services as the physician of first contact, this policy identifies a significant need to modify the existing curriculum. A need-based, skill-oriented syllabus, with a more significant component of practical training, would make fresh doctors useful immediately after graduation. The Policy also recommends a period skill-updating of working health professionals through a system of continuing medical education.

4.8.2 The Policy emphasises the need to expose medical students, through the under-graduate syllabus, to the emerging concerns for geriatric disorders, as also to the cutting edge disciplines of contemporary medical research. The policy also envisages that the creation of additional seats for post-graduate courses should reflect the need for more manpower in the deficient specialities.

4.9 Need for Specialists in 'Public Health' and 'Family Medicine'

4.9.1 In order to alleviate the acute shortage of medical personnel with specialization in the disciplines of 'public health' and 'family medicine', the Policy envisages the progressive implementation of mandatory norms to raise the proportion of post-graduate seats in these discipline in medical training institutions, to reach a stage wherein 1/4th of the seats are earmarked for these disciplines. It is envisaged that in the sanctioning of post-graduate seats in future, it shall be insisted upon that a certain reasonable number of seats be allocated to 'public health' and 'family medicine'. Since the 'public health' discipline has an interface with many other developmental sectors, specialization in public health may be encouraged not only for medical doctors, but also for non-medical graduates from the allied fields of public health engineering, microbiology and other natural sciences.

4.10 Nursing Personnel

4.10.1.1 In the interest of patient care, the policy emphasizes the need for an improvement in the ratio of nurses *vis-a-vis* doctors/beds. In order to discharge their responsibility as model providers of health services, the public health delivery centres need to make a beginning by increasing the number of nursing personnel. The Policy anticipates that with the increasing aspiration for improved health care amongst the citizens, private health facilities will also improve their ratio of nursing personnel *vis-a-vis* doctors/beds.

4.10.1.2 The Policy lays emphasis on improving the skill-level of nurses, and on increasing the ratio of degree-holding nurses *vis-a-vis* diploma-holding nurses. NHP-2002 recognizes a need for the Central Government to subsidize the setting up, and the running of, training facilities for nurses on a decentralized basis. Also, the Policy recognizes the need for establishing training courses for super-speciality nurses required for tertiary care institutions.

4.11 Use of Generic Drugs and Vaccines

4.11.1.1 This Policy emphasizes the need for basing treatment regimens, in both the public and private domain, on a limited number of essential drugs of a generic nature. This is a prerequisite for cost-effective public health care. In the public health system, this would be enforced by prohibiting the use of proprietary drugs, except in special circumstances. The list of essential drugs would no doubt have to be reviewed periodically. To encourage the use of only essential drugs in the private sector, the imposition of fiscal disincentives would be resorted to. The production and sale of irrational combinations of drugs would be prohibited through the drug standards statute.

4.11.1.2 The National Programme for Universal Immunization against Preventable Diseases requires to be assured of an uninterrupted supply of vaccines at an affordable price. To minimize the danger arising from the volatility of the global market, and thereby to ensure long-term national health security, NHP-2002 envisages that not less than 50% of the requirement of vaccines/sera be sourced from public sector institutions.

4.12 Urban Health

4.12.1.1 NHP-2002 envisages the setting up of an organised urban primary health care structure. Since the physical features of urban settings are different from those in rural areas, the policy envisages the adoption of appropriate population norms for the urban public health infrastructure. The structure conceived under NHP-2002 is a two-tiered one: the primary centre is seen as the first-tier, covering a population of one lakh, with a dispensary providing an OPD facility and essential drugs, to enable access to all the national health programmes; and a second-tier of the urban health organisation at the level of the Government general hospital, where reference is made from the primary centre. The Policy envisages that the funding for the urban primary health system will be jointly borne by the local self-government institutions and State and Central Governments.

4.12.1.2 The Policy also envisages the establishment of fully-equipped 'hub-spoke' trauma care networks in large urban agglomerations to reduce accident mortality.

4.13 Mental Health

4.13.1.1 NHP-2002 envisages a network of decentralised mental health services for ameliorating the more common categories of disorders. The programme outline for such a disease would involve the diagnosis of common disorders, and the prescription of common therapeutic drugs, by general duty medical staff.

4.13.1.2 In regard to mental health institutions for in-door treatment of patients, the Policy envisages the upgrading of the physical infrastructure of such institutions at Central Government expense so as to secure the human rights of this vulnerable segment of society.

4.14 Information, Education and Communication

4.14.1 NHP-2002 envisages an IEG policy, which maximizes the dissemination of information to those population groups which cannot be effectively approached by using only the mass media. The focus would therefore be on the inter-personal communication of information and on folk and other traditional media to bring about behavioural change. The IEC programme would set specific targets for the association of PRIs/ NGOs/Trusts in such activities. In several public health programmes, where behavioural change is an essential component, the success of the initiatives is crucially dependent on dispelling myths and misconceptions pertaining to religious and ethical issues. The community leaders, particularly religious leaders, are effective in imparting knowledge which facilitates such behavioural change. The programme will also have the component of an annual evaluation of the performance of the non-Governmental agencies to monitor the impact of the programmes on the targeted groups. The Central/State Government initiative will also focus on the development of modules for information dissemination in such population groups, who do not normally benefit from the more common media forms.

4.14.2 NHP-2002 envisages giving priority to school health programmes which aim at preventive-health education, providing regular health check-ups, and promotion of health-seeking behaviour among children. The school health programmes can gainfully adopt specially designed modules in order to disseminate information relating to 'health' and 'family life'. This is expected to be the most cost-effective intervention as it improves the level of awareness, not only of the extended family, but the future generation as well.

4.15 Health Research

4.15.1 This Policy envisages an increase in Government-funded health research to a level of 1 percent of the total health spending by 2005; and thereafter, up to 2 percent by 2010. Domestic medical research would be focused on new therapeutic drugs and vaccines for tropical diseases, such as TB and Malaria, as also on the sub-types of HIV/AIDS prevalent in the country. Research programmes taken up by the Government in these priority areas would be conducted in a mission mode. Emphasis would also be laid on time-bound applied research for developing operational applications. This would ensure the cost-effective dissemination of existing/future therapeutic drugs/vaccines in the general population. Private entrepreneurship will be encouraged in the field of medical research for new molecules/vaccines, *inter alia*, through fiscal incentives.

4.16 Role of the Private Sector

4.16.1.1 In principle, this Policy welcomes the participation of the private sector in all areas of health activities—primary, secondary or tertiary. However, looking to past experience of the private sector, it can reasonably be expected that its contribution would be substantial in the urban primary sector and the tertiary sector, and moderate in the secondary sector. This Policy envisages the enactment of suitable legislation for regulating minimum infrastructure and quality standards in clinical establishments/medical institutions by 2003. Also, statutory guidelines for the conduct of clinical practice and delivery of medical services are targeted to be developed over the same period. With the acquiring of experience in the setting and enforcing of minimum quality standards, the Policy envisages graduation to a scheme of quality accreditation of clinical establishments/medical institutions, for the information of the citizenry. The regulatory/accreditation mechanisms will no doubt also cover public health institutions. The Policy also encourages the setting up of private insurance instruments for increasing the scope of the coverage of the secondary and tertiary sector under private health insurance packages.

4.16.1.2 In the context of the very large number of poor in the country, it would be difficult to conceive of an exclusive Government mechanism to provide health services to this category. It has sometimes been felt that a social health insurance scheme, funded by the Government, and with service delivery through the private sector, would be the appropriate solution. The administrative and financial implications of such an initiative are still unknown. As a first step, this policy envisages the introduction of a pilot scheme in a limited number of representative districts, to determine the administrative features of such an arrangement, as also the requirement of resources for it. The results obtained from these pilot projects would provide material on which future public health policy can be based.

4.16.2 NHP-2002 envisages the co-option of the non-governmental practitioners in the national disease control programmes so as to ensure that standard treatment protocols are followed in their day-to-day practice.

4.16.3 This Policy recognizes the immense potential of information technology applications in the area of tele-medicine in the tertiary health care sector. The use of this technical aid will greatly enhance the capacity for the professionals to pool their clinical experience.

4.17 The Role of Civil Society

4.17.1 NHP-2002 recognizes the significant contribution made by NGOs and other institutions of the civil society in making available health services to the community. In order to utilize their high motivational skills on an increasing scale, this Policy envisages that the disease control programmes should earmark not less than 10% of the budget in respect of identified programme components, to be exclusively implemented through these institutions. The policy also emphasizes the need to simplify procedures for government-civil society interfacing in order to enhance the involvement of civil society in public health programmes. In principle, the state would encourage the handing over of public health service, outlets at any level for management by NGOs and other institutions of civil society, on an 'as-is-where-is' basis, along with the normative funds earmarked for such institutions.

4.18 National Disease Surveillance Network

4.18.1 This Policy envisages the full operationalization of an integrated disease control network from the lowest rung of public health administration to the Central Government, by 2005. The programme for setting up this network will include components relating to the installation of data-base handling hardware; IT inter-connectivity between different tiers of the network; and in-house training for data collection and interpretation for undertaking timely and effective response. This public health surveillance network will also encompass information from private health care institutions and practitioners. It is expected that real-time information from outside the government system will greatly strengthen the capacity of the public health system to counter focal outbreaks of seasonal diseases.

4.19 Health Statistics

4.19.1.1 The Policy envisages the completion of baseline estimates for the incidence of the common diseases—TB, Malaria, Blindness—by 2005. The Policy proposes that statistical methods be put in place to enable the periodic updating of these baseline estimates through representative sampling, under an appropriate statistical methodology. The policy also recognizes the need to establish, in a longer time-frame, baseline estimates for non-communicable diseases, like CVD, Cancer, Diabetes; and accidental injuries, and communicable diseases, like Hepatitis and JE. NHP-2002 envisages that, with access to such reliable data on the incidence of various diseases, the public health system would move closer to the objective of evidence-based policy-making.

4.19.1.2 Planning for the health sector requires a robust information system, *inter-alia,* covering data on service facilities available in the private sector. NHP-2002 emphasises the need for the early completion of an accurate data-base of this kind.

4.19.2 In an attempt at consolidating the data base and graduating from a mere estimation of the annual health expenditure, NHP-2002 emphasises the need to establish national health accounts, conforming to the 'source-to-users' matrix structure. Also, the policy envisages the estimation of health costs on a continuing basis. Improved and comprehensive information through national health accounts and accounting systems would pave the way for decision-makers to focus on relative priorities, keeping in view the limited financial resources in the health sector.

4.20 Women's Health

4.20.1 NHP-2002 envisages the identification of specific programmes targeted at women's health. The Policy notes that women, alongwith other under-privileged groups, are significantly handicapped due to a disproportionately low access to health care. The various Policy recommendations of NHP-2002, in regard to the expansion of primary health sector infrastructure, will facilitate the increased access of women to basic health care. The Policy commits the highest priority of the Central Government to the funding of the identified programmes relating to women's health. Also, the policy recognizes the need to review the staffing norms of the public health administration to meet the specific requirements of women in a more comprehensive manner.

4.21 Medical Ethics

4.21.1.1 NHP-2002 envisages that, in order to ensure that the common patient is not subjected to irrational or profit-driven medical regimens, a contemporary code of ethics be notified and rigorously implemented by the Medical Council of India.

4.21.1.2 By and large, medical research within the country in the frontier disciplines, such as gene-manipulation and stem cell research, is limited. However, the policy recognises that a vigilant watch will have to be kept so that the existing guidelines and statutory provisions are constantly reviewed and updated.

4.22 Enforcement of Quality Standards for Food

4.22.1 NHP-2002 envisages that the food and drug administration will be progressively strengthened, in terms of both laboratory facilities and technical expertise. Also, the policy envisages that the standards of food items will be progressively tightened up at a pace which will permit domestic food handling/manufacturing facilities to undertake the necessary upgradation of technology so that they are not shut out of this production sector. The Policy envisages that ultimately food standards will be close, if not equivalent, to Codex specifications; and that drug standards will be at par with the most rigorous ones adopted elsewhere.

4.23 Regulation of Standards in Paramedical Disciplines

4.23.1 NHP-2002 recognises the need for the establishment of statutory professional councils for paramedical disciplines to register practitioners, maintain standards of training, and monitor performance.

4.24 Environmental and Occupational Health

4.24.1 This Policy envisages that the independently-stated policies and programmes of the environment-related sectors be smoothly interfaced with the policies and the programmes of the health sector, in order to reduce the health risk to the citizens and the consequential disease burden.

4.24.2 NHP-2002 envisages the periodic screening of the health conditions of the workers, particularly for high-risk health disorders associated with their occupation.

4.25 Providing Medical Facilities to Users from Overseas

4.25.1 To capitalize on the comparative cost advantage enjoyed by domestic health facilities in the secondary and tertiary sectors, NHP-2002 strongly encourages the providing of such health services on a payment basis to service seekers from overseas. The providers of such services to patients from overseas will be encouraged by extending to their earnings in foreign exchange, all fiscal incentives, including the status of "deemed exports", which are available to other exporters of goods and services.

4.26 Impact of Globalisation on the Health Sector

4.26.1 The Policy takes into account the serious apprehension, expressed by several health experts, of the possible threat to health security in the post-TRIPs era, as a result of a sharp increase in the prices of drugs and vaccines. To protect the citizens of the country from such a threat, this policy envisages a national patent regime for the future, which, while being consistent with TRIPs, avails of all opportunities to secure for the country, under its patent laws, affordable access to the latest medical and other therapeutic discoveries. The policy also sets out that the Government will bring to bear its full influence in all international fora—UN, WHO, WTO, etc.—to secure commitments on the part of the Nations of the Globe, to lighten the restrictive features of TRIPs in its application to the health care sector.

5. Summation

5.1 The crafting of a National Health Policy is a rare occasion in public affairs when it would be legitimate, indeed valuable, to allow our dreams to mingle with our understanding of ground realities. Based purely on the clinical facts defining the current status of the health sector, we would have arrived at a certain policy formulation; but, buoyed by our dreams, we have ventured slightly beyond that in the shape of NHP-2002, which, in fact, defines a vision for the future.

5.2 The health needs of the country are enormous and the financial resources and managerial capacity available to meet them, even on the most optimistic projections, fall somewhat short. In this situation, NHP-2002 has had to make hard choices between various priorities and operational options. NHP-2002 does not claim to be a road-map for meeting all the health needs of the populace of the country. Further, it has to be recognized that such health needs are also dynamic, as threats in the area of public health keep changing over time. The Policy, while being holistic, undertakes the necessary risk of recommending differing emphasis on different policy components. Broadly speaking, NHP-2002 focuses on the need for enhanced funding and an organizational restructuring of the national public health initiatives in order to facilitate more equitable access to the health facilities. Also, the Policy is focused on those diseases which are principally contributing to the disease burden—TB, Malaria and Blindness from the category of historical diseases; and HIV/AIDS from the category of 'newly emerging diseases'. This is not to say that other items contributing to the disease burden of the country will be ignored; but only that the resources, as also the principal focus of the public health administration, will recognize certain relative priorities. It is unnecessary to labour the point that under the umbrella of the macro-policy prescriptions in this document, governments and private sector programme planners will have to design separate schemes, tailor-made to the health needs of women, children, geriatrics, tribals and other socio-economically under-served sections. An adequately robust disaster management plan has to be in place to effectively cope with situations arising from natural and man-made calamities.

5.3 One nagging imperative, which has influenced every aspect of this Policy, is the need to ensure that 'equity' in the health sector stands as an independent goal. In any future evaluation of its success or failure, NHP-2002 would wish to be measured against this equity norm, rather than any other aggregated financial norm for the health sector. Consistent with the primacy given to 'equity', a marked emphasis has been provided in the policy for expanding and improving the primary health facilities, including the new concept of the provisioning of essential drugs through Central funding. The Policy also commits the Central Government to an increased under-writing of the resources for meeting the minimum health needs of the people. Thus, the Policy attempts to provide guidance for prioritizing expenditure, thereby facilitating rational resource allocation.

5.4 This Policy broadly envisages a greater contribution from the Central Budget for the delivery of Public Health services at the State level. Adequate appropriations, steadily rising over the years, would need to be ensured. The possibility of ensuring this by imposing an earmarked health cess has been carefully examined. While it is recognized that the annual budget must accommodate the increasing resource needs of the social sectors, particularly in the health sector, this Policy does not specifically recommend an earmarked health cess, as that would have a tendency of reducing the space available to Parliament in making appropriations looking to the circumstances prevailing from time to time.

5.5 The Policy highlights the expected roles of different participating groups in the health sector. Further, it recognizes the fact that, despite all that may be guaranteed by the Central Government for assisting public health programmes, public health services would actually need to be delivered by the State administration, NGOs and other institutions of civil society. The attainment of improved health levels would be significantly dependent on population stabilisation, as also on complementary efforts from other areas of the social sectors—like improved drinking water supply, basic sanitation, minimum nutrition, etc.—to ensure that the exposure of the populace to health risks is minimized.

5.6 Any expectation of a significant improvement in the quality of health services, and the consequential improved health status of the citizenry, would depend not only on increased financial and material inputs, but also on a more empathetic and committed attitude in the service providers, whether in the private or public sectors. In some measure, this optimistic policy document is based on the understanding that the citizenry is increasingly demanding more by way of quality in health services, and the health delivery system, particularly in the public sector, is being pressed to respond. In this backdrop, it needs to be recognized that any policy in the social sector is critically dependent on the service providers treating their responsibility not as a commercial activity, but as a service, albeit a paid one. In the area of public health, an improved standard of governance is a prerequisite for the success of any health policy.

Bibliography

Anita, N.H. and Bhatia, Kavita, People's Health in People's Hand—A Model for Panchayati Raj, FRCH, Mumbai, 1993.

Basch, P.E., Vaccines and World Health, New York, Oxford University Press, 1994.

Bhatnagar, S. and Goel, S.L., Development Planning and Administration, New Delhi, Deep & Deep Publications (P) Ltd., 1992.

Bhattacharjee, P.I. and G.N. Shastri, Population in India, A Study of Interstate Variation, New Delhi, Vikas, 1976.

Bosh, Ashish, From Population to People, Delhi, B.R. Publication, 1988.

Brown, Esther, Newer Dimensions of Patient Care, Russell Sage Foundation, New York, 1961.

Cartwright, A., Patients and their Doctors, A Study of General Practice, Routledge Kegan Paul, London, 1961.

Chanawongse Krasal, Rural Development Management, Research and Development Institute, Khon Kaen University, Thailand.

Chandra, R.C., A Geography of Population, Concepts, Determinents and Patterns, New Delhi, Kalyani, 1987.

Chauhan, Devraj, Anaita, N.H. & Ramdan, Sangita, Health Care in India: A Profile, FRCH, Mumbai, 1996.

Das, K., Civil Service Reforms and Structural Adjustment, Oxford, Delhi 1998.

Duggal, R., Nandaraj, S. & Shetty, Sahana, State Sector Health Expenditure—A Database: All India, FRCH, Mumbai, 1992.

P. Jurfelds, O. & Lindbergs, Pills against Poverty—A Study of Introduction of Western Medicine in a Tamil Village, Curzon Press, London, 1975.

FRCH, Panchayati Raj: Information Resource Book, Mumbai, 1996.

Ghai, Sandhya, Bursing Services Administration: A Case Study of Nehru Hospital, PGI, Chandigarh (Doctoral Thesis, Panjab University, 1998).

Ghosh, Brindra Nath, A Treatise on Hygiene and Public Health, Scientific Publishing Company, 1970, Calcutta.

Gill, Sonya, Health Status of the Indian People, FRCH, Mumbai, 1987.

Goel, S.L., Health Care Administration: Policy-making and Planning, Sterling, Delhi, 1981.

———, Health Care Administration: Levels and Aspects, Sterling, Delhi, 1981.

Goel, S.L., Health Care Administration: Ecology, Principles and Modern Trends, Sterling, Delhi, 1981.
———, Family Planning Programme and Beyond, New Delhi, Deep & Deep Publications Pvt. Ltd., 1990.
———, International Administration: WHO, South-East Asia Regional Office, Sterling, New Delhi, 1977.
———, Modern Management Techniques, Deep & Deep Publications Pvt. Ltd., Delhi, 1987.
———, Public Health Administration, Sterling, New Delhi, 1984.
———, Public Personnel Administration, Sterling, New Delhi, 1984.
———, Hospital Administration and Management, Deep & Deep Publications Pvt. Ltd., New Delhi, 1993.
———, Distance Education in 21st Century, Deep & Deep Publications Pvt. Ltd., New Delhi, 2000.
Hanlon, John, Principles of Public Health Administration, C.V. Mobsy, Sthouis, 1969.
ICSSR & ICMR, Health for All—An Alternative Strategy—Report of a Study Group set-up Jointly by ICSSR & ICMR, Pune, Indian Institute of Education, 1981.
Government of India, Annual Reports of the Ministry of Health and Family Welfare, Delhi.
——— Committee on Multi-purpose Workers under Health and Family Welfare Programme (Kartar Singh Report), Delhi, Ministry of Health and Family Welfare, Delhi, 1973.
———, Health in Independent India (G. Borkar Report), Delhi, 1961.
———, Health Survey and Development Committee (Bhore Committee), Delhi, 1946.
———, Lok Sabha Secretariat, Estimates Committees and Public Accounts Committees Reports.
———, Planning Commission, Five Year Plans, New Delhi.
———, Report of Health Survey and Planning Committee (Mudaliar Committee), Ministry of Health, August 1959-October, 1961.
———, Ministry of Information and Broadcasting, India, 1999, A Refresher Manual, New Delhi, 1999.
———, Initiatives and Best Practices of Government of India for Effective and Responsive Administration, New Delhi, Ministry of Personnel, Public Grievances and Pensions, 1997.
———, Deptt. of Family Welfare, Reproductive and Child Health (World Bank Component), Vols. I and II, New Delhi, 1997.
———, Report of the Working Group on Health for All by 2000 AD, New Delhi, Ministry of Health and Welfare, 1981.
Gunaratne Herat, V.T., Challenges and Response Health in South-East Asia Region, New Delhi, McGraw Hill, 1977.
Hardon, A., *et. al.*, Monitoring Family Planning and Reproductive Rights: A Manual for Empowerment, London, Zed Books, 1997.
Indian Society of Health Administrators, Bangalore.

Annual Conference Reports

Health for all by 2000 (AD 1980).
The Role of Hospitals in Health Care (1981).
Health Manpower Requirements for 2000 (1982).
Role of the Health Administrator in India (1983).
Financing of Health Services in India (1984).
On Growing Needs of Urban Health Management (1985).
Cost Reduction in Hospitals and Health Care (1986).
Health of the High Risk Groups: Mothers, Children and Elderly (1985).
Health of Women and Children for Development (1988).
Health Care for the Villages and Urban Slums (1989-90).
Health of the Youth and the Female Child.
Role of Voluntary Organizations in Health Care in India (1992).

Books

Stress and Health of Executives and Professionals.
Hospital and Health Administration.
Modern Technology for Hospitals and Health Care.
Management for Nursing Administrators.
Community Participation in Health and Family Welfare—Indian Experiences.
Health of the Metropolis, Bangalore, A Guide to Health.
Planning and Development of Urban Cities in India.
Leadership and Human Resources Development for Health Care.
Managerial Effectiveness for Organizational Excellence.
Computer Applications to Hospitals, Health Care and Medical Education.
Health and Development of the Tribal People in India—A Guide for Professionals and Administrators.
Retirement Planning, Adjustment and Health.
Janovsky, K., Health Policy and Systems Development: An Agenda for Research, WHO/SHS/NHP/96.1, Geneva, 1996.
Jesani, Amar & Ganguly, Shilpi, Some Issues in Community Participation in Health Services, FRCH, Mumbai, 1993.
Khandewale, Shreekant V., Health Administration and the Weaker Sections in an Indian Metropolis, Devika Publications, Delhi, 1996.
Klinoboul Krienkrai, Health and Family Welfare Administration in Thailand—A Case Study of Lampang Province (Doctoral Thesis).
Kumar, R., Child Development in India, Ashish, New Delhi, 1988.
——— Environment Pollution and Health Hazards in India, Ashish, New Delhi (Year not mentioned).
Youth Health, Problem, Planning and Development, Deep and Deep Publications Pvt. Ltd., New Delhi, 1986.
Lane, S.D., From Population Control to Reproductive Health: An Emerging Policy Agenda, Social Science and Medicine, 1994.
Lush, L., Integrating Services, from Rhetroic to Action, Development Research Insights, 1997.

Mattoo, P.K., Project Formulation in Developing Countries, Macmillan, Delhi, 1978.

Meher C. Nanavaty and P.D. Kulkarni, NGO's in the Changing Scenario, New Delhi, Uppal, 1998.

Miller George E. and Tamas Fulop, Educational Strategies for the Health Professionals, Geneva, WHO, 1974.

Mishra, R.P., Medical Geography of India, NBT, Delhi, 1970.

Murray, C.J.L., Lopez, A.D., The Global Burden of Diseases, WHO, Geneva, Switzerland, 1996.

Myrdal Gunnar, Asian Drama, An Enquiry into the Poverty of Nations, Vol. III, Penguis, London, 1968.

Naik, J.P., An Alternative System of Health Care Service in India: Some Proposals, Allied, Bombay, 1988.

National Institute of Health and Family Welfare, New Delhi

Management Training Modules for District Health Offices.

Management Training Modules for Health Offices.

Management Training Modules for Health Assistants (Male and Female).

Management Training Modules for Health Workers (Male and Female).

Management Training Modules for TBA.

Management Training Modules for Health Guide.

Park, J.E. and K. Park (1990), Textbook on Preventive and Social Medicine, Banarasidas Bhanot Publishers, Jabalpur.

Pai Panadiker, V.A., *et. al.*, Organizational Policy for Family Planning, New Delhi, Uppal, 1983.

Pathak, Shankar, Social Welfare, Health and Family Planning in India, Marwah Publications, Delhi, 1979.

Rao, C. Hayavandana, Mysore Gazetteer, Vol. IV: B.R. Publishing Corporation, Delhi, 1984.

Ramanathan, S. (ed.), Landmarks in Karnataka Administration, New Delhi, Uppal, 1998 (Published for Indian Institute of Public Administration, Karnataka, Regional Branch, Bangalore).

Rafei, Dr. Uton M., Primary Health Care in Changing World: South-East Asia Regional Perspectives, WHO Regional Office for South-East Asia, Delhi, India, 1993.

Ranga, R.K., Admn. of Family Planning Programmes in India: A Case Study of Haryana (Doctoral Thesis, Panjab University, 1998).

Rao, V.K.R.V., Food, Nutrition and Poverty in India, Vikas, New Delhi, 1982.

Riffkin, S.B., Health Planning and Community Participation, Crown Helm, London, 1985.

Sahni, Ashok, The Third Force in Health Care—Voluntary Sector, Bangalore: Indian Society of Health Administrators (1992).

Scott-Samuel A., Total Participation, Total Health, Scottish Academic Press, 1990.

Sarjivi, K.S., Planning India's Health, Orient Longman, Delhi, 1971.

Shenoi, P.V. (ed.), Contours of Social and Economic Development: Political Issues, Concept, New Delhi, 1997.

Sharma, R.D., Advanced Public Administration, New Delhi, H.K. Publishers, 1994.

Singh, Sarabjit, Management Information System in a Hospital—A Case Study of General Hospital, Chandigarh (Doctoral Thesis, Panjab University, 1991).

Taori, Kamal, People's Participation in Sustainable Human Development (A Unified Approach), New Delhi, Concept, 1998.

Vaeth, R.M., A Theory of Medical Ethics, New York, Basic Books, 1981.

Vettivel, S.K., People's Participation in Social Development, Role of NGO, New Delhi, Vetri Publishers, 1992.

World Health Organisation, Alma Ata Revisited, WHO/SHS/CC/94.2, WHO, Geneva, 1994.

Werner, D., Where there is no doctor, The Voluntary Health Association of India, Delhi, 1984.

World Bank: Financing of Health Services in Developing Countries, Washington, 1987.

World Bank, Development Report, 1993, New York, Oxford University Press.

World Bank, World Development Report, 1997, New York, Oxford University Press, 1997.

World Health Organisation, Annual Report of South-East Asia Regional Office, Delhi, 1997.

——— Bulletin of Regional Health Information, Regional Office for South-East Asia, Delhi, 1980, 1981, 1982, 1983, 1984-85, 1986-87, 1988-90, and 1991-93.

———, Collaboration in Health Development in South-East Asia, 1948-88, Fortieth Anniversary Volume (Revised), Delhi, 1992.

———, Community Action for Health, SEA/HSD/185, Regional Office for South-East Asia, Delhi, 1993.

———, Development of Indicator for Monitoring Progress towards Health for All by the Year 2000, Geneva, 1981.

———, Eighth General Programme of Work—Covering the period 1990-95, Geneva, 1987.

———, Evaluation of the Strategy for Health for All by the year 2000, Regional Office for South-East Asia, Delhi, 1986.

———, Formulating Strategies for Health for All by the year 2000, Geneva, 1979.

———, Global Strategy for Health for All by the year 2000, Geneva, 1981.

———, Health in Development—Prospects for 21st Century, WHO, DGH/94.5, Geneva, 1994.

———, Health Situation in the South-East Asia Region, 1991-93.

———, Regional Office for South-East Asia, Delhi, 1995.

———, Implementation of the Global Strategy for Health for All by the year 2000, Second Evaluation, Regional Office for South-East Asia, Delhi, 1993.

World Health Organisation, Inter-sectoral Action for Health in South-East Asia Region, SEA/HSD/107, Regional Office for South-East Asia, Delhi, 1987.

———, Monitoring of Strategies for Health for All by the year 2000, WHO/SEA/RC41/15 Rev. 1, Regional Office for South-East Asia, Delhi, 1988.

———, National Decision-making for Primary Health Care, Geneva, 1981.

———, New Challenges for Public Health, WHO/HRH/96.4, Geneva, 1996.

———, Ninth General Programme of Work—Covering the period 1996-2001, Geneva, 1994.

———, Primary Health Care, Geneva, 1978.

———, Regional Health Report, 1996, Regional Office for South-East Asia, Delhi, 1996.

Regional Summary of Progress, Impediments and Further Actions Needed in Implementing National HFA Strategies, WHO/SEA/RC47/20, Regional Office for South-East Asia, Delhi, 1994.

World Health Organization, Renewing the Health for All Strategy, WHO/PAC/95.1, Geneva, 1995.

Report on Monitoring of Progress in Implementing Strategies for Health for All by the year 2000 in the South-East Asia Region, WHO/SEA/RC36/14, Regional Office for South-East Asia, Delhi, 3983.

Strategies for Health for All by the year 2000, SEA/HSD/43, Rev. 1, Regional Office for South-East Asia, Delhi, 1983.

——— The World Health Report, 1995, Geneva, 1995, The World Health Report, 1996, Geneva, 1996, The World Health Report, 1997, Geneva, 1997.

WHO Declaration on Health Development in the South-East Asia Region in the 21st Century, WHO, Delhi, 1997.

WHO Quality Assurance in Health Care, Report of a WHO, Introductory Meeting, Surahaya, Indonesia, 16-20 Dec., 1996, WHO, Delhi.

WHO Health Sector Reform, Delhi, 1997.

WHO South-East Asia Regional Committee Report, WHO, Delhi, 1997.

WHO Sixth Consultative Committee on Organization of Health Systems Based on Primary Health Care, Geneva, 7-10 November, 1994.

WHO Role of Health Centres in the Development of Urban Health Systems, Report of a WHO Study Group on Primary Health Care in Urban Areas, WHO Technical Report Series, No. 827, 1992, (42 pages).

WHO Community Involvement in Health Development Challenging Health Services, Report of a WHO Study Group, WHO Technical Report Series, No. 809, 1991 (56 pages).

WHO Coordinated Health and Human Resources Development, Report of a WHO Study Group, WHO Technical Report Series, No. 801,

1990.

WHO Health System Decentralization: Concept, Issues and Country Experience, A. Mills, J.P. Vaughan, D.L. Smith, I. Tabibzadehg, eds., 1990.

WHO Information Support for New Public Health Action at District-Level, Report of a WHO Expert Committee, WHO Technical Report Series, No. 845, 1994.

WHO Strengthening Health Management in Districts and Provisions, Handbook for Facilitators, A. Cassels and K. Janovsky, 1991.

WHO towards a Healthy District, Organizing and Managing District Health Systems based on Primary Health Care, E. Tarimo, 1991.

WHO Integration of Health Care Delivery, Report of a WHO Study Group, WHO Technical Report Series, No. 861, 1996.

WHO Primary Health Care Reviews, Guidance and Methods, A. El Bindari-Hammad and D.L. Smith, 1992.

WHO Health Promotion and Community Action for Health in Developing Countries, H.S. Dhillon and L. Philip, 1994.

WHO Achieving Health for All by the year 2000, Midway Reports of Country Experiences, E. Tarimo, A. Creese, eds., (1990).

Young Paul V., Scientific Social Surveys and Research, Englewood Cliffs, New Jersey, 1966.

Index

Absence of Comprehensive Health Legislation, 351
Absence of Referral System, 68
Accelerated Rural Water Supply Programme, 103
Ackoff, 223
Administrative Improvement, 543
  Strategies and Policies, 543
Air (Prevention and Control of Pollution) Act, 1981, 95
Akhtar, M., 113
Allied Programmes, 106
  Need of Cooperation and Coordination, 106
Alma Ata Declaration, 1978, 298
Auxiliary Nurse Midwives, 242

Bailey, Maureen A., 499
Balaraman, C.S., 407
Bal, A.S., 111
Bandaranaike, S.W.R.D., 461
Banerji, D., 8
Bankowski, Zbigniew, 112
Barton, W.L., 34
Basu, R.N., 11
Beard, Charles, 24
Berlin, Isaiah, 543
Bernard, Chester, 276, 459
Berthet, E., 19, 194, 522
Bharara, S.S., 199
Bhore Committee, 1946, 292
Big Size of Ward, 258
Block Extension Educator, 429
  Role, 429
Block Level Health Care Administration, 397
  Organisational Structure, 399
  Buildings, 401
  Equipment, 401
  Facilities, 402
  Norms and Services, 402
  Functions, 402
Bogue, Donald J., 187
Bonamour, P., 22
Borlaug, Norman, 139
Boyer, Martin, 102
Brahmachari, S.K., 84
B.Sc. Nursing Degree Course, 243
Buddha, 17

Categories of Nurses and their Education, 242
Central Government Health Scheme, 331
Central Health Education Bureau, 524
Central Pollution Control Board, 94
Central Sterile Supply Services Management, 479
Chadah Committee, 294
Challenges of Public Health Care in the New Millennium, 47
Channels of Communication, 191
  Radio, 191
  Television, 191
  Films, 191
  Advertising, 192
  Song, 192
  Press Information, 192
  Personal Communication, 193
  Local Community Group, 195
Charaka, 17
Charlesworth, J.C., 194, 365
Chaturvedi, T.N., 91
CHC Services, 403
  Aspects, 403
Chest Disease Institute, 486
  Organisation, 486
Chhuttani, P.N., 503
Chidambaram, R., 76
Child Health and Survival, 587
Community Health Care, 400
  Organisational Structure, 400
Control of Drugs Standards, 328
Creation of Women Club, 531
Crude Death Rate, 39

Day Hammers Kjold Report, 5
Dale, Ernest, 263
Dandekar, V.M., 145

Davis, Keith, 262
Davis, Likert, 262
Davis, R.C., 35
Dayal, Ishwar, 24
Decentralisation Generates Interest among Employees, 365
Decentralisation Lightens the Works, 365
Decentralisation Promotes:
  Effective Supervision and Control, 365
  Quick Disposal of Work, 365
  Effective Supervision and Control, 365
Declining Professional Ethics among Specialists, 66
Democratic Decentralisation, 385
Department of Family Planning, 131
  Organisation Chart, 131
Department of Indian Systems of Medicine and Homeopathy, 324
Deshpande, Nirmal, 112
Development, 5
  Meaning and Goals, 5
Devashayam, M.G., 391
Development of Medical Science, 31
Devi, P.K., 247
Diarrhoea Disease Control Programme, 328
Dietary Services, 502
  Poor Management, 502
Dieterich, B.H., 107
Diet Management, 480
Director General of Health Services, 327
  Organisational Structure, 327
Director of Health Services, 350
  Status and Role, 350
Disease, 39
  Incidence and Prevalence, 39
District Health Care Administration, 363
District Health Department, 373
District Health Officer, 376
  Administrative Function, 376
    Health Planning, 376
    Implementation, 377
    Intersectoral Action, 377
    Leadership, 377
    Supervision, 378
    Communication, 378
    Co-ordination, 378
    Control, 379
    Finances, 379
    Monitoring, 379
District Health System, 367-68, 380
  Functioning, 380
    Headquarter-Field Relationship, 380
    Field Reports, 380
  Organisational Structure, 368
  Government Responsibility, 367
Dodzie, K.S., 7
Dolgor, P., 461
Draft Health Policy, 576
Drucker, 36
Drugs and Medical Supplies, 498
  Unsatisfactory System, 498
Drugs, 314
  Insufficient Supply, 314
Dubey, Dinesh Chandra, 199

Education, Awareness and Information, 94
Effective Maternal and Child Health, 166
Efficiency of a Hospital, 475
  Indices for Measuring, 475
Emergency Services, 477
Employees' State Insurance Scheme, 357
  Unsatisfactory Management, 357
Empowering Women for Improved Health Nutrition, 583
Environmental Administration in India, 93
Environmental Education, 110
Environmental Health, 97
  Aspects, 97
Environmental Health Programmes, 91
  Administration, 91
Environment (Protection) Act, 1986, 95
Environment *vis-a-vis* Development, 96
Essential Reproductive and Child Health Service, 162
Existing Health Policy, 215
Experiments of PHC, 305
Expectation of Life, 40
Exploitation by Community Health Workers, 312

Family Planning Education, 199
  Impart Training, 199
Family Planning Programme, 121
  Administration, 121
Family Welfare,
  Policy-making and Planning, 126
Family Welfare Services, 138
  Monitoring, 138
    Training, 138
Field Organisation, 383
  Supervision and Inspection, 383
Forest (Conservation) Act, 1980, 95
Fragmentation of Sectoral Responsibilities at National Level, 334

Gandhi, Indira, 231
Gandhi, Mahatma, 387
Gastrin, Gisela, 522
General Hospital, 472, 483
General Nursing, 243
Goals and Objectives, 228
  Definition, 228
Goddard, H.A., 499
Gross, Bertram M., 66

Haire, Mason, 277
Harwood, 271
Hoseltine, William, 82
Health Administration, 38
Research and Monitoring, 38
Monitoring and Surveillence, 38
Limitations, 40
Health and Development, 91
A Good Environment is the Key, 91
Health Care Administration at the Union Level, 319
Role of the Union Government, 320
Health Care Administration, 39
Indicators Measuring Impact, 39
Health Care System Administration at the State Level, 347
Health Care System, 364
Decentralisation, 364
Health Education and Health Development, 511
Health Information System in Relation to Primary Health Care, 303
Health Insurance, 572
Health, 19
Meaning, 19
Health Administration, 7, 22
Meaning, 22
Health Care Administration, 7, 21
Principles, 21
Scope, 30
Challenges, 48
Health Care, 386, 387
Poor Quality, 386
Lack of Equity, 387
Health Department, 374
Organisational Structure, 374
Health Education, 434, 470, 515-16, 521, 523, 571
Essentials, 516
Methods, 521
Training Personnel, 523
Meaning, Nature and Scope, 515
Health Education in Hospitals, 527
Health Education Programme, 517
Functions, 517
Health Experts Lack Commitment, 309
Health, 20
Factor Influencing, 20
Health Guide Scheme in India, 309
Critical Appraisal, 309
Health Intelligence, 330
Health, 358
Lack of Community Participation, 358
Health Organisation of the League of Nations, 443
Health Planning, 231
Constraints, 231
Health Plans, 224
Development, 224
Pre-planning, 224
Health Policy, 212
Definition, 212
Health Problems, 227
Identifying, 227
Health Situation, 224
Analysis, 224
Hiremath, Shivayogi P., 76
Homoeopathic System of Medicine, 488
Working of a Hospital. 488
Hospital Administration, 63
Hospital Nursing, 250
Indices, 250
Hospitals, 471
Classification, 471
Hospital Services, 79, 469, 477, 482
Aspects, 477, 482
Line Services, 477
Supportive Services, 479
Auxiliary Services, 481
Administration, 469
Nature, 469
Functions, 469
Deteriorating Quality, 79
Hospital Waste causing Environmental Pollution, 69

ILO, 460
Implementation of Programmes, 428
India, 3, 232, 308
Formulation of Health Plan, 232
Synoptic View of Health Systme, 321
Primary Health Care, 308
Indian Medical Council Act, 1956, 329
Indoor Beds, 434
Infant Mortality Rate, 39
Information, Education and Communication, 187
Information System, 303
Design, 303
Institutions Responsible for the Provision of RCH Services, 172
Lack of Adequate Facilities, 172
Insufficient Training to Community Health Workers, 310
Intensive Care Unit, 479
International Cooperation for Health and Family Welfare, 332
International Council of Nurses, 255
International Health Care Administration, 441
Role of WHO, 441
Activities, 446
Organisational Structure and Functions, 447

Health Assembly, 447
Executive Boards, 449
Secretariat, 447
Regionalisation, 449
Finances, 454

Jolly, D., 22
Jungalwalla Committee, 1967, 295
Jungalwalla, N., 295

Kaplan, Martin, 114
Karnataka Panchayat Raj Act, 1993, 369
Kartar Committee, 1973, 296
Kaul, K., 491
Kaur, Raj Kumari Amrit, 321
Kennedy, D.A., 408
Kessler, Alexander, 121
Khan, A.N., 111
Kulkarni, Manu N., 193
Kurup, P.N.Y., 37

Lack of Sound Health Manpower Policy, 58
Lack of Team Work in Family Planning, 148
Lady Health Visitors' Course, 243
Lal, P., 350
Lambo, T. Adeoye, 20
Life Style Causing many Health Problems, 338
Linkage between Community and PHC, 435

Mahila Swasthya Sangh, 196
Mahler, H., 28, 101, 124, 287, 513
Management Improvement, 543
Scope, 543
Management Information System, 552, 571
Management Techniques, 544, 547-48, 557
Critical Appraisal, 557
Functional Classification, 548
Nature, 547
Need, 544
Managerial Planning, 231
Mani, C., 459
Mar Del Plata Conference, 107
Martinez, Norberto, 306
Mashelkar, R.A., 76
Mass Motivation Campaign, 190
Essentials and Aspects, 190
Masters in Nursing, 243
McCany, J.L., 270
McFarland, 35
Medical and Health Education, 563
Medical Education is Urban Oriented, 311
Medical Education not Oriented to Rural Needs, 351
Medical Education, 329, 337
Unsuitable System, 337
Medical Industry, 571
Medical Record Keeping, 410
Poor Keeping, 410
Medical Research, 470
Medical Termination of Pregnancy Act, 1971, 127
Meetings between the District and Field Staff, 384
Mental Health Programme, 328
Millett, John D., 273, 275
Modernise Health Education Institutes, 530
Modernizing Health and Hospital Administration, 539
Montaya, 224
Morley, David, 52
Mortuary, 482
MTP Services, 136
Mudaliar Committee, 1962, 293
Mukherjee, B., 294
Mukherjee Committee,
1965, 294
1966, 294
Mukherjee, Ramakrishna, 123
Mushroom Growth of Private Hospitals with No Norms, 73
Mutalik, Gururajl, 288
Myrdal, 8, 121, 236

Nagpal, Narinder, 246
Nakajima, Hiroshi, 91
Nanavatty, C., 143
Nanjudiah, Y.N., 100
Napulbow, Nikolas, 101
National AIDS Control Progamme, 328
National Assessment and Acreditation Council, 81
National Cholera Control Programme, 328
National Diabetes Control Programme, 328
National Environment Appellate Authority Act, 1977, 95
National Environment Tribunal Act, 1995
National Family Welfare Programme, 128, 349
Achievements, 128
National Filaria Control Programme, 328
National Goitre Control Programme, 328
National Health Policy, 217, 219, 298, 560
Five Dimensions, 217, 219
National Health Programme, 318
National Institute of Health and Family Welfare, 168
History, 168
Organisation, 168
Structure, 168
Actitivites, 169
Objectives, 169

National Iodine Deficiency Disorder Control Programme, 328
National Leprosy Control Programme, 328
National Malaria Eradication Programme, 328
National Medical Library, 331
National Population Policy, 126, 581
National Programme for Control of Blindness, 328
National Tuberculosis Control Programme, 328
Neglect of Hospital Maintenance, 81
Neki, J.S., 29, 67
Newman, 275
New Millennium, 47
  Challenges of Health and Hospital Administration, 47
Nicklas, Charles F., 28
Ninth Five Year Plan, 61
Non-availability and Non-judicious Utilisation of Blood, 502
Non-availability of Balanced Diet, 511
Non-availability of Dedicated Doctors, 355
Non-nursing Duties by Nursing Personnel, 260
Nurses and Primary Health Care, 255
Nurse-Teacher Supply, 252
  Indices, 252
Nurse Technician, 244
Nursing Aides, 244
Nursing Care, 249
  Indices, 249
Nursing, 241
  Definition, 241
Nursing Education, 246
  Critical Appraisal, 246
Nursing Personnel, 241, 260
  Nature and Classification, 241
    Significance, 241
  Low Morale, 260
Nursing Service Administration, 249
  Meaning, 249
Nursing Staff Pattern, 250
  Indices, 250
Nursing Unit, 254
  Administration, 254

O'Donell, 35
Office of International O'Hygiene Publique, 443
OPD, 404, 479
  Problems, 404
  Procedure, 479
Operation Theatres, 479
Opposition from Local Practitioner, 310
Oral Dehydration Therapy, 155
Organisation for Family Planning:
  in a Block, 135
  a District, 134
  in State, 133
Out-Patient Services, 478

Package of Reproductive and Child Health Services, 158
  For the Mothers, 158
  For the Children, 159
  For Eligible Couples, 159
  RTI/STD, 159
Palmer, D., 270
Pan American Sanitary Bureau, 443
Panchayat Raj Institutions, 370, 372
  Committee System, 370
  Administrative Structure, 372
  Organisational Structure, 370
Parameters of Assessment of Primary Health Care, 299
  Availability of Health Services, 299
  Acessibility of Health Services, 299
  Acceptability, 299
Participative Management and Organizational Development, 551
Pathak, R.S., 68, 356
Patient Care, 469
Patients to the Hospitals in the Area, 40
  Admission Rate, 40
Personnel Administrations, 551
Personnel Management, 277
Person Responsible for Implementation of RCH Programme, 173
  Lack of Clarity, 173
Petty, William, 9
Pharmaceutical Services Management, 480
PHC, 426
  Organisational Structure, 426
Planning a Nursing Unit of a Hospital, 253
  Need, 253
Planning for Health Care Administration, 223
Planning Machinery at Various Levels, 232
Planning Nursing Education and Administration, 241
Planning Nursing Organisation and Administration, 261
Planning Nursing Services, 249
Planning Public Health Nursing, 255
Planning Nursing Services, 252
Policy-making and Decision-making, 214
  Relationship, 214
Policy-making for Health Administration, 211
  Nature, 211
Policy-making and Planning, 213
  Relationship, 213
Pollution, 93

Prevention and Control of Pollution, 93
Poor Financial Allocation to the Health Care Delivery, 54
Poor Accessibility for Disadvantaged Groups, 334
Poor Nutritional Status of the People, 357
Population Growth in India, 125
Decadal Variations, 125
Population Stabilisation, 563
Post-Certificate B.Sc. Degree Course, 243
Present Health Situation, 226
Assessment, 226
Prevention of Food Adulteration, 328
Prevention of Pregnancy, 136
Primary Health Care Infrastructure of District Level, 375
Primary Health Care, 285-86, 300, 419, 427
Need, 286
Meaning, 287
Nature, 288
Essentials, 289
Principles, 290
Equitable Distribution, 290
Community Involvement, 290
Multi-sectoral Approval, 291
Appropriate Technologies, 291
Prevention of Disease, 291
Development of Effective Referral Support, 291
Medical and Health Services Research, 291
Health Manpower Development, 291
Administration, 285
Organisation and Working, 419
Strengthening of Infrastructure, 423
General Principles, 300
Organisational Structure, 427
Principles and Approach of Existing MCH/FP Programme, 160
Promotion of Health Education in India, 524
Role of Union and State Government, 524
Public Accounts Committee, 1977-78, 498
Public Health Administration, 17, 25
Objectives, 25
Nature and Scope, 17
Public Health Facilities, 433
Public Health Nursing, 251
Indices, 251
Public Liability Insurance Act, 1991, 95
Punjab Mental Hospital, 485

Quality and Availability of Medical Facilities, 409
Quality of Behaviour, 408

Raina, B.L., 198
Rajan, W.V., 490
Rajeshwar, I.V., 103
Ramalingaswami, V., 302
Rao, K.N., 497
Rao, Radhakrishna, 178
Ragcha, T., 442
Ratnasingham, P.K., 459
Ray, C.N., 408
Ray, Prodipto, 146
Registration and Indoor Case Records, 481
Reproductive and Child Health Programme, 155
Rogers, E.M., 190, 197
Role of:
DHO, 373
the Doctor, 426
Pharmacist, 429
Rural and Urban Areas, 349
Serious Imbalance, 349

Sahay, K.B., 139
Saigal, M.D., 430
Sanga, Kulwinder, 408
Sanitary Conferences and Conventions, 442
Sapru, R.K., 215
Sarma, J.V.R., 310
Saroda, P.R., 111
Seal, S.C., 19
Sen, A.S., 11
Senior Health Assistants, 429
Role, 429
Sexually Transmitted Disease Control Programme, 328
Shah, K.K., 461
Shanks, Mary D., 408
Sharp, Walter R., 428
Shrivastava Group Report, 1975, 297
Shrivastava, J.B., 297
Sharma, S.K., 191
Siegel, M., 56
Simon, Herbert A., 261
Singh, Joginder, 539
Singh, Karan, 219
Singh, Kartar, 296
Singh, S.P., 73, 138, 151
Social Education, Social Services and Health Care, 5
South-East Asia, 462
Future Assistance Policy of WHO, 462
Special Hospitals, 472
State Health Department, 343
Organisation, 343
Political Head, 343
Administrative Head, 345
Technical Health, 346
Sterotyped Health Management System, 391

Stockholm Conference, 1972, 110

Tatochenko, V., 520
Teaching-*cum*-Research Hospitals, 483
Thahane, T.T., 12
Thierry, E.J., 9
Total Nursing Supply, 250
    Indices, 250

Under-utilisation of Indigenous System of Medicine, 356
UNDP, 460
UNICEF, 460
United Nations Environment Programme, 95
Untied Nations Relief and Rehabilitation Administration, 443
Unscientific Manpower Planning, 175
Universal Immunisation Programme, 155

Vacant Posts, 413
Village Community not Educated, 311
Village Health Guide Scheme, 308
Viraavaidya, Mechai, 389
Vuthipongse, Prakron, 75

Waldheim, Kurt, 101, 461
Ward, 258
    Defective Construction, 258
Water (Prevention and Control of Pollution) Act, 1974, 95
Whang, Joung, 197
WHO and India, 460
WHO, 461
    Assessment of the Functioning, 461
    Birth, 444
Working of an Ayurvedic Hospital Dispensary, 489
Working of Hospitals, 489
World without WHO, 463
Wildlife (Protection) Act, 1972, 95
William, H., 351
Williamson, Margaret, 275
Wilson, Frank A., 176
Winslow, C.E.A., 23
Wolman, Abel, 106
Working of WHO, 455
World Health Organisation, 332
Write-up Formulated Plan, 229
Wu, Chi-Yuen, 146, 539

Yadav, Jagdambi Prasad, 289

ZP, 372
    Role of Chief Executive Officer, 372